DOSAGE CALCULATIONS

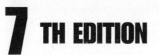

7 TH EDITION

Gloria D. Pickar, EdD, RN

Chief Education Officer
Compass Knowledge Group
Orlando, Florida
Former Academic Dean
Seminole Community College
Sanford, Florida

THOMSON

DELMAR LEARNING

Australia Canada Mexico Singapore Spain United Kingdom United States

THOMSON

DELMAR LEARNING

Dosage Calculations, seventh edition

by Gloria D. Pickar

Vice President, Health Care Business Unit:
William Brottmiller

Editorial Director:
Cathy L. Esperti

Acquisitions Editor:
Matthew Kane

Senior Developmental Editor:
Marah Bellegarde

Marketing Director:
Jennifer McAvey

Channel Manager:
Tamara Caruso

Editorial Assistant:
Erin Silk

Technology Project Manager:
Laurie Davis

Art/Design Coordinator:
Robert Plante/Jay Purcell

Project Editor:
Shelley Esposito

Production Editor:
Anne Sherman

Library of Congress Cataloging-in-Publication Data

Pickar, Gloria D., 1946–
    Dosage calculations / Gloria D. Pickar. -- 7th ed.
        p.   cm.
    Includes index.
    ISBN 0-7668-6286-0
    1. Pharmaceutical arithmetic.
    [DNLM: 1. Pharmaceutical Preparations--administration & dosage. 2. Mathematics. QV 748 P594d 2004] I. Title
RS57.P53 2004
615′.14--dc21
        2003007831

NOTICE TO THE READER

CONTENTS

PREFACE

Introduction

Dosage Calculations, seventh edition, offers a clear and concise method of calculating drug dosages. The text is directed to the student or professional who feels uncomfortable with mathematics. The first through sixth editions have been classroom tested and reviewed by well over 600,000 faculty and students, who report that it helped them allay math anxiety and promoted confidence in their ability to perform accurate calculations. As one reviewer noted, "I have looked at others [texts] and I don't feel they can compare."

The only math prerequisite is the ability to do basic arithmetic. For those who need a review, Chapters 1 and 2 offer an overview of basic arithmetic calculations with extensive exercises for practice. The student is encouraged to use a three-step method for calculating dosages:

1. convert measurements to the same system and same size units;

2. consider what dosage is reasonable; and

3. calculate using the formula method $\frac{D}{H} \times Q = X$ (*desired* over *have* times *quantity* equals *amount* to give) or the ratio-proportion method.

The seventh edition is based upon feedback from users of the previous editions and users of other dosage calculations texts. The revision also responds to changes in the health care field and includes the introduction of new drugs, replacement of outdated drugs, and new or refined methods of administering medications. The importance of avoiding medication errors is highlighted by the incorporation of applied critical thinking skills based on patient care situations.

Organization of Content

The text is organized in a natural progression of basic to more complex information. Learners gain self-confidence as they master content in small increments with ample review and reinforcement. Many learners claim that while using this text, they did not fear math, for the very first time.

The sixteen chapters are divided into four sections. *Section 1* includes a mathematics diagnostic evaluation and a mathematics review in Chapters 1 and 2. The *mathematics diagnostic evaluation* allows learnes to determine their computational strengths and weaknesses to guide them through the review of the Section 1 chapters. *Chapters 1* and *2* provide a review of basic arithmetic procedures, with numerous examples and practice problems to ensure that students can apply the procedures.

Section 2 includes Chapters 3 through 8. This section provides a foundation of information essential for measuring drug dosages and understanding drug orders and labels. *Chapters 3* and *4* introduce the three systems of measurement (metric, apothecary, and household) and conversion from one system of measurement to another. The metric system of measurement is stressed because of its increased standardization in the health care field. The use of the apothecary and household system is further deemphasized. The ratio-proportion method of performing conversions is also included. International or 24-hour time and Fahrenheit and Celsius temperature conversions are presented in *Chapter 5*.

In *Chapter 6*, users learn to recognize and select appropriate equipment for the administration of medications based on the drug, dosage, and the method of administration. Emphasis is placed on interpreting syringe calibrations to ensure that the dosage to be administered is accurate. All photos and drawings have been enhanced for improved clarity.

Chapter 7 presents the common abbreviations used in health care so that learners can become proficient in interpreting medical orders. Additionally, the content on computerized medication administration records has been updated.

It is essential that learners are able to read medication labels to calculate dosages accurately. This ability is developed by having students interpret the medication labels provided beginning in *Chapter 8*. These labels represent current commonly prescribed medications and are presented in full color and actual size (except in a few instances where the label is enlarged to improve readability).

In *Section 3*, the user learns and practices the skill of dosage calculations applied to patients across the life span. *Chapters 9* and *10* guide the learner to apply all the skills mastered to achieve accurate oral and injectable drug dosage calculations. Users learn to think through the problem logically for the right answer and then to apply a simple formula to double-check their thinking. When this logical but unique system is applied every time to every problem, experience has shown that decreased math anxiety and increased accuracy result.

Insulin content (types, species, and manufacturers) has been expanded with a description of insulin action time. The 70-30 and 50-50 insulins are also thoroughly explained.

A new *Chapter 11* introduces the concepts of solutions. Users learn the calculations associated with diluting solutions and reconstitution of injectable drugs. This chapter provides a segue to intravenous calculations by fully describing the preparation of solutions. With the expanding role of the nurse and other health care workers in the home setting, clinical calculations for home care, such as nutritional feedings, are also emphasized.

Chapter 12 introduces the ratio-proportion method of calculating dosages. Ample review sets and practice problems provide the opportunity to apply this method. Ratio-proportion is also applied in *Chapters 13* through *16*.

Chapter 13 covers the calculation of pediatric and adult dosages and concentrates on the body weight method. Emphasis is placed on verifying safe dosages and applying concepts across the life span.

Advanced clinical calculations applicable to both adults and children are presented in *Section 4*. Intravenous administration calculations are presented in Chapters *14* through *16*. Coverage reflects the greater application of IVs in drug therapy. Shortcut calculation methods are presented and explained fully. More electronic infusion devices are included. Heparin and saline locks, types of IV solutions, IV monitoring, IV administration records, and IV push drugs are included in *Chapter 14*. Pediatric IV calculations are presented in *Chapter 15* and obstetric, heparin, and critical care IV calculations are covered in *Chapter 16*. Ample problems help students master the necessary calculations.

Procedures in the text are introduced using several examples. Key concepts are summarized and highlighted in quick review boxes before each set of review problems to give learners an opportunity to review major concepts prior to working through the problems. Math tips provide memory joggers to assist learners in accurately solving problems. Learning is reinforced by practice problems that conclude each chapter. The importance of calculation accuracy and patient safety are emphasized by patient scenarios that apply critical thinking skills. Critical thinking skill scenarios have also been added to chapter practice problems and comprehensive exams to further emphasize accuracy and safety.

Information to be memorized is identified in remember boxes, and caution boxes alert learners to critical procedures.

Section Self-Evaluations found at the end of each section provide learners with an opportunity to test their mastery of chapter objectives prior to proceeding to the next section. Two *posttests* at the conclusion of the text serve to evaluate the learner's overall skill in dosage calculations. The first posttest covers essential skills commonly tested by employers, and the second serves as a comprehensive examination. Both are presented in a case study format to simulate actual clinical calculations.

An *answer key* at the back of the text provides all answers and selected solutions to problems in the Review Sets, Practice Problems, Section Self-Evaluations, and posttests.

Features of the Seventh Edition

- Content is divided into four main sections to help learners better organize their studies.
- More than 2050 problems for learners to practice their skills and reinforce their learning reflect current drugs and protocols.
- Critical thinking skills are applied to real-life patient care situations to emphasize the importance of accurate dosage calculations and the avoidance of medication errors.
- Full color is used to make the text user friendly. Chapter elements such as rules, math tips, cautions, remember boxes, quick reviews, and examples are color-coded for easy recognition and use. Color also highlights review sets and practice problems.
- All syringes and measuring devices are drawn to full size to provide accurate scale renderings to help learners master the measurement and reading of dosages.
- An amber color has been added to selected syringe drawings throughout the text to *simulate a specific amount of medication,* as indicated in the example or problem. Because the color used may not correspond to the actual color of the medications named, *it must not be used as a reference for identifying medications.*
- Photos and drug labels are presented in full color; color is used to highlight and enhance the visual presentation of content to improve readability. Special attention is given to visual clarity with some labels enlarged to ensure legibility.
- The math review has been expanded to bring learners up to the required level of basic math competence.
- Measurable objectives at the beginning of each chapter emphasize the content to be learned.

- SI conventional metric system notation is used (apothecary and household system of measurement are deemphasized but are still included).
- RULE boxes draw the learner's attention to pertinent instructions.
- REMEMBER boxes highlight information to be memorized.
- QUICK REVIEW boxes summarize critical information throughout the chapters before Review Sets are solved.
- CAUTION boxes alert learners to critical information.
- MATH TIPS serve to point out math short cuts and reminders.
- Content is presented from simple to complex concepts in small increments followed by Review Sets and chapter Practice Problems for better understanding and to reinforce learning.
- Many problems involving the interpretation of syringe scales are included to ensure that the proper dosage is administered. Once the dosage is calculated, the learner is directed to draw an arrow on a syringe at the proper value. Syringe photos and illustrations have been updated.
- Many more labels of current and commonly prescribed medications are included to help users learn how to select the proper information required to determine correct dosage. There are over 375 labels included.
- More solved examples are included to demonstrate the $\frac{D}{H} \times Q = X$ and the ratio-proportion method of calculating dosages.
- The ratio-proportion method is included and expanded by popular demand, giving learners and instructors a choice of which method they prefer to use.
- The IV equipment and calculations content has been expanded.
- Clear instructions are included for calculating IV medications administered in mg per kilogram per minute.
- Clinical situations are simulated using actual medication labels, syringes, physician order forms, and medication administration records.
- Case study format of posttests simulates actual clinical calculations and scenarios.
- Essential skills posttest simulates exams commonly administered by employers for new-hires.
- The index facilitates learner and instructor access to content and skills.

New to the Edition

- New labels have been added throughout the book to reflect current drugs on the market.
- New questions have been added throughout to reflect current drugs and protocols.
- Photographs of syringes have been replaced to make them more legible.
- Illustrations of 1, 3, 5, and 10 mL syringes have all been updated to accurately reflect actual needle-length. Measurements have been changed from cc to mL to reflect what is being used in health care practice today.
- *Right of documentation* has been added to the *Rights of Medication Administration* discussion.
- *Chapter 11, Reconstitution of Solutions*, has been created from content that appeared in the sixth edition's *Chapter 10, Parenteral Dosage of Drugs*, and *Chapter 13, Reconstitution of Non-injectable Solutions*. This new chapter puts all the reconstitution information within one chapter to make it easier for the student to connect concepts.
- The sixth edition's *Chapter 12, Pediatric Dosages*, has been expanded to include dosage calculations applied to patients across the life span in the new *Chapter 13, Pediatric and Adult Dosages Based on Body Weight*.
- Sequencing problems and answers better guides the user's understanding of complex concepts.
- Practice with IV push medications calculated in incremental solutions prepare users for this critical skill.

Instructor Resources

Electronic Classroom Manager

For the first time in *Dosage Calculations*, instructor supplements will be available in CD-ROM format! The *Electronic Classroom Manager to Accompany Dosage Calculations*, seventh edition, contains a variety of tools to successfully prepare lectures and teach within this subject area. The following components are all free to adopters of *Dosage Calculations*:

Instructor's Manual—locate solutions for the review sets, practice problems, section evaluations, and posttests from the book

Computerized Test Bank—additional questions not found in the book are available for further assessment. The software also allows for the creation of test items, tests, and coding for difficulty level.

PowerPoint Slides—depiction of administration tools and inclusion of calculation tips helpful to classroom lecture of dosage calculations

ISBN # 0-7668-6287-9

Learner Resources

Tutorial Software

An electronic study aid is available FREE to each user of Dosage Calculations! The CD-ROM packaged within the book features:

- A bank of over 2,000 questions from *Dosage Calculations*
- A clean menu structure to immediately access the program's items
- Enhanced short-answer functionality that will accept several variations of correct answers
- Interactive question navigator displays what questions you have answered correctly and incorrectly
- Review Sets and Practice Problems that operate within a tutorial mode, which allows two tries before the correct solution is provided. The Quick Review link offers tips for giving an accurate response
- Self-Evaluation Tests and posttests operate as a true testing environment that allow only one opportunity for correct answers
- Drop-down calculator available at a click of a button, as used on the NCLEX-RN™ examination

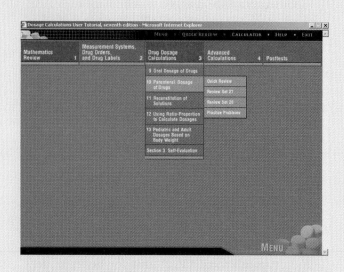

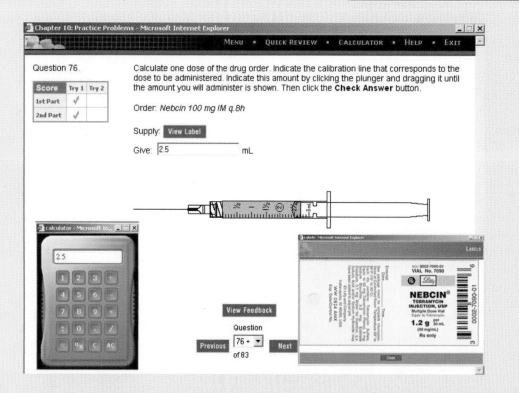

ACKNOWLEDGMENTS

Contributors

Lou Ann Boose, RN, MSN
Gladdi Tomlinson, RN, MSN
Harrisburg Area Community College
Harrisburg Pennsylvania

Lou Ann and Gladdi expertly contributed to the research, updating, and expansion of the seventh edition. Lou Ann was also a major contributor to the Instructor's Manual.

Reviewers

Ann Bello, RN, MSN, MA
Professor of Nursing
Norwalk Community College
Norwalk, CT

Marilyn M. Collins, RN, BSN
Director of Health Occupations
Citrus College
Glendora, CA

Lisa D. Ezzell, BA
Instructor
Park Community College
Workforce Development Program
Lakeland, FL

Susan Harrell, MSN, RN
Associate Professor and Interim Program
Coordinator
Dona Ana Branch Community College
Las Cruces, NM

Ms. Susan T. Mitchell-Sanders, RN, MSN, CNAA
Director of Nursing Education and Allied Health
Motlow State Community College
Tullahoma, TN

Beverly Meyers, MEd, MAT
Professor, Mathematics
Jefferson College
Hillsboro, MO

Linda D. O'Boyle, RNC, EdD
Associate Professor, School of Nursing
Barton College
Wilson, NC

Carol Rafferty, RN, MSN
Staff RN
Berlin Health Systems
Green Bay, WI

Patricia A. Roper, RN, MS
Professor in Nursing
Columbus State Community College
Columbus, OH

Susan Sienkiewicz, MA, RN, CS
Associate Professor of Nursing
Community College of Rhode Island
Lincoln, RI

Maureen Tremel, MSN, ARNP
Professor of Nursing
Seminole Community College
Sanford, FL

Manufacturers

The following companies provided technical data, photographs, syringes, drug labels, package inserts, package labels, or packaging to illustrate examples, problems, and posttests.

Abbott Laboratories, Abbott Park, IL 60064
> Calcijex, Sterile Water for Injection, Bacteriostatic Sodium, 0.9% Sodium Chloride, Various IV Solutions, Synthroid

Akorn, Inc., Buffalo Grove, IL
> Inapsine

Alaris Medical Systems, San Diego, CA

American Pharmaceutical Partners, Schaumberg, IL
> Potassium Chloride, Sodium Bicarbonate, Heparin Sodium, Furosemide, Dexamethasone Sodium Phosphate, Calcium Gluconate Injection

Amgen, Inc., Thousand Oaks, CA
> Cyanocobalamin, Furosemide, Levothyroxine Sodium, Gentamicin Sulfate Injection, Epogen, Neupogen

Apothecon, Princeton, NJ
> Kantrex, Mesna, Stadol

Astra Zeneca LP, Wilmington, DE
> Toprol, Nexium

Aventis Pharmaceuticals, Bridgewater, NJ
> Lasix, Diabeta

Baxter Healthcare Corporation, Round Lake, IL
(Baxter and Continu-Flo are trademarks of Baxter International, Inc.)
> 5% Dextrose Injection, 0.45% Sodium Chloride Injection, Continu-Flo Solution Set, Morphine Sulfate Injection, Lidocaine HCL Injection, Methotrexate Injection, Meperidine HCl Injection

Bayer Corporation, West Haven, CT
> Cipro

Becton-Dickinson and Company, Franklin Lake, NJ
> Insulin Syringes, Tuberculin Syringe, Intravenous Syringes, Needleless Syringe System

Bristol-Myers-Squibb Company, Princeton, NJ
> Cytoxan, Megace

Eisai, Inc., Teaneck, NJ
> Aricept

Eli Lilly and Company, Indianapolis, IN
  Humulin R, Humulin L, Humulin N, Humalog, Ceclor, Keflex, Tazidime, Oncovin, V-Cillin K, Nebcin

Endo Pharmaceutical, Chadds Ford, PA
  Percocet, Narcan, Nubain

ESI Lederle, Division of Wyeth, Philadelphia, PA (Labels courtesy of ESI Lederle, A Business Unit of Wyeth Pharmaceuticals)
  Robinul, Reglan, Hep-Lock, Heparin

Genetics Institute, L.L.C., Cambridge, MA
  Neumega

GlaxoSmithKline, Research Triangle Park, NC (Labels reproduced with permission of GlaxoSmithKline)
  Digoxin Dropper, Dyazide, Thorazine, Tagamet, Augmentin, Eskalith, Amoxil, Stelazine, Tazicef, Ticar, Ancef, Lanoxin, Zantac, Fortaz

Hoechst Marion Roussel, Inc, Cincinnati, OH
  Allegra

Hoffman-La Roche, Inc., Nutley, NJ
  Klonopin, Bactrim, Bumex, Versed, Naprosyn, Rocephin

ICN Pharmaceuticals, Inc., Costa Mesa, CA (The following drugs are distributed by ICN Pharmaceuticals, Inc.)
  Librium, Special Muscular Diluent

Janssen Pharmaceuticals
  Propulsid

King Pharmaceuticals, Inc.
  Cortisporin Otic Suspension, Bicillin C-R 900/300, Pencillin G Procaine, Injection Suspension

KV Pharmaceutical Co, St Louis, MO
  Nitroglycerin Extended-Release Capsules

Luitpold Pharmaceuticals, Shirley, NJ
  Epinephrine Injection, Furosemide Injection

McNeil Consumer Health, Raritan, NJ (Courtesy of McNeil Consumer and Specialty Pharmaceuticals)
  Tylenol

Mead Johnson Nutritionals, Evansville, IN
  Enfamil Infant Formula

Merck & Co. Inc., North Wales, PA (Labels used with permission of Merck & Co., Inc.)
  Prinivil, Vasotec

Mylan Pharmaceuticals, Inc., Morgantown, WV
  Thiothixene Capsules, Erythromycin Ehtylsuccinate, Allopurinol, Indomethacin

Novartis Pharmaceuticals Corporation, Summit, NJ
  Syntocinon Injection, Tegretol, Ritalin, Lopressor, Brethine

Novo Nordisk Pharmaceuticals, Inc., Princeton, NJ
  Novolin 70/30, Novolin R, Novolin L, Novolin, N NPH

Ortho-McNeil Pharmaceuticals, Raritan, NJ
  Tylenol with Codeine, Haldol

Pfizer, Inc., New York, NY (Label reproduced with permission of Pfizer, Inc.)
  Antivert, Vistaril, Pfizerpen, Zithromax, Unasyn, Lopid, Nitrostat, Theramycin, Dilantin

Pharmaceutical Associates, Inc., Tampa, FL
  Potassium Chloride Solution

Pharmacia Corporation, Peapack, NJ and Kalamazoo, MI
  Solu-Medrol, Micronase, Calan, Xanax, Halcion, Cleocin Phosphate, Lomotil, Theo-24, Flagyl, Aldactone, Heparin Sodium, Depo-Provera, Vantin, Bacitracin for Injection, Amphocin

Proctor & Gamble Company, Cincinnati, OH
  Metamucil

Purdue Pharma L.P., Stamford, CT
  OxyFAST

Roxane Laboratories, Inc., Columbus, OH (Labels used with permission of Roxane Laboratories, Inc.)
  Furosemide Oral Solution, Codeine Sulfate Injection

Schering Laboratories, Kenilworth, NJ
  Proventil, Claritin D

Schwarz Pharma, Inc., Milwaukee, WI
  Dilatrate-SR

G.D. Searle & Co., Chicago, IL
  Lomotil, Lactulose

Syntex Corporation, Palo Alto, CA
  Naprosyn

UCB Pharma, Inc. Smyrna, GA
  Lortab

W.B. Saunders, Philadelphia, PA

Wyeth-Ayerst Laboratories, St. Davids, PA (Courtesy of Wyeth Pharmaceuticals)
  Robitussin, Robinul, Inderal, Phenergan

Zeneca Pharmaceuticals, Wilmington, DE
  Nolvadex

From the Author

I wish to thank my many students and colleagues who have provided inspiration and made contributions to the production of the text. I am particularly grateful to Professors Lou Ann Boose, Gladdi Tomlinson, and Maureen Tremel for their careful attention to researching and updating information, to Professor Beverly Meyers for her careful attention to accuracy, to Marah Bellegarde, Matthew Kane, Erin Silk, Shelley Esposito, Anne Sherman, Robert Plante, Jay Purcell, and Laurie Davis for their careful attention to deadlines and details, and to Roger Pickar for his careful attention to me and our children.

Gloria D. Pickar, EdD, RN

INTRODUCTION TO THE LEARNER

The accurate calculation of drug dosages is an essential skill in health care. Serious harm to the patient can result from a mathematical error during the calculation and subsequent administration of a drug dosage. It is the responsibility of those administering drugs to precisely and efficiently carry out medical orders.

Learning to calculate drug dosages need not be a difficult or burdensome process. *Dosage Calculations, seventh edition,* provides an uncomplicated, easy-to-learn, easy-to-recall three-step method of dosage calculations. Once you master this method, you will be able to consistently compute dosages with accuracy, ease, and confidence.

The text is a self-study guide that is divided into four main sections. The only mathematical prerequisite is the basic ability to add, subtract, multiply, and divide whole numbers. A review of fractions, decimals, percents, ratios, and proportions is included. You are encouraged to work at your own pace and seek assistance from a qualified instructor as needed.

Each procedure in the text is introduced by several examples. Key concepts are summarized and highlighted before the practice problems. This gives you an opportunity to review the concepts before working the problems. Ample review and practice problems are given to reinforce your skill and confidence.

Before calculating the dosage, you are asked to consider the reasonableness of the computation. More often than not, the correct amount can be estimated in your head. Many errors can be avoided if you approach dosage calculation in this logical fashion. The mathematical computation can then be used to double-check your thinking. Answers to all problems and step-by-step solutions to selected problems are included at the back of the text.

Many photos and drawings are included to demonstrate key concepts and equipment. Drug labels and measuring devices (for example, syringes) are included to give a simulated "hands-on" experience outside of the clinical setting or laboratory. Critical thinking skills emphasize the importance of dosage calculation accuracy.

This text has helped hundreds of thousands of learners just like you to feel at ease about math and to master dosage calculations. I am interested in your feedback. Please write to me to share your reactions and success stories.

Gloria D. Pickar, EdD, RN
gpickar@cfl.rr.com

DEDICATION

In loving memory of my mother, my personal hero.
MONTANA JUNE RISH
1919–2003
"It's a great life, if you don't weaken." She never did.

USING THIS BOOK...

■ Content is presented from simple to complex concepts in small increments followed by a quick review and solved examples. Review sets and practice problems provide opportunities to reinforce learning.

■ All syringes are drawn to full size to provide accurate scale renderings to help learners master the reading of injectable dosages.

Draw an arrow to point to the calibration that corresponds to the dose to be administered.

11. Administer 0.75 mL

12. Administer 1.33 mL

13. Administer 2.2 mL

14. Administer 1.3 mL

15. Administer 0.33 mL

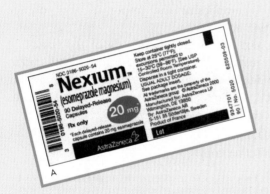

■ Photos and drug labels are presented in full color; color is used to highlight and enhance the visual presentation of content and to improve readability. Special attention is given to visual clarity.

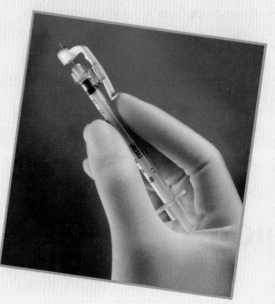

■ *Math tip* boxes provide clues to essential computations.

■ *Caution* boxes alert learners to critical information and safety concerns.

MATH TIP
When converting pounds to kilograms, round kilogram weight to one decimal place (tenths).

CAUTION
Those who administer drugs to patients are legally responsible for recognizing incorrect and unsafe dosages and for alerting the prescribing practitioner.

■ *Critcal Thinking Skills* are applied to real-life patient care situations to emphasize the importance of accurate dosage calculations and the avoidance of medication errors. As an added benefit, critical thinking scenarios that allow learners to present their own prevention strategy are included in end-of-chapter tests.

CRITICAL THINKING SKILLS

Many insulin errors occur when the nurse fails to clarify an incomplete order. Let's look at an example of an insulin error when the order did not include the type of insulin to be given.

error

Failing to clarify an insulin order when the type of insulin is not specified.

possible scenario

Suppose the physician wrote an insulin order this way:

Humulin U-100 insulin 50 U ā breakfast

Because the physician did not specify the type of insulin, the nurse assumed it was Regular insulin and noted that on the medication administration record. Suppose the patient was given the Regular insulin for three days. On the morning of the third day, the patient developed signs of hypoglycemia (low blood glucose), including shakiness, tremors, confusion, and sweating.

potential outcome

A stat blood glucose would likely reveal a dangerously low glucose level. The patient would be given a glucose infusion to increase the blood sugar. The nurse may not realize the error until she and the doctor check the original order and find that the incomplete order was filled in by the nurse. When the doctor did not specify the type of insulin, the nurse assumed the physician meant Regular, which is short-acting, when in fact intermediate-acting NPH insulin was desired.

prevention

This error could have been avoided by remembering all the essential components of an insulin order: species, type of insulin (such as Regular or NPH), supply dosage, the amount to give in units, and the frequency. When you fill in an incomplete order, you are essentially practicing medicine without a license. This would be a clear malpractice incident. It does not make sense to put you and your patient in such jeopardy. A simple phone call would clarify the situation for everyone involved. Further, the nurse should have double-checked the dosage with another licensed practitioner. Had the nurse done so, the error could have been discovered prior to administration.

RULE

Ratio for recommended drug dilution equals ratio for desired drug dilution.

■ *Rule* boxes highlight and draw the learners' attention to pertinent instructions.

REMEMBER

1 kg = 2.2 lb and 1 lb = 16 oz
Simply stated, weight in pounds is approximately twice the metric weight in kg; or weight in kg is approximately $\frac{1}{2}$ of weight in pounds. You can estimate kg by halving the weight in lb.

■ *Remember* boxes highlight information to be memorized.

QUICK REVIEW

■ To solve parenteral dosage problems, apply the three steps to dosage calculations:

STEP 1   CONVERT
STEP 2   THINK
STEP 3   CALCULATE $\frac{D \text{ (desired)}}{H \text{ (have)}} \times Q \text{ (quantity)} = X \text{ (amount)}$

■ Prepare a maximum of 3 mL per intramuscular injection site for an average-size adult, 2 mL per site for children ages 6 through 12, and 0.5 to 1 mL for children under age 6.

■ Calculate dose volumes and prepare injectable fractional doses in a syringe using these guidelines:

● Standard doses more than 1 mL: Round to *tenths* and measure in a 3 mL syringe. The 3 mL syringe is calibrated to 0.1 mL increments. Example: 1.53 mL is rounded to 1.5 mL and drawn up in a 3 mL syringe.

● Small (less than 0.5 mL) doses: Round to *hundredths* and measure in a 1 mL syringe. Critical care and children's doses less than 1 mL calculated in hundredths should also be measured in a 1 mL syringe. The 1 mL syringe is calibrated in 0.01 mL increments. Example: 0.257 mL is rounded to 0.26 mL and drawn up in a 1 mL syringe.

● Amounts of 0.5–1 mL calculated in tenths, can be accurately measured in either a 1 mL or 3 mL syringe.

■ *Quick review* boxes summarize critical information.

Illustrations simulate critical dosage calculation and dose preparation skills.

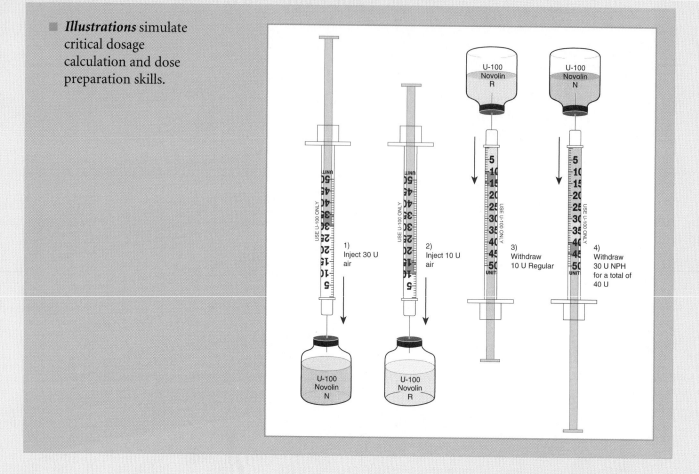

Mathematics Review

Mathematics Diagnostic Evaluation

As a prerequisite objective, *Dosage Calculations* takes into account that you can add, subtract, multiply, and divide whole numbers. You should have a working knowledge of fractions, decimals, ratios, percents, and basic problem solving as well. This text reviews these important mathematical operations, which support all dosage calculations in health care.

Set aside $1\frac{1}{2}$ hours in a quiet place to complete the 50 items in the following diagnostic evaluation. You will need scratch paper and a pencil to work the problems.

Use your results to determine your current computational strengths and weaknesses to guide your review. A minimum score of 86 is recommended as an indicator of readiness for dosage calculations. If you achieve that score, you may proceed directly to Chapter 3. However, note any problems that you answered incorrectly, and use the related review materials in Chapters 1 and 2 to refresh your skills.

This mathematics diagnostic evaluation and the review that follows are provided to enhance your confidence and proficiency in arithmetic skills, thereby helping you to avoid careless mistakes later when you perform dosage calculations.

Good luck!

Directions:

1. Carry answers to three decimal places and round to two places.

    (Examples: 5.175 = 5.18; 5.174 = 5.17)

2. Express fractions in lowest terms.

    (Example: $\frac{6}{10} = \frac{3}{5}$)

Mathematics Diagnostic Evaluation

1. $1517 + 0.63 =$ _____

2. Express the value of $0.7 + 0.035 + 20.006$ rounded to two decimal places.   _____

3. $9.5 + 17.06 + 32 + 41.11 + 0.99 =$ _____

4. $\$19.69 + \$304.03 =$ _____

5. $93.2 - 47.09 =$ _____

6. $1005 - 250.5 =$ _____

7. Express the value of $17.156 - 0.25$ rounded to two decimal places.   _____

8. $509 \times 38.3 =$ _____

9. $\$4.12 \times 42 =$ _____

10. $17.16 \times 23.5 =$ _____

11. $972 \div 27 =$ _____

12. $2.5 \div 0.001 =$ _____

13. Express the value of $\frac{1}{4} \div \frac{3}{8}$ as a fraction reduced to lowest terms. _____

14. Express $\frac{1500}{240}$ as a decimal. _____

15. Express 0.8 as a fraction. _____

16. Express $\frac{2}{5}$ as a percent. _____

17. Express 0.004 as a percent. _____

18. Express 5% as a decimal. _____

19. Express $33\frac{1}{3}\%$ as a ratio in lowest terms. _____

20. Express 1:50 as a decimal. _____

21. $\frac{1}{2} + \frac{3}{4} =$ _____

22. $1\frac{2}{3} + 4\frac{7}{8} =$ _____

23. $1\frac{5}{6} - \frac{2}{9} =$ _____

24. Express the value of $\frac{1}{100} \times 60$ as a fraction. _____

25. Express the value of $4\frac{1}{4} \times 3\frac{1}{2}$ as a mixed number. _____

26. Identify the fraction with the greatest value: $\frac{1}{150}, \frac{1}{200}, \frac{1}{100}$ _____

27. Identify the decimal with the least value: 0.009, 0.19, 0.9 _____

28. $\frac{6.4}{0.02} =$ _____

29. $\frac{0.02 + 0.16}{0.4 - 0.34} =$ _____

30. Express the value of $\frac{3}{12 + 3} \times 0.25$ as a decimal. _____

31. 8% of 50 = _____

32. $\frac{1}{2}\%$ of 18 = _____

33. 0.9% of 24 = _____

Find the value of "X." Express your answer as a decimal.

34. $\frac{1:1000}{1:100} \times 250 = X$ _____

35. $\frac{300}{150} \times 2 = X$ _____

36. $\frac{2.5}{5} \times 1.5 = X$ _____

37. $\frac{1,000,000}{250,000} \times X = 12$ _____

38. $\frac{0.51}{1.7} \times X = 150$ _____

39. $X = (82.4 - 52)\frac{3}{5}$ _____

40. $\frac{\frac{1}{150}}{\frac{1}{300}} \times 1.2 = X$ _____

41. Express 2:10 as a fraction in lowest terms.   _____

42. Express 2% as a ratio in lowest terms.   _____

43. If 5 equal medication containers contain 25 tablets total, how many tablets are in each container?   _____

44. A person is receiving 0.5 milligrams of a medication four times a day. What is the total amount of medication in milligrams given each day?   _____

45. If 1 kilogram equals 2.2 pounds, how many kilograms does a 66 pound child weigh?   _____

46. If 1 kilogram equals 2.2 pounds, how many pounds are in 1.5 kilograms? (Express your answer as a decimal.)   _____

47. If 1 centimeter equals $\frac{3}{8}$ inch, how many centimeters are in $2\frac{1}{2}$ inches? (Express your answer as a decimal.)   _____

48. If 2.5 centimeters equal 1 inch, how long in centimeters is a 3 inch wound?   _____

49. This diagnostic test has a total of 50 problems. If you incorrectly answer 5 problems, what percentage will you have answered correctly?   _____

50. For every 5 female student nurses in a nursing class, there is 1 male student nurse. What is the ratio of female to male student nurses?   _____

After completing these problems, see page 463 to check your answers. Give yourself two points for each correct answer.

Perfect score = 100   My score = _____

Minimum readiness score = 86 (43 correct)

Fractions and Decimals

OBJECTIVES

Upon mastery of Chapter 1, you will be able to perform basic mathematical computations that involve fractions and decimals. Specifically, you will be able to:

- Compare the values of fractions and decimals.
- Convert between mixed numbers and improper fractions, and between reduced and equivalent forms of fractions.
- Add, subtract, multiply, and divide fractions and decimals.
- Round a decimal to a given place value.
- Read and write out the value of decimal numbers.

FRACTIONS

Health care professionals need to understand fractions to be able to interpret and act on medical orders, read prescriptions, and understand patient records and information in health care literature. You will see fractions used in apothecary and household measures in dosage calculations. Proficiency with fractions will add to your success with medical applications.

A *fraction* indicates a portion of a whole number. There are two types of fractions: *common fractions,* such as $\frac{1}{2}$ (usually referred to simply as fractions) and *decimal fractions,* such as 0.5 (usually referred to simply as decimals).

A fraction is an expression of division, with one number placed over another number ($\frac{1}{4}, \frac{2}{3}, \frac{4}{5}$). The bottom number, or *denominator,* indicates the total number of parts into which the whole is divided. The top number, or *numerator,* indicates how many of those parts are considered. The fraction may also be read as the "numerator *divided* by the denominator."

Example:

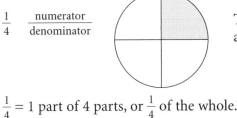

$\frac{1}{4}$ $\frac{\text{numerator}}{\text{denominator}}$

The whole is divided into four equal parts (denominator), and one part (numerator) is considered.

$\frac{1}{4}$ = 1 part of 4 parts, or $\frac{1}{4}$ of the whole.

The fraction $\frac{1}{4}$ may also be read as "1 divided by 4."

> **MATH TIP**
>
> The *d*enominator begins with *d* and is *d*own below the line in a fraction.

Types of Fractions

There are four types of common fractions: proper, improper, mixed, and complex.

Proper Fractions

Proper fractions are fractions in which the value of the numerator is less than the value of the denominator. The value of the proper fraction is also less than 1.

> **RULE**
>
> Whenever the numerator is less than the denominator, the value of the fraction must be less than 1.

Example:

$\frac{5}{8}$ 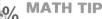 $= $ less than 1; $\frac{5}{8} < 1$

> **MATH TIP**
>
> The symbol < denotes "is less than," and the symbol > denotes "is greater than." Notice that the point of the symbol always points toward the smaller number.

Examples:

3 < 10 means 3 "is less than" 10

20 > 5 means 20 "is greater than" 5

Improper Fractions

Improper fractions are fractions in which the value of the numerator is greater than or equal to the value of the denominator. The value of the improper fraction is greater than or equal to 1.

> **RULE**
>
> Whenever the numerator is greater than the denominator, the value of the fraction must be greater than 1.

Example:

$\frac{8}{5} > 1$

> **RULE**
>
> Whenever the numerator and denominator are equal, the value of the improper fraction is always equal to 1; a nonzero number divided by itself is equal to 1.

Example:

$\frac{5}{5} = 1$

Mixed Numbers

When a whole number and a proper fraction are combined, the result is referred to as a *mixed number*. The value of the mixed number is always greater than 1.

Example:

$1\frac{5}{8} = 1 + \frac{5}{8}; 1\frac{5}{8} > 1$

Complex Fractions

Complex fractions include fractions in which the numerator, the denominator, or both may be a proper fraction, improper fraction, or mixed number. The value may be less than, greater than, or equal to 1.

Examples:

$\frac{\frac{5}{8}}{\frac{1}{2}} > 1 \qquad \frac{\frac{5}{8}}{2} < 1 \qquad \frac{1\frac{5}{8}}{\frac{1}{5}} > 1 \qquad \frac{\frac{1}{2}}{\frac{2}{4}} = 1$

To perform dosage calculations that involve fractions, you must be able to convert among these different types of fractions and reduce them to lowest terms. You must also apply the operations of addition, subtraction, multiplication, and division. Review these simple rules of working with fractions. Continue to practice until the concepts are crystal clear and automatic.

Equivalent Fractions

The value of a fraction can be expressed in several ways. This is called *finding an equivalent fraction*. In finding an equivalent fraction, both terms of the fraction (numerator and denominator) are either multiplied or divided by the *same nonzero number*.

> **MATH TIP**
>
> In an equivalent fraction, the form of the fraction is changed, but the value of the fraction remains the same.

Examples:

$\frac{2}{4} = \frac{2 \div 2}{4 \div 2} = \frac{1}{2} \qquad \frac{1}{3} = \frac{1 \times 3}{3 \times 3} = \frac{3}{9}$

Reducing Fractions to Lowest Terms

When calculating dosages, it is usually easier to work with fractions using the smallest numbers possible. Finding these equivalent fractions is called *reducing the fraction to the lowest terms* or *simplifying the fraction.*

> **RULE**
>
> To reduce a fraction to lowest terms, *divide* both the numerator and denominator by the *largest nonzero whole number* that will go evenly into both the numerator and the denominator.

Example:

Reduce $\frac{6}{12}$ to lowest terms.

6 is the largest number that will divide evenly into both 6 (numerator) and 12 (denominator).

$\frac{6}{12} = \frac{6 \div 6}{12 \div 6} = \frac{1}{2}$ in lowest terms

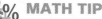 **MATH TIP**

If *both* the numerator and denominator *cannot* be divided evenly by a nonzero number other than 1, then the fraction is in lowest terms.

Enlarging Fractions

> **RULE**
>
> To find an equivalent fraction in which both terms are larger, *multiply both* the numerator and the denominator by the *same nonzero number.*

Example:

Enlarge $\frac{3}{5}$ to the equivalent fraction in tenths.

$\frac{3}{5} = \frac{3 \times 2}{5 \times 2} = \frac{6}{10}$

Conversion

It is important to be able to convert among different types of fractions. Conversion allows you to perform various calculations with greater ease and permits you to express answers in simplest terms.

Converting Mixed Numbers to Improper Fractions

> **RULE**
>
> To change or convert a mixed number to an improper fraction with the same denominator, *multiply the whole number by the denominator and add the numerator.* Place that value in the numerator, and use the denominator of the fraction part of the mixed number.

Example:

$1\frac{5}{8} = \frac{1 \times 8 + 5}{8} = \frac{13}{8}$

Converting Improper Fractions to Mixed Numbers

> **RULE**
>
> To change or convert an improper fraction to an equivalent mixed number or whole number, *divide the numerator by the denominator.* Any remainder is expressed as a proper fraction and reduced to lowest terms.

Examples:

$$\frac{8}{5} = 8 \div 5 = 1\frac{3}{5}$$

$$\frac{10}{4} = 10 \div 4 = 2\frac{2}{4} = 2\frac{1}{2}$$

Comparing Fractions

In calculating some drug dosages, it is helpful to know when the value of one fraction is greater or less than another. The relative sizes of fractions can be determined by comparing the numerators when the denominators are the same or comparing the denominators if the numerators are the same.

> **RULE**
>
> If the numerators are the same, the fraction with the smaller denominator has the greater value.

Example:

Compare $\frac{1}{2}$ and $\frac{1}{4}$.

Numerators are both 1.

Denominators: $2 < 4$.

$\frac{1}{2}$ has a greater value.

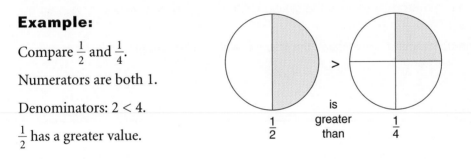

$$\frac{1}{2} \quad \text{is greater than} \quad \frac{1}{4}$$

> **RULE**
>
> If the denominators are both the same, the fraction with the smaller numerator has the lesser value.

Example:

Compare $\frac{2}{5}$ and $\frac{3}{5}$

Denominators are both 5.

Numerators: $2 < 3$.

$\frac{2}{5}$ has as a lesser value.

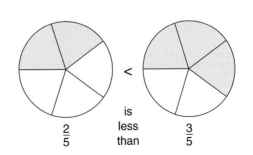

$$\frac{2}{5} \quad \text{is less than} \quad \frac{3}{5}$$

QUICK REVIEW

- Proper fraction: numerator < denominator; value is < 1. Example: $\frac{1}{2}$
- Improper fraction: numerator > denominator; value is > 1. Example: $\frac{4}{3}$. Or numerator = denominator; value = 1. Example: $\frac{5}{5}$
- Mixed number: whole number + a fraction; value is > 1. Example: $1\frac{1}{2}$
- Complex fraction: numerator and/or denominator composed of fractions; value is >, <, or = 1. Example: $\frac{\frac{1}{2}}{\frac{1}{50}}$
- Any nonzero number divided by itself = 1. Example: $\frac{3}{3} = 1$
- To reduce a fraction to lowest terms, divide both terms by the largest nonzero whole number that will divide both the numerator and denominator evenly. Value remains the same. Example: $\frac{6}{10} = \frac{6 \div 2}{10 \div 2} = \frac{3}{5}$
- To enlarge a fraction, multiply both terms by the same nonzero number. Value remains the same. Example: $\frac{1}{12} = \frac{1 \times 2}{12 \times 2} = \frac{2}{24}$
- To convert a mixed number to an improper fraction, multiply the whole number by the denominator and add the numerator; use original denominator in the fractional part. Example: $1\frac{1}{3} = \frac{4}{3}$
- To convert an improper fraction to a mixed number, divide the numerator by the denominator. Express any remainder as a proper fraction reduced to lowest terms. Example: $\frac{21}{9} = 2\frac{3}{9} = 2\frac{1}{3}$
- When numerators are equal, the fraction with the smaller denominator is greater. Example: $\frac{1}{2} > \frac{1}{3}$
- When denominators are equal, the fraction with the larger numerator is greater. Example: $\frac{2}{3} > \frac{1}{3}$

REVIEW SET 1

1. Circle the *improper* fraction(s).

   $\frac{2}{3}$ $1\frac{3}{4}$ $\frac{6}{6}$ $\frac{7}{5}$ $\frac{16}{17}$ $\frac{\frac{1}{9}}{\frac{2}{3}}$

2. Circle the *complex* fraction(s).

   $\frac{4}{5}$ $3\frac{7}{8}$ $\frac{2}{2}$ $\frac{9}{8}$ $\frac{8}{9}$ $\frac{\frac{1}{100}}{\frac{1}{150}}$

3. Circle the *proper* fraction(s).

   $\frac{1}{4}$ $\frac{1}{14}$ $\frac{14}{1}$ $\frac{14}{14}$ $\frac{144}{14}$

4. Circle the *mixed* number(s) *reduced to the lowest terms.*

   $3\frac{4}{8}$ $\frac{2}{3}$ $1\frac{2}{9}$ $\frac{1}{3}$ $1\frac{1}{4}$ $5\frac{7}{8}$

5. Circle the pair(s) of *equivalent* fractions.

   $\frac{3}{4} = \frac{6}{8}$ $\frac{1}{5} = \frac{2}{10}$ $\frac{3}{9} = \frac{1}{3}$ $\frac{3}{4} = \frac{4}{3}$ $1\frac{4}{9} = 1\frac{2}{3}$

Change the following mixed numbers to improper fractions.

6. $6\frac{1}{2} =$ _____

9. $7\frac{5}{6} =$ _____

7. $1\frac{1}{5} =$ _____

10. $102\frac{3}{4} =$ _____

8. $10\frac{2}{3} =$ _____

Change the following improper fractions to whole numbers or mixed numbers; reduce to lowest terms.

11. $\frac{24}{12} =$ _____

14. $\frac{100}{75} =$ _____

12. $\frac{8}{8} =$ _____

15. $\frac{44}{16} =$ _____

13. $\frac{30}{9} =$ _____

Enlarge the following fractions to the number of parts indicated.

16. $\frac{3}{4}$ to eighths _____

19. $\frac{2}{5}$ to tenths _____

17. $\frac{1}{4}$ to sixteenths _____

20. $\frac{2}{3}$ to ninths _____

18. $\frac{2}{3}$ to twelfths _____

Circle the correct answer.

21. Which is larger? $\frac{1}{150}, \frac{1}{100}$

22. Which is smaller? $\frac{1}{1000}, \frac{1}{10,000}$

23. Which is larger? $\frac{2}{9}, \frac{5}{9}$

24. Which is smaller? $\frac{3}{10}, \frac{5}{10}$

25. A patient is supposed to drink a 10 ounce bottle of magnesium citrate prior to his x-ray study. He has been able to drink 6 ounces. What portion of the bottle remains? (Express your answer as a fraction reduced to lowest terms.) _____

26. If 1 medicine bottle contains 12 doses, how many bottles are used up for 18 doses?

_____

27. A respiratory therapy class consists of 3 men and 57 women. What fraction of the students in the class are men? (Express your answer as a fraction reduced to lowest terms.)

_____

28. A nursing student answers 18 out of 20 questions correctly on a test. Write a proper fraction (reduced to lowest terms) to represent the portion of the test questions that were answered correctly. _____

29. A typical dose of Children's Tylenol contains 160 milligrams of Tylenol per teaspoonful. Each 80 milligrams is what part of a typical dose? _____

30. In question 29, how many teaspoons of Tylenol would you need to give 80 milligrams?

_____

After completing these problems, see page 463–464 to check your answers.

If you answered question 30 correctly, you can already calculate dosages!

Addition and Subtraction of Fractions

To add or subtract fractions, all the denominators must be the same. You can determine the least common denominator by finding the smallest whole number into which all denominators will divide evenly. Once the least common denominator is determined, convert the fractions to equivalent fractions with the least common denominator. This operation involves *enlarging the fractions,* which we examined in the last section. Let's look at an example of this important operation.

Example:

Find the equivalent fractions with the least common denominator for $\frac{3}{8}$ and $\frac{1}{3}$.

1. Find the smallest whole number into which the denominators 8 and 3 will divide evenly. The least common denominator is 24.

2. Convert the fractions to equivalent fractions with 24 as the denominator.

$$\frac{3}{8} = \frac{3 \times 3}{8 \times 3} = \frac{9}{24} \qquad \frac{1}{3} = \frac{1 \times 8}{3 \times 8} = \frac{8}{24}$$

You have enlarged $\frac{3}{8}$ to $\frac{9}{24}$ and $\frac{1}{3}$ to $\frac{8}{24}$. Now both fractions have the same denominator. Finding the least common denominator is the first step in adding or subtracting fractions.

RULE

To add or subtract fractions:
1. Convert all fractions to equivalent fractions with the least common denominators; then
2. Add or subtract the numerators, place that value in the numerator, and use the least common denominator as the denominator; and
3. Convert to a mixed number and/or reduce the fraction to lowest terms.

MATH TIP
To *add or subtract fractions*, no calculations are performed on the denominators. Once they are all converted to least common denominators, perform the mathematical operation (addition or subtraction) on the *numerators* only, and use the least common denominator as the denominator.

Adding Fractions

Example 1:

$\frac{3}{4} + \frac{1}{4} + \frac{2}{4}$

1. Find the least common denominator. This step is not necessary in this example, because the fractions already have the same denominator.

2. Add the numerators: $\frac{3+1+2}{4} = \frac{6}{4}$

3. Convert to a mixed number and reduce to lowest terms: $\frac{6}{4} = 1\frac{2}{4} = 1\frac{1}{2}$

Example 2:

$\frac{1}{3} + \frac{3}{4} + \frac{1}{6}$

1. Find the least common denominator: 12. The number 12 is the least common denominator that 3, 4, and 6 will all equally divide into.

   Convert to equivalent fractions in twelfths. This is the same as enlarging the fractions.

   $$\frac{1}{3} = \frac{1 \times 4}{3 \times 4} = \frac{4}{12}$$

   $$\frac{3}{4} = \frac{3 \times 3}{4 \times 3} = \frac{9}{12}$$

   $$\frac{1}{6} = \frac{1 \times 2}{6 \times 2} = \frac{2}{12}$$

2. Add the numerators, and use the common denominator: $\frac{4 + 9 + 2}{12} = \frac{15}{12}$

3. Convert to a mixed number, and reduce to lowest terms: $\frac{15}{12} = 1\frac{3}{12} = 1\frac{1}{4}$

Subtracting Fractions

Example 1:

$\frac{15}{18} - \frac{8}{18}$

1. Find the least common denominator. This is not necessary in this example, because the denominators are the same.

2. Subtract the numerators, and use the common denominator: $\frac{15 - 8}{18} = \frac{7}{18}$

3. Reduce to lowest terms. This is not necessary. No further reduction is possible.

Example 2:

$1\frac{1}{10} - \frac{3}{5}$

1. Find the least common denominator: 10. The number 10 is the least common denominator that both 10 and 5 will equally divide into.

   Convert to equivalent fractions in tenths:

   $$1\frac{1}{10} = \frac{11}{10}$$

   $$\frac{3}{5} = \frac{3 \times 2}{5 \times 2} = \frac{6}{10}$$

2. Subtract the numerators, and use the common denominator: $\frac{11 - 6}{10} = \frac{5}{10}$

3. Reduce to lowest terms: $\frac{5}{10} = \frac{1}{2}$

Let's review one more time how to add and subtract fractions.

QUICK REVIEW

To add or subtract fractions:
- Convert to equivalent fractions with least common denominators.
- Add or subtract the numerators; place that value in the numerator. Use the least common denominator as the denominator.
- Convert the answer to a mixed number and/or reduce to lowest terms.

REVIEW SET 2

Add, and reduce the answers to lowest terms.

1. $7\frac{4}{5} + \frac{2}{3} =$ _____

2. $\frac{3}{4} + \frac{2}{3} =$ _____

3. $4\frac{2}{3} + 5\frac{1}{24} + 7\frac{1}{2} =$ _____

4. $\frac{3}{4} + \frac{1}{8} + \frac{1}{6} =$ _____

5. $12\frac{1}{2} + 20\frac{1}{3} =$ _____

6. $\frac{1}{4} + 5\frac{1}{3} =$ _____

7. $\frac{1}{7} + \frac{2}{3} + \frac{11}{21} =$ _____

8. $\frac{4}{9} + \frac{5}{8} + 4\frac{2}{3} =$ _____

9. $34\frac{1}{2} + 8\frac{1}{2} =$ _____

10. $\frac{12}{17} + 5\frac{2}{7} =$ _____

11. $\frac{6}{5} + 1\frac{1}{3} =$ _____

12. $\frac{1}{4} + \frac{5}{33} =$ _____

Subtract, and reduce the answers to lowest terms.

13. $\frac{3}{4} - \frac{1}{4} =$ _____

14. $8\frac{1}{12} - 3\frac{1}{4} =$ _____

15. $\frac{1}{8} - \frac{1}{12} =$ _____

16. $100 - 36\frac{1}{3} =$ _____

17. $355\frac{1}{5} - 55\frac{2}{5} =$ _____

18. $\frac{1}{3} - \frac{1}{6} =$ _____

19. $2\frac{3}{5} - 1\frac{1}{5} =$ _____

20. $14\frac{3}{16} - 7\frac{1}{8} =$ _____

21. $25 - 17\frac{7}{9} =$ _____

22. $4\frac{7}{10} - 3\frac{9}{20} =$ _____

23. $48\frac{6}{11} - 24 =$ _____

24. $1\frac{2}{3} - 1\frac{1}{12} =$ _____

25. A patient weighs 50 pounds on admission and 48 pounds on day 3 of his hospital stay. Write a fraction, reduced to lowest terms, to express the weight he has lost. _____

26. A patient is on strict recording of fluid intake and output, including measurement of liquid medications. A nursing student gave the patient $\frac{1}{4}$ ounce of medication at 8 AM and $\frac{1}{3}$ ounce of medication at 12 noon. What is the total amount of medication to be recorded on the Intake and Output sheet? _____

27. An infant has grown $\frac{1}{2}$ inch during his first month of life, $\frac{1}{4}$ inch during his second month, and $\frac{3}{8}$ inch during his third month. How much did he grow during his first 3 months? _____

28. The required margins for your term paper are $1\frac{1}{2}$ inches at the top and bottom of a paper that has 11 inches of vertical length. How long is the vertical area available for written information? _____

29. The central supply stock clerk finds there are $34\frac{1}{2}$ pints of hydrogen peroxide on the shelf. If the fully stocked shelf held 56 pints of hydrogen peroxide, how many pints were used? _____

30. Your 1-year-old patient weighs $30\frac{1}{8}$ pounds. At birth, she weighed $10\frac{1}{16}$ pounds. How much weight has she gained in one year? _____

After completing these problems, see page 464 to check your answers.

Multiplication of Fractions

To multiply fractions, multiply numerators (for the numerator of the answer), and multiply denominators (for the denominator of the answer).

When possible, *cancellation of terms* simplifies and shortens the process of multiplication of fractions. Cancellation (like reducing to lowest terms) is based on the fact that the division of both the numerator and denominator by the same whole number does not change the value of the resulting number. In fact, it makes the calculation simpler, because you are working with smaller numbers.

Example:

$\frac{1}{3} \times \frac{250}{500}$ (numerator and denominator of $\frac{250}{500}$ are both divisible by 250)

$$= \frac{1}{3} \times \frac{\overset{1}{\cancel{250}}}{\underset{2}{\cancel{500}}} = \frac{1}{3} \times \frac{1}{2} = \frac{1}{6}$$

Also, a numerator and a denominator of any of the fractions involved in the multiplication may be cancelled when they can be divided by the same whole number. This is called *cross-cancellation*.

Example:

$$\frac{1}{8} \times \frac{8}{9} = \frac{1}{\underset{1}{\cancel{8}}} \times \frac{\overset{1}{\cancel{8}}}{9} = \frac{1}{1} \times \frac{1}{9} = \frac{1}{9}$$

> **RULE**
>
> To multiply fractions:
> 1. Cancel terms, if possible;
> 2. Multiply numerators for the numerator of the answer, multiply denominators for the denominator of the answer; and
> 3. Reduce the result (*product*) to lowest terms.

Example 1:

$\frac{3}{4} \times \frac{2}{6}$

1. Cancel terms: Divide 2 and 6 by 2

    $$\frac{3}{4} \times \frac{\overset{1}{\cancel{2}}}{\underset{3}{\cancel{6}}} = \frac{3}{4} \times \frac{1}{3}$$

    Divide 3 and 3 by 3

    $$\frac{\overset{1}{\cancel{3}}}{4} \times \frac{1}{\underset{1}{\cancel{3}}} = \frac{1}{4} \times \frac{1}{1}$$

2. Multiply numerators and denominators:

    $$\frac{1}{4} \times \frac{1}{1} = \frac{1}{4}$$

3. Reduce to lowest terms: not necessary. Product is in lowest terms.

Example 2:

$\frac{15}{30} \times \frac{2}{5}$

1. Cancel terms: Divide 15 and 30 by 15

    $\frac{\overset{1}{\cancel{15}}}{\underset{2}{\cancel{30}}} \times \frac{2}{5} = \frac{1}{2} \times \frac{2}{5}$

    Divide 2 and 2 by 2

    $\frac{1}{\underset{1}{\cancel{2}}} \times \frac{\overset{1}{\cancel{2}}}{5} = \frac{1}{1} \times \frac{1}{5}$

2. Multiply numerators and denominators:

    $\frac{1}{1} \times \frac{1}{5} = \frac{1}{5}$

3. Reduce to lowest terms: not necessary. Product is in lowest terms.

MATH TIP

When multiplying a fraction by a nonzero whole number, the same rule applies as for multiplying fractions. First convert the whole number to a fraction with a denominator of 1; the value of the number remains the same.

Example 3:

$\frac{2}{3} \times 4$

1. No terms to cancel. (You cannot cancel 2 and 4, because both are numerators. To do so would change the value.) Convert the whole number to a fraction.

    $\frac{2}{3} \times 4 = \frac{2}{3} \times \frac{4}{1}$

2. Multiply numerators and denominators:

    $\frac{2}{3} \times \frac{4}{1} = \frac{8}{3}$

3. Convert to a mixed number.

    $\frac{8}{3} = 8 \div 3 = 2\frac{2}{3}$

MATH TIP

To multiply mixed numbers, first convert them to improper fractions, and then multiply.

Example 4:

$3\frac{1}{2} \times 4\frac{1}{3}$

1. Convert: $3\frac{1}{2} = \frac{7}{2}$

    $4\frac{1}{3} = \frac{13}{3}$

    Therefore, $3\frac{1}{2} \times 4\frac{1}{3} = \frac{7}{2} \times \frac{13}{3}$

2. Cancel: not necessary. No numbers can be cancelled.

3. Multiply: $\frac{7}{2} \times \frac{13}{3} = \frac{91}{6}$

4. Convert to a mixed number: $\frac{91}{6} = 15\frac{1}{6}$

Division of Fractions

The division of fractions uses three terms: *dividend, divisor,* and *quotient.* The *dividend* is the fraction being divided or the first number. The *divisor,* the number to the right of the division sign, is the fraction the dividend is divided by. The *quotient* is the result of the division. To divide fractions, the divisor is inverted, and the operation is changed to multiplication. Once inverted, the calculation is the same as for multiplication of fractions.

Example:

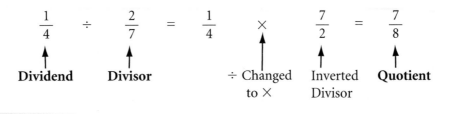

| Dividend | Divisor | ÷ Changed to × | Inverted Divisor | Quotient |

| **RULE** |

To divide fractions,
1. Invert the terms of the divisor, change ÷ to ×,
2. Cancel terms, if possible,
3. Multiply the resulting fractions, and
4. Convert the result (quotient) to a mixed number, and/or reduce to lowest terms.

Example 1:

$\frac{3}{4} \div \frac{1}{3}$

1. Invert divisor, and change ÷ to ×: $\frac{3}{4} \div \frac{1}{3} = \frac{3}{4} \times \frac{3}{1}$

2. Cancel: not necessary. No numbers can be cancelled.

3. Multiply: $\frac{3}{4} \times \frac{3}{1} = \frac{9}{4}$

4. Convert to mixed number: $\frac{9}{4} = 2\frac{1}{4}$

Example 2:

$\frac{2}{3} \div 4$

1. Invert divisor, and change ÷ to ×: $\frac{2}{3} \div \frac{4}{1} = \frac{2}{3} \times \frac{1}{4}$

2. Cancel terms: $\frac{\overset{1}{2}}{3} \times \frac{1}{\underset{2}{4}} = \frac{1}{3} \times \frac{1}{2}$

3. Multiply: $\frac{1}{3} \times \frac{1}{2} = \frac{1}{6}$

4. Reduce: not necessary; already reduced to lowest terms.

| **MATH TIP** |

To divide mixed numbers, first convert them to improper fractions.

Example 3:

$1\frac{1}{2} \div \frac{3}{4}$

1. Convert: $\frac{3}{2} \div \frac{3}{4}$

2. Invert divisor, and change $\div$ to $\times$: $\frac{3}{2} \times \frac{4}{3}$

3. Cancel: $\frac{\overset{1}{\cancel{3}}}{\underset{1}{2}} \times \frac{\overset{2}{\cancel{4}}}{\underset{1}{\cancel{3}}} = \frac{1}{1} \times \frac{2}{1}$

4. Multiply: $\frac{1}{1} \times \frac{2}{1} = \frac{2}{1}$

5. Reduce: $\frac{2}{1} = 2$

MATH TIP

Multiplying complex fractions also involves the division of fractions. Study this carefully.

Example 4:

$\dfrac{\frac{1}{150}}{\frac{1}{100}} \times 2$

1. Convert: Express 2 as a fraction. $\dfrac{\frac{1}{150}}{\frac{1}{100}} \times \frac{2}{1}$

2. Rewrite complex fraction as division: $\frac{1}{150} \div \frac{1}{100} \times \frac{2}{1}$

3. Invert divisor and change $\div$ to $\times$: $\frac{1}{150} \times \frac{100}{1} \times \frac{2}{1}$

4. Cancel: $\frac{1}{\underset{3}{\cancel{150}}} \times \frac{\overset{2}{\cancel{100}}}{1} \times \frac{2}{1} = \frac{1}{3} \times \frac{2}{1} \times \frac{2}{1}$

5. Multiply: $\frac{1}{3} \times \frac{2}{1} \times \frac{2}{1} = \frac{4}{3}$

6. Convert to mixed number: $\frac{4}{3} = 1\frac{1}{3}$

This example appears difficult at first, but when solved logically, one step at a time, it is just like the others.

QUICK REVIEW

- *To multiply fractions*, cancel terms, multiply numerators, and multiply denominators.
- *To divide fractions*, invert the divisor, cancel terms, and multiply.
- Convert results to a mixed number and/or reduce to lowest terms.

REVIEW SET 3

Multiply, and reduce the answers to lowest terms.

1. $\frac{3}{10} \times \frac{1}{12} =$ _____

3. $\frac{5}{8} \times 1\frac{1}{6} =$ _____

2. $\frac{12}{25} \times \frac{3}{5} =$ _____

4. $\frac{1}{100} \times 3 =$ _____

5. $\dfrac{\frac{1}{6}}{\frac{1}{4}} \times \dfrac{3}{\frac{2}{3}} =$ _____

6. $\dfrac{\frac{1}{150}}{\frac{1}{100}} \times 2\frac{1}{2} =$ _____

7. $\dfrac{30}{75} \times 2 =$ _____

8. $9\frac{4}{5} \times \frac{2}{3} =$ _____

9. $\dfrac{3}{4} \times \dfrac{2}{3} =$ _____

10. $4\frac{2}{3} \times 5\frac{1}{24} =$ _____

11. $\dfrac{3}{4} \times \dfrac{1}{8} =$ _____

12. $12\frac{1}{2} \times 20\frac{1}{3} =$ _____

Divide, and reduce the answers to lowest terms.

13. $\dfrac{3}{4} \div \dfrac{1}{4} =$ _____

14. $6\frac{1}{12} \div 3\frac{1}{4} =$ _____

15. $\dfrac{1}{8} \div \dfrac{7}{12} =$ _____

16. $\dfrac{1}{33} \div \dfrac{1}{3} =$ _____

17. $5\frac{1}{4} \div 10\frac{1}{2} =$ _____

18. $\dfrac{1}{60} \div \dfrac{1}{2} =$ _____

19. $2\frac{1}{2} \div \dfrac{3}{4} =$ _____

20. $\dfrac{\frac{1}{20}}{\frac{1}{3}} =$ _____

21. $\dfrac{1}{150} \div \dfrac{1}{50} =$ _____

22. $\dfrac{7}{8} \div 1\frac{1}{2} =$ _____

23. $\dfrac{\frac{3}{5}}{\frac{3}{4}} \div \dfrac{\frac{4}{5}}{1\frac{1}{9}} =$ _____

24. The nurse is maintaining calorie counts (or counting calories) for a patient who is not eating well. The patient ate $\frac{3}{4}$ of an apple. If one large apple contains 80 calories, how many calories did he consume? _____

25. How many seconds are there in $9\frac{1}{3}$ minutes? _____

26. A bottle of Children's Tylenol contains 20 teaspoons of liquid. If each dose for a 2-year-old child is $\frac{1}{2}$ teaspoon, how many doses are available in this bottle? _____

27. You need to take $1\frac{1}{2}$ tablets of medication 3 times per day for 7 days. Over the 7 days, how many tablets will you take? _____

28. The nurse aide observes that the patient's water pitcher is still $\frac{1}{3}$ full. If he drank 850 milliliters of water, how many milliliters does the pitcher hold? (Hint: The 850 milliliters does not represent $\frac{1}{3}$ of the pitcher.) _____

29. A pharmacist weighs a tube of antibiotic eye ointment and discovers it weighs $\frac{7}{10}$ of an ounce. How much would 75 tubes weigh? _____

30. A patient is taking a liquid antacid from a 16 ounce bottle. If she takes $\frac{1}{2}$ ounce every 4 hours while awake beginning at 7 AM and ending with a final dose at 11 PM, how many full days would this bottle last? (Hint: First, draw yourself a clock.) _____

After completing these problems, see pages 464–465 to check your answers.

DECIMALS

Decimal Fractions and Decimal Numbers

Decimal fractions are fractions with a denominator of 10, 100, 1000, or any multiple or power of 10. At first glance, they appear to be whole numbers because of the way they are written. But the numeric value of a decimal fraction is *always less than one.*

Examples:

$$0.1 = \frac{1}{10}$$

$$0.01 = \frac{1}{100}$$

$$0.001 = \frac{1}{1000}$$

These incremental multiples of 10 define the decimal system.

Decimal numbers are numeric values that include a whole number, a decimal point, and a decimal fraction.

Examples:

4.67 and 23.956

Generally, decimal fractions and decimal numbers are referred to simply as *decimals,* while common fractions are referred to as *fractions.*

Nurses and other health care professionals must have an understanding of decimals to be competent at dosage calculations. Medication orders and other measurements in health care primarily use metric measure, which is based on the decimal system. Decimals are a special shorthand for designating fractional values. They are simpler to read and faster to use when performing mathematical computations.

> **MATH TIP**
>
> When dealing with decimals, think of the decimal point as the *center* that separates whole and fractional amounts. The position of the numbers in relation to the decimal point indicates the place value of the numbers.

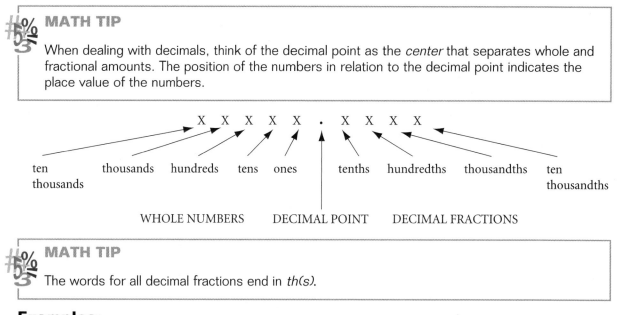

> **MATH TIP**
>
> The words for all decimal fractions end in *th(s).*

Examples:

0.001 = one thousand*th*

0.02 = two hundred*ths*

0.7 = seven ten*ths*

RULE

The decimal number is read by stating the whole number first, the decimal point as *and*, and then the decimal fraction by naming the value of the last decimal place.

Example:

Look carefully at the decimal number 4.125. The last decimal place is thousandths. Therefore, the number is read as "four and one hundred twenty-five thousandths."

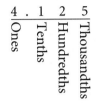

Examples:

The number 6.2 is read as "six and two tenths."

The number 10.03 is read as "ten and three hundredths."

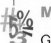 **MATH TIP**

Given a decimal fraction (whose value is always less than one), the decimal number is read alone, without stating the zero. However, the zero is written to emphasize the decimal point.

Example:

0.125 is read as "one hundred twenty-five thousandths."

A set of rules governs the decimal system of notation.

RULE

The whole number value is controlled by its position to the *left* of the decimal point.

Examples:

10.1 = ten and one tenth. The whole number is *ten.*

1.01 = one and one hundredth. The whole number is *one.*

Notice that the decimal point's position completely changes the numeric value.

RULE

The decimal fraction value is controlled by its position to the *right* of the decimal point.

Examples:

25.1 = twenty-five and one tenth. The decimal fraction is *one tenth.*

25.01 = twenty-five and one hundredth. The decimal fraction is *one hundredth.*

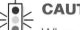

MATH TIP

Each decimal place is counted off as a multiple of 10 to tell you which denominator is expected.

Example 1:

437.5 = four hundred thirty-seven and **five tenths** $(437 + \frac{5}{10})$

One decimal place indicates *tenths*.

Example 2:

43.75 = forty three and **seventy-five hundredths** $(43 + \frac{75}{100})$

Two decimal places indicate *hundredths*.

Example 3:

4.375 = four and **three hundred seventy-five thousandths** $(4 + \frac{375}{1000})$

Three decimal places indicate *thousandths*.

RULE

Zeros added *after* the last digit of a decimal fraction *do not* change its value.

Example:

0.25 = 0.25**0**

Twenty-five hundredths equals two hundred fifty thousandths.

CAUTION

When writing decimals, eliminate unnecessary zeros at the end of the number to avoid confusion.

Although the last zero does not change the value of the decimal, it is not necessary. The preferred notation is 0.25 rather than 0.250.

RULE

Zeros added before or after the decimal point of a decimal number *do* change its value.

Examples:

0.125 $\neq$ (is not equal to) 0.**0**125

1.025 $\neq$ **10**.025

Comparing Decimals

It is important to be able to compare decimal amounts, noting which has a greater or lesser value.

CAUTION

A common error in comparing decimals is to overlook the decimal place values and misinterpret higher numbers for greater amounts and lower numbers for lesser amounts.

MATH TIP

You can accurately compare decimal amounts by aligning the decimal points and adding zeros, so that the numbers to be compared have the same number of decimal places. Remember that adding zeros at the end of a decimal fraction does not change the original value.

Example 1:

Compare 0.125, 0.05, and 0.2 to find which decimal fraction is largest.

Align decimal points and add zeros.

$0.125 = \frac{125}{1000}$ or one hundred twenty-five thousandths

$0.050 = \frac{50}{1000}$ or fifty thousandths

$0.200 = \frac{200}{1000}$ or two hundred thousandths

Now it is easy to see that 0.2 is the greater amount and 0.05 is the least. But at first glance, you might have been tricked into thinking that 0.2 was the least amount and 0.125 was the greater amount. This kind of error can have dire consequences in dosage calculations and health care.

Example 2:

Suppose 0.5 microgram of a drug has been ordered. The recommended maximum dosage of the drug is 0.25 microgram, and the minimum recommended dosage is 0.125 microgram. Comparing decimals, you can see that the ordered dosage is not within the allowable range.

0.125 microgram (recommended minimum dosage)

0.2**50** microgram (recommended maximum dosage)

0.5**00** microgram (ordered dosage)

Now you can see that 0.5 microgram is outside the allowable limits of the safe dosage range of 0.125 to 0.25 microgram for this medication. In fact, it is twice the allowable maximum dosage.

CAUTION

It is important to eliminate possible confusion and avoid errors in dosage calculation. To avoid overlooking a decimal point in a decimal fraction and thereby reading the numeric value as a whole number, *always place a zero to the left of the decimal point* to emphasize that the number has a value less than one.

Example:

0.425, **0.**01, or **0.**005

Conversion between Fractions and Decimals

For dosage calculations, you may need to convert decimals to fractions and vice versa.

> **RULE**
>
> To convert a fraction to a decimal, divide the numerator by the denominator.

Example 1:

Convert $\frac{1}{4}$ to a decimal.

$$\frac{1}{4} = 4\overline{)1.00} = 0.25$$
$$\begin{array}{r}.25\\\underline{8}\\20\\\underline{20}\end{array}$$

Example 2:

Convert $\frac{2}{5}$ to a decimal.

$$\frac{2}{5} = 5\overline{)2.0} = 0.4$$
$$\begin{array}{r}.4\\\underline{20}\end{array}$$

> **RULE**
>
> To convert a decimal to a fraction:
> 1. Express the decimal number as a whole number in the numerator of the fraction,
> 2. Express the denominator of the fraction as the number 1 followed by as many zeros as there are places to the right of the decimal point, and
> 3. Reduce the resulting fraction to lowest terms.

Example 1:

Convert 0.125 to a fraction.

1. Numerator: 125
2. Denominator: 1 followed by 3 zeros = 1000
3. Reduce: $\frac{125}{1000} = \frac{1}{8}$

Example 2:

Convert 0.65 to a fraction.

1. Numerator: 65
2. Denominator: 1 followed by 2 zeros = 100
3. Reduce: $\frac{65}{100} = \frac{13}{20}$

> **QUICK REVIEW**
>
> - In a decimal number, whole number values are to the left of the decimal point, and fractional values are to the right.
> - Zeros added to a decimal fraction before the decimal point of a decimal number less than 1 or at the end of the decimal fraction *do not* change the value. Example: .5 = **0**.5 = 0.5**0**. 0.5 is the preferred notation.
> - In a decimal number, zeros added before or after the decimal point *do* change the value. Example: 1.5 ≠ 1.**0**5 and 1.5 ≠ **1**0.5

- To avoid overlooking the decimal point in a decimal fraction, *always* place a zero to the left of the decimal point. Example: .5 ← Avoid writing a decimal fraction this way; it could be mistaken for the whole number 5. Example: **0.5** ← Preferred method of writing a decimal fraction.
- The number of places in a decimal fraction indicates the power of 10.

  Examples:
  0.5 = five tenths
  0.05 = five hundredths
  0.005 = five thousandths

- Compare decimals by aligning decimal points and adding zeros.

  Example:
  Compare 0.5, 0.05, and 0.005
  0.500 = five-hundred thousandths (greatest)
  0.050 = fifty thousandths
  0.005 = five thousandths (least)

- To convert a fraction to a decimal, divide the numerator by the denominator.
- To convert a decimal to a fraction, express the decimal number as a whole number in the numerator and the denominator as the correct power of ten. Reduce the fraction to lowest terms.

  Example:

  $$0.04 = \frac{4 \text{ (numerator is a whole number)}}{100 \text{ (denominator is 1 followed by two zeros)}} = \frac{\overset{1}{\cancel{4}}}{\underset{25}{\cancel{100}}} = \frac{1}{25}$$

REVIEW SET 4

Complete the following table of equivalent fractions and decimals. Reduce fractions to lowest terms.

	Fraction	Decimal	The decimal number is read as:
1.	$\frac{1}{5}$	_____	_____
2.	_____	_____	eighty-five hundredths
3.	_____	1.05	_____
4.	_____	0.006	_____
5.	$10\frac{3}{200}$	_____	_____
6.	_____	1.9	_____
7.	_____	_____	five and one tenth
8.	$\frac{4}{5}$	_____	_____
9.	_____	250.5	_____
10.	$33\frac{3}{100}$	_____	_____
11.	_____	0.95	_____
12.	$2\frac{3}{4}$	_____	_____
13.	_____	_____	seven and five thousandths
14.	$\frac{21}{250}$	_____	_____
15.	_____	12.125	_____

	Fraction	Decimal	The decimal number is read as:
16.	_____	20.09	_____
17.	_____	_____	twenty-two and twenty-two thousandths
18.	_____	0.15	_____
19.	$1000\frac{1}{200}$	_____	_____
20.	_____	_____	four thousand eighty-five and seventy-five thousandths

21. Change 0.017 to a four-place decimal. _____

22. Change 0.2500 to a two-place decimal. _____

23. Convert $\frac{75}{100}$ to a decimal. _____

24. Convert 0.045 to a fraction reduced to lowest terms. _____

Circle the correct answer.

25. Which is largest?   0.012   0.120   0.021

26. Which is smallest?   0.635   0.6   0.063

27. True or false?   0.375 = 0.0375

28. True or false?   2.2 grams = 2.02 grams

29. True or false?   6.5 ounces = 6.500 ounces

30. For a certain medication, the safe dosage should be greater than or equal to 0.5 gram but less than or equal to 2 grams. Circle each dosage that falls within this range.

    0.8 gram   0.25 gram   2.5 grams   1.25 grams

After completing these problems see page 465 to check your answers.

Addition and Subtraction of Decimals

The addition and subtraction of decimals is very similar to addition and subtraction of whole numbers. There are only two simple but essential rules that are different. Health care professionals must use these two rules to perform accurate dosage calculations for some medications.

> **RULE**
>
> To add and subtract decimals, line up the decimal points.

> **CAUTION**
>
> In final answers, eliminate unnecessary zeros at the end of a decimal to avoid confusion.

Example 1:

$1.25 + 1.75 = $
$$
\begin{array}{r}
1.25 \\
+\ 1.75 \\
\hline
3.00 = 3
\end{array}
$$

Example 2:

$1.25 - 0.13 = $
$$
\begin{array}{r}
1.25 \\
-\ 0.13 \\
\hline
1.12
\end{array}
$$

Example 3:

$3.54 + 1.26 = $
$$
\begin{array}{r}
3.54 \\
+\ 1.26 \\
\hline
4.80 = 4.8
\end{array}
$$

Example 4:

$2.54 - 1.04 = $
$$
\begin{array}{r}
2.54 \\
-\ 1.04 \\
\hline
1.50 = 1.5
\end{array}
$$

> ### RULE
>
> To add and subtract decimals, add zeros at the end of decimal fractions if necessary to make all decimal numbers of equal length.

Example 1:

$3.75 - 2.1 = $
$$
\begin{array}{r}
3.75 \\
-\ 2.10 \\
\hline
1.65
\end{array}
$$

Example 2:

Add 0.9, 0.65, 0.27, 4.712
$$
\begin{array}{r}
0.900 \\
0.650 \\
0.270 \\
+\ 4.712 \\
\hline
6.532
\end{array}
$$

Example 3:

$5.25 - 3.6 = $
$$
\begin{array}{r}
5.25 \\
-\ 3.60 \\
\hline
1.65
\end{array}
$$

Example 4:

$66.96 + 32 = $
$$
\begin{array}{r}
66.96 \\
+\ 32.00 \\
\hline
98.96
\end{array}
$$

> ### QUICK REVIEW
>
> ■ To add or subtract decimals, align the decimal points and add zeros, making all decimals of equal length. Eliminate unnecessary zeros in the final answer.

Examples:

$1.5 + 0.05 = 1.50$

$$\begin{array}{r} 1.50 \\ +\ 0.05 \\ \hline 1.55 \end{array}$$

$7.8 + 1.12 = 7.80$

$$\begin{array}{r} 7.80 \\ +\ 1.12 \\ \hline 8.92 \end{array}$$

$0.725 - 0.5 = 0.725$

$$\begin{array}{r} 0.725 \\ -\ 0.500 \\ \hline 0.225 \end{array}$$

$12.5 - 1.5 = 12.5$

$$\begin{array}{r} 12.5 \\ -\ 1.5 \\ \hline 11.0 = 11 \end{array}$$

REVIEW SET 5

Find the result of the following problems.

1. $0.16 + 5.375 + 1.05 + 16 =$ _____
2. $7.517 + 3.2 + 0.16 + 33.3 =$ _____
3. $13.009 - 0.7 =$ _____
4. $5.125 + 6.025 + 0.15 =$ _____
5. $175.1 + 0.099 =$ _____
6. $25.2 - 0.193 =$ _____
7. $0.58 - 0.062 =$ _____
8. $\$10.10 - \$0.62 =$ _____
9. $\$19 - \$0.09 =$ _____
10. $\$5.05 + \$0.17 + \$17.49 =$ _____
11. $4 + 1.98 + 0.42 + 0.003 =$ _____
12. $0.3 - 0.03 =$ _____
13. $16.3 - 12.15 =$ _____
14. $2.5 - 0.99 =$ _____
15. $5 + 2.5 + 0.05 + 0.15 + 2.55 =$ _____
16. $0.03 + 0.16 + 2.327 =$ _____
17. $700 - 325.65 =$ _____
18. $645.32 - 40.9 =$ _____
19. $18 + 2.35 + 7.006 + 0.093 =$ _____
20. $13.529 + 10.09 =$ _____

21. A dietitian calculates the sodium in a patient's breakfast: raisin bran cereal = 0.1 gram, 1 cup 2% milk = 0.125 gram, 6 ounces orange juice = 0.001 gram, 1 corn muffin = 0.35 gram, and butter = 0.121 gram. How many grams of sodium did the patient consume? _____

22. In a 24-hour period, an infant drank 3.6 oz, 4.2 oz, 3.9 oz, 3.15 oz, and 3.7 oz of formula. How many ounces did the infant drink in 24 hours? _____

23. A patient has a hospital bill for $16,709.43. Her insurance company pays $14,651.37. What is her balance due? _____

24. A patient's hemoglobin was 16.8 grams before surgery. During surgery, his hemoglobin dropped 4.5 grams. What is his hemoglobin value after it dropped? _____

25. A home health nurse accounts for her day of work. If she spent 3 hours and 20 minutes at the office, 40 minutes traveling, $3\frac{1}{2}$ hours caring for patients, 24 minutes for lunch, and took a 12-minute break, what is her total number of hours including the break? Express your answer as a decimal. (HINT: First convert each time to hours and minutes.) _____

After completing these problems, see page 465 to check your answers.

Multiplying Decimals

The procedure for multiplication of decimals is very similar to that used for whole numbers. The only difference is the decimal point, which must be properly placed in the product or answer. Use the following simple rule.

> **RULE**
>
> To multiply decimals:
>   1. Multiply the decimals without concern for decimal point placement,
>   2. Count off the number of decimal places in the decimals multiplied, and
>   3. Place the decimal point in the product to the left of the total number of places counted.

Example 1:

$1.5 \times 0.5 =$ 1.5   (1 decimal place)

    $\times$ 0.5   (1 decimal place)
    _____

    0.75   (The decimal point is located 2 places to the left, because a total of 2 decimal places are counted.)

Example 2:

$1.72 \times 0.9 =$ 1.72   (2 decimal places)

    $\times$ 0.9   (1 decimal place)
    _____

    1.548   (The decimal point is located 3 places to the left, because a total of 3 decimal places are counted.)

Example 3:

$5.06 \times 1.3 =$ 5.06   (2 decimal places)

$\underline{\times\ 1.3}$ (1 decimal place)

1518

$\underline{506}$

6.578   (The decimal point is located 3 places to the left, because a total of 3 decimal places are counted.)

Example 4:

$1.8 \times 0.05 =$ 1.8   (1 decimal place)

$\underline{\times\ 0.05}$ (2 decimal places)

0.090   (The decimal point is located 3 places to the left. Notice that a zero has to be inserted between the decimal point and the 9 to allow for enough decimal places.)

0.090   = 0.09 (Eliminate unnecessary zero.)

RULE

When multiplying a decimal by a power of ten, move the decimal point as many places to the right as there are zeros in the multiplier.

Example 1:

1.25×10

The multiplier 10 has 1 zero; move the decimal point 1 place to the right.

$1.25 \times 10 = 1.2.5 = 12.5$

Example 2:

2.3×100

The multiplier 100 has 2 zeros; move the decimal point 2 places to the right. (Note: Add zeros as necessary to complete the operation.)

$2.3 \times 100 = 2.30. = 230$

Example 3:

0.001×1000

The multiplier 1000 has 3 zeros; move the decimal point 3 places to the right.

$0.001 \times 1000 = 0.001. = 1$

Dividing Decimals

When dividing decimals, set up the problem the same as for the division of whole numbers. Follow the same procedure for dividing whole numbers after you apply the following rule.

RULE

To divide decimals:
1. Move the decimal point in the *divisor* (number divided by) and the *dividend* (number divided) the number of places needed to make the *divisor* a *whole number*, and
2. Place the decimal point in the *quotient* (answer) above the *new* decimal point place in the *dividend*.

Example 1:

$$100.75 \div 2.5 = 2.5\overline{)100.75} = 40.3$$

(dividend) (divisor)   40.3 (quotient)

$$
\begin{array}{r}
40.3 \\
2.5\overline{)100.75} \\
\underline{100} \\
07 \\
\underline{00} \\
75 \\
\underline{75}
\end{array}
$$

Example 2:

$$56.5 \div 0.02 = 0.02\overline{)56.50} = 2825$$

$$
\begin{array}{r}
2825. \\
0.02\overline{)56.50} \\
\underline{4} \\
16 \\
\underline{16} \\
5 \\
\underline{4} \\
10 \\
\underline{10}
\end{array}
$$

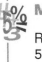

MATH TIP

Recall that adding a zero at the end of a decimal number does not change its value (56.5 = 56.50). Adding a zero was necessary in the last example to complete the operation.

RULE

When dividing a decimal by a power of ten, move the decimal point to the left as many places as there are zeros in the divisor.

Example 1:

$0.65 \div 10$

The divisor 10 has 1 zero; move the decimal point 1 place to the left.

$0.65 \div 10 = .0.65 = 0.065$

(Note: Place the zero to the left of the decimal point to avoid confusion and to emphasize that this is a decimal.)

Example 2:

$7.3 \div 100$

The divisor 100 has 2 zeros; move the decimal point 2 places to the left.

$7.3 \div 100 = .07.3 = 0.073$

(Note: Add zeros as necessary to complete the operation.)

Example 3:

$0.5 \div 1000$

The divisor 1000 has 3 zeros; move the decimal point 3 places to the left.

$0.5 \div 1000 = .000.5 = 0.0005$

Rounding Decimals

For many dosage calculations, it will be necessary to compute decimal calculations to *thousandths* (*three* decimal places) and round back to *hundredths* (*two* places) for the final answer. For example, pediatric care and critical care require this degree of accuracy. At other times, you will need to round to *tenths* (*one* place). Let's look closely at this important math skill.

> ### RULE
>
> To round a decimal to hundredths, drop the number in thousandths place, and
> 1. Do not change the number in hundredths place, if the number in thousandths place is 4 or less;
> 2. Increase the number in hundredths place by 1, if the number in thousandths place is 5 or more.

When rounding for dosage calculations, unnecessary zeros can be dropped. For example, 5.20 rounded to hundredths place could be written as 5.2 because the 0 is not needed to clarify the number.

Examples:

All rounded to hundredths (two places)

$0.123 = 0.12$

$1.744 = 1.74$

$5.325 = 5.33$

$0.666 = 0.67$

$0.30 = 0.3$ (When this is rounded to hundredths, the final zero can be dropped. It is not needed to clarify the number.)

RULE

To round a decimal to tenths, drop the number in hundredths place, and

1. Do not change the number in tenths place, if the number in hundredths place is 4 or less;
2. Increase the number in tenths place by 1, if the number in hundredths place is 5 or more.

Examples:

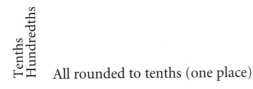

All rounded to tenths (one place)

0 . 1 3   = 0.1

5 . 6 4   = 5.6

0 . 7 5   = 0.8

1 . 6 6   = 1.7

0 . 9 5   = 1.0 = 1   (Zero at the end of a decimal is unnecessary.)

QUICK REVIEW

■ To multiply decimals, place the decimal point in the product to the *left* as many decimal places as there are in the total of the number of places counted in the two decimals multiplied.

Example:

0.25 × 0.2 = 0.050 = 0.05 (Zeros at the end of the decimal is unnecessary.)

■ To divide decimals, move the decimal point in the divisor and dividend the number of decimal places that will make the divisor a whole number and align it in the quotient.

Example:

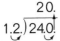

■ To multiply or divide decimals by a power of 10, move the decimal point to the *right* (to *multiply*) or to the *left* (to *divide*) the number of decimal places as there are zeros in the power of 10.

Examples:

5.06 × 10 = 5.0̲6 = 50.6

2.1 ÷ 100 = .0̲2̲.1 = 0.021

■ When rounding decimals, add 1 to the place value considered if the next decimal place is 5 or greater.

Examples:

Rounded to hundredths: 3.054 = 3.05; 0.566 = 0.57. Rounded to tenths: 3.05 = 3.1; 0.54 = 0.5

REVIEW SET 6

Multiply, and round your answers to two decimal places.

1. $1.16 \times 5.03 =$ _____

2. $0.314 \times 7 =$ _____

3. $1.71 \times 25 =$ _____

4. $3.002 \times 0.05 =$ _____

5. $16.1 \times 25.04 =$ _____

6. $75.1 \times 1000.01 =$ _____

7. $16.03 \times 2.05 =$ _____

8. $55.50 \times 0.05 =$ _____

9. $23.2 \times 15.025 =$ _____

10. $1.14 \times 0.014 =$ _____

Divide, and round your answers to two decimal places.

11. $16 \div 0.04 =$ _____

12. $25.3 \div 6.76 =$ _____

13. $0.02 \div 0.004 =$ _____

14. $45.5 \div 15.25 =$ _____

15. $515 \div 0.125 =$ _____

16. $73 \div 13.40 =$ _____

17. $16.36 \div 0.06 =$ _____

18. $0.375 \div 0.25 =$ _____

19. $100.04 \div 0.002 =$ _____

20. $45 \div 0.15 =$ _____

Multiply or divide by the power of 10 indicated. Draw an arrow to demonstrate movement of the decimal point.

21. $562.5 \times 100 =$ _____

22. $16 \times 10 =$ _____

23. $25 \div 1000 =$ _____

24. $32.005 \div 1000 =$ _____

25. $0.125 \div 100 =$ _____

26. $23.25 \times 10 =$ _____

27. $717.717 \div 10 =$ _____

28. $83.16 \times 10 =$ _____

29. $0.33 \times 100 =$ _____

30. $14.106 \times 1000 =$ _____

After completing these problems, see page 466 to check your answers.

PRACTICE PROBLEMS—CHAPTER 1

1. Convert 0.35 to a fraction in lowest terms. _____

2. Convert $\frac{3}{8}$ to a decimal. _____

Find the least common denominator for the following pairs of fractions.

3. $\frac{5}{7}; \frac{2}{3}$ _____

4. $\frac{1}{5}; \frac{4}{11}$ _____

5. $\frac{4}{9}; \frac{5}{6}$ _____

6. $\frac{1}{3}; \frac{3}{5}$ _____

Perform the indicated operation, and reduce fractions to lowest terms.

7. $1\frac{2}{3} + \frac{9}{5} =$ _____

8. $4\frac{5}{12} + 3\frac{1}{15} =$ _____

9. $\frac{7}{9} - \frac{5}{18} =$ _____

10. $5\frac{1}{6} - 2\frac{7}{8} =$ _____

11. $\frac{4}{9} \times \frac{7}{12} =$ _____

12. $1\frac{1}{2} \times 6\frac{3}{4} =$ _____

13. $7\frac{1}{5} \div 1\frac{7}{10} =$ _____

18. $\dfrac{\frac{1}{10}}{\frac{2}{3}} =$ _____

14. $\frac{3}{16} + \frac{3}{10} =$ _____

19. $\frac{1}{125} \times \frac{1}{25} =$ _____

15. $8\frac{4}{11} \div 1\frac{2}{3} =$ _____

20. $\dfrac{\frac{7}{8}}{\frac{1}{3}} \div \dfrac{3\frac{1}{2}}{\frac{1}{3}} =$ _____

16. $\dfrac{9\frac{1}{2}}{1\frac{4}{5}} =$ _____

21. $\frac{20}{35} \times 3 =$ _____

17. $\dfrac{13\frac{1}{3}}{4\frac{6}{13}} =$ _____

22. $2\frac{1}{4} \times 7\frac{1}{8} =$ _____

Perform the indicated operation, and round the answer to two decimal places.

23. $11.33 + 29.16 + 19.78 =$ _____

24. $93.712 - 26.97 =$ _____

25. $43.69 - 0.7083 =$ _____

26. $66.4 \times 72.8 =$ _____

27. $360 \times 0.53 =$ _____

28. $268.4 \div 14 =$ _____

29. $10.10 - 0.62 =$ _____

30. $5 + 2.5 + 0.05 + 0.15 =$ _____

31. $1.71 \times 25 =$ _____

32. $45 \div 0.15 =$ _____

33. $2974 \div 0.23 =$ _____

34. $51.21 \div 0.016 =$ _____

35. $0.74 \div 0.37 =$ _____

36. $1.5 + 146.73 + 1.9 + 0.832 =$ _____

Multiply or divide by the power of 10 indicated. Draw an arrow to demonstrate movement of the decimal point.

37. $9.716 \times 1000 =$ _____

38. $50.25 \div 100 =$ _____

39. $0.25 \times 100 =$ _____

40. $5.75 \times 1000 =$ _____

41. $0.25 \div 10 =$ _____

42. $11.525 \times 10 =$ _____

43. A 1-month-old infant drinks $3\frac{1}{2}$ ounces of formula every four hours. How many ounces will the infant drink in one week on this schedule? _____

44. There are 368 people employed at Riverview Clinic. If $\frac{3}{8}$ of the employees are nurses, $\frac{1}{8}$ are maintenance/cleaners, $\frac{1}{4}$ are technicians, and $\frac{1}{4}$ are all other employees, calculate the number of employees that each fraction represents. _____

45. True or false? A specific gravity of urine of $1\frac{2}{32}$ falls within the normal range of 1.01 to 1.025 for an adult patient. _____

46. Last week a nurse earning $17.43 per hour gross pay worked 40 hours plus 6.25 hours overtime, which is paid at twice the hourly rate. What is the total regular and overtime gross pay for last week? _____

47. The instructional assistant is ordering supplies for the nursing skills laboratory. A single box of 12 urinary catheters costs $98.76. A case of 12 boxes of these catheters costs $975. Calculate the savings per catheter when a case is purchased. _____

48. If each ounce of a liquid laxative contains 0.065 gram of a drug, how many grams of the drug would be contained in 4.75 ounces? (Round answer to the nearest hundredth.)_____

49. A patient is to receive 1200 milliliters of fluid in a 24 hour period. How many milliliters should the patient drink between the hours of 7:00 AM and 7:00 PM if he is to receive $\frac{2}{3}$ of the total amount during that time? _____

50. A baby weighed 3.7 kilograms at birth. The baby now weighs 6.65 kilograms. How many kilograms did the baby gain? _____

After completing these problems, see page 466 to check your answers.

Ratios, Percents, Simple Equations, and Ratio-Proportion

OBJECTIVES

Upon mastery of Chapter 2, you will be able to perform basic mathematical computations that involve ratios, percents, simple equations, and proportions. Specifically, you will be able to:

- Interpret values expressed in ratios.
- Convert among fractions, decimals, ratios, and percents.
- Compare the size of fractions, decimals, ratios, and percents.
- Determine the value of "X" in simple equations.
- Set up proportions for solving problems.
- Cross-multiply to find the value of "X" in a proportion.
- Calculate the percentage of a quantity.

Health care professionals need to understand ratios and percents to be able to accurately interpret, prepare, and administer a variety of medications and treatments. Let's take a look at each of these important ways of expressing ratios and percents and how they are related to fractions and decimals. It is important for you to be able to convert quickly and accurately between equivalent ratios, percents, decimals, and fractions.

RATIOS AND PERCENTS

Ratios

Like a fraction, a *ratio* is used to indicate the relationship of one part of a quantity to the whole. When written, the two quantities are separated by a colon (:). The use of the colon is a traditional way to write the division sign within a ratio.

Example:

On an evening shift, if there are 5 nurses and 35 patients, what is the ratio of nurses to patients? 5 nurses to 35 patients = 5 nurses per 35 patients = $\frac{5}{35} = \frac{1}{7}$. This is the same as a ratio of 5:35 or 1:7.

> **MATH TIP**
>
> The terms of a ratio are the *numerator* (always to the left of the colon) and the *denominator* (always to the right of the colon) of a fraction. Like fractions, ratios should be stated in lowest terms.

If you think back to the discussion of fractions and parts of a whole, it is easy to see that a ratio is *actually the same as* a fraction and its equivalent decimal. It is just a different way of *expressing the same quantity*. Recall from Chapter 1 that to convert a fraction to a decimal, you simply divide the numerator by the denominator.

Example:

Adrenalin 1:1000 for injection = 1 part Adrenalin to 1000 total parts of solution. It is a fact that 1:1000 is the same as $\frac{1}{1000}$ and 0.001.

In some drug solutions such as Adrenalin 1:1000, the ratio is used to indicate the drug's concentration. This will be covered in more detail later.

Percents

A type of ratio is a percent. *Percent* comes from the Latin phrase *per centum,* translated *per hundred.* This means per hundred parts or hundredth part.

> **MATH TIP**
>
> To remember the value of a given percent, replace the % symbol with "/" for *per* and "100" for *cent.* THINK: *Percent* (%) means "/100."

Example:

$3\% = 3$ percent $= 3/100 = \frac{3}{100} = 0.03$

Converting between Ratios, Percents, Fractions, and Decimals

When you understand the relationship of ratios, percents, fractions, and decimals, you can readily convert from one to the other. Let's begin by converting a percent to a fraction.

> **RULE**
>
> To convert a percent to a fraction:
> 1. Delete the % sign,
> 2. Write the remaining number as the numerator,
> 3. Write 100 as the denominator, and
> 4. Reduce the result to lowest terms.

Example:

$5\% = \frac{5}{100} = \frac{1}{20}$

It is also easy to express a percent as a ratio.

> **RULE**
>
> To convert a percent to a ratio:
> 1. Delete the % sign,
> 2. Write the remaining number as the numerator,
> 3. Write "100" as the denominator,
> 4. Reduce the result to lowest terms, and
> 5. Express the fraction as a ratio.

Example:

$$25\% = \frac{25}{100} = \frac{1}{4} = 1{:}4$$

Because the denominator of a percent is always 100, it is easy to find the equivalent decimal. Recall that to divide by 100, you move the decimal point two places to the left, the number of places equal to the number of zeros in the denominator. This is the hundredths place.

> **RULE**
>
> To convert a percent to a decimal:
> 1. Delete the % sign, and
> 2. Divide the remaining number by 100, which is the same as moving the decimal point 2 places to the left.

Example:

$$25\% = \frac{25}{100} = 25 \div 100 = .25. = 0.25$$

Conversely, it is easy to change a decimal to a percent.

> **RULE**
>
> To convert a decimal to a percent:
> 1. Multiply the decimal number by 100 (move the decimal point 2 places to the right), and
> 2. Add the % sign.

Example:

$$0.25 \times 100 = 0.25. = 25\%$$

Now you know all the steps to change a ratio to the equivalent percent.

> **RULE**
>
> To convert a ratio to a percent:
> 1. Convert the ratio to a fraction,
> 2. Convert the fraction to a decimal, and
> 3. Convert the decimal to a percent.

Example:

Convert 1:1000 Adrenalin solution to the equivalent concentration expressed as a percent.

1. $1{:}1000 = \frac{1}{1000}$ (ratio converted to fraction)

2. $\frac{1}{1000} = .001. = 0.001$ (fraction converted to decimal)

3. $0.001 = 0.00.1 = 0.1\%$ (decimal converted to percent)

Thus, 1:1000 Adrenalin solution = 0.1% Adrenalin solution.

Review the preceding example again slowly until it is clear. Ask your instructor for assistance, as needed. If you go over this one step at a time, you can master these important calculations. You need never fear fractions, decimals, ratios, and percents again.

Comparing Percents and Ratios

Nurses and other health care professionals frequently administer solutions with the concentration expressed as a percent or ratio. Consider two intravenous solutions given directly into a person's vein: one that is 0.9%; the other 5%. It is important to be clear that 0.9% is *smaller* than 5%. A 0.9% solution means that there are 0.9 parts of the solid per 100 total parts (0.9 parts is less than one whole part, so it is less than 1%). Compare this to the 5% solution, with 5 parts of the solid (or more than 5 times 0.9 parts) per 100 total parts. Therefore, the 5% solution is much more concentrated, or stronger, than the 0.9% solution. A misunderstanding of these numbers and the quantities they represent can have dire consequences.

Likewise, you may see a solution concentration expressed as $\frac{1}{3}$% and another expressed as 0.45%. Convert these amounts to equivalent decimals to clarify values and compare concentrations.

$$\frac{1}{3}\% = \frac{\frac{1}{3}}{100} = \frac{1}{3} \div \frac{100}{1} = \frac{1}{3} \times \frac{1}{100} = \frac{1}{300} = 0.003\overline{3}$$

$$0.45\% = \frac{0.45}{100} = 0.0045 \text{ (greater value, stronger concentration)}$$

Compare solution concentrations expressed as a ratio, such as 1:1000 and 1:100.

$$1:1000 = \frac{1}{1000} = 0.001$$

$$1:100 = \frac{1}{100} = 0.01 \text{ or } 0.010 \text{ (add zero for comparison) } 1:100 \text{ is a stronger}$$
concentration.

QUICK REVIEW

- Fractions, decimals, ratios, and percents are related equivalents.
  Example: $1:2 = \frac{1}{2} = 0.5 = 50\%$
- Like fractions, ratios should be reduced to lowest terms.
  Example: $2:4 = 1:2$
- To express a ratio as a fraction, the number to the left of the colon becomes the numerator, and the number to the right of the colon becomes the denominator. The colon in a ratio is equivalent to the division sign in a fraction.
  Example: $2:3 = \frac{2}{3}$
- To change a ratio to a decimal, convert the ratio to a fraction, and divide the numerator by the denominator.
  Example: $1:4 = \frac{1}{4} = 1 \div 4 = 0.25$
- To change a percent to a fraction, drop the % sign and place the remaining number as the numerator over the denominator 100. Reduce the fraction to lowest terms. THINK: per (/) cent (100)
  Example: $75\% = \frac{75}{100} = \frac{3}{4}$
- To change a percent to a ratio, first convert the percent to a fraction in lowest terms. Then, place the numerator to the left of a colon and the denominator to the right of that colon.
  Example: $35\% = \frac{35}{100} = \frac{7}{20} = 7:20$
- To change a percent to a decimal, drop the % sign, and divide by 100.
  Example: $4\% = .04. = 0.04$

■ To change a decimal to a percent, multiply by 100, and add the % sign.

Example: $0.5 = 0.50. = 50\%$

■ To change a ratio to a percent, first convert the ratio to a fraction. Convert the resulting fraction to a decimal and then to a percent.

Example: $1:2 = \frac{1}{2} = 1 \div 2 = 0.5 = 0.50. = 50\%$

REVIEW SET 7

Change the following ratios to fractions that are reduced to lowest terms.

1. $3 : 150 =$ _____

2. $6 : 10 =$ _____

3. $0.05 : 0.15 =$ _____

4. $4 : 7 =$ _____

5. $6 : 8 =$ _____

Change the following ratios to decimals; round to two decimal places, if needed.

6. $20 : 40 =$ _____

7. $\frac{1}{1000} : \frac{1}{150} =$ _____

8. $0.12 : 0.88 =$ _____

9. $0.3 : 4.5 =$ _____

10. $1\frac{1}{2} : 6\frac{2}{9} =$ _____

Change the following ratios to percents; round to two decimal places, if needed.

11. $12 : 48 =$ _____

12. $2 : 5 =$ _____

13. $0.08 : 0.64 =$ _____

14. $7 : 10 =$ _____

15. $50 : 100 =$ _____

Change the following percents to fractions that are reduced to lowest terms.

16. $45\% =$ _____

17. $60\% =$ _____

18. $0.5\% =$ _____

19. $1\% =$ _____

20. $66\frac{2}{3}\% =$ _____

Change the following percents to decimals; round to two decimal places, if needed.

21. $2.94\% =$ _____

22. $4.5\% =$ _____

23. $6.32\% =$ _____

24. $33\% =$ _____

25. $0.9\% =$ _____

Change the following percents to ratios that are reduced to lowest terms.

26. $16\% =$ _____

27. $25\% =$ _____

28. $50\% =$ _____

29. $45\% =$ _____

30. $6\% =$ _____

Which of the following is largest? Circle your answer.

31. 0.9% 0.9 $1:9$ $\frac{1}{90}$

32. 0.05 $\frac{1}{5}$ 0.025 $1:25$

33. 0.0125% 0.25% 0.1% 0.02%

34. $\frac{1}{150}$ $\frac{1}{300}$ 0.5 $\frac{2}{3}\%$

35. $1:1000$ 0.0001 $\frac{1}{100}$ 0.1%

After completing these problems, see pages 466–467 to check your answers.

SOLVING SIMPLE EQUATIONS FOR "X"

The dosage calculations you will perform can be set up and solved in different ways. One way is to use a simple equation form. The following examples demonstrate the various forms of this equation. Learn to express your answers in decimal form, because decimals will be used most often in dosage calculations and administration. Round decimals to hundredths or to two places.

> **MATH TIP**
>
> The unknown quantity is represented by "X."

Example 1:

$$\frac{100}{200} \times 1 = X$$

> **MATH TIP**
>
> You can drop the 1, because a number multiplied by 1 is the same number.

$\frac{100}{200} \times 1 = X$ is the same as $\frac{100}{200} = X$.

1. Reduce to lowest terms: $\frac{100}{200} = \frac{\overset{1}{\cancel{100}}}{\underset{2}{\cancel{200}}} = \frac{1}{2} = X$

2. Convert to decimal form: $\frac{1}{2} = 0.5 = X$

3. You have your answer. $X = 0.5$

Example 2:

$$\frac{3}{5} \times 2 = X$$

> **MATH TIP**
>
> Dividing a number by 1 does not change its value.

1. Convert: Express 2 as a fraction: $\frac{3}{5} \times \frac{2}{1} = X$

2. Multiply fractions: $\frac{3}{5} \times \frac{2}{1} = \frac{6}{5} = X$

3. Convert to a mixed number: $\frac{6}{5} = 1\frac{1}{5} = X$

4. Convert to decimal form: $1\frac{1}{5} = 1.2 = X$

5. You have your answer. $X = 1.2$

Example 3:

$$\frac{\frac{1}{6}}{\frac{1}{4}} \times 5 = X$$

1. Convert: Express 5 as a fraction: $\dfrac{\frac{1}{6}}{\frac{1}{4}} \times \dfrac{5}{1} = X$

2. Divide fractions: $\dfrac{1}{6} \div \dfrac{1}{4} \times \dfrac{5}{1} = X$

3. Invert the divisor, and multiply: $\dfrac{1}{6} \times \dfrac{4}{1} \times \dfrac{5}{1} = X$

4. Cancel terms: $\dfrac{1}{\cancel{6}_{3}} \times \dfrac{\cancel{4}^{2}}{1} \times \dfrac{5}{1} = \dfrac{1}{3} \times \dfrac{2}{1} \times \dfrac{5}{1} = \dfrac{10}{3} = X$

5. Convert to a mixed number: $\dfrac{10}{3} = 3\dfrac{1}{3} = X$

6. Convert to decimal form: $3\dfrac{1}{3} = 3.33\overline{3} = X$

7. Round to hundredths place: $3.33\overline{3} = 3.33 = X$

8. Easy, when you take it one step at a time. $X = 3.33$

MATH TIP

The line over the last 3 in steps 6 and 7 ($3.33\overline{3}$) indicates that the number repeats indefinitely.

Example 4:

$$\frac{\frac{1}{100}}{\frac{1}{150}} \times 2.2 = X$$

1. Convert: Express 2.2 in fraction form: $\dfrac{\frac{1}{100}}{\frac{1}{150}} \times \dfrac{2.2}{1} = X$

2. Divide fractions: $\dfrac{1}{100} \div \dfrac{1}{150} \times \dfrac{2.2}{1} = X$

3. Invert the divisor, and multiply: $\dfrac{1}{100} \times \dfrac{150}{1} \times \dfrac{2.2}{1} = X$

4. Cancel terms: $\dfrac{1}{\cancel{100}_{2}} \times \dfrac{\cancel{150}^{3}}{1} \times \dfrac{2.2}{1} = \dfrac{1}{\cancel{2}_{1}} \times \dfrac{3}{1} \times \dfrac{\cancel{2.2}^{1.1}}{1} = \dfrac{1}{1} \times \dfrac{3}{1} \times \dfrac{1.1}{1} = X$

5. Multiply: $\dfrac{1}{1} \times \dfrac{3}{1} \times \dfrac{1.1}{1} = \dfrac{3.3}{1} = 3.3 = X$

6. That's it! $X = 3.3$

Example 5:

$$\frac{0.125}{0.25} \times 1.5 = X$$

1. Convert: Express 1.5 in fraction form: $\frac{0.125}{0.25} \times \frac{1.5}{1} = X$

2. Convert: Add a zero to thousandths place for 0.25 for easier comparison: $\frac{0.125}{0.250} \times \frac{1.5}{1} = X$

3. Cancel terms: $\frac{\overset{1}{\cancel{0.125}}}{\underset{2}{\cancel{0.250}}} \times \frac{1.5}{1} = \frac{1}{2} \times \frac{1.5}{1} = X$

4. Multiply: $\frac{1}{2} \times \frac{1.5}{1} = \frac{1.5}{2} = X$

5. Divide: $\frac{1.5}{2} = 0.75 = X$

6. You've got it! $X = 0.75$

Example 5 can also be solved by computing with fractions instead of decimals.

Try this: $\frac{0.125}{0.25} \times 1.5 = X$

1. Convert: Express 1.5 in fraction form: $\frac{0.125}{0.25} \times \frac{1.5}{1} = X$

2. Convert: Add zeros for easier comparison, making *both* decimals of equal length:

   $$\frac{0.125}{0.250} \times \frac{1.5}{1.0} = X$$

3. Cancel terms: $\frac{\overset{1}{\cancel{0.125}}}{\underset{2}{\cancel{0.250}}} \times \frac{\overset{3}{\cancel{1.5}}}{\underset{2}{\cancel{1.0}}} = \frac{1}{2} \times \frac{3}{2} = X$ (It is easier to work with whole numbers.)

4. Multiply: $\frac{1}{2} \times \frac{3}{2} = \frac{3}{4} = X$

5. Convert: $\frac{3}{4} = 0.75 = X$

6. You've got it again! $X = 0.75$

Which way do you find easier?

Example 6:

$$\frac{3}{4} \times 45\% = X$$

1. Convert: Express 45% as a fraction reduced to lowest terms: $45\% = \frac{45}{100} = \frac{9}{20}$

2. Multiply fractions: $\frac{3}{4} \times \frac{9}{20} = X$

   $$\frac{27}{80} = X$$

3. Divide: $\frac{27}{80} = 0.337 = X$

4. Round to hundredths place: $0.34 = X$

5. You have your answer. $X = 0.34$

QUICK REVIEW

- To solve simple equations, perform the mathematical operations indicated to find the value of the unknown "X."
- Express the result (value of X) in decimal form.

REVIEW SET 8

Solve the following problems for "X." Express answers as decimals rounded to two places.

1. $\dfrac{75}{125} \times 5 = X$ _____

2. $\dfrac{\frac{3}{4}}{\frac{1}{2}} \times 2.2 = X$ _____

3. $\dfrac{150}{300} \times 2.5 = X$ _____

4. $\dfrac{40\%}{60\%} \times 8 = X$ _____

5. $\dfrac{0.35}{2.5} \times 4 = X$ _____

6. $\dfrac{0.15}{0.1} \times 1.2 = X$ _____

7. $\dfrac{0.4}{2.5} \times 4 = X$ _____

8. $\dfrac{1,200,000}{400,000} \times 4.2 = X$ _____

9. $\dfrac{\frac{2}{3}}{\frac{1}{6}} \times 10 = X$ _____

10. $\dfrac{30}{50} \times 0.8 = X$ _____

11. $\dfrac{200,000}{300,000} \times 1.5 = X$ _____

12. $\dfrac{0.08}{0.1} \times 1.2 = X$ _____

13. $\dfrac{7.5}{5} \times 3 = X$ _____

14. $\dfrac{250,000}{2,000,000} \times 7.5 = X$ _____

15. $\dfrac{600}{150} \times 2.5 = X$ _____

16. $\dfrac{600,000}{750,000} \times 0.5 = X$ _____

17. $\dfrac{75\%}{60\%} \times 1.2 = X$ _____

18. $\dfrac{0.25}{0.125} \times 5 = X$ _____

19. $\dfrac{1,000,000}{250,000} \times 5 = X$ _____

20. $\dfrac{\frac{1}{100}}{\frac{1}{150}} \times 1.2 = X$ _____

After completing these problems, see pages 467–468 to check your answers.

RATIO-PROPORTION: CROSS-MULTIPLYING TO SOLVE FOR "X"

A *proportion* is two ratios that are equal or an equation between two equal ratios.

> **#5%3%** **MATH TIP**
>
> A proportion is written as two ratios separated by an equal sign, such as 5:10 = 10:20. The two ratios in a proportion may also be separated by a double colon sign, such as 5:10 :: 10:20.

Some of the calculations you will perform will have the unknown "X" as a different term in the equation. To determine the value of the unknown "X," you must apply the rule for cross-multiplying used in a proportion.

In a proportion, the product of the *means* (the two inside numbers) equals the product of the *extremes* (the two outside numbers). Finding the product of the means and the extremes is called *cross-multiplying*.

Example:

Extremes

$5:10 \ = \ 10:20$

Means

$5 \times 20 = 10 \times 10$

$100 = 100$

Because ratios are the same as fractions, the same proportion can be expressed like this: $\frac{5}{10} = \frac{10}{20}$. The fractions are *equivalent,* or equal. The numerator of the first fraction and the denominator of the second fraction are the extremes, and the denominator of the first fraction and the numerator of the second fraction are the means.

Example:

Extreme $\quad \frac{5}{10} \quad \frac{10}{20} \quad$ Mean

Mean $\qquad\qquad\qquad$ Extreme

Cross-multiply to find the equal products of the means and extremes.

If two fractions are *equivalent*, or equal, their cross-products are also equal.

Example:

$\frac{5}{10} \ \frac{10}{20}$

$5 \times 20 = 10 \times 10$

$100 = 100$

When one of the quantities in a proportion is unknown, a letter, such as "*X*," may be substituted for this unknown quantity. You would solve the equation to find the value of "X." In addition to cross-multiplying, there is one more rule you need to know to solve for "X" in a proportion.

Dividing or multiplying each side (*member*) of an equation by the same nonzero number produces an equivalent equation.

MATH TIP

Dividing each side of an equation by the same nonzero number is the same as reducing or simplifying the equation. Multiplying each side by the same nonzero number enlarges the equation.

Let's examine how to simplify an equation.

Example:

$25X = 100$ (25X means $25 \times X$)

Simplify the equation to find "X." Divide both sides by 25, the number before "X." Reduce to lowest terms.

$$\frac{\overset{1}{\cancel{25X}}}{\underset{1}{\cancel{25}}} = \frac{\overset{4}{\cancel{100}}}{\underset{1}{\cancel{25}}}$$

$\frac{1X}{1} = \frac{4}{1}$ (Dividing or multiplying a number by 1 does not change its value. "1X" is understood to be simply "X.")

$X = 4$

Replace "X" with 4 in the same equation, and you can prove that the calculations are correct.

$25 \times 4 = 100$

Now you are ready to apply the concepts of cross-multiplying and simplifying an equation to solve for "X" in a proportion.

Example 1:

$$\frac{90}{2} = \frac{45}{X}$$

You have a proportion with an unknown quantity "X" in the denominator of the second fraction. Find the value of "X."

1. Cross-multiply: $\frac{90}{2} \bowtie \frac{45}{X}$

2. Multiply terms: $90 \times X = 2 \times 45$

   $90X = 90$ (90X means $90 \times X$)

3. Simplify the equation: Divide both sides of the equation by the number before the unknown "X." You are equally reducing the terms on both sides of the equation.

$$\frac{\overset{1}{\cancel{90X}}}{\underset{1}{\cancel{90}}} = \frac{\overset{1}{\cancel{90}}}{\underset{1}{\cancel{90}}}$$

   $X = 1$

Try another one. The unknown "X" is a different term.

Example 2:

$$\frac{80}{X} \times 60 = 20$$

1. Convert: Express 60 as a fraction.

    $$\frac{80}{X} \times \frac{60}{1} = 20$$

2. Multiply fractions: $\frac{80}{X} \times \frac{60}{1} = 20$

    $$\frac{4800}{X} = 20$$

3. Convert: Express 20 as a fraction.

    $$\frac{4800}{X} = \frac{20}{1}$$

    You now have a proportion.

4. Cross-multiply: $\frac{4800}{X} \diagup\!\!\!\diagdown \frac{20}{1}$

    $$20X = 4800$$

5. Simplify: Divide both sides of the equation by the number before the unknown "X."

    $$\frac{\overset{1}{\cancel{20}X}}{\underset{1}{\cancel{20}}} = \frac{\overset{240}{\cancel{4800}}}{\underset{1}{\cancel{20}}}$$

    $$X = 240$$

Example 3:

$$\frac{X}{160} = \frac{2.5}{80}$$

1. Cross-multiply: $\frac{X}{160} \diagup\!\!\!\diagdown \frac{2.5}{80}$

    $$80 \times X = 2.5 \times 160$$

    $$80X = 400$$

2. Simplify: $\frac{\overset{1}{\cancel{80}X}}{\underset{1}{\cancel{80}}} = \frac{\overset{5}{\cancel{400}}}{\underset{1}{\cancel{80}}}$

    $$X = 5$$

Example 4:

$$\frac{40}{100} = \frac{X}{2}$$

1. Cross-multiply: $\frac{40}{100} \diagup\!\!\!\diagdown \frac{X}{2}$

2. Multiply terms: $100 \times X = 40 \times 2$

    $$100X = 80$$

3. Simplify the equation: $\frac{\overset{1}{\cancel{100}X}}{\underset{1}{\cancel{100}}} = \frac{\cancel{80}}{\cancel{100}}$

    $$X = 0.8$$

Calculations that result in an amount less than 1 should be expressed as a decimal. Most medications are ordered and supplied in metric measure. Metric measure is a decimal-based system.

QUICK REVIEW

- A *proportion* is an equation of two equal ratios. The ratios may be expressed as fractions.

  Example: 1:4 = X:8 or $\frac{1}{4} = \frac{X}{8}$

- In a proportion, the product of the means equals the product of the extremes.

  Extremes

  Example: 1:4   =   X:8   Therefore, 4 × X = 1 × 8

  Means

- If two fractions are equal, their cross-products are equal. This operation is referred to as cross-multiplying.

  Example: $\frac{1}{4} \times\!\!\!\!\times \frac{X}{8}$ Therefore, 4 × X = 1 × 8 or 4X = 8

- Dividing each side of an equation by the same number produces an equivalent equation. This operation is referred to as *simplifying the equation*.

  Example: If 4X = 8, then $\frac{4X}{4} = \frac{8}{4}$, and X = 2

REVIEW SET 9

Find the value of "X." Express answers as decimals rounded to two places.

1. $\frac{1000}{2} = \frac{125}{X}$ _____

2. $\frac{500}{2} = \frac{250}{X}$ _____

3. $\frac{500}{1} = \frac{280}{X}$ _____

4. $\frac{0.5}{2} = \frac{250}{X}$ _____

5. $\frac{75}{1.5} = \frac{35}{X}$ _____

6. $\frac{1200}{X} \times 12 = 28$ _____

7. $\frac{1000}{X} \times 60 = 28$ _____

8. $\frac{2}{2000} \times X = 0.5$ _____

9. $\frac{15}{500} \times X = 6$ _____

10. $\frac{5}{X} = \frac{10}{21}$ _____

11. $\frac{250}{1} = \frac{750}{X}$ _____

12. $\frac{80}{5} = \frac{10}{X}$ _____

13. $\frac{5}{20} = \frac{X}{40}$ _____

14. $\frac{\frac{1}{100}}{1} = \frac{\frac{1}{150}}{X}$ _____

15. $\frac{2.2}{X} = \frac{8.8}{5}$ _____

16. $\frac{60}{15} = \frac{125}{X}$ _____

17. $\frac{60}{10} = \frac{100}{X}$ _____

18. $\frac{80}{X} \times 60 = 20$ _____

19. $\frac{X}{0.5} = \frac{6}{4}$ _____

20. $\frac{5}{2.2} = \frac{X}{1}$ _____

21. $\frac{\frac{1}{4}}{15} = \frac{X}{60}$ _____

22. $\frac{25\%}{30\%} = \frac{5}{X}$ _____

23. In any group of 100 nurses, you would expect to find 45 nurses who will specialize in a particular field of nursing. In a class of 240 graduating nurses, how many would you expect to specialize? _____

24. Low-fat cheese has 48 calories per ounce. A client who is having his caloric intake measured has eaten $1\frac{1}{2}$ ounces of cheese. How many calories has he eaten? _____

25. If a patient receives 450 milligrams of a medication given evenly over 5.5 hours, how many milligrams did the patient receive per hour? _____

After completing these problems, see page 468 to check your answers.

FINDING THE PERCENTAGE OF A QUANTITY

An important computation that health care professionals use for dosage calculations is to find a given percentage or part of a quantity. *Percentage* is a term that describes a *part* of a whole quantity. A *known percent* determines the part in question. Said another way, the percentage (or part in question) is equal to some known percent multiplied by the whole quantity.

> **RULE**
>
> Percentage (Part) = Percent × Whole Quantity
> To find a percentage or part of a whole quantity:
>   1. Change the percent to a decimal, and
>   2. Multiply the decimal by the whole quantity.

Example:

A patient reports that he drank 75% of his 8 ounce cup of coffee for breakfast. To record the amount he actually drank in his chart, you must determine what amount is 75% of 8 ounces.

> **MATH TIP**
>
> In a mathematical expression, the word *of* means *times* and indicates that you should multiply.

To continue with the example:

Percentage (Part) = Percent × Whole Quantity

Let X represent the unknown.

1. Change 75% to a decimal: $75\% = \frac{75}{100} = .75. = 0.75$

2. Multiply 0.75 × 8 ounces: $X = 0.75 \times 8 = 6$ ounces

Therefore, 75% of 8 ounces is 6 ounces.

QUICK REVIEW

- Percentage (Part) = Percent $\times$ Whole Quantity

  Example: What is 12% of 48? X = 12% $\times$ 48 = 0.12 $\times$ 48 = 5.76

REVIEW SET 10

Perform the indicated operation; round decimals to hundredths place.

1. What is 0.25% of 520? _____
2. What is 5% of 95? _____
3. What is 40% of 140? _____
4. What is 0.7% of 62? _____
5. What is 3% of 889? _____

6. What is 20% of 75? _____
7. What is 4% of 20? _____
8. What is 7% of 34? _____
9. What is 15% of 250? _____
10. What is 75% of 150? _____

11. A patient has an order for an anti-infective in the amount of 500 milligrams by mouth twice a day for 10 days to treat pneumonia. He received a bottle of 20 pills. How many pills has this patient taken if he has used 40% of the 20 pills? _____

12. The patient is on oral fluid restrictions of 1200 milliliters for a 24 hour period. For breakfast and lunch he has consumed 60% of the total fluid allowance. How many milliliters has he had? _____

13. A patient's hospital bill for surgery is $17,651.07. Her insurance company pays 80%. How much will the patient owe? _____

14. Table salt (sodium chloride) is 40% sodium by weight. If a box of salt weighs 18 ounces, how much sodium is in the box of salt? _____

15. A patient has an average daily intake of 3500 calories. At breakfast she eats 20% of the total daily caloric allowance. How many calories did she ingest? _____

After completing these problems, see pages 468–469 to check your answers.

PRACTICE PROBLEMS—CHAPTER 2

Find the equivalent decimal, fraction, percent, and ratio forms. Reduce fractions and ratios to lowest terms; round decimals to two places.

	Decimal	Fraction	Percent	Ratio
1.	_____	$\frac{2}{5}$	_____	_____
2.	0.05	_____	_____	_____
3.	_____	_____	17%	_____
4.	_____	_____	_____	1:4
5.	_____	_____	6%	_____

Decimal	Fraction	Percent	Ratio
6. _____	$\frac{1}{6}$	_____	_____
7. _____	_____	50%	_____
8. _____	_____	_____	1:100
9. 0.09	_____	_____	_____
10. _____	$\frac{3}{8}$	_____	_____
11. _____	_____	_____	2:3
12. _____	$\frac{1}{3}$	_____	_____
13. 0.52	_____	_____	_____
14. _____	_____	_____	9:20
15. _____	$\frac{6}{7}$	_____	_____
16. _____	_____	_____	3:10
17. _____	$\frac{1}{50}$	_____	_____
18. 0.6	_____	_____	_____
19. 0.04	_____	_____	_____
20. _____	_____	10%	_____

Convert as indicated.

21. 1:25 to a decimal _____

22. $\frac{10}{400}$ to a ratio _____

23. 0.075 to a percent _____

24. 17:34 to a fraction _____

25. 75% to a ratio _____

Perform the indicated operation. Round decimals to hundredths.

26. What is 35% of 750? _____

27. What is 7% of 52? _____

28. What is 8.2% of 24? _____

Identify the strongest solution in each of the following:

29. 1:40   1:400   1:4   _____

30. 1:10   1:200   1:50   _____

Find the value of X in the following equations. Express your answers as decimals rounded to the nearest hundredth.

31. $\dfrac{20}{400} = \dfrac{X}{1680} =$ _____

36. $\dfrac{3}{9} = \dfrac{X}{117}$ _____

32. $\dfrac{75}{X} = \dfrac{\frac{1}{300}}{4}$ _____

37. $\dfrac{\frac{1}{8}}{\frac{1}{3}} \times 2 = X$ _____

33. $\dfrac{X}{5} = \dfrac{3}{15}$ _____

38. $\dfrac{X}{7} = \dfrac{12}{4}$ _____

34. $\dfrac{500}{250} = \dfrac{2.2}{X}$ _____

39. $\dfrac{X}{8} = \dfrac{9}{0.6}$ _____

35. $\dfrac{0.6}{1.2} = \dfrac{X}{200}$ _____

40. $\dfrac{0.4}{0.1} \times 22.5 = X$ _____

41. A portion of meat totaling 125 grams contains 20% protein and 5% fat. How many grams each of protein and fat does the meat contain? __25__ protein __6.25__ fat

42. The total points for a course in a nursing program is 308. A nursing student needs to achieve 75% of the total points to pass the semester. How many points are required to pass? __231__

43. To work off 90 calories, Angie must walk for 27 minutes. How many minutes would she need to walk to work off 200 calories? _____60_____

44. The doctor orders a record of the patient's fluid intake and output. The patient drinks 25% of a bowl of broth. How many milliliters of intake will be recorded if the bowl holds 200 milliliters? _____50_____

45. The recommended daily allowance (RDA) of a particular vitamin is 60 milligrams. If a multivitamin tablet claims to provide 45% of the RDA, how many milligrams of the particular vitamin would a patient receive from the multivitamin tablet? __27__

46. A label on a dinner roll wrapper reads, "2.7 grams of fiber per $\frac{3}{4}$ ounce serving." If you eat 1.5 ounces of dinner rolls, how many grams of fiber will you consume? __3.04__ __5.4__

47. A patient received an intravenous medication at a rate of 6.75 milligrams per minute. After 42 minutes, how much medication had she received? __283.5__

48. A person weighed 130 pounds at his last doctor's office visit. At this visit the patient has lost 5% of his weight. How many pounds has the patient lost? __6.5 lbs__

49. The cost of a certain medication is expected to decrease by 17% next year. If the cost is $12.56 now, how much would you expect it to cost at this time next year? __10.42__

50. A patient is to be started on 150 milligrams of a medication and then decreased by 10% of the original dose for each dose until he is receiving 75 milligrams. When he takes his 75 milligram dose, how many total doses will he have taken? HINT: Be sure to count his first (150 milligrams) and last (75 milligrams) doses. _____6_____

After completing these problems, see pages 469–470 to check your answers.

SECTION 1 SELF-EVALUATION

Directions:

1. Round decimals to two places, as needed.
2. Express fractions in lowest terms.

Section 1 Mathematics Review for Dosage Calculations

Multiply or divide by the power of 10 indicated. Draw an arrow to demonstrate movement of the decimal point.

1. $30.5 \div 10 =$ _____

3. $63 \div 100 =$ _____

2. $40.025 \times 100 =$ _____

4. $72.327 \times 10 =$ _____

Identify the least common denominator for the following sets of numbers.

5. $\frac{1}{6}, \frac{2}{3}, \frac{3}{4}$ _____

6. $\frac{2}{5}, \frac{3}{10}, \frac{3}{11}$ _____

Complete the operations indicated.

7. $\frac{1}{4} + \frac{2}{3} =$ _____

13. $80.3 - 21.06 =$ _____

8. $\frac{6}{7} - \frac{1}{9} =$ _____

14. $0.3 \times 0.3 =$ _____

9. $1\frac{3}{5} \times \frac{5}{8} =$ _____

15. $1.5 \div 0.125 =$ _____

10. $\frac{3}{8} \div \frac{3}{4} =$ _____

16. $\frac{1}{150} \div \frac{1}{100} =$ _____

11. $13.2 + 32.55 + 0.029 =$ _____

17. $\dfrac{\frac{1}{120}}{\frac{1}{60}} =$ _____

12. 20% of $0.09 =$ _____

18. $\dfrac{16\%}{\frac{1}{4}} =$ _____

Arrange in order from smallest to largest.

19. $\frac{1}{3} \quad \frac{1}{2} \quad \frac{1}{6} \quad \frac{1}{10} \quad \frac{1}{5}$ _____

20. $\frac{3}{4} \quad \frac{7}{8} \quad \frac{5}{6} \quad \frac{2}{3} \quad \frac{9}{10}$ _____

21. $0.25 \quad 0.125 \quad 0.3 \quad 0.009 \quad 0.1909$ _____

22. $0.9\% \quad \frac{1}{2}\% \quad 50\% \quad 500\% \quad 100\%$ _____

23. Identify the strongest solution of the following: 1:3, 1:60, 1:6 _____

24. Identify the weakest solution of the following: 1:75, 1:600, 1:60 _____

Convert as indicated.

25. 1:100 to a decimal   _____

26. $\frac{6}{150}$ to a decimal   _____

27. 0.009 to a percent   _____

28. $33\frac{1}{3}\%$ to a fraction   _____

29. $\frac{5}{9}$ to a ratio   _____

30. 0.05 to a fraction   _____

31. $\frac{1}{2}\%$ to a ratio   _____

32. 2:3 to a fraction   _____

33. 3:4 to a percent   _____

34. $\frac{2}{5}$ to a percent   _____

35. $\frac{1}{6}$ to a decimal   _____

Find the value of "X" in the following equations. Express your answers as decimals; round to the nearest hundredth.

36. $\frac{0.35}{1.3} \times 4.5 = X$ _____

37. $\frac{0.3}{2.6} = \frac{0.15}{X}$ _____

38. $\frac{1,500,000}{500,000} \times X = 7.5$ _____

39. $\frac{\frac{1}{6}}{\frac{1}{4}} \times 1 = X$ _____

40. $\frac{1:100}{1:4} \times 2500 = X$ _____

41. $\frac{0.25}{0.125} \times 2 = X$ _____

42. $\frac{10\%}{\frac{1}{2}\%} \times 1000 = X$ _____

43. $\frac{\frac{1}{100}}{\frac{1}{150}} \times 2.2 = X$ _____

44. X:15 = 150:7.5   _____

45. $\frac{1,000,000}{600,000} \times 5 = X$ _____

46. In a drug study, it was determined that 4% of the participants developed the *headache* side effect. If there were 600 participants in the study, how many developed headaches?   _____

47. You are employed in a health care clinic where each employee must work 25% of 8 major holidays. How many holidays will you expect to work?   _____

48. If the value of 1 roll of guaze is $0.69, what is the value of $3\frac{1}{2}$ rolls?   _____

49. To prepare a nutritional formula from frozen concentrate, you mix 3 cans of water to every 1 can of concentrate. How many cans of water will you need to prepare formula from 4 cans of concentrate?   _____

50. If 1 centimeter equals $\frac{3}{8}$ inch, how many centimeters is a laceration that measures 3 inches?   _____

After completing these problems, see page 470 to check your answers. Give yourself two points for each correct answer.

Perfect score = 100   My score = _____

Minimum mastery score = 86 (43 correct)

For more practice, go back to the beginning of this section and repeat the Mathematics Diagnostic Evaluation.

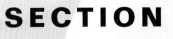

Measurement Systems, Drug Orders, and Drug Labels

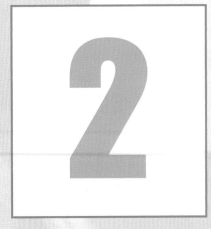

SECTION

2

Systems of Measurement

OBJECTIVES

Upon mastery of Chapter 3, you will be able to recognize and express the basic systems of measurement used to calculate dosages. To accomplish this you will also be able to:

- Interpret and properly express metric, apothecary, and household notation.
- Recall metric, apothecary, and household equivalents.
- Explain the use of milliequivalent (mEq), international unit (IU), unit (U), and milliunit (mU) in dosage calculation.

To administer the correct amount of the prescribed medication to the patient, you must have a thorough knowledge of the weights and measures used in the prescription and administration of medications. The three systems used by health professionals are the metric, the apothecary, and the household systems.

It is necessary for you to understand each system and how to convert from one system to another. Most prescriptions are written using the metric system, and all U.S. drug labels today provide metric measurements. The household system uses measurement found in familiar containers such as teaspoons, cups, and quarts. Prescriptions for older drugs may still be written in the apothecary system, usually by physicians trained in this system. Until the metric system completely replaces the apothecary and household systems, health care professionals must be familiar with each system.

Three essential parameters of measurement are associated with the prescription and administration of drugs within each system of measurement: weight, volume, and length. *Weight* is the most utilized parameter. It is very important as a dosage unit. Most drugs are ordered and supplied by the weight of the drug. Keep in mind that the metric weight units, such as gram and milligram, are the most accurate and are preferred for health care applications. Occasionally you will also use the apothecary unit of weight referred to as the *grain*.

Think of capacity, or how much a container holds, as you contemplate *volume*, which is the next most important parameter. Volume usually refers to liquids. Volume also adds two additional parameters to dosage calculations: *quantity* and *concentration*. The milliliter is the most common metric volume unit for dosage calculations. Much less frequently you will use household and apothecary measures, such as teaspoon and ounce.

Length is the least utilized parameter for dosage calculations, but linear measurement is still essential to learn for health care situations. A person's height, the circumference of an infant's head, body surface area, and the size of lacerations and tumors are examples of important length measurements. You are probably familiar with the household measurements of inches and feet. Typically in the health care setting, length is measured in millimeters and centimeters.

THE METRIC SYSTEM

The metric system was first adopted in 1799 in France. It is the most widely used system of measurement in the world today and is preferred for prescribing and administering medications.

The metric system is a decimal system, which means it is based on multiples of ten. The base units (the primary units of measurement) of the metric system are *gram* for weight, *liter* for volume, and *meter* for length. In this system, prefixes are used to show which portion of the base unit is being considered. It is important that you learn the most commonly used prefixes.

REMEMBER

Metric Prefixes

micro	=	one millionth or 0.000001 or $\frac{1}{1,000,000}$ of the base unit
milli	=	one thousandth or 0.001 or $\frac{1}{1000}$ of the base unit
centi	=	one hundredth or 0.01 or $\frac{1}{100}$ of the base unit
deci	=	one tenth or 0.1 or $\frac{1}{10}$ of the base unit
kilo	=	one thousand or 1000 times the base unit

Figure 3-1 demonstrates the relationship of metric units. Notice that the values of most of the common prefixes used in health care and the ones applied in this text are highlighted: **kilo-, base, milli-,** and **micro-.** These units are three places away from the next place. Often you can either multiply or divide by 1000 to calculate an equivalent quantity. The only exception is **centi-.** Centi- is easy to remember, though, if you think of the relationship between one cent and one U.S. dollar as a clue to the relationship of centi- to the base, $\frac{1}{100}$. **Deci-** is one tenth ($\frac{1}{10}$) of the base. See Chapter 1 to review the rules of multiplying and dividing decimals by a power of ten.

PREFIX	KILO-	hecto-	deca-	BASE	DECI-	CENTI-	MILLI-	decimilli-	centimilli-	MICRO-
Weight	kilogram			gram			milligram			microgram
Volume				liter	deciliter		milliliter			
Length				meter		centimeter	millimeter			
Value to Base	1000	100	10	1.0	0.1	0.01	0.001	0.0001	0.00001	0.000001

FIGURE 3-1 Relationship and Value of Metric Units, with Comparison of Common Metric Units Used in Health Care

---

MATH TIP

Try this to remember the order of six of the metric units—<u>k</u>ilo-, <u>h</u>ecto-, <u>d</u>eca-, (BASE), <u>d</u>eci-, <u>c</u>enti-, and <u>m</u>illi-: "**K**ing **H**enry **D**ied from a **D**isease **C**alled **M**umps."

			gram			
			liter			
			meter			
kilo	hecto	deca	BASE	deci	centi	milli
K	**H**	**D**	Δ	**D**	**C**	**M**
"King	Henry	Died	from a	Disease	Called	Mumps"

The international standardization of metric units was adopted throughout much of the world in 1960 with the International System of Units or SI (from the French *Système International*). The abbreviations of this system of metric notation are the most widely accepted. The metric units of measurement and the SI abbreviations most often used for dosage calculations and measurements of health status are given in the following units of weight, volume, and length. Other acceptable abbreviations are given in parentheses. Although these alternate abbreviations are still in use, they are considered confusing. This text uses SI standardized abbreviations throughout. It is recommended that you learn and practice these notations primarily.

SI METRIC SYSTEM			
	Unit	Abbreviation	Equivalents
Weight	**gram** (base unit)	g	1 g = 1000 mg
	milligram	mg	1 mg = 1000 mcg = 0.001 g
	microgram	mcg (or μg)	1 mcg = 0.001 mg = 0.000001 g
	kilogram	kg	1 kg = 1000 g
Volume	**liter** (base unit)	L (or ℓ)	1 L = 1000 mL
	milliliter	mL (or mℓ)	1 mL = 1 cc = 0.001 L
	cubic centimeter	cc	1 cc = 1 mL = 0.001 L
Length	**meter** (base unit)	m	1 m = 100 cm = 1000 mm
	centimeter	cm	1 cm = 0.01 m = 10 mm
	millimeter	mm	1 mm = 0.001 m = 0.1 cm

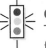

MATH TIP

A cubic centimeter is the amount of space occupied by one milliliter of liquid. 1 cc = 1 mL

CAUTION

You may see gram abbreviated as *Gm* or *gm,* liter as lowercase *l,* or milliliter as *ml.* These abbreviations are considered obsolete and too easily misinterpreted. You should only use the standardized SI abbreviations. Use *g* for gram, *L* for liter, and *mL* for milliliter.

CAUTION

The SI abbreviations for milligram (*mg*) and milliliter (*mL*) appear to be somewhat similar, but in fact mg is a weight unit and mL is a volume unit. Confusing these two units can have dire consequences in dosage calculations. Learn to clearly differentiate them now.

In addition to learning the metric units, their equivalent values, and their abbreviations, it is important to use the following rules of metric notation.

The metric system is the most common and the only standardized system of measurement in health care. Take a few minutes to review these essential points.

QUICK REVIEW

In the metric system:
- The metric base units are gram, liter, and meter.
- Subunits are designated by the appropriate prefix and the base unit (such as *milli*gram) and standardized abbreviations (such as *mg*).
- The unit or abbreviation always follows the amount.
- Decimals are used to designate fractional amounts.
- Use a zero to emphasize the decimal point for fractional amounts of less than 1.
- Omit unnecessary zeros.
- Multiply or divide by 1000 to derive most equivalents needed for dosage calculations.
- 1 cc = 1 mL.
- When in doubt about the exact amount or the abbreviation used, do not guess. Ask the writer to clarify.

REVIEW SET 11

1. The system of measurement most commonly used for prescribing and administering medications is the ___metric___ system.
2. Liter and milliliter are metric units that measure ___volume___.
3. Gram and milligram are metric units that measure ___weight___.
4. Meter and millimeter are metric units that measure ___length___.
5. 1 mg is ___.001___ of a g.
6. There are ___1000___ mL in a liter.
7. 10 mL = ___10___ cc
8. Which is largest—kilogram, gram, or milligram? ___Kilo___
9. Which is smallest—kilogram, gram, or milligram? ___milligram___
10. 1 liter = ___1000___ cc
11. 1000 mcg = ___1___ mg
12. 1 kg = ___1000___ g
13. 1 cm = ___10___ mm

Select the *correct* metric notation.

14. .3 g, 0.3 Gm, 0.3 g, .3 Gm, 0.30 g   *0.3 g*

15. $1\frac{1}{3}$ ml, 1.33 mL, 1.33 ML, $1\frac{1}{3}$ ML, 1.330 mL   *1.33 mL*

16. 5 Kg, 5.0 kg, kg 05, 5 kg, 5 kG   *5 kg*

17. 1.5 mm, $1\frac{1}{2}$ mm, 1.5 Mm, 1.50 MM, $1\frac{1}{2}$ MM   *1.5 mm*

18. mg 10, 10 mG, 10.0 mg, 10 mg, 10 MG   *10 mg*

Interpret these metric abbreviations.

19. mcg   *micrograms*   23. mm   *millimeter*

20. mL   *milliliter*   24. kg   *kilogram*

21. cc   *cubic centimeter*   25. cm   *centimeter*

22. g   *gram*

After completing these problems, see page 470 to check your answers.

THE APOTHECARY AND HOUSEHOLD SYSTEMS

Within a few years, the metric system will probably be used exclusively in the ordering and measurement of medicines. However, as long as prescriptions are being written with apothecary notation, it is necessary that health care professionals be knowledgeable about this system. Likewise, the household system persists, and nurses and other health care providers need to be familiar with the equivalent measurements that patients or clients use at home.

The historic interconnection between the apothecary and household systems is interesting. The apothecary system was the first system of medication measurement used by pharmacists (apothecaries) and physicians. It originated in Greece and made its way to Europe via Rome and France. The English used it during the late 1600s, and the colonists brought it to America. A modified system of measurement for everyday use evolved; it is now recognized as the household system. Large liquid volumes were based on familiar trading measurements, such as *pints, quarts,* and *gallons,* which originated as apothecary measurements. Vessels to accommodate each measurement were made by craftspersons and widely circulated in colonial America.

Units of weight, such as the *grain, ounce,* and *pound,* also are rooted in the apothecary system. The grain originated as the standard weight of a single grain of wheat, which happens to be approximately 60 milligrams. This one equivalency of weight (1 grain = 60 milligrams) is recognized in drug orders. After more than 100 years as the world's most popular pill, aspirin is still prescribed and dispensed in grains.

The Apothecary System

Apothecary notation is unusual. Exercise caution when using this system. The apothecary system utilizes Roman numerals. The ability to interpret Roman numerals is therefore essential. The letters **I**, **V**, and **X** are the basic symbols of this system that you will use in dosage calculations. In medical notation, lowercase letters are typically used to designate Roman numerals (**i, v,** and **x**).

In addition to Roman numerals, apothecary notation also uses common fractions, special symbols, and units of measure that precede numeric values. The common units are grain (**gr**) and ounce (℥). Let's outline the rules and examine what this notation looks like.

> **RULE**
>
> To accurately write apothecary notation:
> 1. The unit or abbreviation precedes the amount. Example: gr v, NOT v gr
> 2. Lowercase Roman numerals are used to express whole numbers, 1–10, 15, 20, and 30. Arabic numbers are used for other quantities. Examples: ℥ iii (three ounces), gr 12 (twelve grains), and gr xx (twenty grains)
> 3. Fractions are used to designate amounts less than 1. Example: gr $\frac{1}{4}$, NOT 0.25 gr
> 4. The fraction $\frac{1}{2}$ is designated by the symbol *ss*. Example: ℥ iiss (two and one-half ounces)

MATH TIP

To decrease errors in interpretation of medical notation, a line can be drawn over the lowercase Roman numerals to distinguish them from other letters in a word or phrase. The lowercase *i* is dotted above, not below, the line.

Example:

3 = iii or iii

Learn the following common Roman numerals and their Arabic equivalents. These are the values that you will use most frequently to interpret drug orders and read drug labels.

REMEMBER

Arabic Number	Roman Numeral	Apothecary Notation	Arabic Number	Roman Numeral	Apothecary Notation
1	I	i, ī	8	VIII	viii, v̄īīī
2	II	ii, īī	9	IX	ix, īx̄
3	III	iii, īīī	10	X	x, x̄
4	IV	iv, īv̄	15	XV	xv, x̄v̄
5	V	v, v̄	20	XX	xx, x̄x̄
6	VI	vi, v̄ī	25	XXV	xxv, x̄x̄v̄
7	VII	vii, v̄īī	30	XXX	xxx, x̄x̄x̄

The apothecary units of measurement and essential equivalents for volume are given in the following table. There are no essential equivalents of weight or length to learn for this system.

REMEMBER

Unit	APOTHECARY Abbreviation	Equivalents
grain	gr	
quart	qt	qt i = pt ii
pint	pt	pt i = ℥ 16
ounce or fluid ounce	℥	qt i = ℥ 32
dram	ʒ	
minim	♏	

NOTE: The minim (♏) and fluid dram (ʒ) are given only so that you will be able to recognize them. Some syringes may have the minim scale identified, and the medicine cup continues to show the dram scale. However, their use is discouraged.

#5% **MATH TIP**

The ounce (℥) is a larger unit, and its symbol has one more loop than the dram (ℨ), or there is "more bounce to the ounce."

CAUTION

Notice that the abbreviations for the apothecary grain (**gr**) and the metric gram (**g**) can be confusing. The rule of indicating the abbreviation or symbol before the quantity in apothecary measurement further distinguishes it from a metric measurement. If you are ever doubtful about the meaning that is intended, be sure to ask the writer for clarification.

QUICK REVIEW

In the apothecary system:

- The common units for dosage calculation are grain (gr) and ounce (℥).
- The quantity is best expressed in lowercase Roman numerals. Amounts greater than ten may be expressed in Arabic numbers, *except* 15 (xv), 20 (xx), and 30 (xxx).
- Quantities of less than one are expressed as fractions, *except* $\frac{1}{2}$. One-half ($\frac{1}{2}$) is expressed by the symbol *ss*.
- The abbreviation or unit symbol is clearly written *before* the quantity.
- If you are unsure about the exact meaning of any medical notation, do not guess or assume. Ask the writer for clarification.

REVIEW SET 12

Interpret the following apothecary symbols.

1. ℨ   Dram

2. ℥   ounce

3. ♏   minim

4. ss   half

5. gr   grain

Write the following quantities in the apothecary system.

6. one-half ounce   _____

7. one sixth grain   _____

8. four ounces   _____

9. two pints   pt ii

10. one and one fourth quarts   _____

11. ten grains   _____

12. eight and one-half ounces   _____

13. two grains   ii gr

14. sixteen pints   _____

15. three grains   iii gr

16. thirty-two ounces   _____

17. seven and one-half grains   _____

Give the equivalent units.

18. qt i = ℥   32

19. ℥ 16 = pt   1

20. qt i = pt   2

After completing these problems, see page 470 to check your answers.

The Household System

Household units are likely to be used by the patient at home where hospital measuring devices are not usually available. You should be familiar with the household system of measurement so that you can explain take-home prescriptions to your patient at the time of discharge. There is no standardized system of notation, but it is preferred to express the quantity in Arabic numbers and common fractions with the abbreviation following the amount. The common household units and abbreviations are given in the following table.

REMEMBER

HOUSEHOLD

Unit	Abbreviation	Equivalents
drop	gtt	
teaspoon	t (or tsp)	
tablespoon	T (or tbs)	1 T = 3 t
ounce (fluid)	oz (ʒ)	2 T = 1 oz
ounce (weight)	oz	1 pound (lb) = 16 oz
cup	cup	1 cup = 8 oz
pint	pt	1 pt = 2 cups
quart	qt	1 qt = 4 cups = 2 pt

NOTE: Like the minim (♏) and dram (ʒ), the drop (gtt) unit is given only for the purpose of recognition. There are no standard equivalents for *drop* to learn. The amount of each drop varies according to the diameter of the utensil used for measurement. (See Figure 6-2 Calibrated Dropper and Figure 14-16 Intravenous Drip Chambers.)

MATH TIP

Tablespoon is the larger unit, and the abbreviation is expressed with a capital *T*. Teaspoon is the smaller unit, and the abbreviation is expressed with a lowercase or small *t*.

CAUTION

There is wide variation in household measures and common household measuring devices, such as tableware teaspoons. Therefore, using the household system or household measures for dosage measurement can constitute a safety risk. Advise your patients and their families to use the measuring devices packaged with the medication or provided by the pharmacy, rather than using common household measuring devices.

QUICK REVIEW

In the household system:

- The common units used in health care are teaspoon, tablespoon, ounce, cup, pint, quart, and pound.
- The quantity is typically expressed in Arabic numbers with the unit abbreviation following the amount. Example: 5 t
- Quantities of less than one are preferably expressed as common fractions. Example: $\frac{1}{2}$ cup
- When in doubt about the exact amount or the abbreviation used, do not guess or assume. Ask the writer to clarify.

OTHER COMMON DRUG MEASUREMENTS: UNITS AND MILLIEQUIVALENTS

Four other measurements may be used to indicate the quantity of medicine prescribed: international unit (IU), unit (U), milliunit (mU), and milliequivalent (mEq). The quantity is expressed in Arabic numbers with the symbol following. The *international unit* (IU) represents a unit of potency used to measure such things as vitamins and chemicals. The *unit* (U) is a standardized amount needed to produce a desired effect. Medications such as penicillin, heparin, and insulin have their own meaning and numeric value related to the type of unit. One thousandth ($\frac{1}{1000}$) of a unit (U) is a *milliunit* (mU). The equivalent of 1 U is 1000 mU. Pitocin is a drug measured in mU. The *milliequivalent* (mEq) is one thousandth ($\frac{1}{1000}$) of an equivalent weight of a chemical. The mEq is the unit used when referring to the concentration of serum electrolytes, such as calcium, magnesium, potassium, and sodium.

It is not necessary to learn conversions for the international unit, unit, or milliequivalent because medications prescribed in these measurements are also prepared and administered in the same system.

Example 1:

Heparin 800 U is ordered, and *heparin 1000 units/1 mL* is the stock drug.

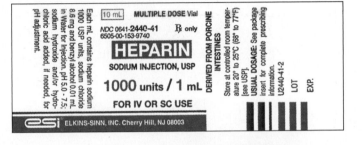

Example 2:

Potassium chloride 10 mEq is ordered, and *potassium chloride 20 mEq per 15 mL* is the stock drug.

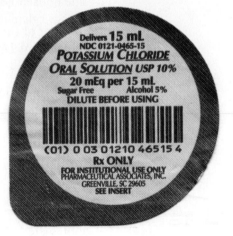

Example 3:

Syntocinon 2 mU (0.002 IU) intravenous per minute is ordered and *Syntocinon 10 IU/1 mL* to be added to 1000 mL intravenous solution is available.

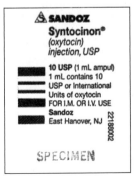

QUICK REVIEW

■ The international unit (IU), unit (U), milliunit (mU), and milliequivalent (mEq) are special measured quantities expressed in Arabic numbers followed by the unit symbol.
■ No conversion is necessary for U, IU, and mEq, because the ordered dosage and supply dosage are in the same system.
■ 1 U = 1000 mU.

REVIEW SET 13

Interpret the following notations.

1. 20 gtt   _Drop_   4. 4 t   _4 tsp_

2. 1000 U   _____   5. 10 T   _____

3. 10 mEq   _milliequivalents_

Express the following using correct notation.

6. four drops   _____

7. 30 milliequivalents _____

8. 5 tablespoons   _____

9. 1500 units   _____

10. 10 teaspoons   _____

11. The household system of measurement is commonly used in hospital dosage calculations.   (True) (False)

12. The drop is a standardized unit of measure.   (True) (False)

13. Fluid ounce is equivalent to the ounce that measures weight.   (True) (False)

14. Drugs such as heparin and insulin are commonly measured in _____, and is abbreviated _____.

15. 1 T = _____ t   18. 2 T = _____ oz

16. 1 oz = _____ T   19. 8 oz = _____ cup

17. 16 oz = _____ lb

20. The unit of potency used to measure vitamins and chemicals is the _____ and is abbreviated _____.

After completing these problems, see page 471 to check your answers.

CRITICAL THINKING SKILLS

The importance of the placement of the decimal point cannot be overemphasized. Let's look at some examples of potential medication errors related to placement of the decimal point.

error 1

Not placing a zero before a decimal point on medication orders.

(continues)

(continued)

possible scenario

An emergency room physician wrote an order for the bronchodilator terbutaline for a patient with asthma. The order was written as follows:

Terbutaline .5 mg subcutaneously now, repeat dose in 30 minutes if no improvement

Suppose the nurse, not noticing the faint decimal point, administered 5 mg of terbutaline subcutaneously instead of 0.5 mg. The patient would receive ten times the dose intended by the physician.

potential outcome

Within minutes of receiving the injection the patient would likely complain of headache, and develop tachycardia, nausea, and vomiting. The patient's hospital stay would be lengthened due to the need to recover from the overdose.

prevention

This type of medication error is avoided by remembering the rule to place a 0 in front of a decimal to avoid confusion regarding the dosage: 0.5 mg. Further, remember to question orders that are unclear or seem unreasonable.

CRITICAL THINKING SKILLS

Many medication errors occur by confusing mg and mL. Remember that mg is the weight of the medication, and mL is the volume of the medication preparation.

error 2

Confusing mg and mL.

possible scenario

Suppose a physician ordered Prelone (prednisolone, a steroid) 15 mg by mouth twice a day for a patient with cancer. Prelone syrup is supplied in a concentration of 15 mg in 5 mL. The pharmacist supplied a bottle of Prelone containing a total volume of 240 mL with 15 mg of Prelone in every 5 mL. The nurse, in a rush to give her medications on time, misread the order as 15 mL and gave the patient 15 mL of Prelone instead of 5 mL. Therefore, the patient received 45 mg of Prelone, or three times the correct dosage.

potential outcome

The patient could develop a number of complications related to a high dosage of steroids: gastrointestinal bleeding, headaches, seizures, and hypertension, to name a few.

prevention

The mg is the weight of a medication, and mL is the volume you prepare. Do not allow yourself to get rushed or distracted so that you would confuse milligrams with milliliters. When you know you are distracted or stressed, have another nurse double-check the calculation of the dose.

PRACTICE PROBLEMS—CHAPTER 3

Give the metric prefix for the following parts of the base units.

1. 0.001 _____   3. 0.01 _____

2. 0.000001 _____   4. 1000 _____

Identify the equivalent unit with a value of 1 that is indicated by the following amounts (such as 1000 mU-1 U).

5. 0.001 gram _____   7. 0.001 milligram _____

6. 1000 grams _____   8. 0.01 meter _____

Identify the metric base unit for the following.

9. length _____   11. volume _____

10. weight _____

Interpret the following notations.

12. gtt _____   23. cc _____

13. ʒ _____   24. pt _____

14. oz _____   25. T _____

15. gr _____   26. mm _____

16. mg _____   27. g _____

17. mcg _____   28. cm _____

18. U _____   29. L _____

19. mEq _____   30. m _____

20. t _____   31. kg _____

21. mU _____   32. IU _____

22. mL _____

Express the following amounts in proper notation.

33. one-half grain _____   37. one-half liter _____

34. two teaspoons _____   38. one fourth dram _____

35. one third ounce _____   39. one two-hundredths of a grain _____

36. five hundred milligrams _____   40. five hundredths of a milligram _____

Express the following numeric amounts in words.

41. $8\frac{1}{4}$ oz _____   45. 20 mEq _____

42. 375 IU _____   46. 0.4 L _____

43. gr $\frac{1}{125}$ _____   47. gr ivss _____

44. 2.6 mL _____   48. 0.17 mg _____

49. Critical Thinking Skill: Describe the strategy that would prevent the medication error.

possible scenario

Suppose a physician ordered oral Coumadin (an anticoagulant) for a patient with a history of phlebitis. The physician wrote an order for 1 mg, but while writing the order placed a decimal point after the 1 and added a 0:

Coumadin 1.0 mg orally once per day

Coumadin 1.0 mg was transcribed on the medication record as Coumadin 10 mg. The patient received ten times the correct dosage.

potential outcome

The patient would likely begin hemorrhaging. An antidote, such as vitamin K, would be necessary to reverse the effects of the overdose. However, it is important to remember that not all drugs have antidotes.

prevention

_____

_____

50. Critical Thinking Skill: Describe the strategy that would prevent a medication error or the need to notify the prescribing practitioner.

possible scenario

Suppose a physician ordered oral codeine (a potent narcotic analgesic) for an adult patient recovering from extensive nasal surgery. The physician wrote the following order for 1 grain (equivalent to about 60 mg), but while writing the order placed the 1 before the abbreviation gr. The gr smeared and the abbreviation gr is unclear. Is it _grains_ or _grams_?

Codeine 1 gr orally every four to six hours as needed for pain

Codeine 1 gram was transcribed on the medication record. Because 1 gram is equivalent to 1000 mg or about 15 grains, this erroneous dosage is about 15 times more than the intended amount.

potential outcome

Even though the nurse was in a rush to help ease the patient's pain, she realized that the available codeine pills would not be dispensable in this amount. She would have to give the patient 15 tablets to equal the 1 gram amount. The nurse saw the questionable order and called the physician for clarification. The nurse correctly concluded it was unlikely that the physician would have ordered such an excessive number of pills or dosage.

prevention

_____

_____

After completing these problems, see page 471 to check your answers.

Conversions: Metric, Apothecary, and Household Systems

OBJECTIVES

Upon mastery of Chapter 4, you will be able to complete step 1, conversion, in the three-step process of dosage calculations. To accomplish this, you will also be able to:

● Recall from memory the metric, apothecary, and household approximate equivalents.
● Convert between units of measurement within the same system.
● Convert units of measurement from one system to another.

Medications are usually prescribed or ordered in a unit of weight measurement such as grams or grains. The nurse must interpret this order and administer the correct number of tablets, capsules, teaspoons, milliliters, or some other unit of volume or capacity measurement in order to deliver the prescribed amount of medication.

Example 1:

A prescription notation may read:

Aldactone 100 mg to be given orally

The nurse has on hand a 100 tablet bottle of *Aldactone labeled 50 mg in each tablet.* To administer the correct amount of the drug, the nurse must convert the prescribed weight of 100 mg to the correct number of tablets. In this case, the nurse gives the patient two of the 50 mg tablets, which equals 100 mg of *Aldactone*. To give the prescribed dosage, the nurse must be able to calculate the order in weight to the correct amount of tablets of the drug on hand or in stock. THINK: If one tablet equals 50 mg, then two tablets equal 100 mg.

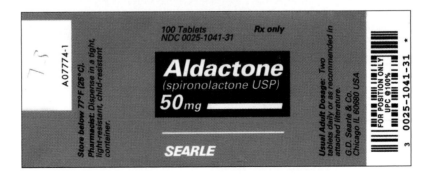

Example 2:

A prescription notation may read:

Versed 2.5 mg by intravenous injection

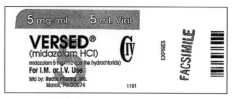

The nurse has on hand a vial of *Versed* labeled *5 mg/mL*. To administer the correct amount of the drug, the nurse must be able to fill the injection syringe with the correct number of milliliters. As the nurse, how many milliliters would you give? THINK: If 5 mg = 1 mL, then 2.5 mg = 0.5 mL. Therefore, 0.5 mL should be administered.

Sometimes a drug order may be written in a unit of measurement that is different from the supply of drugs the nurse has on hand.

Example 1:

Medication order: *Solu-Medrol 500 mg by intramuscular injection*

Supply on hand: *Solu-Medrol injection 1 g*

The drug order is written in milligrams, but the drug is supplied in grams.

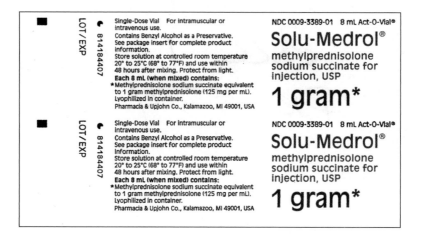

Example 2:

Medication order: *Codeine gr ss orally*

Supply on hand: *Codeine 30 mg tablets*

The drug order is written in grains (apothecary measurement), but the drug is supplied in milligrams (metric measurement).

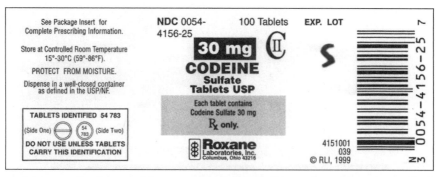

In such cases, the prescribed quantities must be converted into the units as supplied. The nurse or health care professional can then calculate the correct dosage to prepare and administer to the patient. Thus, conversion is the first step in the calculation of dosages.

In this chapter you will learn two methods to do conversions: the *conversion factor* method and the *ratio-proportion* method. Study them both and then choose to use whichever one is easier and more logical to you.

CONVERTING FROM ONE UNIT TO ANOTHER USING THE CONVERSION FACTOR METHOD

After learning the systems of measurement common for dosage calculations and their equivalents (Chapter 3), the next step is to learn how to use them. First, you must be able to convert or change from one unit to another within the same measurement system. To accomplish this simple operation you need to:

- recall the equivalents, and
- multiply or divide.

The following information will help you remember when to multiply and when to divide.

The *conversion factor* is a number used with either multiplication or division to change a measurement from one unit of measurement to its *equivalent* in another unit of measurement.

RULE

To convert from a larger to a smaller unit of measurement, multiply by the conversion factor. THINK: Larger → Smaller: (×)

Stop and think about this. You know this is true because it takes *more* parts of a *smaller* unit to make an equivalent amount of a larger unit. To get *more* parts, *multiply*.

Example 1:

Let's examine units already familiar to you. How many cups are in 3 quarts? In units of measurement, 1 quart = 4 cups. It takes 4 of the cup units to equal 1 of the quart units. Cups are *smaller* than quarts. THINK: Larger → Smaller: (×). The conversion factor for the cup and quart units is 4. Multiply by the conversion factor.

Therefore, 3 quarts (the larger unit) = 3 × 4 = 12 cups (the smaller unit).

Example 2:

How many inches are in 2 feet?

To convert 2 feet to the equivalent number of inches, multiply by the conversion factor of 12, because 1 foot = 12 inches. Multiplication is used because it takes *more* inches to represent the same amount in feet. Inches are smaller units than feet. THINK: Larger → Smaller: (×)

Therefore, 2 feet = 2 × 12 = 24 inches.

RULE

To convert from a smaller to a larger unit of measurement, divide by the conversion factor. THINK: Smaller → Larger: (÷)

You know this is true because it takes *fewer* parts of the *larger* unit to make an equivalent amount of a smaller unit. To get *fewer* parts, *divide*.

Example 1:

How many feet are in 36 inches?

1 foot = 12 inches. Feet are larger units than inches. To convert 36 inches to the equivalent number of feet, divide by the conversion factor of 12. Division is used because it takes *fewer* feet to represent the same amount in inches. THINK: Smaller → Larger: ($\div$)

Therefore, 36 inches (the smaller unit) = 36 $\div$ 12 = 3 feet (the larger unit).

Example 2:

How many quarts are in 8 cups?

You know that 1 quart = 4 cups. The conversion factor is 4. Quarts are larger units than cups.

Divide by the conversion factor because it takes *fewer* of the quart units to equal the same amount in the cup units. THINK: Smaller → Larger: ($\div$)

Therefore, 8 cups = 8 $\div$ 4 = 2 quarts.

QUICK REVIEW

Use the conversion factor method to convert from one unit of measurement to another.
- Recall the equivalents.
- Identify the conversion factor.
- MULTIPLY by the conversion factor to convert to a smaller unit. THINK: Larger → Smaller: ($\times$)
- DIVIDE by the conversion factor to convert to a larger unit. THINK: Smaller → Larger: ($\div$)

REVIEW SET 14

Use the following common household equivalents to answer these items. Express amounts that are less than one as common fractions.

1 gallon = 4 quarts   1 foot = 12 inches

1 quart = 2 pints = 4 cups   1 yard = 3 feet

1. To convert from a smaller unit of measurement (such as inches) to a larger unit of measurement (such as feet), you would _____. (multiply or divide?)

2. To convert from gallons to quarts, you would _____. (multiply or divide?)

3. 12 cups =	_____ quarts		12. 10 yards =	_____ feet	
4. 36 inches =	_____ feet		13. 10 feet =	_____ yards	
5. 14 quarts =	_____ gallons		14. $3\frac{1}{2}$ quarts =	_____ cups	
6. 32 cups =	_____ pints		15. 3 cups =	_____ quart	
7. 6 feet =	_____ inches		16. 1 inch =	_____ foot	
8. $\frac{1}{2}$ yard =	_____ feet		17. 2 feet =	_____ yard	
9. 8 inches =	_____ foot		18. 1 cup =	_____ quart	
10. $3\frac{1}{4}$ gallons =	_____ cups		19. $2\frac{1}{2}$ gallons =	_____ cups	
11. 3 inches =	_____ foot		20. 126 inches =	_____ yards	

21. A fruit punch recipe requires 2 quarts of orange juice, $\frac{1}{2}$ gallon of soda water, and 4 cups of cranberry juice. How many 1 cup servings will this make? _____

22. If you have 16 pints, you have the equivalent of how many quarts? _____

23. Milk costs $1.56 per $\frac{1}{2}$ gallon at Store A; at Store B, milk costs $0.94 per quart. How much do you save by buying 1 gallon of milk at Store A? _____

Using the prices in question 23, calculate the cost of 1 cup of milk bought at Store A and at Store B.

24. Store A cost = _____ 25. Store B cost = _____

After completing these problems, see page 471 to check your answers.

CONVERTING WITHIN THE METRIC SYSTEM USING THE CONVERSION FACTOR METHOD

The most common conversions in dosage calculations are within the metric system. As you recall, most metric conversions are simply derived by multiplying or dividing by 1000. Recall from Chapter 1 that multiplying by 1000 is the same as moving the decimal point three places to the right. Also recall that dividing by 1000 is the same as moving the decimal point three places to the left.

To convert 2 grams to the equivalent number of milligrams, you would first determine that gram is the larger unit. Therefore, you would multiply to convert to milligrams, the smaller unit. THINK: Larger → Smaller: (×)

The equivalent is: 1 g = 1000 mg. Multiply 2 by the conversion factor of 1000.

1 g = 1000 mg (equivalent). Therefore,

2 g = 2 × 1000 = 2000 mg (multiplying by 1000) or

2.000. = 2000 mg (moving decimal 3 places to the right)

Thus, you know that a medicine container labeled *2 grams per tablet* is the same as *2000 milligrams per tablet*. Let's look at more examples.

Example 1:

Convert: 0.3 g to mg

Equivalent: 1 g = 1000 mg. Conversion factor is 1000.

THINK: Larger → Smaller: (×)

Multiply by 1000: 0.3 g = 0.3 × 1000 = 300 mg

or move decimal point 3 places to the right: 0.3 g = 0.300. = 300 mg (add 0s to complete operation)

Example 2:

Convert: 2.5 g to mg

Equivalent: 1 g = 1000 mg. Conversion factor is 1000.

THINK: Larger → Smaller: (×)

Multiply by 1000: 2.5 g = 2.5 × 1000 = 2500 mg

or move decimal point 3 places to the right: 2.5 g = 2.500. = 2500 mg

Example 3:

Convert: 0.15 kg to g

Equivalent: 1 kg = 1000 g. Conversion factor is 1000.

THINK: Larger → Smaller: (×)

Multiply by 1000: 0.15 kg = 0.15 × 1000 = 150 g

or move decimal point 3 places to the right: 0.15 kg = 0.150. = 150 g

Example 4:

Convert: 0.04 L to mL

Equivalent: 1 L = 1000 mL. Conversion factor is 1000.

THINK: Larger → Smaller: (×)

Multiply by 1000: 0.04 L = 0.04 × 1000 = 40 mL

or move decimal point 3 places to the right: 0.04 L = 0.040. = 40 mL

Example 5:

An infant's head circumference is 40.5 cm. How many millimeters is that?

Convert: 40.5 cm to mm

Equivalent: 1 cm = 10 mm. Conversion factor is 10.

THINK: Larger → Smaller: (×)

Notice that, in this example, you are multiplying by 10 (not 1000).

40.5 cm = 40.5 × 10 = 405 mm

or move decimal point 1 place to the right: 40.5 cm = 40.5. = 405 mm

To convert a smaller unit to its equivalent larger unit, such as *milliliters to liters*, divide. THINK: Smaller → Larger: (÷). Recall the equivalent of 1 L = 1000 mL and then divide the number of milliliters by 1000. Thus, if you have a bottle that contains 2000 milliliters of boric acid solution, you know that this is the same as 2 liters. Dividing by 1000 is the same as moving the decimal point three places to the left.

Example 1:

Convert: 5000 mL to L

Equivalent: 1 L = 1000 mL. Conversion factor is 1000.

THINK: Smaller → Larger: (÷)

Divide by 1000: 5000 mL = 5000 ÷ 1000 = 5 L

or move decimal point 3 places to the left: 5000 mL = 5.000. = 5 L (eliminate unnecessary 0s)

Example 2:

Convert: 500 mL to L

Equivalent: 1 L = 1000 mL. Conversion factor is 1000.

THINK: Smaller → Larger: (÷)

Divide by 1000: 500 mL = 500 ÷ 1000 = 0.5 L (one 0 added for emphasis)

or move decimal point 3 places to the left: 500 mL = 0.500. = 0.5 L

Example 3:

Convert: 50 mL to L

Equivalent: 1 L = 1000 mL. Conversion factor is 1000.

THINK: Smaller → Larger: (÷)

Divide by 1000: 50 mL = 50 ÷ 1000 = 0.05 L

or move decimal point 3 places to the left: 50 mL = 0.050. = 0.05 L

Example 4:

Convert: 5 mL to L

Equivalent: 1 L = 1000 mL. Conversion factor is 1000.

THINK: Smaller → Larger: (÷)

Divide by 1000: 5 mL = 5 ÷ 1000 = 0.005 L

or move decimal point 3 places to the left: 5 mL = 0.005. = 0.005 L

Example 5:

A patient's wound measures 31 millimeters. How many centimeters is that? Convert 31 mm to cm.

Equivalent: 1 cm = 10 mm. Conversion factor is 10.

THINK: Smaller → Larger: (÷)

Notice that in this example, you are dividing by 10 (not 1000).

31 mm = 31 ÷ 10 = 3.1 cm

or move decimal point 1 place to the left: 31 mm = 3.1. = 3.1 cm

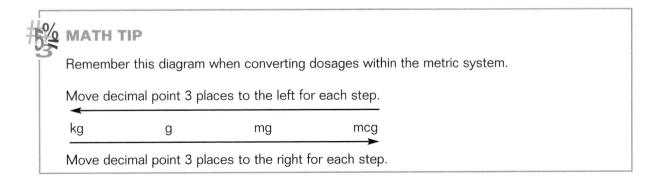

MATH TIP

Remember this diagram when converting dosages within the metric system.

Move decimal point 3 places to the left for each step.

| kg | g | mg | mcg |

Move decimal point 3 places to the right for each step.

Examples:

1 mcg = 0.001 mg (moved decimal point to the left 3 places)

2 g = 2000 mg (moved decimal point to the right 3 places)

2 g = 2,000,000 mcg (moved decimal point to the right 6 places, as the conversion required 2 steps)

   In time you will probably do these calculations in your head with little difficulty. If you feel you do not understand the concept of conversions within the metric system, review the decimal section in Chapter 1 and the metric section in Chapter 3 again. Get help from your instructor before proceeding further.

QUICK REVIEW

To use the conversion factor method to convert between units in the metric system:
- Recall the metric equivalents and appropriately multiply or divide by the conversion factor.
- MULTIPLY to convert from a *larger unit to a smaller unit,* or move the decimal point to the right. Example: 3 L = ? mL
      THINK: Larger → Smaller: (×)
      Equivalent: 1 L = 1000 mL
      3 L = 3 × 1000 or 3.000. = 3000 mL
- DIVIDE to convert from a *smaller unit to a larger unit,* or move the decimal point to the left. Example: 400 mg = ? g
      THINK: Smaller → Larger: (÷)
      Equivalent: 1 g = 1000 mg
      400 mg = 400 ÷ 1000 or .400. = 0.4 g

REVIEW SET 15

Convert each of the following to the equivalent unit indicated.

1. 500 cc = _____ L	16. 56.08 cc = _____ mL
2. 0.015 g = _____ mg	17. 5000 mL = _____ L
3. 8 mg = _____ g	18. 1 L = _____ mL
4. 10 mg = _____ g	19. 1 g = _____ mg
5. 60 mg = _____ g	20. 1 mL = _____ L
6. 300 mg = _____ g	21. 23 mcg = _____ mg
7. 0.2 mg = _____ g	22. 1.05 g = _____ kg
8. 1.2 g = _____ mg	23. 18 mcg = _____ mg
9. 0.0025 kg = _____ g	24. 0.4 mg = _____ mcg
10. 0.065 g = _____ mg	25. 25 g = _____ kg
11. 0.005 L = _____ mL	26. 50 cm = _____ m
12. 1.5 L = _____ mL	27. 10 L = _____ mL
13. 2 mL = _____ cc	28. 450 cc = _____ L
14. 250 cc = _____ L	29. 5 mL = _____ L
15. 2 kg = _____ g	30. 30 mg = _____ mcg

After completing these problems, see pages 471–472 to check your answers.

Approximate Equivalents

Fortunately, the use of the apothecary and household systems is becoming less and less frequent. But until they are obsolete, the nurse must be familiar with conversions between the metric, apothecary, and household systems of measurement.

Approximate equivalents are used for conversions from one system to another. Exact equivalents are not practical and, therefore, rarely used by health care workers. For example, the exact equivalent of one gram as measured in grains is: 1 gram = 15.432 grains. This is rounded to give the approximate equivalent of 1 g = gr 15. The exact equivalent of one grain is 64.8 milligrams. This is rounded to give the approximate equivalent of gr i = 60 mg. This is the conversion most frequently used; however, there will be a few instances in calculations of some common oral medications (such as acetaminophen, aspirin, and iron) where gr i = 65 mg will be more convenient. This points out the true meaning of "approximate" equivalents.

Approximate equivalents that are used for dosage calculations are listed in the following Remember box. Learn the equivalents so that you can change from one system to another quickly and accurately. Commit the equivalents to memory. Review them often. When you learn these essential equivalents in addition to the other equivalents you learned in Chapter 3, you are on your way to mastering the skill of dosage calculations.

REMEMBER

Approximate Equivalents

1 g = gr xv

gr i = 60 mg or gr i = 65 mg (in select instances)

1 t = 5 mL

1 T = 3 t = 15 mL = ʒ ss

ʒ i = 30 mL = 6 t

1 L = qt i = ʒ 32 = pt ii = 4 cups

pt i = 500 mL = ʒ 16 = 2 cups

1 cup = 240 mL = ʒ viii

1 kg = 2.2 lb

1 in = 2.5 cm

Look at the "Conversion Clock" (Figure 4-1) for an easy-to-remember method for converting between common metric and apothecary weight measures. It is based on the approximate equivalent of gr i = 60 mg, with 15 mg increments around the "clock" (similar to the 15 minute, 30 minute, 45 minute, 60 minute increments equivalent to $\frac{1}{4}, \frac{1}{2}, \frac{3}{4}$, and 1 hour).

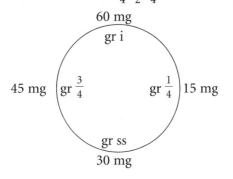

FIGURE 4-1 Metric–Apothecary Approximate Equivalent Conversion Clock

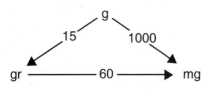

FIGURE 4-2 Weight Equivalents

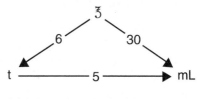

FIGURE 4-3 Volume Equivalents

Figures 4-2 and 4-3 are visual aids that associate most of the base equivalents. You may find these diagrams easier to remember than the tables.

Look at the first triangle of weight equivalents (Figure 4-2). Beginning at the top of the triangle, use your finger to trace the arrow from *g* (gram) down to *gr* (grain). The arrow indicates that *1 g = gr xv*. On the other side, trace down from *g* (gram) to *mg* (milligram). This arrow indicates that *1 g = 1000 mg*. Likewise, the bottom arrow goes from *gr* to *mg* to remind you that *gr i = 60 mg*. In summary, the triangle simply says:

$$1 \text{ g} = \text{gr xv, } 1 \text{ g} = 1000 \text{ mg, and gr i} = 60 \text{ mg}$$

Look at the second triangle of volume equivalents (Figure 4-3). Beginning at the top of the triangle, use your finger to trace the arrow from ʒ (ounce) down to *t* (teaspoon). The arrow indicates that *ʒ i = 6 t*. On the other side, trace down from ʒ (ounce) to *mL* (milliliter). This arrow reminds you that *ʒ i = 30 mL*. Likewise, the bottom arrow goes from *t* (teaspoon) to *mL* (milliliter). This arrow reminds you that *1 t = 5 mL*. In summary this triangle simply says:

$$\text{ʒ i} = 6 \text{ t, ʒ i} = 30 \text{ mL, and } 1 \text{ t} = 5 \text{ mL}$$

CONVERTING BETWEEN SYSTEMS OF MEASUREMENT USING THE CONVERSION FACTOR METHOD

Now let's convert units between systems of measurement using approximate equivalents and the conversion factor method. Recall that to convert from a larger to a smaller unit of measure, you must multiply by the conversion factor. Larger → Smaller: (×)

Example 1:

Convert: 0.5 g to gr

Approximate equivalent: 1 g = gr xv = gr 15. Conversion factor is 15.

THINK: Larger → Smaller: (×)

0.5 g = 0.5 × 15 = gr 7.5 = gr viiss

Example 2:

Convert: ʒ ii to mL

Approximate equivalent: ʒ i = 30 mL. Conversion factor is 30.

THINK: Larger → Smaller: (×)

ʒ ii = 2 × 30 = 60 mL

Example 3:

Convert: $\text{gr}\ \frac{1}{300}$ to mg

Approximate equivalent: gr i = 60 mg. The conversion factor is 60.

THINK: Larger → Smaller: (×)

$\text{gr}\ \frac{1}{300} = \frac{1}{300} \times \frac{60}{1} = \frac{1}{5}\ \text{mg} = 0.2\ \text{mg}$

Example 4:

The scale weighs the child at 40 kilograms. The mother wants to know her child's weight in pounds.

Convert: 40 kg to lb

Approximate equivalent: 1 kg = 2.2 lb. The conversion factor is 2.2.

THINK: Larger → Smaller: (×)

$40\ \text{kg} = 40 \times 2.2 = 88\ \text{lb}$

Recall that to convert from a smaller to a larger unit of measure, you must divide by the conversion factor. THINK: Smaller → Larger: (÷)

Example 1:

Convert: 120 mg to gr

Approximate equivalent: gr i = 60 mg. Conversion factor is 60.

THINK: Smaller → Larger: (÷)

$120\ \text{mg} = 120 \div 60 = \text{gr}\ 2 = \text{gr}\ \text{ii}$

Example 2:

Convert: 45 mL to t

Approximate equivalent: 1 t = 5 mL. Conversion factor is 5.

THINK: Smaller → Larger: (÷)

$45\ \text{mL} = 45 \div 5 = 9\ \text{t}$

Example 3:

Convert: 66 lb to kg

Approximate equivalent: 1 kg = 2.2 lb. Conversion factor is 2.2.

THINK: Smaller → Larger: (÷)

$66\ \text{lb} = 66 \div 2.2 = 30\ \text{kg}$

Example 4:

Convert: 40 cm to in (inches)

Approximate equivalent: 1 in = 2.5 cm. Conversion factor is 2.5.

THINK: Smaller → Larger: (÷)

40 cm = 40 ÷ 2.5 = 16 in

NOTE: Because inches are a household measurement, amounts less than 1 are preferably expressed in fractions.

Try this: Convert your weight in pounds to kilograms rounded to hundredths or two decimal places.

MATH TIP

A clue to remember the approximate equivalent 1 kg = 2.2 lb is to realize that there are about 2 pounds for every kilogram, so the number of kilograms you weigh is about half the number of pounds you weigh. (This could almost make getting on a metric scale pleasant.)

QUICK REVIEW

To perform dosage calculations, you must be able to convert between systems of measurement. To use the *conversion factor method*, recall the approximate equivalent, identify the conversion factor, and

- MULTIPLY by the conversion factor to convert to a SMALLER unit.
  THINK: Larger → Smaller: (×)
- DIVIDE by the conversion factor to convert to a LARGER UNIT.
  THINK: Smaller → Larger: (÷)

REVIEW SET 16

Use the conversion factor method to convert each of the following amounts to the unit indicated. Indicate the approximate equivalent(s) used in the conversion.

	Approximate Equivalent			Approximate Equivalent
1. gr ss = _____ mg _____		7. 13 t = _____ mL _____	
2. gr $\frac{3}{4}$ = _____ mg _____		8. 15 cc = ℥ _____ _____	
3. 3 g = _____ kg _____		9. ℥ iiss = _____ mL _____	
4. gr $\frac{1}{150}$ _____ mg _____		10. 750 mL = pt _____ _____	
5. gr viiss = _____ g _____		11. 20 mL = _____ t _____	
6. 15 mg = gr _____ _____		12. 4 T = _____ mL _____	

	Approximate Equivalent				Approximate Equivalent		
13. 9 kg =	_____ lb	_____		27. 90 mg =	gr _____	_____	
14. qt iv =	pt _____	_____		28. 60 mL =	℥ _____	_____	
15. 3 L =	℥ _____	_____		29. gr $\frac{1}{6}$ =	_____ mg	_____	
16. 55 kg =	_____ lb	_____		30. 65 mg =	gr _____	_____	
17. 12 in =	_____ cm	_____		31. 32 in =	_____ cm	_____	
18. qt ii =	_____ L	_____		32. 350 mm =	_____ in	_____	
19. 3 t =	_____ mL	_____		33. 7.5 cm =	_____ in	_____	
20. 99 lb =	_____ kg	_____		34. 2 in =	_____ mm	_____	
21. gr v =	_____ mg	_____		35. 40 kg =	_____ lb	_____	
22. 0.6 mg =	gr _____	_____		36. 7.16 kg =	_____ g	_____	
23. pt i =	_____ mL	_____		37. 110 lb =	_____ kg	_____	
24. gr x =	_____ mg	_____		38. 3.5 kg =	_____ lb	_____	
25. 300 mg =	gr _____	_____		39. 63 lb =	_____ kg	_____	
26. 30 cm =	_____ in	_____					

40. A newborn infant is $21\frac{1}{2}$ inches long. Her length is _____ cm.

41. The label for a granular medicine recommends mixing it with at least 120 mL of water or juice. At the time of discharge, the nurse should advise the patient to mix the medicine with _____ ounce(s) or _____ cup(s) of water or juice.

42. A patient starts an exercise program and walks 0.75 kilometer on the first day. Each day he increases his distance by 500 meters. How many total kilometers does he walk in seven days? _____ kilometers

43. Calculate the total fluid intake in mL for 24 hours.

Breakfast	8 ounces milk
	6 ounces orange juice
	4 ounces water with medication
Lunch	8 ounces iced tea
Snack	10 ounces coffee
	4 ounces gelatin dessert
Dinner	8 ounces water
	6 ounces tomato juice
	6 ounces beef broth
Snack	5 ounces pudding
	12 ounces diet soda
	4 ounces water with medication

Total = _____ mL

44. A child who weighs 55 lb is to receive 0.05 mg of a drug per kg of body weight per dose. How much of the drug should the child receive for each dose? _____ mg

45. A child is taking 12 mL of a medication four times per day. If the full bottle contains 16 ounces of the medication, how many days will the bottle last? _____ day(s)

46. The doctor prescribes 10 mL of Betadine concentrate in 500 mL of warm water as a soak for a finger infection. Using measures commonly found in the home, how would you instruct the patient to prepare the solution? _____

47. The patient is to receive 10 mL of a drug. How many teaspoonsful should the patient take? _____ t

48. An infant is taking a ready-to-feed formula. The formula comes in quart containers. If the infant usually takes 4 ounces of formula every 3 hours during the day and night, how many quarts of formula should the mother buy for a 3 day supply? _____ qt

49. An infant's head circumference is 40 cm. The parents ask for the equivalent in inches. You tell the parents their infant's head circumference is _____ in.

50. The patient tells you he was weighed in the doctor's office and was told he is 206 pounds. What is his weight in kilograms? _____ kg

After completing these problems, see pages 472–473 to check your answers.

Shortcut Conversion Factor Method

By using a simple formula, you can use a conversion factor shortcut to convert within and between systems of measurement. With this method you do not have to remember when to multiply or when to divide. You simply align units and multiply.

> **RULE**
>
> $$\frac{\text{Desired amount}}{\text{Matching conversion}} \times \textbf{Equivalent} \text{ that matches the unknown} = \textbf{Quantity}$$
>
> $$\frac{\textbf{D}}{\textbf{M}} \times \text{E} = \text{Q}$$

The desired amount—the numerator of the fraction—is always the amount you desire to convert. Insert the conversion factor into the formula so you always multiply by the part of the conversion equivalent that has the same unit of measurement as the unknown or desired answer.

Example 1:

Convert: $\text{gr} \frac{1}{4}$ to mg

Approximate equivalent: gr i = 60 mg

$$\frac{\cancel{\text{gr}} \frac{1}{4}}{\cancel{\text{gr}} \text{ i}} \times 60 \text{ mg} = 15 \text{ mg}$$

In this example you are essentially multiplying by the conversion factor. You know this is true because you are converting from a larger to a smaller unit. Notice that the numerator of the fraction is the amount you want to convert and that the units of this fraction match. Also, the units of the equivalent amount you multiply by match the desired answer or unknown. *Each of these factors is critical for the shortcut to be accurate.*

Example 2:

Convert: 250 mg to g

Approximate equivalent: 1 g = 1000 mg

$\dfrac{250 \text{ mg}}{1000 \text{ mg}} \times 1 \text{ g} = 0.250 \text{ g} = 0.25 \text{ g}$ (eliminate the unnecessary 0)

Now notice what has happened. You are converting from a smaller to a larger unit, and must divide by the conversion factor. By aligning the units you are essentially dividing by the conversion factor of 1000 (1 g = 1000 mg). Again, the numerator of the fraction in the equation is the amount you want to convert and the units of this fraction match. Also, the units of the equivalent amount you multiply by match the desired answer or unknown.

QUICK REVIEW

Align units and you can use the shortcut conversion factor method to quickly convert within and between units of measurement.

$\dfrac{\text{Desired amount}}{\text{Matching conversion}} \times \text{Equivalent that matches the unknown} = \text{Quantity}$

REVIEW SET 17

Use the shortcut conversion factor method to convert each of the following amounts to the unit indicated. Indicate the approximate equivalent used in the conversion.

Approximate
Equivalent

1. 0.03 g = _____ mg _____
2. 8 in = _____ cm _____
3. 100 kg = _____ lb _____
4. 45 mg = gr _____ _____
5. 175 mcg = _____ mg _____
6. 10 lb = _____ kg _____
7. 3 t = _____ mL _____
8. qt ii = _____ L _____
9. 3500 g = _____ kg _____
10. 30 cm = _____ in _____
11. gr $\dfrac{1}{100}$ = _____ mg _____
12. 150 mcg = _____ g _____
13. 10 mg = gr _____ _____
14. 10 mL = _____ t _____
15. 5 lb = _____ g _____
16. 0.375 mg = _____ mcg _____
17. $\dfrac{1}{2}$ t = _____ mL _____
18. ʒ ss = _____ mL _____
19. 75 mL = ʒ _____ _____

After completing these problems, see page 473 to check your answers.

If you like this shortcut conversion factor method and you want more practice, go back to Review Set 16 and solve those problems using this method.

CONVERTING USING THE RATIO-PROPORTION METHOD

An alternate method of performing conversions is to set up a proportion of two ratios expressed as fractions. Refer to Chapter 2 to review ratio-proportion, if needed.

> **RULE**
>
> In a proportion, the ratio for a known equivalent equals the ratio for an unknown equivalent. To use ratio-proportion to convert from one unit to another, you need to:
> 1. recall the equivalents,
> 2. set up a proportion of two equivalent ratios, and
> 3. cross-multiply to solve for an unknown quantity, X.

Each ratio in a proportion must have the same relationship and follow the same sequence. A proportion compares like things to like things. Be sure the units in the numerators match and the units in the denominators match. Label the units in each ratio.

Example 1:

How many grams are equivalent to 3.5 kg?

The first ratio of the proportion contains the *known equivalent,* for example 1 kg : 1000 g. The second ratio contains the *desired unit of measure* and the *unknown equivalent* expressed as "X," for example 3.5 kg : X g. This proportion in fractional form looks like this:

$$\frac{1 \text{ kg}}{1000 \text{ g}} = \frac{3.5 \text{ kg}}{\text{X g}}$$

> **CAUTION**
>
> Notice that the ratios follow the same sequence. **THIS IS ESSENTIAL.** The proportion is set up so that like units are across from each other. The units in the numerators match (kg) and the units in the denominators match (g).

Cross-multiply to solve the proportion for "X." Refer to Chapter 2 to review this skill if needed.

$$\frac{1 \text{ kg}}{1000 \text{ g}} \times = \times \frac{3.5 \text{ kg}}{\text{X g}}$$

X = 3.5 × 1000 = 3500 g

You know the answer is in grams, because grams is the unknown equivalent.

3.5 kg = 3500 g

In Example 2 the unknown "X" is in the numerator. It doesn't matter, as long as the sequence is the same (numerator units match and denominator units match). Remember, a proportion must compare like things to like things. In the next example it is gr : mg = gr : mg.

Example 2:

Convert: 45 mg to gr

Known approximate equivalent: gr i = 60 mg

$$\frac{\text{gr i}}{60 \text{ mg}} \diagup\kern-1em\diagdown = \frac{\text{gr X}}{45 \text{ mg}}$$

$$60X = 45$$

$$\frac{60X}{60} = \frac{45}{60}$$

$$X = \text{gr } \frac{45}{60} = \text{gr } \frac{3}{4}$$

CAUTION

As is customary, the capital letter "X" is consistently used in this text to denote the unknown quantity in an equation and proportion. It is important that you do not confuse the unknown "X" with the value of gr x, which designates 10 grains.

Example 3:

Convert: 10 mL to t

Known approximate equivalent: 1 t = 5 mL

$$\frac{1 \text{ t}}{5 \text{ mL}} \diagup\kern-1em\diagdown = \frac{X \text{ t}}{10 \text{ mL}}$$

$$5X = 10$$

$$\frac{5X}{5} = \frac{10}{5}$$

$$X = \frac{10}{5} \text{ t} = 2 \text{ t}$$

Example 4:

Convert: 150 lb to kg

Known approximate equivalent: 1 kg = 2.2 lb

$$\frac{1 \text{ kg}}{2.2 \text{ lb}} \diagup\kern-1em\diagdown = \frac{X \text{ kg}}{150 \text{ lb}}$$

$$2.2X = 150$$

$$\frac{2.2X}{2.2} = \frac{150}{2.2}$$

$$X = \frac{150}{2.2} \text{ kg} = 68.18 \text{ kg}$$

QUICK REVIEW

To use the ratio-proportion method to convert from one unit to another or between systems of measurement:
- Recall the equivalent.
- Set up a proportion: Ratio for known equivalent equals ratio for unknown equivalent.
- Label the units and match the units in the numerators and denominators.
- Cross-multiply to find the value of the unknown "X" equivalent.

REVIEW SET 18

Use the ratio-proportion method to convert each of the following amounts to the unit indicated. Indicate the approximate equivalent used in the conversion.

	Approximate Equivalent			Approximate Equivalent	
1. 50 mL = _____ L	_____		11. 2.5 mL = _____ t	_____	
2. 3 g = gr _____	_____		12. gr ss = _____ mg	_____	
3. 84 lb = _____ kg	_____		13. 10 mg = gr _____	_____	
4. gr xx = _____ g	_____		14. 0.6 mg = gr _____	_____	
5. gr $\frac{1}{8}$ = _____ mg	_____		15. 7.5 cm = _____ in	_____	
6. 75 mL = ʒ _____	_____		16. 16 g = _____ mg	_____	
7. 750 mL = pt _____	_____		17. 15 mL = ʒ _____	_____	
8. ʒ iss = _____ mL	_____		18. ʒ 16 = qt _____	_____	
9. 15 mg = gr _____	_____		19. qt ii = _____ L	_____	
10. 625 mcg = _____ mg	_____		20. pt i = qt _____	_____	

21. The medicine order states to administer a potassium chloride supplement added to at least 150 mL of juice. How many ounces of juice should you pour? ʒ _____

22. A child should have 5 mL of liquid Children's Tylenol (acetaminophen) every 4 hours as needed for fever above 100°F. To relate these instructions to the child's mother, you should advise her to give her child _____ teaspoon(s) of Tylenol per dose.

23. The doctor advises his patient to drink at least 2000 mL of fluid per day. The patient should have at least _____ 8 ounce glasses of water per day.

24. A child needs 15 mL of a drug. How many teaspoonsful should he receive? _____ t

25. The doctor orders codeine gr $\frac{1}{4}$. This is equivalent to how many milligrams? _____ mg

After completing these problems, see page 474 to check your answers.
For more practice, rework Review Sets 14–17 using the ratio-proportion method.

CRITICAL THINKING SKILLS

error

Incorrectly interpreting grains as milligrams.

possible scenario

A physician ordered a single dose of 15 grains of aspirin for a patient complaining of a severe headache. Aspirin was available in 500 mg aspirin tablets. While preparing the medication, the nurse was distracted by a visitor who fell by the nurses' station. The nurse returned to read the order as *1.5 grams* and calculated the dose this way:

If: 1 g = 1000 mg and 0.5 g = 0.5 × 1000 = 500 mg
then: 1.5 g = 1000 mg + 500 mg = 1500 mg, so the patient was given 3 tablets.

You know that 15 grains is equivalent to 1 g or 1000 mg. By misreading the dose, the nurse gave 500 mg more than ordered, overdosing the patient.

(continues)

(continued)

potential outcome

The patient received $1\frac{1}{2}$ times, or 150% of the dosage ordered. This larger dose, 1500 mg, could cause nausea, heartburn, and gastric upset. In aspirin-sensitive patients it could result in gastric bleeding.

prevention

This type of medication error is avoided by carefully checking the drug order at least three times: before preparing a medication, once the dose is prepared, and prior to giving the patient the medication. Also, the nurse should recognize that the ordered dose is in *apothecary* measurement, while the supply dosage is in *metric* measurement, and carefully convert between systems.

SUMMARY

At this point, you should be quite familiar with the equivalents for converting within the metric, apothecary, and household systems, and from one system to another. From memory, you should be able to recall quickly and accurately the equivalents for conversions. If you are having difficulty understanding the concept of converting from one unit of measurement to another, review this chapter and seek additional help from your instructor.

Work the practice problems for Chapter 4. Concentrate on accuracy. One error can be a serious mistake when calculating the dosages of medicines or performing critical measurements of health status.

PRACTICE PROBLEMS—CHAPTER 4

Give the following equivalents without consulting conversion tables.

1. 0.5 g = _____ mg

2. 0.01 g = _____ mg

3. 7.5 cc = _____ mL

4. qt iii = _____ L

5. 4 mg = _____ g

6. 500 mL = _____ L

7. 250 mL = pt _____

8. 300 g = _____ kg

9. 28 in = _____ cm

10. 68 kg = _____ lb

11. gr iii = _____ mg

12. ℥ iiiss = _____ mL

13. gr $\frac{1}{200}$ = _____ mg

14. gr $\frac{1}{4}$ = _____ mg

15. gr $\frac{1}{10}$ = _____ mg

16. gr iss = _____ mg

17. $70\frac{1}{2}$ lb = _____ kg

18. 3634 g = _____ lb

19. 8 mL = _____ L

20. gr xxx = _____ g

21. 237.5 cm = _____ in

22. 0.5 g = gr _____

23. 0.6 mg = gr _____

24. gr x = _____ g

25. 150 lb = _____ kg

26. 60 mg = gr _____

27. gr xv = _____ g

28. 2 cups = _____ mL

29. 6 t = _____ T

30. 90 mL = ℥ _____

31. 1 ft = _____ cm

32. 2 T = _____ mL

33. 2.2 lb = _____ kg

34. 5 cc = _____ t

35. 1000 mL = _____ L

36. 1.5 g = _____ mg

37. ℥ iss = _____ mL

38. 1500 mL = qt _____

39. 10 mg = gr _____

40. 25 mg = _____ g

41. 4.3 kg = _____ g

42. 60 mg = _____ g

43. 0.015 g = _____ mg

44. 45 cc = _____ mL

45. gr 12 = _____ g

46. As a camp nurse for 9- to 12-year-old children, you are administering $2\frac{1}{2}$ teaspoonsful of oral liquid Tylenol to 6 feverish campers every 4 hours for oral temperatures above 100°F. You have on hand a 4 ounce bottle of liquid Tylenol. How many complete or full doses are available from this bottle?   _____ full doses

47. At this same camp, the standard dosage of Pepto-Bismol for 9- to 12-year-olds is 1 tablespoonful. How many full doses are available in a 120 mL bottle?   _____ full doses

48. Calculate the total fluid intake in mL of this clear liquid lunch:

    apple juice   4 ounces

    chicken broth   8 ounces

    gelatin dessert   6 ounces

    hot tea   10 ounces

    TOTAL =   _____ mL

49. An ampule contains 10 mg of morphine. The doctor orders *morphine gr $\frac{1}{6}$ intramuscularly every 4 hours as needed for pain.* What percentage of the solution in the ampule should the patient receive?   _____

50. Critical Thinking Skill: Describe the strategy you would implement to prevent this medication error.

    possible scenario

    An attending physician ordered *Claforan 2 g intravenously immediately* for a patient with a leg abscess. The supply dosage available is 1000 mg per 10 mL. The nurse was in a rush to give the medication and calculated the dose this way:

    If: 1 g = 1000 mg

    then: 2 g = 1000 ÷ 2 = 500 mg (per 5 mL)

    Then the nurse administered 5 mL of the available Claforan.

    potential outcome

    The patient received only $\frac{1}{4}$ or 25% of the dosage ordered. The patient should have received 2000 mg or 20 mL of Claforan. The leg abscess could progress to osteomyelitis (a severe bone infection) because of underdosage.

    prevention

    _____

    _____

    After completing these problems, see pages 474–475 to check your answers.

Conversions for Other Clinical Applications: Time and Temperature

Upon mastery of Chapter 5, you will be able to:
● Convert between traditional and international time.
● Convert between Celsius and Fahrenheit temperature.

This chapter focuses on two other conversions applied in health care. *Time* is an essential part of the drug order. *Temperature* is an important measurement of health status.

CONVERTING BETWEEN TRADITIONAL AND INTERNATIONAL TIME

It is becoming increasingly popular in health care settings to keep time with a more straightforward system using the *24-hour clock*. In use around the world and in the U.S. military for many years, this system is known as *international time* or *military time*.

Look at the *24-hour clock* (Figure 5-1). Each time designation is comprised of a unique four-digit number. Notice there is an inner and outer circle of numbers that identify the hours from 0100 to 2400. The inside numbers correlate to traditional AM time (12:00 midnight to 11:59 AM); time periods that are *ante meridian* or "before noon." The outside numbers correlate to traditional PM time (12:00 noon to 11:59 PM); time periods that are *post meridian* or "after noon."

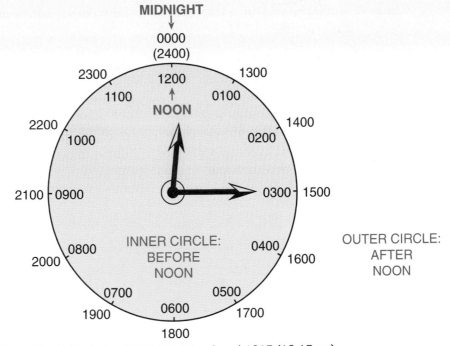

FIGURE 5-1 24-Hour Clock Depicting 0015 (12:15 AM) and 1215 (12:15 PM)

Hours on the 24-hour clock after 0059 minutes ("zero-zero fifty-nine") are stated in hundreds. The word *zero* precedes single-digit hours.

Example 1:

0400 is stated as "zero four hundred."

Example 2:

1600 is stated as "sixteen hundred."

Between each hour, the time is read simply as the hour and the number of minutes, preceded by "zero" as needed.

Example 1:

0421 is stated as "zero four twenty-one."

Example 2:

1659 is stated as "sixteen fifty-nine."

The minutes between 2400 (12:00 midnight) and 0100 (1:00 AM) are written as 0001, 0002, 0003... 0058, 0059. Each zero is stated before stating the number of minutes.

Example 1:

0009 is stated as "zero-zero-zero nine."

Example 2:

0014 is stated as "zero-zero fourteen."

Midnight can be written two different ways in international time:
- 2400 and read as "twenty-four hundred," or
- 0000 (used by the military) and read as "zero hundred."

Use of the 24-hour clock decreases the possibility for error in administering medications and documenting time, because no two times are expressed by the same number. There is less chance for misinterpreting time using the 24-hour clock.

Example 1:

13 minutes after 1 AM is written "0113."

Example 2:

13 minutes after 1 PM is written "1313."

The same cannot be said for traditional time. The AM or PM notations are the only things that differentiate traditional times.

Example 1:

13 minutes after 1 AM is "1:13 AM"

Example 2:

13 minutes after 1 PM is "1:13 PM"

Careless notation in a medical order or in patient records can create misinterpretation about when a therapy is due or actually occurred. Figure 5-2 shows the comparison of traditional and international time. Notice that international time is less ambiguous.

AM	Int'l. Time	PM	Int'l. Time
12:00 midnight	2400	12:00 noon	1200
1:00	0100	1:00	1300
2:00	0200	2:00	1400
3:00	0300	3:00	1500
4:00	0400	4:00	1600
5:00	0500	5:00	1700
6:00	0600	6:00	1800
7:00	0700	7:00	1900
8:00	0800	8:00	2000
9:00	0900	9:00	2100
10:00	1000	10:00	2200
11:00	1100	11:00	2300

FIGURE 5-2 Comparison of Traditional and International Time

RULES

1. Traditional time and international time are the same hours starting with 1:00 AM (0100) through 12:59 PM (1259).
2. Minutes after 12:00 AM (midnight) and before 1:00 AM are 0001 through 0059 in international time.
3. Hours starting with 1:00 PM through 12:00 AM (midnight) are 12:00 hours greater in international time (1300 through 2400).
4. International time is designated by a unique four-digit number.
5. The hour(s) and minute(s) are separated by a colon in traditional time, but no colon is used in international time.

MATH TIP

Between the hours of 1:00 PM (1300) and 12:00 AM (2400), add 1200 to traditional time to find equivalent international time; subtract 1200 from international time to convert to equivalent traditional time.

Let's apply these rules to convert between the two time systems.

Example 1:

3:00 PM = 3:00 + 12:00 = 1500

Example 2:

2212 = 2212 − 1200 = 10:12 PM

Example 3:

12:45 AM = 0045

Example 4:

0004 = 12:04 AM

Example 5:

0130 = 1:30 AM

Example 6:

11:00 AM = 1100

QUICK REVIEW

- International time is designated by 0001 through 1259 for 12:01 AM through 12:59 PM, and 1300 through 2400 for 1:00 PM through 12:00 midnight.
- The hours from 1:00 PM through 12:00 midnight are 12:00 hours greater in international time (1300 through 2400).

REVIEW SET 19

Convert international time to traditional AM/PM time.

1. 0032 = _____
2. 0730 = _____
3. 1640 = _____
4. 2121 = _____
5. 2359 = _____

6. 1215 = _____
7. 0220 = _____
8. 1010 = _____
9. 1315 = _____
10. 1825 = _____

Convert traditional to international time.

11. 1:30 PM = _____
12. 12:04 AM = _____
13. 9:45 PM = _____
14. 12:00 noon = _____
15. 11:15 PM = _____

16. 3:45 AM = _____
17. 12:00 midnight = _____
18. 3:30 PM = _____
19. 6:20 AM = _____
20. 5:45 PM = _____

Fill in the blanks by writing out the words as indicated.

21. 24-hour time 0623 is stated " _____."

22. 24-hour time 0041 is stated " _____."

23. 24-hour time 1903 is stated " _____."

24. 24-hour time 2311 is stated " _____."

25. 24-hour time 0300 is stated " _____."

After completing these problems, see page 475 to check your answers.

CONVERTING BETWEEN CELSIUS AND FAHRENHEIT TEMPERATURE

Another important conversion in health care involves Celsius and Fahrenheit temperatures. Simple formulas are used for converting between the two temperature scales. It is easier to remember the formulas when you understand how they were developed.

The Fahrenheit (F) scale establishes the freezing point of pure water at 32° and the boiling point of pure water at 212°. The Celsius (C) scale establishes the freezing point of pure water at 0° and the boiling point of pure water at 100°.

Look at Figure 5-3. Note that there is 180° difference between the boiling and freezing points on the Fahrenheit thermometer, and 100° between the boiling and freezing points on the Celsius thermometer. The ratio of the difference between the Fahrenheit and Celsius scales can be expressed as 180:100 or $\frac{180}{100}$. When reduced, this ratio is equivalent to 1.8. You will use this constant in temperature conversions.

To convert between Fahrenheit and Celsius temperature, formulas have been developed based on the differences between the freezing and boiling points on each scale.

RULE

To convert a given Fahrenheit temperature to Celsius, first subtract 32 and then divide the result by 1.8.

$$°C = \frac{°F - 32}{1.8}$$

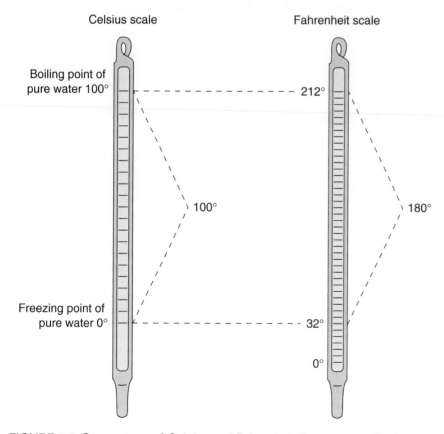

NOTE: Glass thermometers pictured in Figure 5-3 are for demonstration purposes. Electronic digital temperature devices are more commonly used in health care settings. Most electronic devices can instantly convert between the two scales, freeing the health care provider from doing the actual calculations. However, the health care provider's ability to understand the difference between Celsius and Fahrenheit remains important.

FIGURE 5-3 Comparison of Celsius and Fahrenheit Temperature Scales

Example:

Convert 98.6°F to °C

$$°C = \frac{98.6 - 32}{1.8}$$

$$°C = \frac{66.6}{1.8}$$

$$°C = 37°$$

RULE

To convert Celsius temperature to Fahrenheit, multiply by 1.8 and add 32.
$°F = 1.8°C + 32$

Example:

Convert 35°C to °F

$$°F = 1.8 \times 35 + 32$$

$$°F = 63 + 32$$

$$°F = 95°$$

QUICK REVIEW

Use these formulas to convert between Fahrenheit and Celsius temperatures:
- $°C = \frac{°F - 32}{1.8}$
- $°F = 1.8°C + 32$

REVIEW SET 20

Convert these temperatures as indicated. Round your answers to tenths.

1. 0°F =	_____ °C		9. 80°C =	_____ °F
2. 85°C =	_____ °F		10. 36.4°C =	_____ °F
3. 100°C =	_____ °F		11. 100°F =	_____ °C
4. 32°C =	_____ °F		12. 19°C =	_____ °F
5. 72°F =	_____ °C		13. 4°C =	_____ °F
6. 99°F =	_____ °C		14. 94.2°F =	_____ °C
7. 103.6°F =	_____ °C		15. 102.8°F =	_____ °C
8. 40°C =	_____ °F			

For each of the following statements, convert the given temperature in °F or °C to its corresponding equivalent in °C or °F.

16. An infant has a body temperature of 95.5°F. _____ °C

17. Store the vaccine serum at 7°C. _____ °F

18. Do not expose medication to temperatures > 88°F. _____ °C

19. Normal body temperature is 37°C. _____ °F

20. If Mr. Rose's temperature is > 103.5°F, call MD.   _____ °C

After completing these problems, see page 475 to check your answers.

CRITICAL THINKING SKILLS

error

Incorrect interpretation of order due to misunderstanding of traditional time.

possible scenario

A physician ordered a mild sedative for an anxious patient who is scheduled for a sigmoidoscopy in the morning. The order read *"Valium 5 mg orally at 6:00 X 1 dose."* The evening nurse interpreted that single-dose order to be scheduled for 6 o'clock PM along with the enema and other preparations to be given to the patient. The doctor meant for the Valium to be given at 6 o'clock AM to help the patient relax prior to the actual test.

potential outcome

Valium would help the patient relax during the enema and make the patient sleepy. But it is not desirable for the patient to be drowsy or sedated during the evening preparations. Because of the omission of the AM designation, the patient would not benefit from this mild sedative at the intended time, just before the test. The patient would have likely experienced unnecessary anxiety both before and during the test.

prevention

This scenario emphasizes the benefit of the 24-hour clock. If international time had been in use at this facility, the order would have been written as *"Valium 5 mg orally at 0600 X 1 dose"* clearly indicating the exact time of administration. Be careful to verify AM and PM times if your facility uses traditional time.

PRACTICE PROBLEMS—CHAPTER 5

Give the following time equivalents as indicated.

AM/PM Clock	24-Hour Clock	AM/PM Clock	24-Hour Clock
1. _____	0257	11. 7:31 PM	_____
2. 3:10 AM	_____	12. 12:00 midnight	_____
3. 4:22 PM	_____	13. 6:45 AM	_____
4. _____	2001	14. _____	0915
5. _____	1102	15. _____	2107
6. 12:33 AM	_____	16. _____	1823
7. 2:16 AM	_____	17. _____	0540
8. _____	1642	18. 11:55 AM	_____
9. _____	2356	19. 10:12 PM	_____
10. 4:20 AM	_____	20. 9:06 PM	_____

Find the length of each time interval for questions 21 through 30.

21. 0200 to 0600 _____   26. 2316 to 0328 _____

22. 1100 to 1800 _____   27. 8:22 AM to 1:10 PM _____

23. 1500 to 2330 _____   28. 4:35 PM to 8:16 PM _____

24. 0935 to 2150 _____   29. 1:00 AM to 7:30 AM _____

25. 0003 to 1453 _____

30. 10:05 AM Friday to 2:43 AM Saturday _____

31. The 24-hour clock is imprecise and not suited to health care.   (True) (False)

32. Indicate whether these international times would be AM or PM when converted to traditional time.

    a. 1030 _____   c. 0158 _____

    b. 1920 _____   d. 1230 _____

Give the following temperature equivalents as indicated.

33. $99.6°F$ _____ $°C$ 41. $97.8°F$ _____ $°C$

34. $36.5°C$ _____ $°F$ 42. $35.4°C$ _____ $°F$

35. $39.2°C$ _____ $°F$ 43. $103.5°F$ _____ $°C$

36. $100.2°F$ _____ $°C$ 44. $25°C$ _____ $°F$

37. $98°F$ _____ $°C$ 45. $100°C$ _____ $°F$

38. $37.4°C$ _____ $°F$ 46. $42°F$ _____ $°C$

39. $0°C$ _____ $°F$ 47. $18°F$ _____ $°C$

40. $104°F$ _____ $°C$

48. Four temperature readings in $°C$ for Mrs. Baskin are 37.6, 35.5, 38.1, and 37.6. Find her average (or mean) $°C$ temperature and convert it to $°F$.   _____ $°C$, or _____ $°F$

49. The freezing and boiling points of pure water on the Fahrenheit and Celsius temperature scales were used to develop the conversion formulas.   (True) (False)

50. Critical Thinking Skill:

Describe the strategy you would implement to prevent this conversion error.

possible scenario

A nurse takes a child's temperature and finds that it is $38.2°C$. The child's mother asks what that equates to in Fahrenheit temperature. The nurse does a quick calculation in her head and multiplies $38°$ by 2 and adds 32, as she recalls the conversion constant is 1.8 and 2 is close enough. The nurse tells the mother, "Well, about $108°$." The mother replies, "I hope not," and smiles.

potential outcome

The nurse immediately recognizes that she made an error and feels very embarrassed. The mother could have become very alarmed and experienced undue anxiety and a loss of confidence in the nurse. The correct temperature measurement is $100.8°F$. Fever-reducing medical orders often vary the dosage depending on the severity of the elevated temperature. An incorrect conversion could result in over- or under-medication of the child.

prevention

_____

_____

After completing these problems, see page 475 to check your answers.

Equipment Used in Dosage Measurement

OBJECTIVES

Upon mastery of Chapter 6, you will be able to correctly measure the prescribed dosages that you calculate. To accomplish this, you will also be able to:
- Recognize and select the appropriate equipment for the medication, dosage, and method of administration ordered.
- Read and interpret the calibrations of each utensil presented.

Now that you are familiar with the systems of measurement used in the calculation of dosages, let's take a look at the common measuring utensils. In this chapter you will learn to recognize and read the calibrations of devices used in both oral and parenteral (other than gastrointestinal) administration. The oral utensils include the medicine cup, pediatric oral devices, and calibrated droppers. The parenteral devices include the 3 mL syringe, prefilled syringe, a variety of insulin syringes, 1 mL syringe, and special safety and intravenous syringes.

ORAL ADMINISTRATION

Medicine Cup

Figure 6-1 shows the 30 milliliter or 1 ounce medicine cup that is used to measure most liquids for oral administration. Two views are presented to show all of the scales. Notice that the approximate equivalents of the metric, apothecary, and household systems of measurement are indicated on the cup. The medicine cup can serve as a great study aid to help you learn the volume equivalents of the three systems of measurement. Look at the calibrations for milliliters, teaspoons, tablespoons, ounces, and drams. You can see that 30 milliliters equal 1 ounce, 5 milliliters equal 1 teaspoon, and so forth. For volumes less than 2.5 mL, a smaller, more accurate device should be used (see Figures 6-2, 6-3, and 6-4).

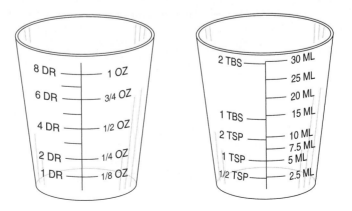

FIGURE 6-1 Medicine Cup with Approximate Equivalent Measures

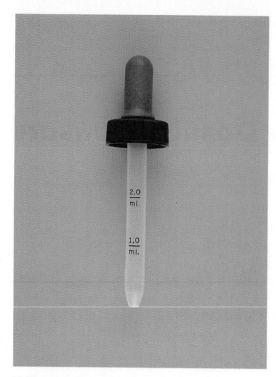

FIGURE 6-2 Calibrated Dropper

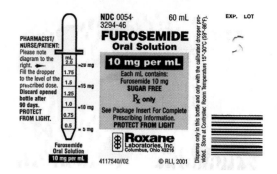

FIGURE 6-3 Furosemide Oral Solution Label (Used with permission of Roxane Laboratories, Inc.)

Calibrated Dropper

Figure 6-2 shows the calibrated dropper, which is used to administer some small quantities. A dropper is used when giving medicine to children, the elderly, and when adding small amounts of liquid to water or juice. Eye and ear medications are also dispensed from a medicine dropper or squeeze drop bottle.

The amount of the drop varies according to the diameter of the hole at the tip of the dropper. For this reason, a properly calibrated dropper usually accompanies the medicine (Figure 6-3). It is calibrated according to the way that drug is prescribed. The calibrations are usually given in milliliters, cubic centimeters, or drops.

> **CAUTION**
>
> To be safe, never interchange packaged droppers between medications, because drop size varies from one dropper to another.

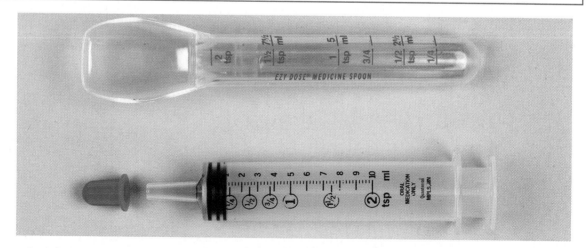

FIGURE 6-4 Devices for Administering Oral Medications to Children

Pediatric Oral Devices

Various types of calibrated equipment are available to administer oral medications to children. Several devices intended only for oral use are shown in Figure 6-4. Parents and child care givers should be taught always to use calibrated devices when administering medications to children. Household spoons vary in size and are not reliable for accurate dosing.

☼ CAUTION

To be safe, do not use syringes intended for injections in the administration of oral medications. Confusion about the route of administration may occur.

You can distinguish oral from parenteral syringes in two ways. Syringes intended for oral use typically do not have a luerlock hub. They also usually have a cap on the tip that must be removed before administering the medication. Syringes intended for parenteral use have a luerlock hub that allows a needle to be secured tightly (see Figure 6-6).

PARENTERAL ADMINISTRATION

The term *parenteral* is used to designate routes of administration other than gastrointestinal. However, in this text, parenteral always means injection routes.

3 mL or 3 cc Syringe

Figure 6-5 shows a 3 mL syringe assembled with needle unit. The parts of the syringe are identified in Figure 6-6. Notice that the black rubber tip of the suction plunger is visible. The nurse pulls back on the plunger to withdraw the medicine from the storage container. The calibrations are read from the top black ring, NOT the raised middle section and NOT the bottom ring. Look closely at the metric scale in Figure 6-5, which is calibrated in milliliters (mL) for each tenth (0.1) of a milliliter. Each $\frac{1}{2}$ (or 0.5) milliliter is marked up to the maximum volume of 3 milliliters.

Standardized to the syringe calibrations, standard drug dosages of 1 mL or greater can be rounded to the nearest tenth (0.1) of a mL and measured on the mL scale. Refer to Chapter 1 to review the rules of decimal rounding. For example, 1.45 mL is rounded to 1.5 mL. Notice that the colored liquid in Figure 6-5 identifies 1.5 mL.

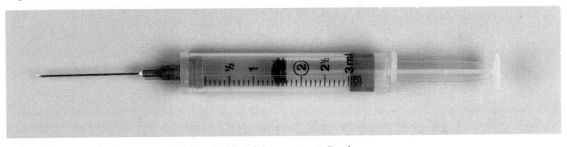

FIGURE 6-5 3 mL Syringe with Needle Unit Measuring 1.5 mL

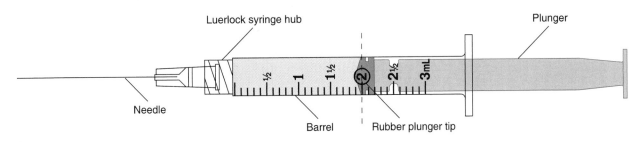

FIGURE 6-6 3 mL Syringe with Needle Unit Measuring 2 mL

Prefilled, Single-Dose Syringe

Figure 6-7 is an example of a *prefilled, single-dose syringe*. Such syringes contain the usual single dose of a medication and are to be used only once. The syringe is discarded after the single use.

If you are to give *less than the full single dose* of a drug provided in a prefilled, single-dose syringe, you should discard the extra amount *before* injecting the patient.

Example:

The drug order prescribes 7.5 mg of Valium to be administered to a patient. You have a prefilled, single-dose syringe of Valium containing 10 mg per 2 mL of solution (as in Figure 6-7). You would discard 2.5 mg (0.5 mL) of the drug solution; then 7.5 mg would remain in the syringe. You will learn more about calculating drug dosages beginning in Chapter 9.

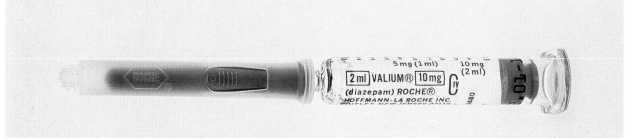

FIGURE 6-7 Prefilled, Single-Dose Syringe (Courtesy of Roche Laboratories, Inc.)

> **MATH TIP**
>
> Some syringes are marked in cubic centimeters (cc), whereas most drugs are prepared and labeled with the strength given per milliliter (mL). Remember that the cubic centimeter and milliliter are equivalent measurements in dosage calculations (1 cc = 1 mL).

Insulin Syringe

Figure 6-8(a) shows *both sides* of a standard U-100 insulin syringe. This syringe is to be used for the measurement and administration of U-100 insulin *only*. It must not be used to measure other medications that are measured in units.

> **CAUTION**
>
> U-100 insulin should be measured only in a U-100 insulin syringe.

Notice that Figure 6-8(a) pictures one side of the insulin syringe calibrated in odd-number two-unit increments and the other side calibrated in even-number two-unit increments. The plunger in Figure 6-9(a) simulates the measurement of 70 units of U-100 insulin. It is important to note that for U-100 insulin, 100 units equal 1 mL.

Figure 6-8(b) shows two Lo-Dose U-100 insulin syringes. The enlarged scale is easier to read and is calibrated for each 1 unit (U) up to 50 units per 0.5 mL or 30 units per 0.3 mL. Every 5 units are labeled. The 30-unit syringe is commonly used for pediatric administration of insulin. The plunger in Figure 6-9(b) simulates the measurement of 19 units of U-100 insulin.

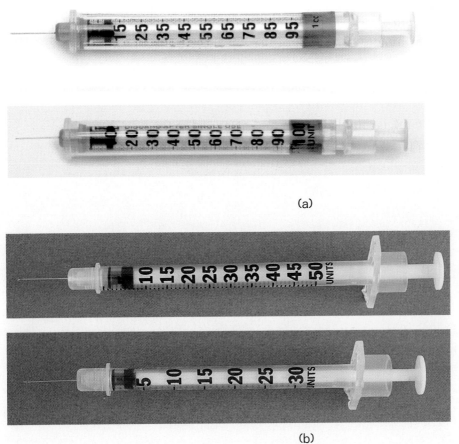

(a)

(b)

FIGURE 6-8 Isulin Syringes (a) Front and Reverse of a Standard U-100 Insulin Syringe; (b) Lo-Dose U-100 Insulin Syringes, 50 and 30 Units

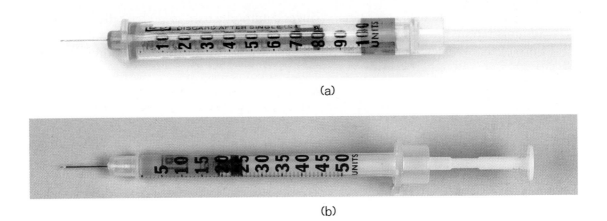

(a)

(b)

FIGURE 6-9 (a) Standard U-100 Insulin Syringe Measuring 70 Units of U-100 Insulin; (b) Lo-Dose U-100 Insulin Syringe Measuring 19 Units of U-100 Insulin

1 mL Syringe

Figure 6-10 shows the 1 mL syringe. This syringe is also referred to as the *tuberculin* or *TB syringe*. It is used when a small dose of a drug must be measured, such as an allergen extract, vaccine, or child's medication. Notice that the 1 mL syringe is calibrated in hundredths (0.01) of a milliliter, with each one tenth (0.1) milliliter labeled on the metric scale. Pediatric and critical care doses of less than 1 mL can be rounded to hundredths and measured in the 1 mL syringe. It is preferable to measure all amounts less than 0.5 mL in a 1 mL syringe.

Example:

The amount 0.366 mL is rounded to 0.37 and measured in the 1 mL syringe.

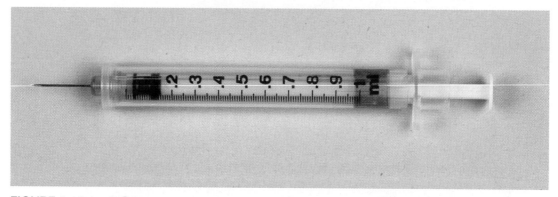

FIGURE 6-10 1 mL Syringe

Safety Syringe

Figure 6-11 shows safety 3 mL, 1 mL, and insulin syringes. Notice that the needle is protected by a shield to prevent accidental needlestick injury to the nurse after administering an injectable medication.

Intravenous Syringe

Figures 6-12 and 6-13 show large syringes commonly used to prepare medications for intravenous administration. The volume and calibration of these syringes vary. To be safe, examine the calibrations of the syringes, and select the one best suited for the volume to be administered.

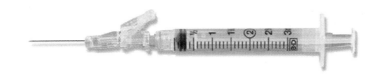

(a)

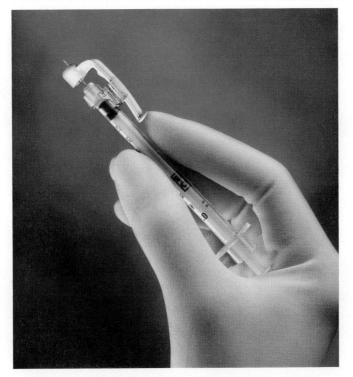

(b)

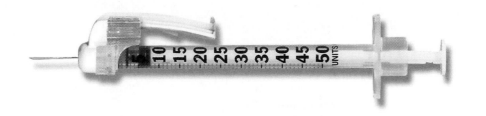

(c)

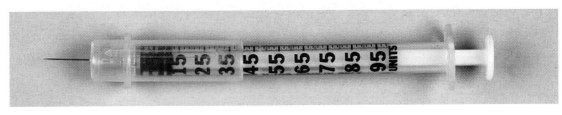

(d)

FIGURE 6-11 Safety Syringes (Courtesy of BD) (a) 3 mL; (b) 1 mL; (c) Lo-Dose U-100 Insulin; (d) Standard U-100 Insulin

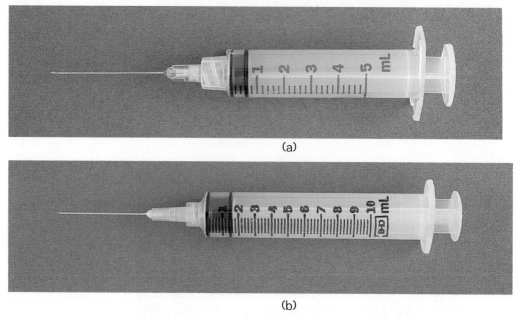

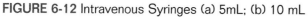

(a)

(b)

FIGURE 6-12 Intravenous Syringes (a) 5mL; (b) 10 mL

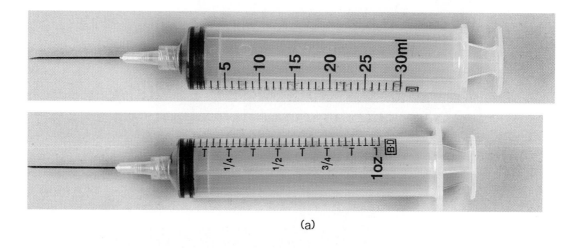

(a)

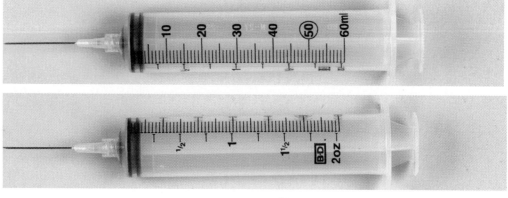

(b)

FIGURE 6-13 Intravenous Syringes (a) Front and Reverse of a 30 mL/1 oz syringe; (b) Front and Reverse of a 60 mL/2 oz syringe.

Needleless Syringe

Figure 6-14 pictures a needleless syringe system designed to prevent accidental needlesticks during intravenous administration.

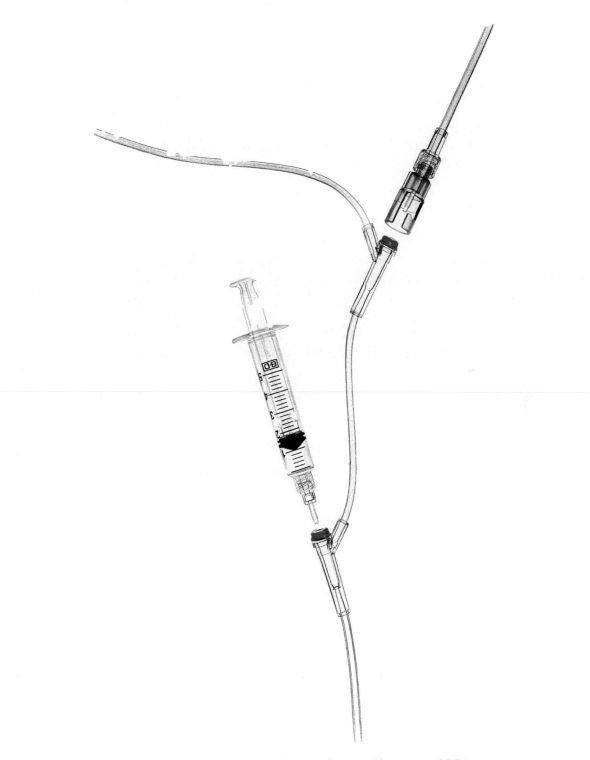

FIGURE 6-14 Example of a Needleless Syringe System (Courtesy of BD)

QUICK REVIEW

- The medicine cup has a 1 ounce or 30 milliliter capacity for oral liquids. It is also calibrated to measure teaspoons, tablespoons, and drams. Amounts less than 2.5 milliliters should be measured in a smaller device, such as an oral syringe.
- The calibrated dropper measures small amounts of oral liquids. The size of the drop varies according to the diameter of the tip of the dropper.
- The standard 3 mL syringe is used to measure most injectable drugs. It is calibrated in tenths of a mL.
- The prefilled, single-dose syringe cartridge is to be used once and then discarded.
- The Standard U-100 insulin syringe is used to measure U-100 insulin only. It is calibrated for a total of 100 units per 1 mL.
- The Lo-Dose U-100 insulin syringe is used for measuring small amounts of U-100 insulin. It is calibrated for a total of 50 units per 0.5 mL or 30 units per 0.3 mL. The smaller syringe is commonly used for administering small amounts of insulin.
- The 1 mL syringe is used to measure small or critical amounts of injectable drugs. It is calibrated in hundredths of a mL.
- Syringes intended for injections should never be used to measure or administer oral medications.

REVIEW SET 21

1. In which syringe should 0.25 mL of a drug solution be measured? _____

2. a. Can 1.25 mL be measured in the regular 3 mL syringe?

   _____

   b. How? _____

3. Should insulin be measured in a 1 mL syringe? _____

4. Fifty (50) units of U-100 insulin equals how many cubic centimeters? _____

5. a. The gtt is considered a consistent quantity for comparisons between different droppers.
   (True) (False)

   b. Why? _____

6. Can you measure 3 mL in a medicine cup? _____

7. How would you measure 3 mL of oral liquid to be administered to a child? _____

   _____

8. The medicine cup indicates that each teaspoon is the equivalent of _____ mL.

9. Describe your action if you are to administer less than the full amount of a drug supplied in a prefilled, single-dose syringe. _____

   _____

10. What is the primary purpose of the safety and needleless syringes? _____

   _____

Note to Learner

The drawings on subsequent pages of the syringes represent actual sizes.

Draw an arrow to point to the calibration that corresponds to the dose to be administered.

11. Administer 0.75 mL

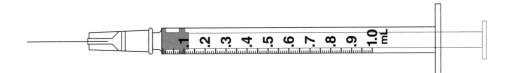

12. Administer 1.33 mL

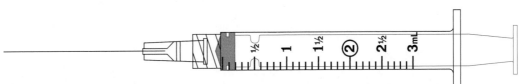

13. Administer 2.2 mL

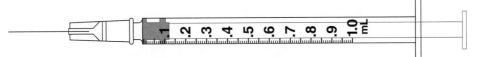

14. Administer 1.3 mL

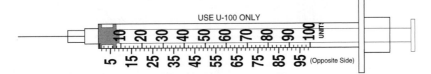

15. Administer 0.33 mL

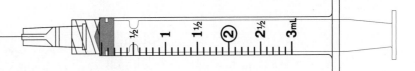

16. Administer 65 U of U-100 insulin

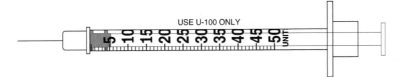

17. Administer 27 U of U-100 insulin

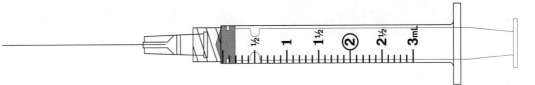

18. Administer 75 U of U-100 insulin

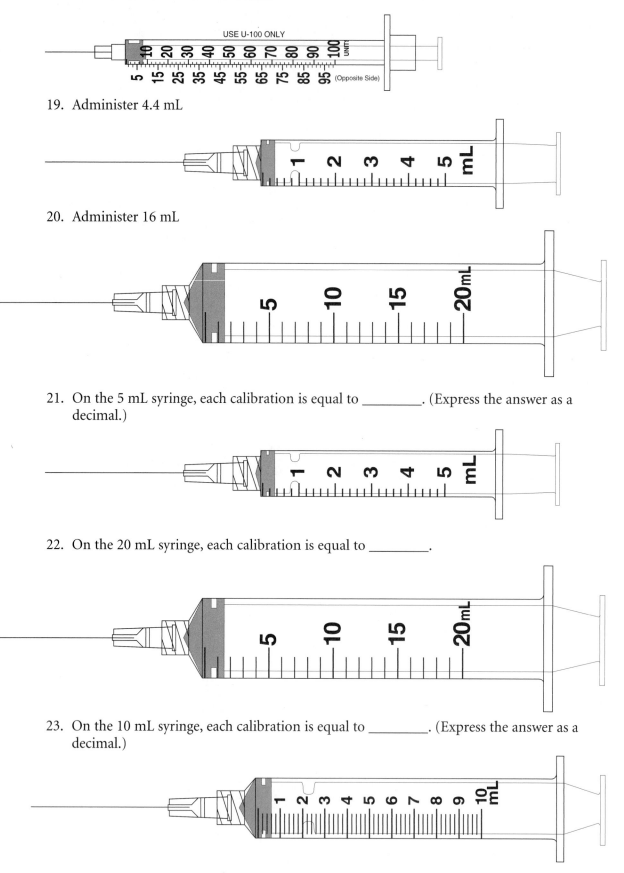

19. Administer 4.4 mL

20. Administer 16 mL

21. On the 5 mL syringe, each calibration is equal to _____. (Express the answer as a decimal.)

22. On the 20 mL syringe, each calibration is equal to _____.

23. On the 10 mL syringe, each calibration is equal to _____. (Express the answer as a decimal.)

After completing these problems, see pages 475–477 to check your answers.

CRITICAL THINKING SKILLS

Select correct equipment to prepare medications. In the following situation, the correct dosage was not given because an incorrect measuring device was used.

error

Using an inaccurate measuring device for oral medications.

possible scenario

Suppose a pediatrician ordered Amoxil suspension (250 mg/5 mL), 1 teaspoon, every 8 hours, to be given to a child. The child should receive the medication for 10 days for otitis media, an ear infection. The pharmacy dispensed the medication in a bottle containing 150 mL, or a 10-day supply. The nurse did not clarify for the mother how to measure and administer the medication. The child returned to the clinic in 10 days for routine follow-up. The nurse asked whether the child had taken all the prescribed Amoxil. The child's mother stated, "No, we have almost half of the bottle left." When the nurse asked how the medication had been given, the mother showed the bright pink plastic teaspoon she had obtained from the local ice cream parlor. The nurse measured the spoon's capacity and found it to be less than 3 mL. (Remember, 1 tsp = 5 mL.) The child would have received only $\frac{3}{5}$, or 60%, of the correct dose.

potential outcome

The child did not receive a therapeutic dosage of the medication and was actually underdosed. The child could develop a super infection, which could lead to a more severe illness like meningitis.

prevention

Teach family members (and patients, as appropriate) to use calibrated measuring spoons or specially designed oral syringes to measure the correct dosage of medication. The volumes of serving spoons may vary considerably, as this situation illustrates.

PRACTICE PROBLEMS—CHAPTER 6

1. In the U-100 insulin syringe, 100 U = _____ mL.

2. The 1 mL syringe is calibrated in _____ of a mL.

3. Can you measure 1.25 mL in a single tuberculin syringe? _____ Explain. _____

   _____

   _____

4. How would you measure 1.33 mL in a 3 mL syringe? _____

5. The medicine cup has a _____ mL or _____ oz capacity.

6. To administer exactly 0.52 mL to a child, select a _____ syringe.

7. 75 U of U-100 insulin equals _____ mL.

8. All droppers are calibrated to deliver standardized drops of equal amounts regardless of the dropper used. (True) (False)

9. The prefilled syringe is a multiple-dose system. (True) (False)

10. Insulin should be measured in an insulin syringe *only*. (True) (False)

11. The purpose of needleless syringes is _____.

12. Medications are measured in syringes by aligning the calibrations with the _____ of the black rubber tip of the plunger. (top ring, raised middle, or bottom ring)

13. The medicine cup calibrations indicate that 2 teaspoons are approximately _____ milliliters.

14. Some syringes are marked in cubic centimeters (cc) rather than milliliters (mL). (True) (False)

15. The _____ syringe(s) is(are) intended to measure parenteral doses of medications. (standard 3 mL, 1 mL, or insulin)

Draw an arrow to indicate the calibration that corresponds to the dose to be administered.

16. Administer 0.45 mL

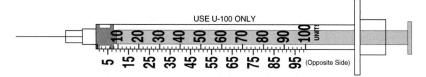

17. Administer 80 U of U-100 insulin

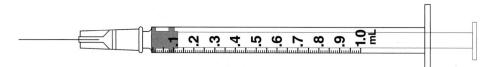

18. Administer ℥ ss

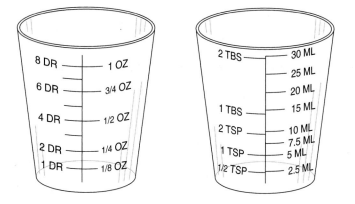

19. Administer 2.4 mL

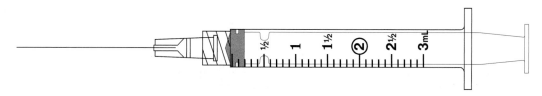

20. Administer 1.1 mL

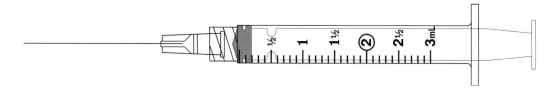

21. Administer 6.2 mL

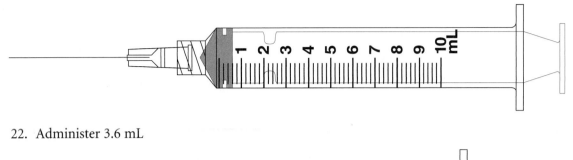

22. Administer 3.6 mL

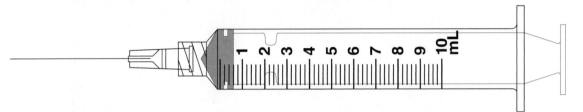

23. Administer 4.8 mL

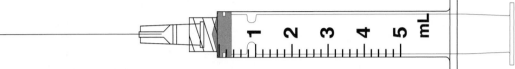

24. Administer 12 mL

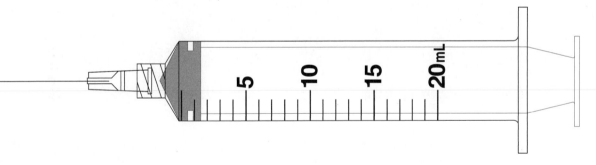

25. Critical Thinking Skill: Describe the strategy that would prevent this medication error.

possible scenario

Suppose a patient with cancer has oral Compazine liquid ordered for nausea. Because the patient has had difficulty taking the medication, the nurse decided to draw up the medication in a syringe without a needle to facilitate giving the medication. The nurse found this to be quite helpful and prepared several doses in syringes without the needles. A nurse from another unit covered for the nurse during lunch, and when the patient complained of nausea, the nurse assumed that the Compazine prepared in an injection syringe was to be given via injection. The nurse attached a needle and injected the oral medication.

potential outcome

The medication would be absorbed systemically, and the patient could develop an abscess at the site of injection.

prevention

_____

_____

26. Critical Thinking Skill: Describe the strategy that would prevent this medication administration error.

possible scenario

A child with ear infections is to receive Ceclor oral liquid as an anti-infective. The medication is received in oral syringes for administration. The nurse fails to remove the cap on the tip of the syringe and attempts to administer the medication.

potential outcome

The nurse would exert enough pressure on the syringe plunger that the protective cap could pop off in the child's mouth and possibly cause the child to choke.

prevention

_____

_____

After completing these problems, see pages 477–479 to check your answers.

Interpreting Drug Orders

OBJECTIVES

Upon mastery of Chapter 7, you will be able to interpret the drug order. To accomplish this you will also be able to:

- Read and write correct medical notation.
- Write the standard medical abbreviation from a list of common terminology.
- Classify the notation that specifies the dosage, route, and frequency of the medication to be administered.
- Interpret physician and other prescribing practitioner orders and medication administration records.

The prescription or medication order conveys the therapeutic drug plan for the patient. It is the responsibility of the nurse to:

- interpret the order
- prepare the exact dosage of the prescribed drug
- identify the patient
- administer the proper dosage by the prescribed route, at the prescribed time intervals
- record the administration of the prescribed drug
- monitor the patient's response for desired (therapeutic) and adverse effects

Before you can prepare the correct dosage of the prescribed drug, you must learn to interpret or read the written drug order. For brevity and speed, the health care professions have adopted certain standards and common abbreviations for use in notation. You should learn to recognize and interpret the abbreviations from memory. As you practice reading drug orders, you will find that this skill becomes second nature to you.

An example of a typical written drug order is:

9/4/XX Amoxil 500 mg p.o. q.i.d. (p.c. & h.s.)
J. Physician, M.D.

This order means the patient should receive 500 milligrams of an antibiotic named Amoxil (or amoxicillin) orally four times a day (after meals and at bedtime). You can see that the medical notation considerably shortens the written-out order.

MEDICAL ABBREVIATIONS

The following table lists common medical abbreviations used in writing drug orders. The abbreviations are grouped according to those that refer to the route (or method) of administration, the frequency (time interval), and other general terms. Commit these to memory, along with the other abbreviations related to systems of measurement presented in Chapter 3.

REMEMBER

Common Medical Abbreviations

Abbreviation	Interpretation	Abbreviation	Interpretation
Route:		**Frequency:**	
IM	intramuscular	t.i.d.	three times a day
IV	intravenous	q.i.d.	four times a day
IV PB	intravenous piggyback	min	minute
SC	subcutaneous	h	hour
SL	sublingual, under the tongue	q.h	every hour
ID	intradermal	q.2h	every two hours
GT	gastrostomy tube	q.3h	every three hours
NG	nasogastric tube	q.4h	every four hours
NJ	nasojejunal tube	q.6h	every six hours
p.o.	by mouth, orally	q.8h	every eight hours
p.r.	per rectum, rectally	q.12h	every twelve hours
O.D.	right eye	**General:**	
O.S.	left eye	$\bar{a}$	before
O.U.	both eyes	$\bar{p}$	after
A.D.	right ear	$\bar{c}$	with
A.S.	left ear	$\bar{s}$	without
A.U.	both ears	q	every
Frequency:		qs	quantity sufficient
a.c.	before meals	aq	water
p.c.	after meals	NPO	nothing by mouth
ad. lib.	as desired, freely	ss	one-half
p.r.n.	when necessary	gtt	drop
h.s.	hour of sleep, at bedtime	tab	tablet
stat	immediately, at once	cap	capsule
q.d.	once a day, every day	et	and
q.o.d.	every other day	noct	night
b.i.d.	twice a day		

THE DRUG ORDER

The drug order consists of seven parts:

1. Name of the *patient*

2. Name of the *drug* to be administered

3. *Dosage* of the drug

4. *Route* by which the drug is to be administered

5. *Frequency,* time, and special instructions related to administration

6. *Date and time* when the order was written

7. *Signature* of the person writing the order

> **CAUTION**
>
> If any of the seven parts is missing or unclear, the order is considered incomplete and is, therefore, not a legal drug order.

Parts 1 through 5 of the drug order are known as the original Five Rights of safe medication administration. They are essential and each one must be faithfully checked every time a medication is prepared and administered. Following safe administration of the medication, the nurse or health care practitioner must accurately document the drug administration. Combined with the original Five Rights, the patient is entitled to *Six Rights* of safe and accurate medication administration and documentation with each and every dose.

> **REMEMBER**
>
> The Six Rights of safe and accurate medication administration:
>
> The *right patient* must receive the *right drug* in the *right amount* by the *right route* at the *right time*, followed by the *right documentation*.

Each drug order should follow a specific sequence. The name of the drug is written first, followed by the dosage, route, and frequency. When correctly written, the brand (or trade) name of the drug begins with a capital or uppercase letter. The generic name begins with a lowercase letter.

Example:

Procan SR 500 mg p.o. q.6h

1. *Procan SR* is the brand name of the drug

2. *500 mg* is the dosage

3. *p.o.* is the route

4. *q.6h* is the frequency

This order means: Give 500 milligrams of Procan SR orally every 6 hours.

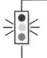

> **CAUTION**
>
> If the nurse has difficulty understanding and interpreting the drug order, the nurse *must* clarify the order with the writer. Usually this person is the physician or another authorized practitioner, such as an advanced registered nurse practitioner.

Let's practice reading and interpreting drug orders.

Example 1:

Dilantin 100 mg p.o. t.i.d.

Reads: "Give 100 milligrams of Dilantin orally 3 times a day."

Example 2:

procaine penicillin G 400,000 U IM q.6h

Reads: "Give 400,000 units of procaine penicillin G intramuscularly every 6 hours."

Example 3:

Demerol 75 mg IM q.4h p.r.n., pain

Reads: "Give 75 milligrams of Demerol intramuscularly every 4 hours when necessary for pain."

CAUTION

The *p.r.n.* frequency designates the minimum time allowed between doses. There is no maximum time other than automatic stops as defined by hospital or agency policy.

Example 4:

Humulin R Regular U-100 insulin 5 U SC stat

Reads: "Give 5 units of Humulin R Regular U-100 insulin subcutaneously immediately."

Example 5:

Ancef 1 g IV PB q.6h

Reads: "Give one gram of Ancef by intravenous piggyback every 6 hours."

The administration times are designated by hospital policy. For example, t.i.d. administration times may be 0900 or 9 AM, 1300 or 1 PM, and 1700 or 5 PM.

QUICK REVIEW

- The *right patient* must receive the *right drug* in the *right amount* by the *right route* at the *right time* followed by the *right documentation*.
- Understanding drug orders requires interpreting common medical abbreviations.
- The drug order must contain (in this sequence): drug name, dosage, route, frequency.
- All parts of the drug order must be stated clearly for accurate, exact interpretation.
- If you are ever in doubt as to the meaning of any part of a drug order, ask the writer to clarify before proceeding.

REVIEW SET 22

Interpret the following medication (drug) orders:

1. *naproxen 250 mg p.o. b.i.d.* _____

_____

2. *Humulin N NPH U-100 insulin 30 U SC q.d. 30 min ā breakfast* _____

_____

3. *Ceclor 500 mg p.o. stat, then 250 mg q.8h* _____

_____

4. *Synthroid 25 mcg p.o. q.d.* _____

_____

5. *Ativan 10 mg IM q.4h p.r.n., agitation* _____

_____

6. *furosemide 20 mg IV stat (slowly)* _____

_____

7. *Gelusil 10 mL p.o. h.s.* _____

_____

8. *atropine sulfate ophthalmic 1% 2 gtt O.D. q.15 min × 4* _____

_____

9. *morphine sulfate gr $\frac{1}{4}$ IM q.3–4h p.r.n., pain* _____

_____

10. *Lanoxin 0.25 mg p.o. q.d.* _____

_____

11. *tetracycline 250 mg p.o. q.i.d.* _____

_____

12. *nitroglycerin gr $\frac{1}{400}$ SL stat* _____

_____

13. *Cortisporin otic suspension 2 gtt A.U. t.i.d. et h.s.* _____

_____

14. Compare and contrast *t.i.d.* and *q.8h* administration times. Include sample administration times for each in your explanation. _____

_____

15. Describe your action if no method of administration is written. _____

_____

16. Do q.i.d. and q.4h have the same meaning? _____ Explain. _____

_____

17. Who determines the medication administration times? _____

_____

18. Name the seven parts of a written medication prescription. _____

_____

19. Which parts of the written medication prescription/order are included in the original Five Rights of medication administration? _____

_____

20. State the Six Rights of safe and accurate medication administration. _____

_____

After completing these problems, see page 479 to check your answers.

Medication Order and Administration Forms

Hospitals have a special form for recording drug orders. Figure 7-1 shows a sample physician's order form. Find and name each of the seven parts of the drug orders listed. Notice that the nurse or other health care professional must verify and initial each order, ensuring that each of the seven parts is accurate. In some places, the pharmacist may be responsible for verifying the order as part of the computerized record.

			ENTERED	FILLED	CHECKED	VERIFIED

NOTE: A NON-PROPRIETARY DRUG OF EQUAL QUALITY MAY BE DISPENSED - IF THIS COLUMN IS NOT CHECKED!

DATE	TIME WRITTEN	PLEASE USE BALL POINT - PRESS FIRMLY	✓	TIME NOTED	NURSES SIGNATURE
11/3/xx	0815	Keflex 250 mg p.o. q.6h	✓		
		Humulin N NPH U-100 Insulin 40 U SC ā breakfast	✓	0830	
		Demerol 75 mg IV q. 3–4 h p.r.n. severe pain	✓		G. Pickar, R.N.
		Codeine 30 mg p.o. q.4h p.r.n. mild–mod pain	✓		
		Tylenol 650 mg p.o. q.4h p.r.n., fever > 101° F	✓		
		Lasix 40 mg p.o. q.d.	✓		
		Slow-K 8 mEq p.o. b.i.d.	✓		
		J. Physician, M.D.			
11/3/xx	2200	Lasix 80 mg IV stat	✓		
		J. Physician, M.D.		2210	M. Smith, R.N.

AUTO STOP ORDERS: UNLESS REORDERED, FOLLOWING WILL BE D/C'D AT 0800 ON:

DATE	ORDER		
		☐ CONT	PHYSICIAN SIGNATURE
		☐ D/C	
		☐ CONT	PHYSICIAN SIGNATURE
		☐ D/C	
		☐ CONT	PHYSICIAN SIGNATURE
		☐ D/C	

CHECK WHEN ANTIBIOTICS ORDERED   ☐ Prophylactic   ☐ Empiric   ☐ Therapeutic

Allergies:
None Known

PATIENT DIAGNOSIS
Diabetes

HEIGHT 5' 5"   WEIGHT 130 lb

PHYSICIANS ORDER

FORM 959-706 (8-XX)   Reynolds + Reynolds LITHO IN U.S.A. K41914 (7-XX) D030060

Patient, Mary Q.
#3-11316-7

①

FIGURE 7-1 Physician's Order

The drug orders from the physician's order form are transcribed to a medication administration record (MAR), Figure 7-2. The nurse or other health care professional uses this record as a guide to:

- check the drug order,
- prepare the correct dosage, and
- record the drug administered.

These three check points help to ensure accurate medication administration.

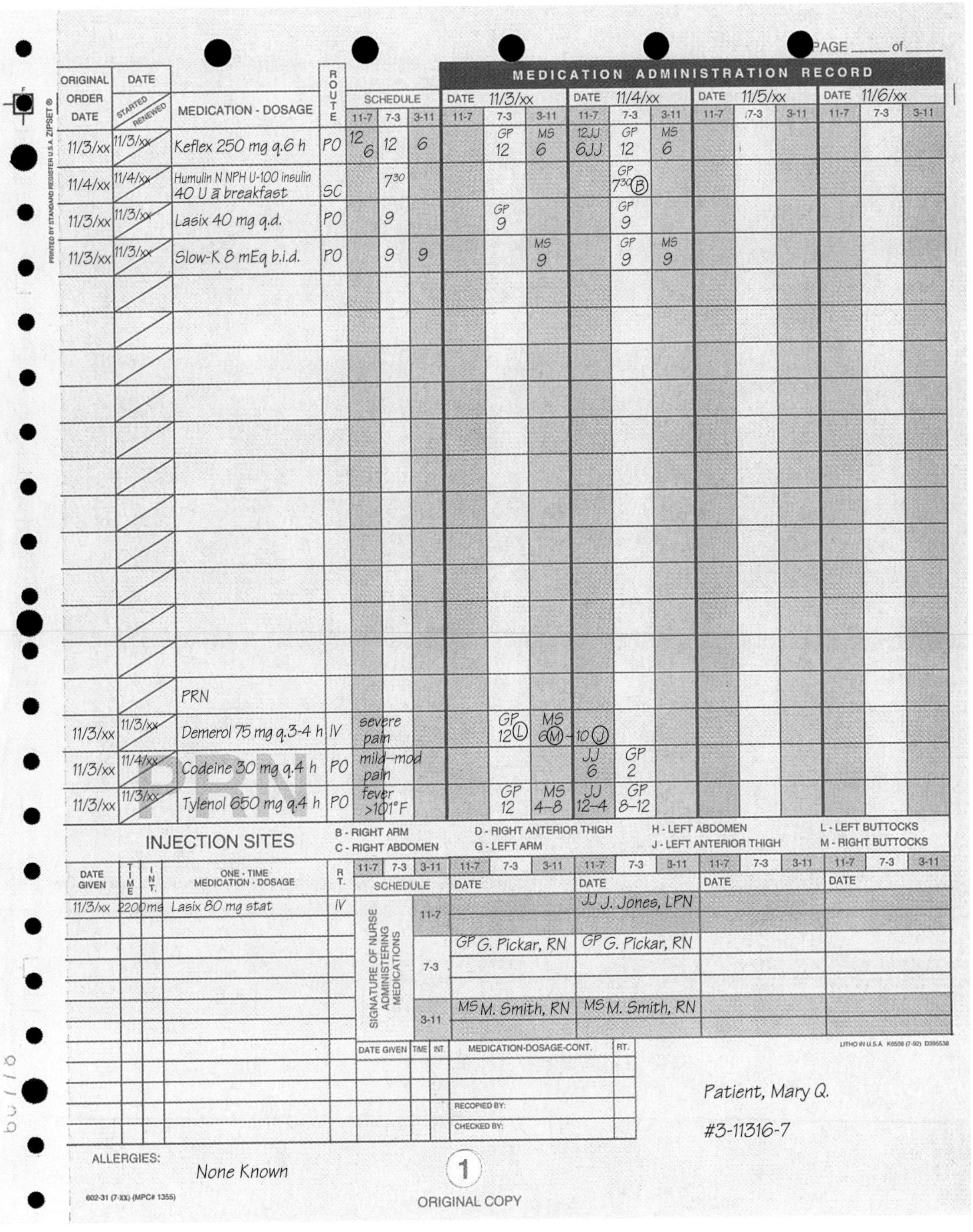

MEDICATION ADMINISTRATION RECORD

PAGE _____ of _____

ORIGINAL ORDER DATE	DATE STARTED / RENEWED	MEDICATION - DOSAGE	ROUTE	SCHEDULE 11-7	7-3	3-11	DATE 11/3/xx 11-7	7-3	3-11	DATE 11/4/xx 11-7	7-3	3-11	DATE 11/5/xx 11-7	7-3	3-11	DATE 11/6/xx 11-7	7-3	3-11
11/3/xx	11/3/xx	Keflex 250 mg q.6 h	PO	12 6	12	6		GP 12	MS 6	12JJ 6JJ	GP 12	MS 6						
11/4/xx	11/4/xx	Humulin N NPH U-100 insulin 40 U ā breakfast	SC		7³⁰						GP 7³⁰ Ⓑ							
11/3/xx	11/3/xx	Lasix 40 mg q.d.	PO		9			GP 9			GP 9							
11/3/xx	11/3/xx	Slow-K 8 mEq b.i.d.	PO		9	9			MS 9		GP 9	MS 9						

PRN

11/3/xx	11/3/xx	Demerol 75 mg q.3-4 h	IV	severe pain				GP 12Ⓛ	MS 6Ⓜ	10 Ⓙ								
11/3/xx	11/4/xx	Codeine 30 mg q.4 h	PO	mild-mod pain							JJ 6	GP 2						
11/3/xx	11/3/xx	Tylenol 650 mg q.4 h	PO	fever >101°F				GP 12	MS 4-8	JJ 12-4	GP 8-12							

INJECTION SITES

B - RIGHT ARM	D - RIGHT ANTERIOR THIGH	H - LEFT ABDOMEN	L - LEFT BUTTOCKS
C - RIGHT ABDOMEN	G - LEFT ARM	J - LEFT ANTERIOR THIGH	M - RIGHT BUTTOCKS

DATE GIVEN	TIME	INT.	ONE - TIME MEDICATION - DOSAGE	RT.	SCHEDULE	11-7	7-3	3-11	DATE 11-7	7-3	3-11	DATE 11-7	7-3	3-11	DATE	DATE
11/3/xx	2200	ms	Lasix 80 mg stat	IV	SIGNATURE OF NURSE ADMINISTERING MEDICATIONS	11-7			JJ J. Jones, LPN							
						7-3			GP G. Pickar, RN	GP G. Pickar, RN						
						3-11			MS M. Smith, RN	MS M. Smith, RN						

DATE GIVEN	TIME	INT.	MEDICATION-DOSAGE-CONT.	RT.

RECOPIED BY:

CHECKED BY:

Patient, Mary Q.

#3-11316-7

ALLERGIES: None Known

602-31 (7-XX) (MPC# 1355)

① ORIGINAL COPY

FIGURE 7-2 Medication Administration Record

COMPUTERIZED MEDICATION ADMINISTRATION SYSTEMS

Many health care facilities now use computers for processing drug orders. Drug orders are either electronically transmitted or manually entered into the computer from an order form, such as Figure 7-3. Through the computer, the nurse or other health care professional can transmit the order within seconds to the pharmacy for filling. The computer can keep track of drug stock and usage patterns and even notify the business office to post charges to the patient's account. Most importantly, it can

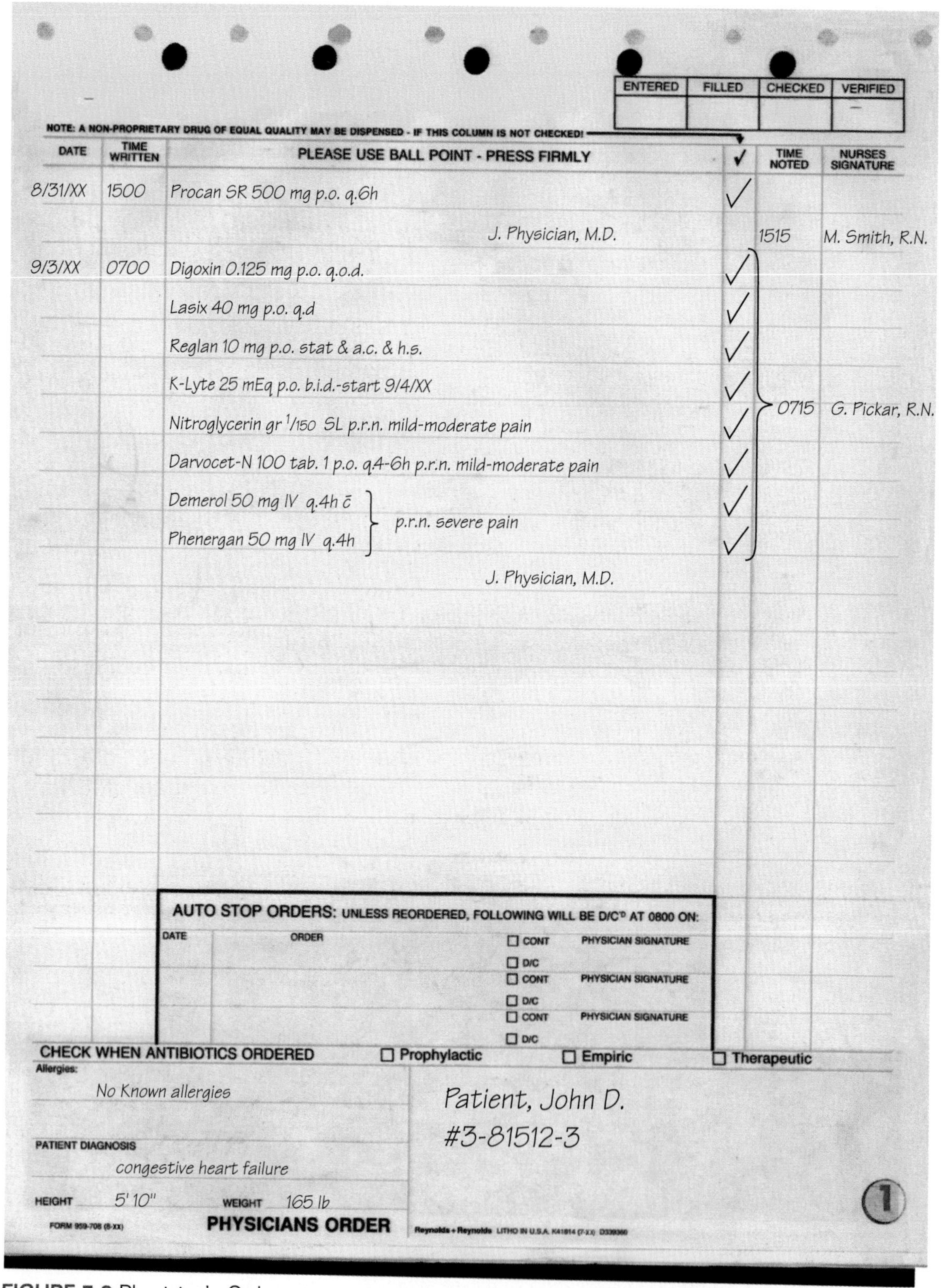

ENTERED	FILLED	CHECKED	VERIFIED
			—

NOTE: A NON-PROPRIETARY DRUG OF EQUAL QUALITY MAY BE DISPENSED - IF THIS COLUMN IS NOT CHECKED!

DATE	TIME WRITTEN	PLEASE USE BALL POINT - PRESS FIRMLY	✓	TIME NOTED	NURSES SIGNATURE
8/31/XX	1500	Procan SR 500 mg p.o. q.6h	✓		
		J. Physician, M.D.		1515	M. Smith, R.N.
9/3/XX	0700	Digoxin 0.125 mg p.o. q.o.d.	✓		
		Lasix 40 mg p.o. q.d	✓		
		Reglan 10 mg p.o. stat & a.c. & h.s.	✓		
		K-Lyte 25 mEq p.o. b.i.d.-start 9/4/XX	✓		
		Nitroglycerin gr $^{1}/_{150}$ SL p.r.n. mild-moderate pain	✓	0715	G. Pickar, R.N.
		Darvocet-N 100 tab. 1 p.o. q.4-6h p.r.n. mild-moderate pain	✓		
		Demerol 50 mg IV q.4h c̄ } p.r.n. severe pain	✓		
		Phenergan 50 mg IV q.4h	✓		
		J. Physician, M.D.			

AUTO STOP ORDERS: UNLESS REORDERED, FOLLOWING WILL BE D/C'D AT 0800 ON:

DATE	ORDER		
		☐ CONT ☐ D/C	PHYSICIAN SIGNATURE
		☐ CONT ☐ D/C	PHYSICIAN SIGNATURE
		☐ CONT ☐ D/C	PHYSICIAN SIGNATURE

CHECK WHEN ANTIBIOTICS ORDERED ☐ Prophylactic ☐ Empiric ☐ Therapeutic

Allergies: No Known allergies

PATIENT DIAGNOSIS: congestive heart failure

HEIGHT 5' 10" WEIGHT 165 lb

Patient, John D.
#3-81512-3

FORM 959-708 (8-XX) PHYSICIANS ORDER

Reynolds + Reynolds LITHO IN U.S.A.

1

FIGURE 7-3 Physician's Order

scan for information previously entered, such as drug incompatibilities, drug allergies, safe dosage ranges, doses already given, or recommended administration times. The health care staff can be readily alerted to potential problems or inconsistencies. The corresponding medication administration record may also be printed directly from the computer, Figure 7-4.

The computerized medication administration record (MAR) may be viewed at the computer or from a printed copy, Figure 7-4. The nurse may be able to look back at the patient's cumulative medication administration record, document administration times and comments at the computer terminal, and then keep a printed copy of the information obtained and entered. The data analysis, storage, and retrieval abilities of computers are making them essential tools for safe and accurate medication administration.

PHARMACY MAR

START	STOP	MEDICATION	SCHEDULED TIMES	OK'D BY	0001 HRS. TO 1200 HRS.	1201 HRS. TO 2400 HRS.
08/31/xx 1800 SCH		PROCAN SR 500 MG TAB-SR 500 MG Q6H PO	0600 1200 1800 2400	JD	0600GP 1200 GP	1800 MS 2400 JD
09/03/xx 0900 SCH		DIGOXIN (LANOXIN) 0.125 MG TAB 1 TAB QOD PO ODD DAYS-SEPT	0900	JD	0900 GP	
09/03/xx 0900 SCH		FUROSEMIDE (LASIX) 40 MG TAB 1 TAB QD PO	0900	JD	0900 GP	
09/03/xx 0730 SCH		REGLAN 10 MG TAB 10 MG AC&HS PO GIVE ONE NOW!!	0730 1130 1630 2100	JD	0730 GP 1130 GP	1630 MS 2100 MS
09/04/xx 0900 SCH		K-LYTE 25 MEQ EFFERVESCENT TAB 1 EFF. TAB BID PO DISSOLVE AS DIR START 9-4	0900 1700	JD	0900 GP	1700 GP
09/03/xx 1507 PRN		NITROGLYCERIN 1/50 GR 0.4 MG TAB-SL 1 TABLET PRN* SL PRN CHEST PAIN		JD		
09/03/xx 1700 PRN		DARVOCET-N 100* 1 TAB Q4-6H PO PRN MILD–MODERATE PAIN		JD		
09/03/xx 2100 PRN		MEPERIDINE* (DEMEROL) INJ 50 MG Q4H IM PRN SEVERE PAIN W PHENERGAN		JD		2200 Ⓗ MS
09/03/xx 2100 PRN		PROMETHAZINE (PHENERGAN) INJ 50 MG Q4H IM PRN SEVERE PAIN W DEMEROL		JD		2200 Ⓗ MS

Gluteus / Thigh
A. Right / H. Right
B. Left / I. Left
Ventro Gluteal
C. Right / J. Right
D. Left / K. Left
E. Abdomen 1|2 3|4
730-13 (12/xx)

NURSE'S SIGNATURE	INITIAL
7–3 G. Pickar, R.N.	GP
3–11 M. Smith, R.N.	MS
11–7 J. Doe, R.N.	JD

ALLERGIES: NKA
DIAGNOSIS: CHF

Patient: Patient, John D.
Patient # 3-81512-3
Admitted: 08/31/xx
Physician: J. Physician, MD
Room: PCU-14 PCU

FIGURE 7-4 Computerized Medication Administration Record

REVIEW SET 23

Refer to the Computerized Medication Administration Record (Figure 7-4) on page 125 to answer questions 1 through 10. Convert the scheduled international time to traditional AM/PM time.

1. Scheduled times for administering Procan SR. _____

2. Scheduled times for administering Lanoxin and Lasix. _____

3. Scheduled times for administering Reglan. _____

4. Scheduled times for administering K-Lyte. _____

5. How often can the Demerol be given? _____

6. If the Lanoxin was last given on 9/5/xx at 0900, when is the next time and date it will be given? _____

7. What is the ordered route of administration for the nitroglycerin? _____

8. How many times a day is furosemide ordered? _____

9. The equivalent dosage of Lanoxin is _____ mcg.

10. Which drugs are ordered to be administered "as necessary"? _____

Refer to the Medication Administration Record (Figure 7-2) on page 123 to answer questions 11 through 20.

11. What is the route of administration for the insulin? _____

12. How many times in a 24-hour period will Lasix be administered? _____

13. What is the only medication ordered to be given routinely at noon? _____

14. What time of day is the insulin to be administered? _____

15. A dosage of 8 mEq of Slow-K is ordered. What does mEq mean? _____

16. You work 3 to 11 PM on November 5. Which routine medications will you administer to Mary Q. Patient during your shift? _____

17. Mary Q. Patient has a fever of 101.4°F. What medication should you administer? _____

18. How many times in a 24-hour period will Slow-K be administered? _____

19. What is the equivalent of the scheduled administration time(s) for the Slow-K as converted to international time? _____

20. What is the equivalent of the scheduled administration time(s) for the Keflex as converted to international time? _____

21. Identify the place on the MAR where the stat IV Lasix was charted. _____

After completing these problems, see page 480 to check your answers.

CRITICAL THINKING SKILLS

It is the responsibility of the nurse to clarify any drug order that is incomplete; that is, an order that does not contain the essential seven parts discussed in this chapter. Let's look at an example in which this error occurred.

error

Failing to clarify incomplete orders.

possible scenario

Suppose a physician ordered *Pepcid tablet p.o. h.s.* for a patient with an active duodenal ulcer. You will note there is no dosage listed. The nurse thought the medication came in only one dosage strength, added 20 mg to the order, and sent it to the pharmacy. The pharmacist prepared the dosage written on the physician's order sheet. Two days later, during rounds, the physician noted that the patient had not responded well to the Pepcid. When asked about the Pepcid, the nurse explained that the patient had received 20 mg at bedtime. The physician informed the nurse that the patient should have received the 40 mg tablet.

potential outcome

Potentially, the delay in correct dosage could result in gastrointestinal bleeding or delayed healing of the ulcer.

prevention

This medication error could have been avoided simply by the physician writing the strength of the medication. When this was omitted, the nurse should have checked the dosage before sending the order to the pharmacy. When you fill in an incomplete order, you are essentially practicing medicine without a license, which is illegal and potentially dangerous.

PRACTICE PROBLEMS—CHAPTER 7

Interpret the following abbreviations and symbols without consulting another source.

1. ℨ	_____	9. q.d.	_____
2. p.r.	_____	10. O.D.	_____
3. a.c.	_____	11. stat	_____
4. p̄	_____	12. ad.lib.	_____
5. t.i.d.	_____	13. h.s.	_____
6. q.4h	_____	14. IM	_____
7. p.r.n.	_____	15. s̄	_____
8. p.o.	_____		

Give the abbreviation or symbol for the following terms without consulting another source.

16. one-half   _____   23. subcutaneous   _____

17. drop   _____   24. teaspoon   _____

18. milliliter   _____   25. twice daily   _____

19. grain   _____   26. every 3 hours   _____

20. gram   _____   27. after meals   _____

21. four times a day   _____   28. before   _____

22. both eyes   _____   29. kilogram   _____

Interpret the following physician's drug orders without consulting another source.

30. *Toradol 60 mg IM stat et q.6h* _____

31. *procaine penicillin G 300,000 U IM q.i.d.* _____

32. *Mylanta 5 mL p.o. 1 h a.c., 1 h p.c., h.s., et q.2h p.r.n. @ noct, gastric upset* _____

_____

33. *Librium 25 mg p.o. q.6h p.r.n., agitation* _____

34. *heparin 5,000 U SC stat* _____

35. *Demerol 50 mg IM q.3–4h p.r.n., pain* _____

36. *digoxin 0.25 mg p.o. q.d.* _____

37. *Neo-Synephrine ophthalmic 10% 2 gtt O.S. q.30 min X 2* _____

_____

38. *Lasix 40 mg IM stat* _____

39. *Decadron 4 mg IV b.i.d.* _____

Refer to the Medication Administration Record in Figure 7-5 on page 129 to answer questions 40 through 44.

40. Convert the scheduled times for Isosorbide SR to traditional AM/PM time.

_____   _____   _____

41. How many units of heparin will the patient receive at 2200? _____

42. What route is ordered for the Humulin R Regular insulin? _____

43. Interpret the order for Cipro. _____

44. If the administration times for the sliding scale insulin are accurate (30 minutes before meals), what times will meals be served? (Use traditional AM/PM time.) _____

Refer to the Computerized Pharmacy MAR in Figure 7-6 on page 130 to answer questions 45 through 49.

45. The physician visited about 5:00 PM on 8/8/xx. What order did the physician write? _____

_____

46. Using the time as a clue, interpret the symbol "w/" in the Zantac order and give the proper medical abbreviation. _____

_____

47. Interpret the order for ranitidine. _____

48. Which of the routine medications is(are) ordered for 6:00 PM? _____

PAGE _1_ of _1_

MEDICATION ADMINISTRATION RECORD

ORIGINAL ORDER DATE	DATE STARTED / RENEWED	MEDICATION - DOSAGE	ROUTE	SCHEDULE 11-7	SCHEDULE 7-3	SCHEDULE 3-11	DATE 11/3/xx 11-7	7-3	3-11	DATE 11/4/xx 11-7	7-3	3-11	DATE 11/5/xx 11-7	7-3	3-11	DATE 11/6/xx 11-7	7-3	3-11
11/3/xx	11/3/xx	Heparin lock Central line flush (10U/cc solution) 2cc	IV b.i.d.		1000	2200												
11/3/xx	11/3/xx	Isosorbide SR 40 mg q.8h	PO	2400	0800	1600												
11/3/xx	11/3/xx	Cipro 500 mg q.12h	PO		1000	2200												
11/3/xx	11/3/xx	Humulin N NPH U-100 insulin 15U q.am	SC	0700														
11/3/xx	11/3/xx	Humulin R Regular U-100 insulin 30 min. ac and hs per sliding scale Blood glucose 0-150 3U 151-250 8U 251-350 13U 351-400 18U >400 call Dr.	SC		0730 1130	1730 2200												
		PRN																
11/3/xx	11/3/xx	Tylenol 1000 mg q.3–4h prn headache	PO															

PRN

INJECTION SITES

B - RIGHT ARM   D - RIGHT ANTERIOR THIGH   H - LEFT ABDOMEN   L - LEFT BUTTOCKS
C - RIGHT ABDOMEN   G - LEFT ARM   J - LEFT ANTERIOR THIGH   M - RIGHT BUTTOCKS

DATE GIVEN	TIME	INT.	ONE - TIME MEDICATION - DOSAGE	RT.	11-7 SCHEDULE	7-3	3-11	11-7 DATE	7-3	3-11	11-7 DATE	7-3	3-11	11-7 DATE	7-3	3-11	11-7 DATE	7-3	3-11
					SIGNATURE OF NURSE ADMINISTERING MEDICATIONS	11-7													
						7-3													
						3-11													

DATE GIVEN	TIME	INT.	MEDICATION-DOSAGE-CONT.	RT.

RECOPIED BY:

CHECKED BY:

LITHO IN U.S.A. K6508 (7-92) D395536

Patient, Pat H.
#6-33725-4

ALLERGIES:
None Known

602-31 (7-XX) (MPC# 1355)

(1) ORIGINAL COPY

FIGURE 7-5 Medication Administration Record for Chapter 7 Practice Problems (Questions 40–44)

START	STOP	MEDICATION			SCHEDULED TIMES	OK'D BY	0701 TO 1500	1501 TO 2300	2301 TO 0700
21:00 8/17/xx SCH		MEGESTROL ACETATE (MEGACE) 40 MG TAB	2 TABS	PO	BID	0900 2100				
12:00 8/17/xx SCH		VANCOMYCIN 250 MG CAP	1 CAPSULE	PO	QID	0800 1200 1800 2200				
9:00 8/13/xx SCH		FLUCONAZOLE (DIFLUCAN) 100 MG TAB	100 MG	PO	QD	0900				
21:00 8/11/xx SCH		PERIDEX ORAL RINSE 480 ML	30 ML ORAL RINSE SWISH & SPIT		BID	0900 2100				
17:00 8/10/xx SCH		RANITIDINE (ZANTAC) 150 MG TAB	1 TABLET PO W/BREAK.&SUPPER		BID	0800 1700				
17:00 8/08/xx SCH		DIGOXIN (LANOXIN) 0.125 MG TAB	1 TAB	PO	QD1700	1700				
0:01 8/27/xx PRN		LIDOCAINE 5% OINT 35 GM TUBE	APPLY TOPICAL TO RECTAL AREA		PRN*					
14:00 8/22/xx PRN		SODIUM CHLORIDE INJ 10 ML	AS DIR IV DILUENT FOR ATIVAN IV		TID					
14:00 8/22/xx PRN		LORAZEPAM (ATIVAN)*2 MG INJ	1 MG IV	PRN ANXIETY	TID					
9:30 8/21/xx PRN		TUCKS 40 PADS APPLY	APPLY TOPICAL TO RECTUM PRN		Q4-6H					
9:30 8/21/xx PRN		ANUSOL SUPP 1 SUPP	1 SUPP	PR	Q4-6H					
16:00 8/18/xx PRN		MEPERIDINE* (DEMEROL) INJ 25 MG	10 MG IV PRN PAIN	IN ADDITION TO PCA	Q1H					

Gluteus	Thigh	STANDARD TIMES	NURSE'S SIGNATURE	INITIAL	ALLERGIES: NAFCILLIN	
A. Right	H. Right	QD = 0900	0701-		BACTRIM	Patient Smith, John
B. Left	I. Left	BID = Q12H = 0900 & 2100	1500 _____		SULFA	Patient # 3-90301-4
		TID = 0800, 1400, 2200	1501-		TRIMETHOPRIM	
Ventro Gluteal	Deltoid	Q8H = 0800, 1600, 2400	2300 _____		CIPROFLOXACIN HCL	Physician: J. Physician, M.D.
C. Right	J. Right	QID = 0800, 1200, 1800, 2200	2301-			Room: 407-4 South
D. Left	K. Left	Q6H = 0600, 1200, 1800, 2400	0700 _____			
E. Abdomen	1|2	Q4H = 0400, 0800, 1200...	Ok'd			
	3|4	QD DIGOXIN = 1700	by _____		FROM: 08/30/xx 0701 TO: 08/31/xx 0700	
Page **1** of **2**	QD	QD WARFARIN = 1600				

FIGURE 7-6 Computerized Pharmacy MAR for Chapter 7 Practice Problems (Questions 45–49)

49. How many hours are between the scheduled administration times for Megace? _____

50. Critical Thinking Skill: Describe the strategy that would prevent this medication error.

possible scenario

Suppose a physician wrote an order for gentamicin 100 mg to be given IV q.8h to a patient hospitalized with meningitis. The unit secretary transcribed the order as:

gentamicin 100 mg IV q.8h

(12 AM–6 AM–12 PM–6 PM)

The medication nurse checked the order without noticing the discrepancy in the administration times. Suppose the patient received the medication every six hours for three days before the error was noticed.

potential outcome

The patient would have received one extra dose each day, which is equivalent to one third more medication daily. Most likely, the physician would be notified of the error, and the medication would be discontinued with serum gentamicin levels drawn. The levels would likely be in the toxic range, and the patient's gentamicin levels would be monitored until the levels returned to normal. This patient would be at risk of developing ototoxicity or nephrotoxicity from the overdose of gentamicin.

prevention

_____

_____

After completing these problems, see page 480 to check your answers.

Understanding Drug Labels

OBJECTIVES

Upon mastery of Chapter 8, you will be able to read and understand the labels of the medications you have available. To accomplish this you will also be able to:

- Find and differentiate the brand and generic names of drugs.
- Determine the dosage strength.
- Determine the form in which the drug is supplied.
- Determine the supply dosage or concentration.
- Identify the total volume of the drug container.
- Differentiate the total volume of the container from the supply dosage.
- Find the directions for mixing or preparing the supply dosage of drugs, as needed.
- Recognize and follow drug alerts.
- Identify the administration route.
- Check the expiration date.
- Identify the lot or control number, National Drug Code, and bar code symbols.
- Recognize the manufacturer's name.
- Differentiate labels for multidose and unit dose containers.
- Identify combination drugs.
- Describe supply dosage expressed as a ratio or percent.

The drug order prescribes how much of a drug the patient is to receive. The nurse must prepare the order from the drugs on hand. The drug label tells how the available drug is supplied. Examine the various preparations, labels, and dosage strengths of Nebcin (tobramycin sulfate) injection, Figure 8-1.

Look at the following common drug labels to learn to recognize pertinent information about the drugs supplied.

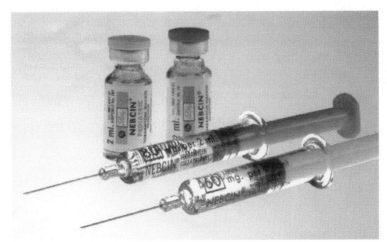

FIGURE 8-1 Various Nebcin Preparations

BRAND AND GENERIC NAMES

The brand, trade, or proprietary name is the manufacturer's name for a drug. Notice that the brand name is usually the most prominent word on the drug label—large type and boldly visible to promote the product. It is often followed by the sign ® meaning that both the name and formulation are registered. The generic or established, nonproprietary name appears directly under the brand name. Sometimes the generic name is also placed inside parentheses. By law, the generic name must be identified on all drug labels.

NDC 63323-280-02   28002

FUROSEMIDE
INJECTION, USP

20 mg/2 mL
(10 mg/mL)
For IM or IV Use   Rx only
2 mL Single Dose Vial
Preservative Free
Discard unused portion.
PROTECT FROM LIGHT.
Do not use if discolored.
American Pharmaceutical Partners, Inc.
Los Angeles, CA 90024

401803A

LOT

EXP

Generic Drug
(furosemide)

NDC 0088-1712-53

Carafate®

Tablets

sucralfate

1 gram

120 Tablets

¥*Aventis*

R̠x ONLY
Each CARAFATE® Tablet contains 1g sucralfate.
Dosage and Administration: See package insert for dosage information.
WARNING: Keep out of reach of children.
Pharmacist: Dispense in light-resistant, tight container with child-resistant closure.
Important: This package is not child-resistant.
Store at controlled room temperature 59–86°F (15–30°C).
Aventis Pharmaceuticals Inc.
Kansas City, MO 64137
USA   ©2000
www.aventispharma-us.com

Exp
50059224

Brand Name (Carafate) and Generic Name (sucralfate)

Generic equivalents of many brand-name drugs are ordered as substitutes by the prescribing practitioner's preference or pharmacy policy. Because only the generic name appears on these labels, nurses need to carefully cross-check all medications. Failure to do so could cause inaccurate drug identification.

DOSAGE STRENGTH

The dosage strength refers to the dosage *weight* or amount of drug provided in a specific unit of measurement. The dosage strength of Lopid tablets is 600 milligrams (the weight and specific unit of measurement) per tablet. Some drugs, like V-cillin K, have two different but equivalent dosage strengths. V-cillin K has a dosage strength of 250 milligrams (per tablet) or 400,000 units (per tablet). This allows prescribers to order the drug using either unit of measurement.

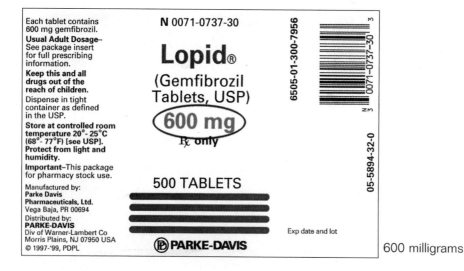

Each tablet contains 600 mg gemfibrozil.
Usual Adult Dosage– See package insert for full prescribing information.
Keep this and all drugs out of the reach of children.
Dispense in tight container as defined in the USP.
Store at controlled room temperature 20°- 25°C (68°- 77°F) [see USP]. Protect from light and humidity.
Important–This package for pharmacy stock use.
Manufactured by:
Parke Davis Pharmaceuticals, Ltd.
Vega Baja, PR 00694
Distributed by:
PARKE-DAVIS
Div of Warner-Lambert Co
Morris Plains, NJ 07950 USA
© 1997-'99, PDPL

N 0071-0737-30

Lopid®

(Gemfibrozil Tablets, USP)

600 mg
R̠x only

500 TABLETS

Ⓟ **PARKE-DAVIS**

Exp date and lot

600 milligrams

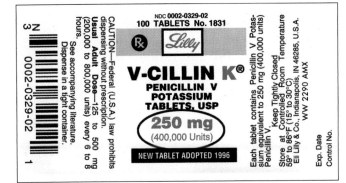

250 milligrams (400,000 units)

FORM

The form identifies the *structure* and *composition* of the drug. Solid dosage forms for oral use include tablets and capsules. Some powdered or granular medications that are not manufactured in tablet or capsule form can be directly combined with food or beverages and administered. Others must be reconstituted (liquefied) and measured in a precise liquid volume, such as milliliters, drops, or ounces. They may be a crystaloid (clear solution) or a suspension (solid particles in liquid that separate when held in a container).

Injectable medications may be supplied in solution or dry powdered form to be reconstituted. Once reconstituted, they are measured in milliliters or cubic centimeters.

Medications are also supplied in a variety of other forms, such as suppositories, creams, and patches.

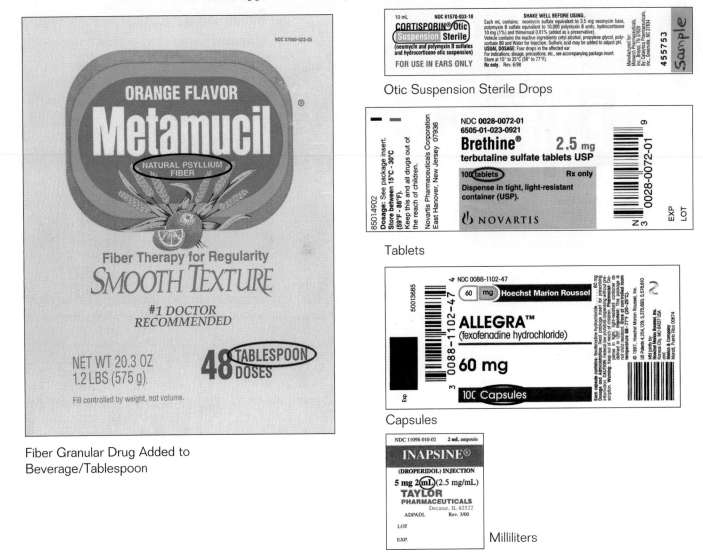

Fiber Granular Drug Added to Beverage/Tablespoon

Otic Suspension Sterile Drops

Tablets

Capsules

Milliliters

SUPPLY DOSAGE

The supply dosage refers to both *dosage strength* and *form.* It is read "X measured units per some quantity." For solid-form medications, such as tablets, the supply dosage is X measured units per tablet. For liquid medications, the supply dosage is the same as the medication's concentration, such as X measured units per milliliter. Take a minute to read the supply dosage printed on the following labels.

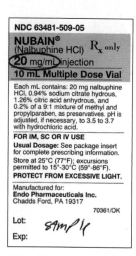

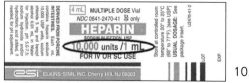

10,000 units per milliliter

20 milligrams per milliliter

TOTAL VOLUME

The total volume refers to the *full quantity* contained in a package, bottle, or vial. For tablets and other solid medications, it is the total number of individual items. For liquids, it is the total fluid volume.

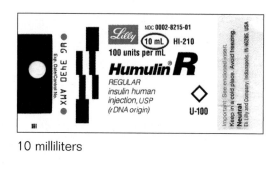

10 milliliters

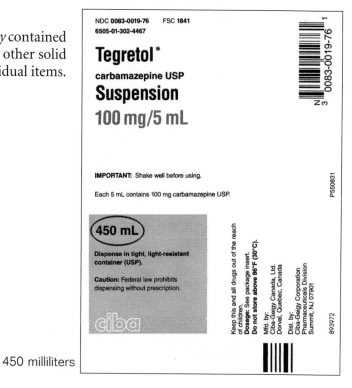

450 milliliters

ADMINISTRATION ROUTE

The administration route refers to the *site* of the body or *method of drug delivery* into the patient. Examples of routes of administration include oral, enteral (into the gastrointestinal tract through a tube), sublingual, injection (IV, IM, SC), otic, optic, topical, rectal, vaginal, and others. Unless specified otherwise, tablets, capsules, and caplets are intended for oral use.

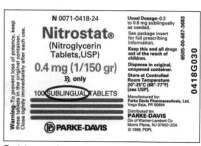

Sublingual

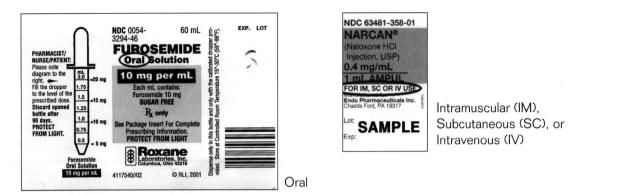

Oral

Intramuscular (IM), Subcutaneous (SC), or Intravenous (IV)

DIRECTIONS FOR MIXING OR RECONSTITUTING

Some drugs are dispensed in *powder form* and must be *reconstituted for use.* (Reconstitution is discussed further in Chapters 9 and 11.)

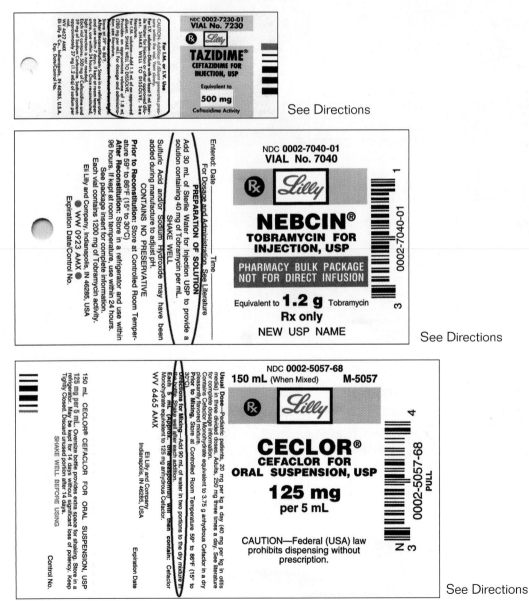

See Directions

See Directions

See Directions

LABEL ALERTS

Manufacturers may print warnings on the packaging or special alerts may be added by the pharmacy before dispensing. Look for special storage alerts such as "refrigerate at all times," "keep in a dry place," "replace cap and close tightly before storing," or "protect from light." Reconstituted suspensions may be dispensed already prepared for use, and directions may instruct the health care professional to "shake well before using" as a reminder to remix the components. Read and follow all label instructions carefully.

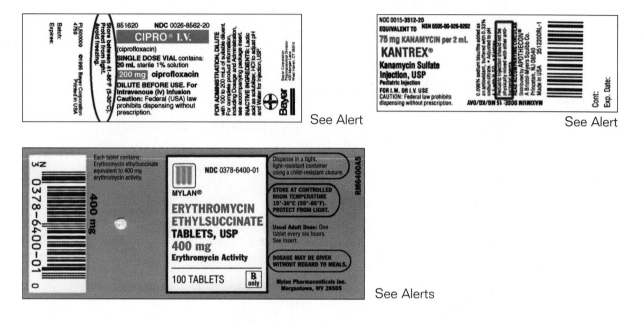

See Alert

See Alert

See Alerts

NAME OF THE MANUFACTURER

The name of the manufacturer is circled on the following labels.

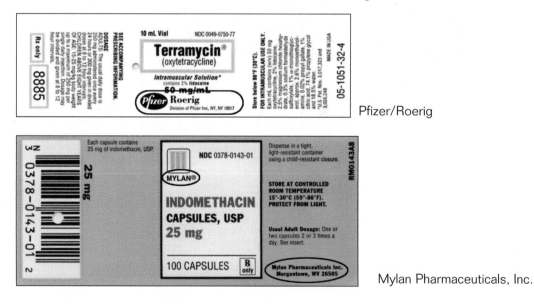

Pfizer/Roerig

Mylan Pharmaceuticals, Inc.

EXPIRATION DATE

The medication should be used, discarded, or returned to the pharmacy by the expiration date. Further, note the special expiration instructions given on labels for reconstituted medications. Refer to the Tazidime, Nebcin, and Ceclor labels on page 137.

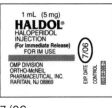

7/06

LOT OR CONTROL NUMBERS

Federal law requires all medication packages to be identified with a lot or control number. If a drug is recalled, for reasons such as damage or tampering, the lot number quickly identifies the particular group of medication packages to be removed from shelves. This number has been invaluable for vaccine and over-the-counter medication recalls.

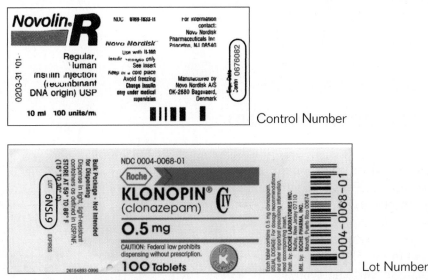

Control Number

Lot Number

NATIONAL DRUG CODE (NDC)

Federal law requires every prescription medication to have a unique identifying number, much like every U.S. citizen has a unique Social Security number. This number must appear on every manufacturer's label and is printed with the letters "NDC" followed by three discrete groups of numbers (e.g., NDC-61570-069-60 for Procanbid).

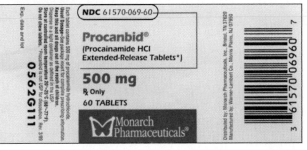

NDC

BAR CODE SYMBOLS

Bar code symbols are commonly used in retail sales. Bar code symbols also document drug dosing for recordkeeping and stock reorder, and may soon automate medication documentation right at the patient's bedside. The horizontal ones look like picket fences and the vertical ones look like ladders.

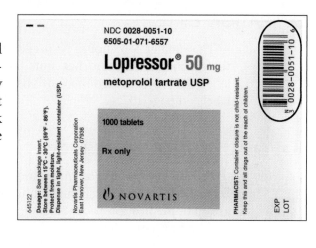

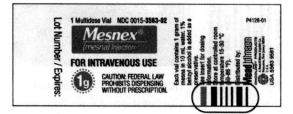

Bar Codes

UNITED STATES PHARMACOPEIA (USP) AND NATIONAL FORMULARY (NF)

These codes are found on many manufacturer-printed medication labels. The USP and NF are the two official national lists of approved drugs. Each manufacturer follows special guidelines that determine when to include these initials on a label. These initials are placed after the generic drug name. Be careful not to mistake these abbreviations for other initials that designate specific characteristics of a drug, such as *SR,* which means "sustained release."

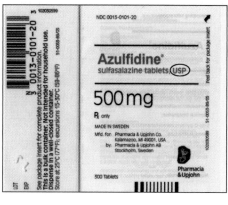

USP

UNIT- OR SINGLE-DOSE LABELS

Most oral medications administered in the hospital setting are available in unit dosage, such as a single capsule or tablet packaged separately in a typical blister pack. The pharmacy provides a 24-hour supply of each drug for the patient. The only major difference in this form of labeling is that the total volume of the container is usually omitted, because the volume is *one* tablet or capsule. Likewise, the dosage strength is understood as *per one.* Further, injectable medicines are packaged in single-dose preparations.

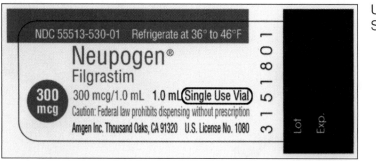

Unit Dose
Single Use Vial

COMBINATION DRUGS

Some medications are a combination of two or more drugs in one form. Read the labels for Percocet and Bactrim and notice the different substances that are combined in each tablet. Combination drugs are usually prescribed by the number of tablets, capsules, or milliliters to be given rather than by the dosage strength.

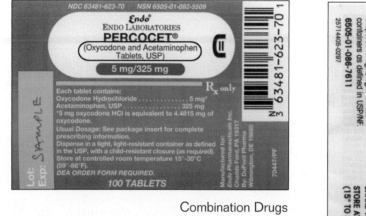
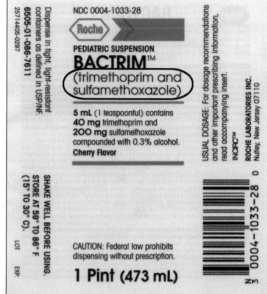

Combination Drugs

SUPPLY DOSAGE EXPRESSED AS A RATIO OR PERCENT

Occasionally, solutions will be ordered and/or manufactured in a supply dosage expressed as a ratio or percent.

RULE

Ratio solutions express the *number of grams* of the drug *per total milliliters of solution.*

Example:

Epinephrine 1:1000 contains 1 g pure drug per 1000 mL solution,
1 g:1000 mL = 1000 mg:1000 mL = 1 mg:1 mL.

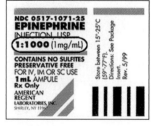

1:1000

RULE

Percentage (%) solutions express the *number of grams* of the drug *per 100 milliliters of solution.*

Example:

Lidocaine 2% contains 2 g pure drug per 100 mL solution, 2 g/100 mL = 2000 mg/100 mL = 20 mg/mL.

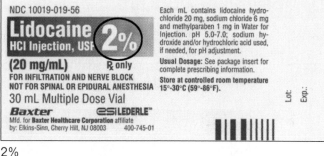

NDC 10019-019-56

Lidocaine 2%
HCl Injection, USP

(20 mg/mL)   ℞ only
FOR INFILTRATION AND NERVE BLOCK
NOT FOR SPINAL OR EPIDURAL ANESTHESIA
30 mL Multiple Dose Vial

Baxter   ⊖SILEDERLE™
Mfd. for **Baxter Healthcare Corporation** affiliate
by: Elkins-Sinn, Cherry Hill, NJ 08003   400-745-01

Each mL contains lidocaine hydro-chloride 20 mg, sodium chloride 6 mg and methylparaben 1 mg in Water for Injection. pH 5.0-7.0; sodium hy-droxide and/or hydrochloric acid used, if needed, for pH adjustment.
Usual Dosage: See package insert for complete prescribing information.
Store at controlled room temperature 15°-30°C (59°-86°F).

Lot: Exp.:

2%

Although these labels look different from many of the other labels, it is important to recognize that the supply dosage can still be determined. Many times the label will have a more commonly identified supply dosage and not just the ratio or percent. Look at the epinephrine and lidocaine labels. On the epinephrine label, the ratio is 1:1000; the supply dosage also can be identified as 1 mg/mL. On the lidocaine label, the percentage is 2%; the supply dosage also can be identified as 20 mg/mL.

CHECKING LABELS

Recall the Six Rights of medication administration: The *right patient* must receive the *right drug* in the *right amount* by the *right route* at the *right time* followed by the *right documentation*. To be absolutely sure the patient receives the right drug, check the label three times.

CAUTION

Before administering a medication to a patient, check the drug label three times:
1. Against the medication order or MAR.
2. Before preparing the medication.
3. After preparing the medication and before administering it.

QUICK REVIEW

Read labels carefully to:
- Identify the drug and the manufacturer.
- Differentiate between dosage strength, form, supply dosage, total container volume, and administration route.
- Recognize that the drug's supply dosage similarly refers to a drug's weight per unit of measure or *concentration*.
- Find the directions for reconstitution, as needed.
- Note expiration date.
- Describe lot or control number.
- Identify supply dosage on labels with ratios and percents.
- Be sure you administer the right drug.

REVIEW SET 24

Use the following labels A through G to find the information requested in questions 1 through 13. Indicate your answer by letter (A through G).

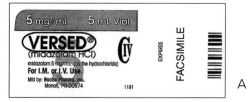

5 mg/mL   5 mL Vial

VERSED® C▐IV
(midazolam HCl)
midazolam 5 mg/mL (as the hydrochloride)
For I.M. or I.V. Use.
Mfd by: Roche Pharma, Inc.
Manati, PR 00674   1191

EXPIRES

FACSIMILE

A

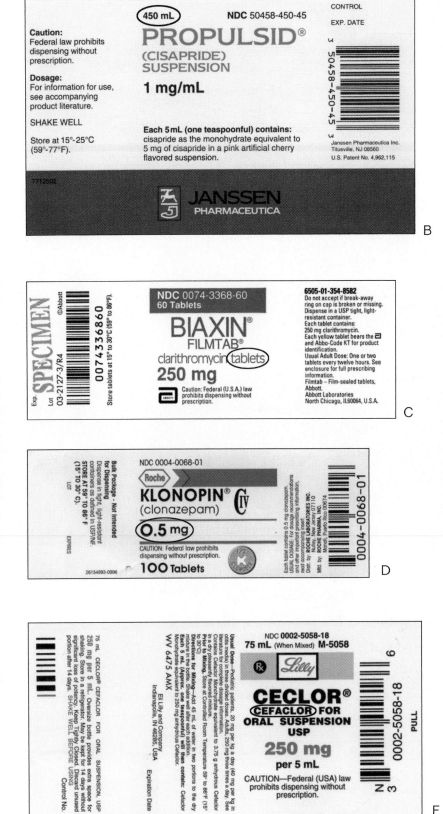

B

450 mL   NDC 50458-450-45

CONTROL
EXP. DATE

PROPULSID®
(CISAPRIDE)
SUSPENSION

1 mg/mL

Caution:
Federal law prohibits dispensing without prescription.

Dosage:
For information for use, see accompanying product literature.

SHAKE WELL

Store at 15°-25°C (59°-77°F).

Each 5 mL (one teaspoonful) contains:
cisapride as the monohydrate equivalent to 5 mg of cisapride in a pink artificial cherry flavored suspension.

50458-450-45

Janssen Pharmaceutica Inc.
Titusville, NJ 08560

U.S. Patent No. 4,962,115

7712502

JANSSEN
PHARMACEUTICA

C

NDC 0074-3368-60
60 Tablets

6505-01-354-8582
Do not accept if break-away ring on cap is broken or missing. Dispense in a USP tight, light-resistant container.
Each tablet contains:
250 mg clarithromycin.
Each yellow tablet bears the ᖯ and Abbo-Code KT for product identification.
Usual Adult Dose: One or two tablets every twelve hours. See enclosure for full prescribing information.
Filmtab – Film-sealed tablets, Abbott.
Abbott Laboratories
North Chicago, IL 60064, U.S.A.

BIAXIN®
FILMTAB®
clarithromycin tablets
250 mg

Caution: Federal (U.S.A.) law prohibits dispensing without prescription.

SPECIMEN
Exp.
Lot
03-2127-3/R4
Store tablets at 15° to 30°C (59° to 86°F).
©Abbott
0074336860

D

NDC 0004-0068-01

Roche

KLONOPIN® C IV
(clonazepam)

0.5 mg

CAUTION: Federal law prohibits dispensing without prescription.

100 Tablets

Bulk Package - Not Intended for Dispensing
Dispense in tight, light-resistant containers as defined in USP/NF.
STORE AT 59° TO 86° F (15° TO 30° C).
LOT
EXPIRES
26154893-0996

Each tablet contains 0.5 mg clonazepam.
USUAL DOSAGE: For dosage recommendations and other important prescribing information, read accompanying insert.
Distr. by: ROCHE LABORATORIES INC. Nutley, New Jersey 07110
Mfd. by: ROCHE PHARMA, INC. Manati, Puerto Rico 00674

0004-0068-01

E

NDC 0002-5058-18
75 mL (When Mixed) M-5058

Rx Lilly

CECLOR®
CEFACLOR FOR
ORAL SUSPENSION
USP

250 mg
per 5 mL

CAUTION—Federal (USA) law prohibits dispensing without prescription.

Usual Dose—Pediatric patients, 20 mg per kg a day (40 mg per kg in otitis media) in three divided doses. Adults, 250 mg three times a day. See literature for complete dosage information. Contains Cefaclor Monohydrate equivalent to 3.75 g anhydrous Cefaclor in a dry, pleasantly flavored mixture.
Prior to Mixing, Store at Controlled Room Temperature 59° to 86°F (15° to 30°C).
Directions for Mixing—Add 45 mL of water in two portions to the dry mixture in the bottle. Shake well after each addition.
Each 5 mL (Approx. one teaspoonful) will then contain: Cefaclor Monohydrate equivalent to 250 mg anhydrous Cefaclor.

Eli Lilly and Company
Indianapolis, IN 46285, USA

Expiration Date
WV 6475 AMX

75 mL CECLOR® CEFACLOR FOR ORAL SUSPENSION, USP 250 mg per 5 mL. Oversize bottle provides extra space for shaking. Store in a refrigerator. May be kept for 14 days without significant loss of potency. Keep Tightly Closed. Discard unused portion after 14 days. SHAKE WELL BEFORE USING.

Control No.

0002-5058-18
PULL

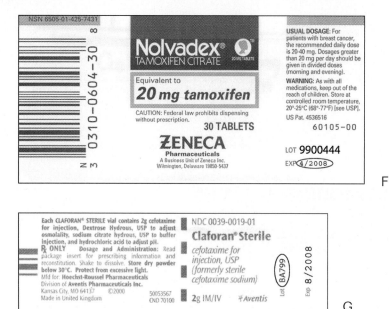

1. The total volume of the liquid container is circled.   _____

2. The dosage strength is circled.   _____

3. The form of the drug is circled.   _____

4. The brand name of the drug is circled.   _____

5. The generic name of the drug is circled.   _____

6. The expiration date is circled.   _____

7. The lot number is circled.   _____

8. Look at label E and determine how much of the supply drug you will administer to the patient per dose for the order *Ceclor 250 mg p.o. q.8h p.r.n.*   _____

9. Look at label A and determine the route of administration.   _____

10. Indicate which labels have an imprinted bar code symbol.   _____

11. Look at label C. What does the word *Filmtab* mean on this label?   _____

12. Look at label B, and determine the supply dosage.   _____

13. Look at label F, and determine how much of the supply drug you will administer to the patient per dose for the order *Tamoxifen 40 mg p.o. q.12h*.

Refer to the following label to identify the specific drug information described in questions 14 through 19.

READ ACCOMPANYING PROFESSIONAL INFORMATION.

RECOMMENDED STORAGE IN DRY FORM.

Store below 86°F (30°C)

Sterile solution may be kept in refrigerator for one (1) week without significant loss of potency.

CAUTION: Federal law prohibits dispensing without prescription.

NDC 0049-0520-83

Buffered

Pfizerpen®

(penicillin G potassium)

For Injection

FIVE MILLION UNITS

Pfizer **Roerig**
Division of Pfizer Inc, NY, NY 10017

USUAL DOSAGE
Average single intramuscular injection: 200,000-400,000 units.
Intravenous: Additional information about the use of this product intravenously can be found in the package insert.

mL diluent added	Units per mL of solution
18.2 mL	250,000
8.2 mL	500,000
3.2 mL	1,000,000

Buffered with sodium citrate and citric acid to optimum pH.

PATIENT: _____
ROOM NO: _____
DATE DILUTED: _____

05-4243-00-3
MADE IN USA

6505-00-958-3305

14. Generic name _____

15. Brand name _____

16. Dosage strength _____

17. Route of administration _____

18. National Drug Code _____

19. Manufacturer _____

Refer to the following label to answer questions 20 through 22.

NDC 10019-017-56

Lidocaine **1**%
HCl Injection, USP

(10 mg/mL) R only

FOR INFILTRATION AND NERVE BLOCK
NOT FOR SPINAL OR EPIDURAL ANESTHESIA

30 mL Multiple Dose Vial

Baxter ⊖Ⓢ|LEDERLE™
Mfd. for **Baxter Healthcare Corporation** affiliate
by: Elkins-Sinn, Cherry Hill, NJ 08003   400-741-01

Each mL contains lidocaine hydrochloride 10 mg, sodium chloride 7 mg
and methylparaben 1 mg in Water for
Injection. pH 5.0-7.0; sodium hydroxide and/or hydrochloric acid used,
if needed, for pH adjustment.

Usual Dosage: See package insert for
complete prescribing information.

Store at controlled room temperature
15°-30°C (59°-86°F).

Lot: Exp.:

20. The supply dosage of the drug is _____ %.

21. The supply dosage of the drug is _____ g per _____ mL.

22. The supply dosage of the drug is _____ mg per mL.

After completing these problems, see page 480 to check your answers.

CRITICAL THINKING SKILLS

Reading the labels of medications is critical. Make sure that the drug you want is what you have on hand before you prepare it. Let's look at an example of a medication error related to reading the label incorrectly.

error

Not checking the label for correct dosage.

possible scenario

A nurse flushed a triple central venous catheter (an IV with three ports). According to hospital policy, the nurse was to flush each port with 10 mL of normal saline followed by 2 mL of heparin flush solution in the concentration of 100 units/mL. The nurse mistakenly picked up a vial of heparin containing heparin 10,000 units/mL. Without checking the label, she prepared the solution for all three ports. The patient received 60,000 units of heparin instead of 600 units.

potential outcome

The patient in this case would be at great risk for hemorrhage, leading to shock and death. Protamine sulfate would likely be ordered to counteract the action of the heparin, but a successful outcome is questionable.

(continues)

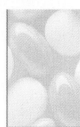

(continued)

prevention

There is no substitute for checking the label before administering a medication. The nurse in this case had three opportunities to catch the error, having drawn three different syringes of medication for the three ports.

PRACTICE PROBLEMS—CHAPTER 8

Look at labels A through G, and identify the information requested.

Label A:

1. The supply dosage of the drug in milliequivalents is _____.

2. The National Drug Code is _____.

3. The supply dosage of the drug in milligrams is _____.

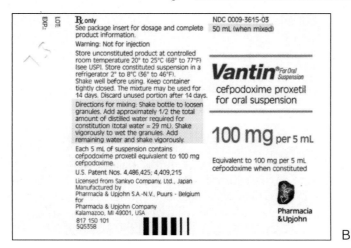

A

Label B:

4. The generic name of the drug is _____.

5. The reconstitution instruction to mix a supply dosage of 100 mg per 5 mL for oral suspension is

_____.

6. The manufacturer of the drug is _____.

B

Label C:

7. The total volume of the medication container is _____.

8. The supply dosage is _____.

9. How much will you administer to the patient per dose for the order *Methotrexate 25 mg IV stat*?

_____.

NDC 10019-940-78

Methotrexate
Injection, USP

PRESERVATIVE FREE R only
250 mg (25 mg/mL)
Sterile Isotonic Liquid
10 mL Single Dose Vial

Mfd. for **Baxter Healthcare Corp.** affiliate
by: Bigmar Pharmaceuticals SA
Barbengo, Switzerland

Lot: Exp. Date:

See package insert for routes of administration.
Usual Dosage: Consult package insert for dosage and full prescribing information.
Each mL contains methotrexate sodium equivalent to 25 mg methotrexate.
Inactive ingredients: Sodium Chloride 0.490% w/v and Water for Injection. Sodium hydroxide and/or hydrochloric acid may be added to adjust pH to 8.5-8.7 during manufacture.
Store at controlled room temperature 15°-30°C (59°-86°F).
PROTECT FROM LIGHT. Retain in carton until time of use. Discard any unused portion.   10-1052A 460-228-00

C

Label D:

10. The brand name of the drug is _____.

11. The generic name is _____.

12. The National Drug Code of the drug is _____.

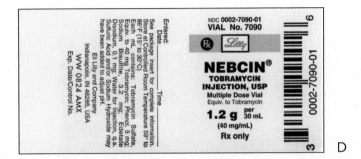

NDC 0002-7090-01
VIAL No. 7090

Ⓡ Lilly

NEBCIN®
TOBRAMYCIN
INJECTION, USP
Multiple Dose Vial
Equiv. to Tobramycin
1.2 g per 30 mL
(40 mg/mL)
Rx only

0002-7090-01

Entered:
Date
Time

See package insert for complete information.
Store at Controlled Room Temperature 59° to 86°F (15° to 30°C).
Each mL contains: Tobramycin, Sulfate, Equiv. to 40 mg Tobramycin; Phenol, 5 mg; Sodium Bisulfite, 3.2 mg; Edetate Disodium, 0.1 mg; Water for Injection, q.s. Sulfuric Acid and/or Sodium Hydroxide may have been added to adjust pH.

Eli Lilly and Company
Indianapolis, IN 46285, USA
WW 0824 AMX
Exp. Date/Control No.

D

Label E:

13. The form of the drug is _____.

14. The total volume of the drug container is _____.

15. The administration route is _____.

FOR INTRAMUSCULAR USE ONLY.
USUAL ADULT DOSE: Intramuscularly: 25 - 100 mg stat; repeat every 4 to 6 hours, as needed.
See accompanying prescribing information.

Each mL contains **50 mg** of hydroxyzine hydrochloride, 0.9% benzyl alcohol and sodium hydroxide to adjust to optimum pH.

To avoid discoloration, protect from prolonged exposure to light.

Rx only

10 mL   NDC 0049-5460-74

Vistaril®
(hydroxyzine hydrochloride)

Intramuscular Solution
50 mg/mL

Pfizer **Roerig**
Division of Pfizer Inc, NY, NY 10017

Store below 86°F (30°C).
PROTECT FROM FREEZING.

PATIENT: _____
ROOM NO.: _____

05-1111-32-4 **9249**
MADE IN USA

E

Label F:

16. The name of the drug manufacturer is _____.

17. The form of the drug is _____.

18. The appropriate temperature for storage of this drug is _____.

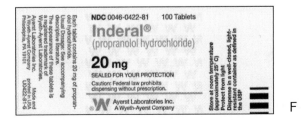

NDC 0046-0422-81   100 Tablets

Inderal®
(propranolol hydrochloride)

20 mg

SEALED FOR YOUR PROTECTION
Caution: Federal law prohibits dispensing without prescription.

Ⓦ Ayerst Laboratories Inc.
A Wyeth-Ayerst Company

Each tablet contains 20 mg of propranolol hydrochloride.
Usual Dosage: See accompanying descriptive literature.
The appearance of these tablets is a registered trademark of Wyeth-Ayerst Laboratories.
Ayerst Laboratories Inc.
A Wyeth-Ayerst Company
Philadelphia, PA 19101

Store at room temperature (approximately 25°C)
Protect from light.
Dispense in well-closed, light-resistant container as defined in the USP

Made and printed in USA
U0422-81-6

F

Label G:

19. The expiration date of the drug is _____.

20. The dosage strength of the drug is _____.

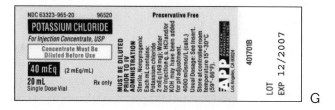

Match label H or I with the correct descriptive statement.

21. This label represents a unit- or single-dose drug.   _____

22. This label represents a combination drug.   _____

23. This label represents a drug usually ordered by the number of tablets or capsules to be administered rather than the dosage strength.   _____

24. The administration route for the drug labeled H is _____.

25. The lot number for the drug labeled I is _____.

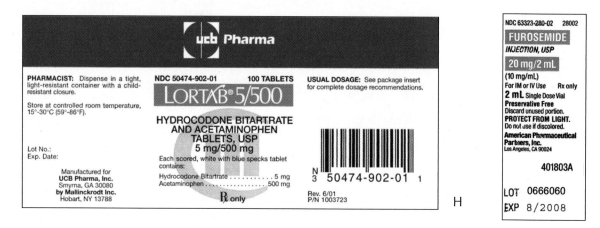

Label J:

26. Expressed as a percentage, the supply dosage of the drug is _____.

27. The supply dosage is equivalent to _____ g per _____ mL or _____ mg/mL.

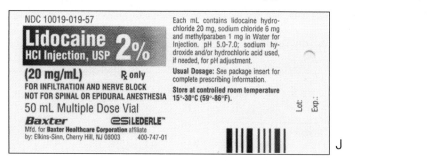

28. Critical Thinking Skill: Describe the strategy you would implement to prevent this medication error.

possible scenario

Suppose a physician ordered an antibiotic *Principen .5 g p.o. q.6h.* The writing was not clear on the order, and Prinivil (an anti-hypertensive medication) 5 mg was sent up by the pharmacy. However, the order was correctly transcribed to the medication administration record (MAR). In preparing the medication, the nurse did not read the MAR or label carefully and administered Prinivil, the wrong medication.

Prinivil® 5 mg
(Lisinopril)

Dist. by
MERCK & CO., INC.
Whitehouse Station, NJ 08889, USA

Store at controlled room temperature,
15 - 30°C (59 - 86°F), and protect from
moisture. Keep container tightly closed.

100 Tablets

Lot

0006-0019-58

Prinivil® 5 mg
(Lisinopril)

NDC 0006-0019-58

USUAL ADULT DOSAGE:
See accompanying circular.
Rx only

100 Tablets

Lot

LIFT HERE

9293910
100| No.3577

potential outcome

A medication error occurred because the wrong medication was given. The patient's infection treatment would be delayed. Furthermore, the erroneous blood pressure drug could have harmful effects.

prevention

_____

_____

Critical Thinking Skill: Describe the strategy you would implement to prevent this medication error.

possible scenario

Suppose a physician wrote the order *Celebrex 100 mg p.o. q.12h* (anti-inflammatory to treat rheumatoid arthritis pain), but the order was difficult to read. The unit secretary and pharmacy interpreted the order as *Celexa* (antidepressant), a medication with a similar spelling. Celexa was written on the MAR.

potential outcome

The nurse administered the Celexa for several days, and the patient began complaining of severe knee and hip pain from rheumatoid arthritis. Also, the patient experienced side effects of Celexa, including drowsiness and tremors. A medication error occurred because several health care professionals misinterpreted the order.

prevention

29. What should have alerted the nurse that something was wrong?

_____

30. What should have been considered to prevent this error?

_____

After completing these problems, see pages 480–481 to check your answers.

SECTION 2 SELF-EVALUATION

Directions:

1. Round decimals to two places. Round temperatures to one decimal place.
2. Reduce fractions to lowest terms.

Chapter 3: Systems of Measurement

Express the following amounts in proper medical notation.

1. two-thirds grain   _____   4. one-half milliliter   _____

2. four teaspoons   _____   5. one-half ounce   _____

3. one three-hundredths grain _____

Interpret the following notations.

6. 4 gtt   _____   9. gr viiss   _____

7. 450 mg   _____   10. 0.25 L   _____

8. gr $\frac{1}{100}$ _____

Chapters 4 and 5: Conversions

Fill in the missing decimal numbers next to each metric unit as indicated.

11.   7.13 kg = _____ g = _____ mg = _____ mcg

12. _____ kg = _____ g = _____ mg = 925 mcg

13. _____ kg = _____ g = 125 mg = _____ mcg

14. _____ kg = 16.4 g = _____ mg = _____ mcg

Convert each of the following to the equivalent units indicated.

15. gr $\frac{1}{6}$ = _____ mg   = _____ g

16. 20 mg   = _____ g   = gr _____

17. 4 T   = _____ t   = _____ mL

18. qt ix   = _____ L   = _____ mL

19. 15 in   = _____ cm   = _____ mm

20. 56.2 mm   = _____ cm   = _____ in

21. 198 lb   = _____ kg   = _____ g

22. 11.59 kg   = _____ g   = _____ lb

23. A patient is told to take 180 mg of a medication. What is the equivalent dosage in grains?   gr _____

24. A patient is being treated for chronic pain with gr $\frac{3}{4}$ of morphine sulphate every 3 hours. How many milligrams will he receive in 24 hours?   _____ mg

25. Your patient uses nitroglycerin for chest pain. The prescription is for gr $\frac{1}{300}$ of nitroglycerin. What is the equivalent dosage in milligrams?   _____ mg

26. Most adults have about 6000 mL of circulating blood volume. This is equivalent to _____ L or qt _____ of blood volume.

27. Your patient drinks the following for breakfast: 3 ounces orange juice, 8 ounces coffee with 1 teaspoon cream, and 4 ounces of water. The total intake is _____ mL.

Convert the following times as indicated. Designate AM or PM where needed.

	Traditional Time	*International Time*
28.	11:35 PM	_____
29.	_____	1844
30.	4:17 AM	_____
31.	_____	0803

Convert the following temperatures as indicated.

	°C	°F
32.	38°C	_____ °F
33.	_____ °C	101.5°F
34.	37.2°C	_____ °F

Chapter 6: Equipment Used in Dosage Measurement

Draw an arrow to demonstrate the correct measurement of the doses given.

35. 1.5 mL

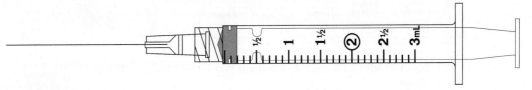

36. 0.33 mL

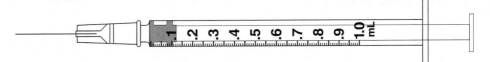

37. 44 U U-100 insulin

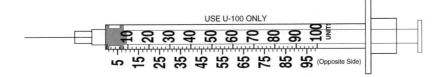

38. 37 U U-100 insulin

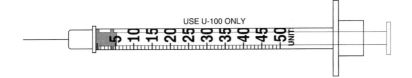

39. $1\frac{1}{2}$ t

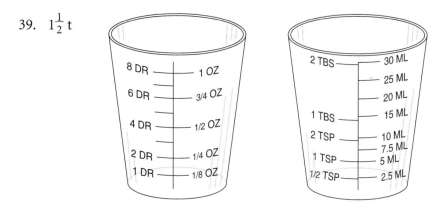

Chapters 7 and 8: Interpreting Drug Orders and Understanding Drug Labels

Use label A to identify the information requested for questions 40 through 43.

40. The generic name is _____.

41. This drug is an otic solution and is intended for _____.

42. The total volume of this container is _____.

43. Interpret: *Cortisporin Otic Solution 2 gtt A.U. q.15 min × 3* _____

---

10 mL	NDC 61570-033-10	SHAKE WELL BEFORE USING.
CORTISPORIN® Otic		Each mL contains: neomycin sulfate equivalent to 3.5 mg neomycin base, polymyxin B sulfate equivalent to 10,000 polymyxin B units, hydrocortisone 10 mg (1%) and thimerosal 0.01% (added as a preservative).

CORTISPORIN® Otic
Suspension Sterile
(neomycin and polymyxin B sulfates
and hydrocortisone otic suspension)
FOR USE IN EARS ONLY

Each mL contains: neomycin sulfate equivalent to 3.5 mg neomycin base, polymyxin B sulfate equivalent to 10,000 polymyxin B units, hydrocortisone 10 mg (1%) and thimerosal 0.01% (added as a preservative). Vehicle contains the inactive ingredients cetyl alcohol, propylene glycol, polysorbate 80 and Water for Injection. Sulfuric acid may be added to adjust pH. **USUAL DOSAGE:** Four drops in the affected ear. For indications, dosage, precautions, etc., see accompanying package insert. Store at 15° to 25°C (59° to 77°F). **Rx only.** Rev. 6/98

Manufactured for:
Monarch Pharmaceuticals,
Inc., Bristol, TN 37620
By: Catalytica Pharmaceuticals,
Inc., Greenville, NC 27834

455753

Sample

A

Use label B to identify the information requested for questions 44 through 46.

44. The supply dosage is _____.

45. The National Drug Code is _____.

46. Interpret: *heparin 3,750 U SC q.8h* _____

_____

Use label C to identify the information requested for questions 47 through 49.

NDC 63323-262-01 926201

HEPARIN SODIUM
INJECTION, USP

5,000 USP Units/mL

(Derived from Porcine
Intestinal Mucosa)
For IV or SC Use   Rx only
1 mL Multiple Dose Vial
Usual Dosage: See insert.
**American Pharmaceutical
Partners, Inc.**
Los Angeles, CA 90024

401810A

LOT
EXP

B

WV 5041 AMX

Mfd by Eli Lilly Industries, Inc.
Carolina, Puerto Rico 00985, a subsidiary of
Eli Lilly & Co. Indianapolis, IN U.S.A.
Expiration Date/Control No.

**PROFESSIONAL PACKAGE
NOT TO BE SOLD**

Usual Dose—Children, 20 mg per kg a day (40 mg per kg in otitis media) in three divided doses. Adults, 250 mg three times a day. See literature for complete dosage information.
Contains Cefaclor Monohydrate equivalent to 3.75 g anhydrous Cefaclor in a dry pleasantly flavored mixture.
Prior to Mixing: Store at Controlled Room Temperature 59° to 86°F (15° to 30°C).
Directions for Mixing—Add 45 mL of water in two portions to the dry mixture in the bottle. Shake well after each addition. **Each 5 mL (Approx. one teaspoonful) will then contain:** Cefaclor Monohydrate equivalent to 250 mg anhydrous Cefaclor.
SHAKE WELL BEFORE USING Oversize bottle provides extra space for shaking. Store in a refrigerator. May be kept for 14 days without significant loss of potency. Discard unused portion after 14 days. Keep Tightly Closed.

75 mL (When Mixed)   M-5058

Lilly

CECLOR®
**CEFACLOR FOR
ORAL SUSPENSION
USP**

250 mg
per 5 mL
CAUTION—Federal (U.S.A.)
law prohibits dispensing
without prescription.

C

47. The trade name is_____.

48. The supply dosage, when reconstituted, is _____.

49. What amount would be given for one dose if the drug order is *Ceclor 125 mg p.o. stat*?
    a. _____ mL   or   b. _____ t
    c. Draw an arrow on the medicine cup to demonstrate the dose volume.

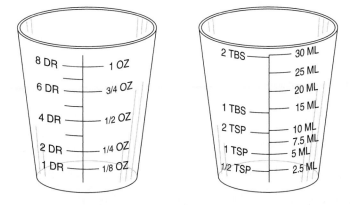

50. Interpret: *Amoxil 250 mg p.o. t.i.d.*_____.

After completing these problems, see pages 481–482 to check your answers. Give yourself two points for each correct answer.

Perfect score = 100   My score = _____

Minimum mastery score = 86 (43 correct)

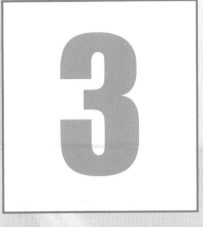

Drug Dosage Calculations

Oral Dosage of Drugs

OBJECTIVES

Upon mastery of Chapter 9, you will be able to calculate oral dosages of drugs. To accomplish this you will also be able to:

- Convert all units of measurement to the same system and same size units.
- Estimate the reasonable amount of the drug to be administered.
- Use the formula $\frac{D}{H} \times Q = X$ to calculate drug dosage.
- Calculate the number of tablets or capsules that are contained in prescribed dosages.
- Calculate the volume of liquid per dose when the prescribed dosage is in solution form.

Medications for oral administration are supplied in a variety of forms, such as tablets, capsules, and liquids. They are usually ordered to be administered by mouth, or *p.o.*, which is an abbreviation for the Latin phrase *"per os."*

When a liquid form of a drug is unavailable, children and many elderly patients may need to have a tablet crushed or a capsule opened and mixed with a small amount of food or fluid to enable them to swallow the medication. Many of these crushed medications and oral liquids also may be ordered to be given enterally, or into the gastrointestinal tract via a specially placed tube. Such tubes and their associated enteral routes include the *nasogastric* (NG) tube from nares to stomach; the *nasojejunal* (NJ) tube from nares to jejunum; the *gastrostomy tube* (GT) placed directly through the abdomen into the stomach; and the *percutaneous endoscopic gastrostomy* (PEG) tube.

It is important to recognize that some solid-form medications are intended to be given whole to achieve a specific effect in the body. For example, enteric-coated medications protect the stomach by dissolving in the duodenum. Sustained-release capsules allow for gradual release of medication over time and should be swallowed whole. Consult a drug reference or the pharmacist if you are in doubt about the safety of crushing tablets or opening capsules.

TABLETS AND CAPSULES

Medications prepared in tablet and capsule form are supplied in the strengths or dosages in which they are commonly prescribed (Figure 9-1). It is desirable to obtain the drug in the same strength as the dosage ordered or in multiples of that dosage. When necessary, scored tablets (those marked for division) can be divided into halves or quarters. Only scored tablets are intended to be divided.

> **CAUTION**
>
> It is safest and most accurate to give the fewest number of whole, undivided tablets possible.

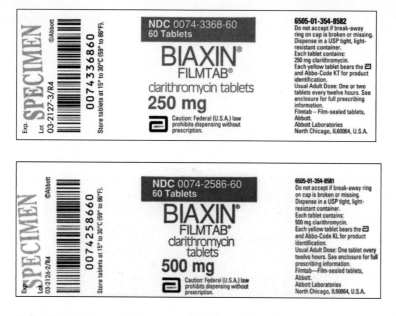

FIGURE 9-1 Biaxin 250 mg and 500 mg tablets

Example 1:

The doctor's order reads: *Biaxin 500 mg p.o. q.12h.*

Biaxin comes in tablet strengths of 250 milligrams per tablet or filmtab and 500 milligrams per tablet. When both strengths are available, the nurse should select the 500 milligram strength, and give one whole tablet for each dose.

Example 2:

The doctor's order reads: *Klonopin 1.5 mg p.o. tid.*

Klonopin comes in strengths of 0.5 mg, 1 mg, and 2 mg tablets (see Figure 9-2). When the three strengths are available, the nurse should select one 1 mg tablet and one 0.5 mg tablet (1 mg + 0.5 mg = 1.5 mg). This provides the ordered dosage of 1.5 mg and is the least number of tablets (2 tablets total) for the patient to swallow.

You might want to halve the 2 mg tablet to obtain two 1 mg parts and pair one-half with a 0.5 mg tablet. This would also equal 1.5 mg and give you $1\frac{1}{2}$ tablets. However, cutting any tablet in half may produce slightly unequal halves. Your patient may not get the ordered dose as a result. It is preferable to give whole, undivided tablets, when they are available.

THREE-STEP APPROACH TO DOSAGE CALCULATIONS

Now you are ready to learn to solve dosage problems. The following simple three-step method has been proven to reduce anxiety about calculations and ensure that your results are accurate. Take notice that you will be asked to think or estimate before you apply a formula. Learn and memorize this simple three-step approach and use it for every dosage calculation every time.

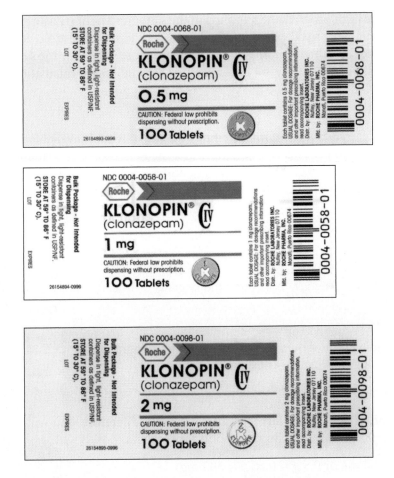

FIGURE 9-2 Klonopin 0.5 mg, 1 mg, and 2 mg tablets

REMEMBER

Three-Step Approach to Dosage Calculations

Step 1	Convert	Ensure that all measurements are in the same system of measurement and the same size unit of measurement. If not, convert before proceeding.
Step 2	Think	Estimate what is a *reasonable amount* of the drug to administer.
Step 3	Calculate	Apply the formula: $\frac{D}{H} \times Q = X$

$$\frac{D \text{ (desired)}}{H \text{ (have)}} \times Q \text{ (quantity)} = X \text{ (amount)}$$

Let's carefully examine each of the three steps as essential and consecutive rules of accurate dosage calculation.

RULE

Step 1	Convert	Be sure that all measurements are in the same system and all units are in the same size, converting when necessary.

Many medications are both ordered and supplied in the same system of measurement and the same size unit of measurement. This makes dosage calculation very easy, because no conversion is necessary. When this is not the case, then you must convert to the same system or the same size units. Let's look at two examples where conversion is a necessary first step in dosage calculation.

Example 1:

The drug order reads: *Keflex 0.5 g p.o. q.6h*. The supply dosage (what is available on hand) is labeled *Keflex 500 mg per capsule*. This is an example of a medication order written and supplied in the same system (metric), but in different size units (g and mg). A drug order written in grams but supplied in milligrams will have to be converted to the same size unit.

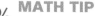

MATH TIP

In most cases, it is more practical to change to the smaller unit (such as g to mg). This requires multiplication and usually eliminates the decimal or fraction, keeping the calculation in whole numbers.

To continue with Example 1, you should convert 0.5 gram to milligrams. Notice that milligrams is the smaller unit and converting eliminates the decimal fraction.

Equivalent: 1 g = 1000 mg

Remember: You are converting from a larger to a smaller unit. Therefore, you will multiply by the conversion factor of 1000 or move the decimal point three places to the right.

0.5 g = 0.5 × 1000 = 500 mg or 0.5 g = 0.500. = 500 mg

Order: *Keflex 500 mg p.o. q.6h*

Supply: *Keflex 500 mg per capsule*

You would give the patient 1 Keflex 500 mg capsule by mouth every 6 hours.

MATH TIP

Convert apothecary and household measurements to their metric equivalents. This will be helpful for your calculations even if the conversion is to a larger unit. The metric system is the predominant system of measurement for drugs.

Example 2:

The drug order reads: *phenobarbital gr ss p.o. q.12h*. The supply dosage (what you have available on hand) is labeled *phenobarbital 15 mg per tablet*. This is an example of the medication ordered in one system but supplied in a different system. The medication order is written in the apothecary system, and the medication is supplied in the metric system. You must recall the approximate equivalents and convert both amounts to the same system. You should convert the apothecary measure to metric.

Approximate equivalent: gr i = 60 mg

Remember: You are converting from a larger to a smaller unit. Therefore, you will multiply by the conversion factor of 60.

gr ss = $\frac{1}{2}$ × 60 = $\frac{60}{2}$ mg = 30 mg

Now the problem looks like this:

Order: *phenobarbital 30 mg p.o. q.12h*

Supply: *phenobarbital 15 mg per tablet*

Now you can probably solve this problem in your head. That's what step 2 is about.

RULE

Step 2	Think	Carefully consider what is the reasonable amount of the drug that should be administered.

Once you have converted all units to the same system and size, step 2 asks you to logically conclude what amount should be given. Before you go on to step 3, you may be able to picture in your mind a reasonable amount of medication to be administered, as was demonstrated in the previous two examples. At least you should be able to estimate a very close approximation, such as more or less than one tablet (or capsule or milliliter). Basically, step 2 asks you to *stop and think before you go any farther.*

In the phenobarbital example, you estimate that the patient should receive more than one tablet. In fact, you realize that you would administer two of the 15 mg tablets to fill the order for gr ss or 30 mg.

RULE

Step 3	Calculate	Apply the dosage calculation formula: $\frac{D}{H} \times Q = X$

Always double-check your estimated amount from step 2 with the simple formula $\frac{D}{H} \times Q = X$.

In this formula, *D* represents the *desired* dosage or the dosage ordered. You will find this in the doctor's or the health care practitioner's order. *H* represents the dosage you *have* on hand per a *quantity, Q*. Both *H* and *Q* constitute the *supply dosage* found on the label of the drug available.

MATH TIP

Follow the rules of math in this order: Multiply, Divide, Add, Subtract.
(You can remember this by: **M**y **D**ear **A**unt **S**ally.)

MATH TIP

When solving dosage problems for drugs supplied in tablets or capsules, Q (quantity) is always 1, because the supply dosage is per one tablet or capsule. Therefore, Q = 1 tablet or capsule.

Let's use the $\frac{D}{H} \times Q = X$ formula to double-check our thinking, and calculate the dosages for the previous phenobarbital example.

Order: *phenobarbital gr ss p.o. q.12h*, converted to phenobarbital 30 mg

Supply: *phenobarbital 15 mg per tablet*

D = desired = 30 mg

H = have = 15 mg

Q = quantity = 1 tablet

$\frac{D}{H} \times Q = \frac{30 \text{ mg}}{15 \text{ mg}} \times 1$ tablet

$\frac{\overset{2}{\cancel{30 \text{ mg}}}}{\underset{1}{\cancel{15 \text{ mg}}}} \times 1$ tablet = 2×1 tablet = 2 tablets   (Notice that mg cancel out.)

Give 2 of the phenobarbital 15 mg tablets orally every 12 hours. The calculations verify your estimate from step 2.

It is wise to get in the habit of always inserting the *Quantity* value in the formula, even when Q is 1. Then you will be prepared to accurately calculate dosages for oral liquid or parenteral injection drugs that may be supplied in a solution strength quantity of more or less than 1 (mL).

Notice that the formula is set up with D (*desired dosage*) as the numerator and H (dosage *strength* you *have* on hand) as the denominator of a fraction. You are calculating for some portion of Q (*quantity* you have on hand). You can see that setting up a dosage calculation like this makes sense. Let's look at two more examples to reinforce this concept.

Example 3:

Order: *Lasix 10 mg p.o. b.i.d.*

Supply: *Lasix 20 mg per tablet*

$\frac{D}{H} \times Q = \frac{10 \text{ mg}}{20 \text{ mg}} \times 1$ tablet

$\frac{\overset{1}{\cancel{10 \text{ mg}}}}{\underset{2}{\cancel{20 \text{ mg}}}} \times 1$ tablet = $\frac{1}{2} \times 1$ tablet = $\frac{1}{2}$ tablet

Notice that you want to give $\frac{1}{2}$ of the Q (quantity of the supply dosage you have on hand, which in this case is 1 tablet). Therefore, you want to give $\frac{1}{2}$ tablet of Lasix 20 mg tablets orally twice daily.

Example 4:

Order: *Tylenol gr x p.o. q.3–4h p.r.n., headache*

Supply: *Tylenol 325 mg per tablet*

Approximate equivalent: gr i = 60 mg

Convert: gr x = gr 10 = 10 × 60 = 600 mg

$\frac{D}{H} \times Q = \frac{600 \text{ mg}}{325 \text{ mg}} \times 1$ tablet = 1.8 tablets

An amount of 1.8 tablets is not reasonable. Remember that gr i = 60 mg, but in some instances gr i = 65 mg is more relevant. This is true because it is an *approximate* equivalent. In this case, gr i = 65 mg is more accurate.

Order: *Tylenol gr x p.o. q.3–4h p.r.n., headache*

Supply: *Tylenol 325 mg per tablet*

Approximate equivalent: gr i = 65 mg

Convert: gr x = gr 10 = 10 × 65 = 650 mg

$$\frac{D}{H} \times Q = \frac{650 \text{ mg}}{325 \text{ mg}} \times 1 \text{ tablet}$$

$$\frac{\overset{2}{\cancel{650 \text{ mg}}}}{\underset{1}{\cancel{325 \text{ mg}}}} \times 1 \text{ tablet} = 2 \times 1 \text{ tablet} = 2 \text{ tablets}$$

Notice that you want to give 2 times the amount of *Q*; that is, you want to give 2 of the Tylenol 325 mg tablets orally every 3–4 hours as needed for headache.

Now you are ready to apply all three steps of this logical approach to dosage calculations. The same three steps will be used to solve both oral and parenteral dosage calculation problems. It is most important that you develop the ability to reason for the answer or estimate before you apply the $\frac{D}{H} \times Q = X$ formula.

Note to Learner

Health care professionals can unknowingly make errors if they rely solely on a formula rather than first asking themselves what the answer should be. As a nurse or allied health professional, you are expected to be able to reason sensibly, problem solve, and justify your judgments rationally. With these same skills you gained admission to your educational program and to your profession. While you sharpen your math skills, your ability to think and estimate are your best resources for avoiding errors. Use the formula as a calculation tool to validate the dose amount you anticipate should be given, rather than the reverse. If your reasoning is sound, you will find the dosages you compute make sense and are accurate. Question any calculation that directs you to administer 15 tablets of any medication.

> ### CAUTION
> The maximum number of tablets or capsules for a single dose is *usually* three. Recheck your calculation if a single dose requires more.

Let's examine more examples of oral dosages supplied in capsules and tablets to reinforce the three basic steps. Then you will be ready to solve problems like these on your own.

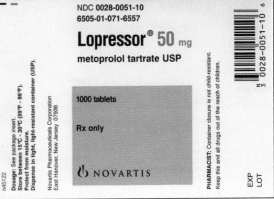

Example 1:

The drug order reads: *Lopressor 100 mg p.o. b.i.d.* The medicine container is labeled *Lopressor 50 mg per tablet*. Calculate one dose.

Step 1	**Convert**	No conversion is necessary. The units are in the same system (metric) and the same size (mg).
Step 2	**Think**	You want to administer 100 milligrams, and you have 50 milligrams in each tablet. You want to give twice the equivalent of each tablet, or you want to administer 2 tablets per dose.
Step 3	**Calculate**	$\frac{D}{H} \times Q = \frac{100 \text{ mg}}{50 \text{ mg}} \times 1 \text{ tablet}$

$$\frac{\overset{2}{\cancel{100 \text{ mg}}}}{\underset{1}{\cancel{50 \text{ mg}}}} \times 1 \text{ tablet} = 2 \times 1 \text{ tablet} = 2 \text{ tablets; given orally twice daily}$$

Double-check to be sure your calculated dosage matches your *reasonable* dosage from step 2. If, for example, you had calculated to give more or less than 2 tablets of Lopressor, you would suspect a calculation error.

Example 2:

The physician prescribes *V-Cillin K 0.5 g p.o. q.i.d.* The dosage available is *V-Cillin K 250 mg per tablet.* How many tablets should the nurse give to the patient per dose?

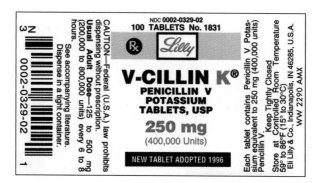

| Step 1 | Convert | To the same size units. Convert 0.5 g to mg. Remember the math tip: Convert larger unit (g) to the smaller unit (mg). |

Equivalent: 1 g = 1000 mg. Conversion factor is 1000.

Larger → Smaller: ($\times$)

0.5 g = 0.5 $\times$ 1000 = 0.500. = 500 mg

Now you have the order and supply measured in the same size units.

Order: *V-Cillin K 0.5 g = 500 mg*

Supply: *V-Cillin K 250 mg tablets*

By now you probably can do conversions like this from memory.

| Step 2 | Think | 500 mg is twice as much as 250 milligrams. You want to give 2 tablets. |

Step 3   Calculate $\dfrac{D}{H} \times Q = \dfrac{500 \text{ mg}}{250 \text{ mg}} \times 1 \text{ tablet}$

$\dfrac{\overset{2}{\cancel{500 \text{ mg}}}}{\underset{1}{\cancel{250 \text{ mg}}}} \times 1 \text{ tablet} = 2 \times 1 \text{ tablet} = 2 \text{ tablets}$; given orally 4 times daily

Example 3:

The drug order reads: *codeine sulfate gr $\frac{3}{4}$ p.o. q.4h p.r.n., pain.* The drug supplied is *codeine sulfate 30 mg per tablet.* Calculate one dose.

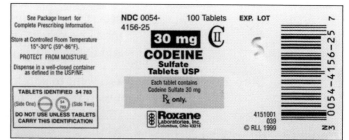

Step 1   Convert   To equivalent units in the same system of measurement. Convert gr to mg. Approximate equivalent: gr i = 60 mg. Conversion factor is 60. Larger → Smaller: (×).

$$\text{gr} \frac{3}{4} = \frac{3}{\overset{}{\underset{1}{4}}} \times \overset{15}{\cancel{60}} = 45 \text{ mg}$$

Order: *codeine gr $\frac{3}{4}$ = 45 mg*

Supply: *codeine 30 mg tablets*

Step 2   Think   You estimate that you want to give more than one tablet but less than two tablets.

Step 3   Calculate $\dfrac{D}{H} \times Q = \dfrac{45 \text{ mg}}{30 \text{ mg}} \times 1$ tablet

$$\frac{\overset{3}{\cancel{45 \text{ mg}}}}{\underset{2}{\cancel{30 \text{ mg}}}} \times 1 \text{ tablet} = \frac{3}{2} \text{ tablets} = 1\frac{1}{2} \text{ tablets; given every 4 hours as needed for pain}$$

Now you can see that a dosage problem that may have seemed difficult on first reading is actually very simple. Approach every dosage calculation just like this: one step at a time.

Example 4:

The order is *Synthroid 0.05 mg p.o. q.d. Synthroid 25 mcg tablets* are available. How many tablets will you give?

Step 1   Convert   To same size units. Remember the math tip: Convert larger unit (mg) to smaller unit (mcg).

Approximate equivalent: 1 mg = 1000 mcg. Conversion factor is 1000.

Larger → Smaller: (×)

0.05 mg = 0.05 × 1000 = 0.050. = 50 mcg

Order: *Synthroid 0.05 mg = 50 mcg*

Supply: *Synthroid 25 mcg tablets*

Step 2   Think   As soon as you convert the ordered dosage of Synthroid 0.05 mg to Synthroid 50 mcg, you realize that you want to give more than 1 tablet for each dose. In fact, you want to give twice the supply dosage, which is the same as 2 tablets.

Avoid getting confused by the way the original problem is presented. Be sure that you recognize which is the dosage ordered (D—desired) and which is the supply dosage (H—have on hand) per the quantity on hand (Q). A common error is to misread the information and mix up the calculations in step 3. This demonstrates the importance of thinking (step 2) before you calculate.

Step 3   Calculate $\frac{D}{H} \times Q = \frac{50 \text{ mcg}}{25 \text{ mcg}} \times 1 \text{ tablet}$

$\frac{\overset{2}{\cancel{50 \text{ mcg}}}}{\underset{1}{\cancel{25 \text{ mcg}}}} \times 1 \text{ tablet} = 2 \times 1 \text{ tablet} = 2 \text{ tablets; given orally once a day}$

Example 5:

Your client is to receive *Nitrostat gr $\frac{1}{400}$ SL p.r.n. for angina pain.* The label on the available Nitrostat bottle tells you that each tablet provides 0.3 mg (gr $\frac{1}{200}$). How much will you give your client?

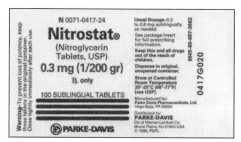

Step 1   Convert   To equivalent units in the same system of measurement. Remember the math tip: Convert apothecary measurement to metric units. Convert the order in grains to milligrams.

Approximate equivalent: gr i = 60 mg. Conversion factor is 60.

Larger → Smaller: (×)

$\text{gr}\frac{1}{400} = \frac{1}{\underset{20}{\cancel{400}}} \times \overset{3}{\cancel{60}} = \frac{3}{20} = 0.15 \text{ mg}$

Order: *Nitrostat gr $\frac{1}{400}$ = 0.15 mg*

Supply: *Nitrostat 0.3 mg tablets*

Step 2   Think   Look at the supply dosage and add a zero at the end of the decimal number: 0.3 mg = 0.30 mg. Now you can compare the ordered dosage of 0.15 mg with the supply dosage of 0.30 mg per tablet. You can reason that you want to give less than 1 tablet. Further, you can see that 0.15 is $\frac{1}{2}$ of 0.30, and you know that you want to give $\frac{1}{2}$ tablet. Check your reasoning in step 3.

Step 3   Calculate $\dfrac{D}{H} \times Q = \dfrac{0.15 \text{ mg}}{0.30 \text{ mg}} \times 1 \text{ tablet}$

$$\dfrac{\overset{1}{\cancel{0.15 \text{ mg}}}}{\underset{2}{\cancel{0.30 \text{ mg}}}} \times 1 \text{ tablet} = \dfrac{1}{2} \times 1 \text{ tablet} = \dfrac{1}{2} \text{ tablet; given sublingually as needed}$$
for angina pain

QUICK REVIEW

Simple Three-Step Approach to Dosage Calculations

Step 1	**Convert**	To units of the same system and the same size.
Step 2	**Think**	Estimate for a reasonable amount to give.
Step 3	**Calculate**	$\dfrac{D}{H} \times Q = X$

$$\dfrac{D \text{ (desired)}}{H \text{ (have)}} \times Q \text{ (quantity)} = X \text{ (amount)}$$

- For most dosage calculation problems:
  - convert to smaller size unit. Example: g → mg
  - convert from the apothecary or household system to the metric system. Example: gr → mg
- Consider the reasonableness of the calculated amount to give. Example: You would question giving more than 3 tablets or capsules per dose for oral administration.

REVIEW SET 25

Calculate the correct number of tablets or capsules to be administered per dose. Tablets are scored.

1. The physician writes an order for *Diabinese 0.1 g p.o. q.d.* The drug container label reads *Diabinese 100 mg tablets.*

   Give: _____ tablet(s)

2. Duricef 500 mg tablets available. The order is for *Duricef 0.5 g p.o. b.i.d.*

   Give: _____ tablet(s)

3. Urecholine 10 mg tablets available. Order: *Urecholine 15 mg p.o. t.i.d.*

   Give: _____ tablet(s)

4. Order: *hydrochlorothiazide 12.5 mg p.o. t.i.d.* Hydrochlorothiazide 25 mg tablets available.

   Give: _____ tablet(s)

5. Order: *Lanoxin 0.125 mg p.o. q.d.*

   Supply: Lanoxin 0.25 mg tablets

   Give: _____ tablet(s)

6. Order: *Motrin 600 mg p.o. b.i.d.*

   Supply: Motrin 300 mg tablets

   Give: _____ tablet(s)

7. Order: *Slow-K 16 mEq p.o. stat*

   Supply: Slow-K 8 mEq tablets

   Give: _____ tablet(s)

8. Cytoxan 25 mg tablets available. Order: *Cytoxan 50 mg p.o. q.d.*

   Give: _____ tablet(s)

9. Zaroxolyn 5 mg tablets available. Order: *Zaroxolyn 7.5 mg p.o. b.i.d.*

   Give: _____ tablet(s)

10. *Coumadin 5 mg p.o. q.d.* ordered. Coumadin 2.5 mg tablets available.

    Give: _____ tablet(s)

11. Levaquin is available in 500 mg tablets. Ordered dose is *Levaquin 0.5 g p.o. q.d.*

    Give _____ tablet(s)

12. Order: *Trandate 150 mg p.o. b.i.d.*

    Supply: Trandate 300 mg tablets

    Give: _____ tablet(s)

13. Order: *Duricef 1 g p.o. b.i.d.*

    Supply: Duricef 500 mg capsules

    Give: _____ capsule(s)

14. Synthroid 50 mcg tablets available. Order: *Synthroid 0.1 mg p.o. q.d.*

    Give: _____ tablet(s)

15. *Tranxene 7.5 mg p.o. q.i.d.* is ordered and you have 3.75 mg Tranxene capsules available.

    Give: _____ capsule(s)

16. Order: *Inderal 15 mg p.o. t.i.d.*

    Supply: Inderal 10 mg tablets

    Give: _____ tablet(s)

17. The doctor orders *Loniten gr $\frac{1}{6}$ p.o. stat* and you have available Loniten 10 mg and 2.5 mg scored tablets. Select _____ mg tablets and give _____ tablet(s).

18. Order: *Reglan 15 mg p.o. 1 h a.c. et h.s.* You have available Reglan 10 mg and Reglan 5 mg scored tablets. Select _____ mg tablets and give _____ tablet(s). How many doses of Reglan will the patient receive in 24 hours? _____ dose(s)

19. Order: *phenobarbital gr $\frac{1}{4}$ p.o. q.d.*

    Supply: phenobarbital 15 mg, 30 mg, and 60 mg scored tablets.

    Select _____ mg tablets and give _____ tablet(s).

20. Order: *Tylenol c̄ codeine gr i p.o. q.4h p.r.n. pain*

    Supply: Tylenol with codeine 7.5 mg, 15 mg, 30 mg, and 60 mg tablets.

    Select _____ mg tablets and give _____ tablet(s).

Calculate one dose for each of the medication orders 21 through 30. The labels lettered A through I are the drugs you have available. Indicate the letter corresponding to the label you select.

21. Order: *verapamil sustained release 240 mg p.o. q.d.*

    Select: _____

    Give: _____

22. Order: *carbamazepine 0.2 g p.o. t.i.d.*

    Select: _____

    Give: _____

23. Order: *Lopressor 50 mg p.o. b.i.d.*

    Select: _____

    Give: _____

24. Order: *potassium chloride 16 mEq p.o. q.d.*

    Select: _____

    Give: _____

25. Order: *Procanbid 1 g p.o. q.6h*

    Select: _____

    Give: _____

26. Order: *cephalexin 0.5 g p.o. q.i.d.*

    Select: _____

    Give: _____

27. Order: *levothyroxine sodium 0.2 mg p.o. q.d.*

    Select: _____

    Give: _____

28. Order: *digoxin 0.5 mg p.o. q.d.*

    Select: _____

    Give: _____

29. Order: *allopurinol 0.1 g p.o. t.i.d.*

    Select: _____

    Give: _____

30. Order: *procainamide hydrochloride 1000 mg q.6h*

    Select: _____

    Give: _____

After completing these problems, see pages 482–483 to check your answers.

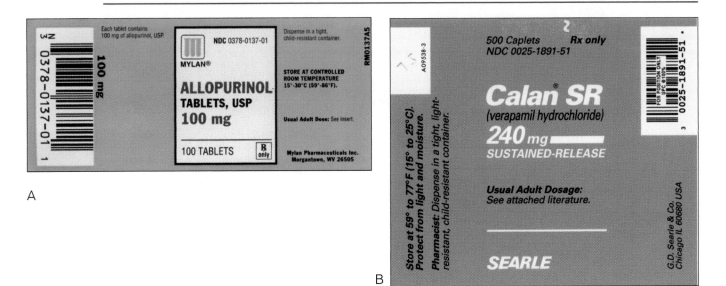

A

Each tablet contains 100 mg of allopurinol, USP.

NDC 0378-0137-01

MYLAN®

ALLOPURINOL
TABLETS, USP
100 mg

100 TABLETS

Rx only

Dispense in a tight, child-resistant container.

STORE AT CONTROLLED ROOM TEMPERATURE 15°-30°C (59°-86°F).

Usual Adult Dose: See insert.

Mylan Pharmaceuticals Inc. Morgantown, WV 26505

0378-0137-01

100 mg

B

Store at 59° to 77°F (15° to 25°C). Protect from light and moisture.

Pharmacist: Dispense in a tight, light-resistant, child-resistant container.

500 Caplets   **Rx only**
NDC 0025-1891-51

Calan® SR
(verapamil hydrochloride)
240 mg
SUSTAINED-RELEASE

Usual Adult Dosage:
See attached literature.

SEARLE

0025-1891-51

G.D. Searle & Co. Chicago IL 60680 USA

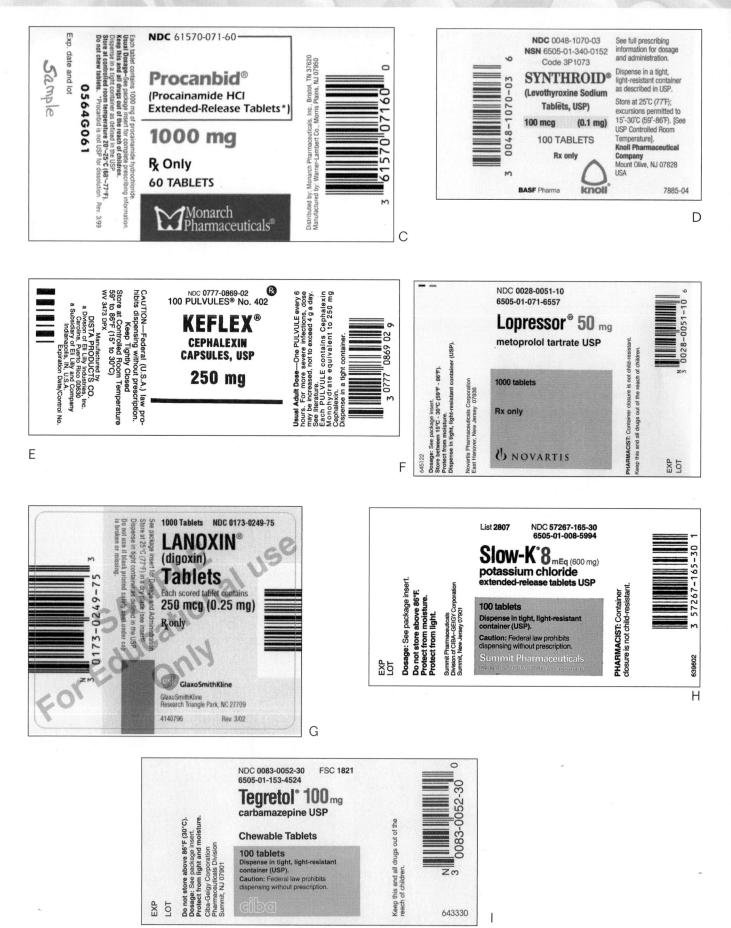

ORAL LIQUIDS

Oral liquids are supplied in solution form and contain a specific amount of drug in a given amount of solution as stated on the label (Figures 9-3a through d).

In solving dosage problems when the drug is supplied in solid form, you calculated the number of tablets or capsules that contained the prescribed dosage. The supply container label indicates the amount of medication per one tablet or one capsule. For medications supplied in liquid form, you must calculate the volume of the liquid that contains the prescribed dosage of the drug. The supply dosage noted on the label may indicate the amount of drug per one milliliter or per multiple milliliters of solution, such as 10 mg per 2 mL, 125 mg per 5 mL, or 1.2 g per 30 mL.

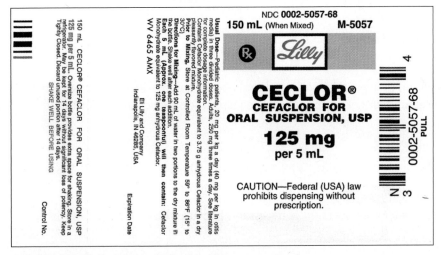

FIGURE 9-3(a) Oral Liquid: Ceclor 125 mg per 5 mL

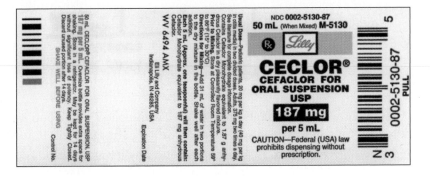

FIGURE 9-3(b) Oral Liquid: Ceclor 187 mg per 5 mL

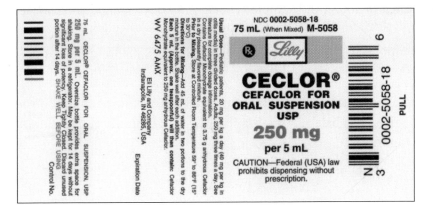

FIGURE 9-3(c) Oral Liquid: Ceclor 250 mg per 5 mL

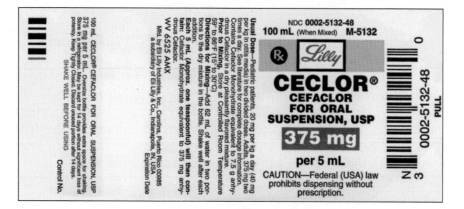

FIGURE 9-3(d) Oral Liquid: Ceclor 375 mg per 5 mL

Steps 1, 2, and 3 can be used to solve liquid oral dosage calculations in the same way that solid-form oral dosages are calculated. Let's apply the three steps to dosage calculations in a few examples.

Example 1:

The doctor orders *Ceclor 100 mg p.o. q.i.d.* Look at the labels of Ceclor available in Figure 9-3. You choose *Ceclor 125 mg per 5 mL.* Follow the three steps to dosage calculations.

Step 1	**Convert**	No conversion is necessary, because the order and supply dosage are both in the same units.
Step 2	**Think**	You want to give less than 125 mg, so you want to give less than 5 mL. Double-check your thinking with the $\frac{D}{H} \times Q = X$ formula.
Step 3	**Calculate**	$\frac{D}{H} \times Q = \frac{100 \text{ mg}}{125 \text{ mg}} \times 5 \text{ mL}$

$$\frac{\overset{4}{\cancel{100 \text{ mg}}}}{\underset{5}{\cancel{125 \text{ mg}}}} \times 5 \text{ mL} = \frac{4}{\cancel{5}} \times \overset{1}{\cancel{5}} \text{ mL} = 4 \text{ mL; given orally 4 times a day}$$

You will give 4 mL of the Ceclor with the dosage strength of 125 mg per 5 mL. Double-check to be sure your calculated dosage is consistent with your *reasonable* dosage from step 2. If, for instance, you calculate to give *more* than 5 mL, then you should suspect a calculation error.

Example 2:

Suppose, using the same drug order in Example 1, *Ceclor 100 mg p.o. q.i.d.*, you choose a stronger solution, *Ceclor 250 mg per 5 mL.* Follow the three steps to dosage calculations.

Step 1	**Convert**	No conversion is necessary, because the order and supply dosage are both in the same units and system.
Step 2	**Think**	You want to give 100 mg, and you have 250 mg per 5 mL so you will give less than half of 5 mL. Double-check your thinking with the $\frac{D}{H} \times Q = X$ formula.
Step 3	**Calculate**	$\frac{D}{H} \times Q = \frac{100 \text{ mg}}{250 \text{ mg}} \times 5 \text{ mL}$

$$\frac{\overset{2}{\cancel{100 \text{ mg}}}}{\underset{5}{\cancel{250 \text{ mg}}}} \times 5 \text{ mL} = \frac{2}{\cancel{5}} \times \overset{1}{\cancel{5}} \text{ mL} = 2 \text{ mL; given orally 4 times a day}$$

Notice that in both Example 1 and Example 2, the supply quantity is the same (5 mL), but the dosage strength (weight) of medication is different (125 mg per 5 mL vs. 250 mg per 5 mL). This results in the calculated dose volume (amount to give) being different (4 mL vs. 2 mL). This difference is the result of each liquid's *concentration*. *Ceclor 125 mg per 5 mL* is half as concentrated as *Ceclor 250 mg per 5 mL*. In other words, there is half as much drug in 5 mL of the *125 mg per 5 mL* supply as there is in 5 mL of the *250 mg per 5 mL* supply. Likewise, *Ceclor 250 mg per 5 mL* is twice as concentrated as *Ceclor 125 mg per 5 mL*. The more concentrated solution allows you to give the patient less volume per dose for the same dosage. This is significant when administering medication to infants and small children when a smaller quantity is needed. Think about this carefully until it is clear.

CAUTION

Think before you calculate. It is important to estimate before you apply any formula. In this way, if you make a careless error in math or if you set up the problem incorrectly, your thinking will alert you to *try again*.

Example 3:

The doctor orders *potassium chloride 40 mEq p.o. q.d.* The label on the package reads *potassium chloride 20 mEq per 15 mL*. How many mL should you administer?

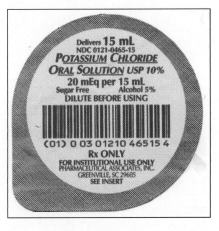

Step 1	Convert	No conversion is necessary.
Step 2	Think	You want to give more than 15 mL. In fact, you want to give exactly twice as much as 15 mL. You know this is true because 40 mEq is twice as much as 20 mEq. Therefore, it will take 2 × 15 mL or 30 mL to give 40 mEq. Continue to step 3 to double-check your thinking.

Step 3 Calculate $\dfrac{D}{H} \times Q = \dfrac{\overset{2}{\cancel{40\ mEq}}}{\underset{1}{\cancel{20\ mEq}}} \times 15\ mL = 30\ mL$; given orally once a day

---

QUICK REVIEW

Look again at steps 1 through 3 as a valuable dosage calculation checklist.

Step 1	Convert	Be sure that all measurements are in the same system, and all units are in the same size.
Step 2	Think	Carefully estimate the reasonable amount of the drug that you should administer.
Step 3	Calculate	$\dfrac{D}{H} \times Q = X$ $\dfrac{D\ \text{(desired)}}{H\ \text{(have)}} \times Q\ \text{(quantity)} = X\ \text{(amount)}$

REVIEW SET 26

Calculate one dose of the drugs ordered.

1. Order: *Demerol syrup 75 mg p.o. q.4h p.r.n. pain*

   Supply: Demerol syrup 50 mg per 5 mL

   Give: _____ mL

2. Order: *Phenergan c̄ codeine gr $\frac{1}{6}$ p.o. q.4–6h p.r.n. cough*

   Supply: Phenergan c̄ codeine solution 10 mg per 5 mL

   Give: _____ mL

3. Order: *Pen-Vee K 1 g p.o. 1h pre-op dental surgery*

   Supply: Pen-Vee K oral suspension 250 mg (400,000 U) per 5 mL

   Give: _____ mL

4. Order: *amoxicillin 100 mg p.o. q.i.d.*

   Supply: 80 mL bottle of Amoxil (amoxicillin) oral pediatric suspension 125 mg per 5 mL

   Give: _____ mL

5. Order: *Tylenol 0.5 g p.o. q.4h p.r.n. pain*

   Supply: Tylenol 500 mg in 5 mL

   Give: _____ t

6. Order: *promethazine HCl 25 mg p.o. h.s. pre-op*

   Supply: Phenergan Plain (promethazine HCl) 6.25 mg per teaspoon

   Give: _____ mL

7. Order: *Pathocil 125 mg p.o. q.6h*

   Supply: Pathocil suspension 62.5 mg per 5 mL

   Give: _____ t

8. Order: *erythromycin suspension 600 mg p.o. q.6h*

   Supply: erythromycin 400 mg/5 mL

   Give: _____ mL

9. Order: *Ceclor suspension 225 mg p.o. b.i.d.*

   Supply: Ceclor suspension 375 mg per 5 mL

   Give: _____ mL

10. Order: *Septra-DS suspension 200 mg p.o. b.i.d.*

    Supply: Septra-DS suspension 400 mg per 5 mL

    Give: _____ mL

11. Order: *Elixophyllin liquid 0.24 g p.o. stat*

    Supply: Elixophyllin liquid 80 mg/7.5 mL

    Give: _____ mL

12. Order: *Trilisate liquid 750 mg p.o. t.i.d.*

    Supply: Trilisate liquid 250 mg/2.5 mL

    Give: _____ mL

13. Order: *Esidrix solution 100 mg p.o. b.i.d.*

    Supply: Esidrix solution 50 mg/5 mL

    Give: _____ t

14. Order: *Pepcid 20 mg p.o. q.i.d.*

    Supply: Pepcid 80 mg/10 mL

    Give: _____ mL

15. Order: *digoxin elixir 0.25 mg p.o. q.d.*

    Supply: digoxin elixir 50 mcg/mL

    Give: _____ mL

16. Order: *nafcillin sodium 0.75 g p.o. q.6h*

    Supply: nafcillin sodium 250 mg/5 mL

    Give: ℥ _____

17. Order: *cephalexin 375 mg p.o. t.i.d.*

    Supply: cephalexin 250 mg/5 mL

    Give: _____ t

18. Order: *lactulose 20 g via gastric tube b.i.d. today*

    Supply: lactulose 10 g/15mL

    Give: ℥ _____

19. Order: *erythromycin 1.2 g p.o. q.8h*

    Supply: erythromycin 400 mg/5 mL

    Give: _____ mL

20. Order: *oxacillin sodium 0.25 g p.o. q.8h*

    Supply: oxacillin sodium 125 mg/2.5 mL

    Give: _____ t

21. Order: *amoxicillin suspension 100 mg p.o. q.6h*

    Supply: amoxicillin suspension 250 mg/ 5 mL

    Give: _____ mL

Use the labels A, B, and C below to calculate one dose of the following orders (22, 23, and 24). Indicate the letter corresponding to the label you select.

22. Order: *erythromycin 125 mg p.o. t.i.d.*

    Select: _____

    Give: _____

24. Order: *Vistaril 10 mg p.o. q.i.d.*

    Select: _____

    Give: _____

23. Order: *Keflex 50 mg p.o. q.6h*

    Select: _____

    Give: _____

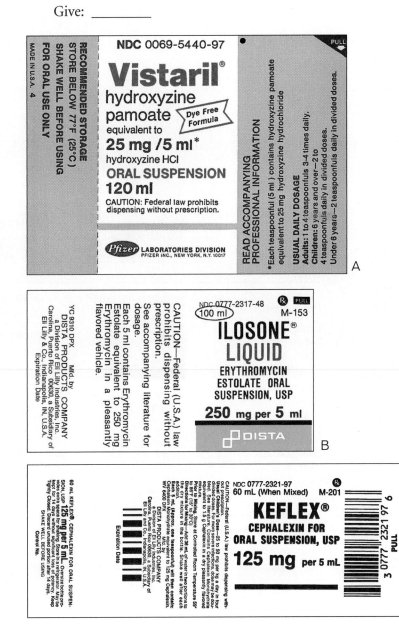

Calculate the information requested based on the drugs ordered. The labels provided are the drugs available.

25. Order: *Lanoxin elixir 0.25 mg p.o. q.d.*

    Give: _____ mL

    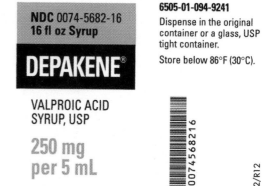

    60 mL   NDC 0173-0264-27

    LANOXIN®
    (digoxin)
    ELIXIR
    PEDIATRIC

    Each mL contains
    50 mcg (0.05 mg)
    PLEASANTLY FLAVORED

    Alcohol 10%, Methylparaben 0.1% (added as a preservative)
    See package insert for Dosage and Administration. excursions permitted to 15 to 30°C (59 to 86°F) [see USP Controlled Room Temperature] and protect from light. Store at 25°C (77°F)

    GlaxoSmithKline   R only
    GlaxoSmithKline
    Research Triangle Park, NC 27709
    Made in Canada   4140729   Rev. 10/01

26. Order: *OxyFast (oral solution concentrate) 15 mg p.o. q.6h p.r.n., pain*

    Give: _____ mL

    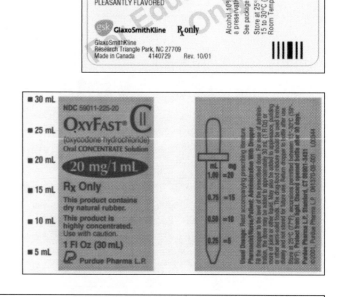

    ■ 30 mL
    ■ 25 mL
    ■ 20 mL
    ■ 15 mL
    ■ 10 mL
    ■ 5 mL

    NDC 59011-225-20
    OxyFast® CII
    (oxycodone hydrochloride)
    Oral CONCENTRATE Solution
    20 mg/1 mL
    Rx Only
    This product contains
    dry natural rubber.
    This product is
    highly concentrated.
    Use with caution.
    1 Fl Oz (30 mL)
    Purdue Pharma L.P.

    mL   mg
    1.00   =20
    0.75   =15
    0.50   =10
    0.25   =5

27. Order: *valproic acid 0.5 g p.o. t.i.d.*

    Give: _____ mL

    How many full doses are available in this bottle? _____ full doses

    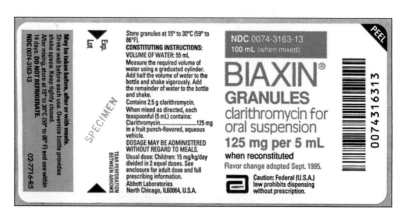

    Do not accept if band on cap is broken or missing.

    Each 5 mL contains equivalent of 250 mg valproic acid as the sodium salt.

    See enclosure for prescribing information.

    ©Abbott

    Abbott Laboratories
    North Chicago,
    IL60064, U.S.A.

    Exp.

    Lot

    NDC 0074-5682-16
    16 fl oz Syrup

    DEPAKENE®

    VALPROIC ACID
    SYRUP, USP

    250 mg
    per 5 mL

    Caution: Federal (U.S.A.) law prohibits dispensing without prescription.

    6505-01-094-9241

    Dispense in the original container or a glass, USP tight container.

    Store below 86°F (30°C).

    0074568216

    02-7538-2/R12

28. Order: *Biaxin 75 mg p.o. q.12h*

    Give: _____ mL

    Store granules at 15° to 30°C (59° to 86°F).
    CONSTITUTING INSTRUCTIONS:
    VOLUME OF WATER: 55 mL.
    Measure the required volume of water using a graduated cylinder. Add half the volume of water to the bottle and shake vigorously. Add the remainder of water to the bottle and shake.
    Contains 2.5 g clarithromycin. When mixed as directed, each teaspoonful (5 mL) contains:
    Clarithromycin................125 mg
    in a fruit punch-flavored, aqueous vehicle.
    DOSAGE MAY BE ADMINISTERED WITHOUT REGARD TO MEALS.
    Usual dose: Children: 15 mg/kg/day divided in 2 equal doses. See enclosure for adult dose and full prescribing information.
    Abbott Laboratories
    North Chicago, IL60064, U.S.A.

    May be taken before, after or with meals. Shake well before each use. Oversize bottle provides shake space. Keep tightly closed. After mixing, store at 15° to 30°C (59° to 86° F) and use within 14 days. DO NOT REFRIGERATE.

    Exp.
    Lot

    SPECIMEN

    PEEL

    NDC 0074-3163-13
    100 mL (when mixed)

    BIAXIN®
    GRANULES
    clarithromycin for
    oral suspension
    125 mg per 5 mL
    when reconstituted
    Flavor change adopted Sept. 1995.

    Caution: Federal (U.S.A.) law prohibits dispensing without prescription.

    0074316313

    NDC 0074-3163-13
    02-7716-R5

29. Order: *Maalox Plus 30 mL p.o. 30 min. p.c. and h.s.*

    How many containers will be needed for a 24-hour period? _____ containers

30. Meals are served at 8 AM, 12 noon, and 6 PM Using international time, what are the administration times for the 30 min p.c. dosages for the order in question 29? (Allow 30 minutes for each meal to be eaten.) _____

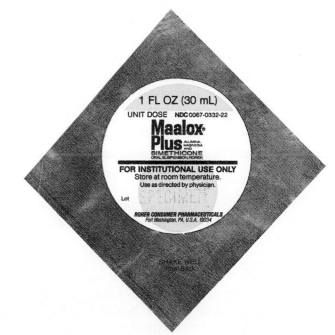

After completing these problems, see pages 483–484 to check your answers.

SUMMARY

Let's examine where you are in mastering the skill of dosage calculations. You have learned to convert equivalent units within systems of measurements and from one system to another. You have also applied this conversion skill to the calculation of oral dosages—both solid and liquid forms. By now, you know that solving dosage problems requires that all units of measurement first be expressed in the same system and same size.

Next, you learned to think through the dosage ordered and dosage supplied to estimate the amount to be given. *To minimize medication errors, it is essential that you consider the reasonableness of the amount before applying a calculation method or formula.*

Finally, you have learned the formula method $\frac{D}{H} \times Q = X$ (*desired* over *have* times *quantity* = *amount to give*). This method is so simple and easy to recall that it will stick with you throughout your career.

Review the Critical Thinking Skills and work the practice problems for Chapter 9. If you are having difficulty, get help from an instructor before proceeding to Chapter 10. Continue to concentrate on accuracy. Keep in mind that one error can be a serious mistake when you are calculating the dosages of medicines. Medication administration is a *legal responsibility.* Remember, when you give a medication, you are legally responsible for your action.

CRITICAL THINKING SKILLS

Inaccuracy in dosage calculation is often attributed to errors in calculating the dosage. By first asking the question, "What is the reasonable amount to give?" many medication errors can be avoided.

error

Incorrect calculation and not assessing the reasonableness of the calculation before administering the medication.

(continues)

(continued)

possible scenario

The physician ordered *phenobarbital 60 mg p.o. b.i.d.* for a patient with seizures. The pharmacy supplied *phenobarbital 30 mg per tablet*. The nurse did not use step 2 to think about the reasonable dosage, and calculated the dosage this way:

$$\frac{\text{DESIRED}}{\text{HAVE}} \times \text{QUANTITY} = \text{AMOUNT}$$

$$\frac{60 \text{ mg}}{30 \text{ mg}} \times 1 \text{ tab} = 20 \text{ tab (incorrect)}$$

Suppose the nurse then gave the patient 20 tablets of the 30 mg per tablet of phenobarbital. The patient would have received 600 mg of phenobarbital, or 10 times the correct dosage. This is a very serious error.

potential outcome

The patient would likely develop signs of phenobarbital toxicity, such as nystagmus (rapid eye movement), ataxia (lack of coordination), central nervous system depression, respiratory depression, hypothermia, and hypotension. When the error was caught and the physician notified, the patient would likely be given doses of charcoal to hasten elimination of the drug. Depending on the severity of the symptoms, the patient would likely be moved to the intensive care unit for monitoring of respiratory and neurological status.

prevention

This medication error could have been prevented if the nurse had used the three-step method and estimated for the reasonable dosage of the drug to give. The order is for 60 mg of phenobarbital and the available drug has 30 mg per tablet, so the nurse should give 2 tablets. The incorrect calculation that indicated such a large amount of tablets to give per dose should have alerted the nurse to a possible error. The formula $\frac{D}{H} \times Q = X$ should be used to verify thinking about the *reasonable* dosage. Further, the nurse should double-check the math to find the error.

$$\frac{D}{H} \times Q = \frac{60 \text{ mg}}{30 \text{ mg}} \times 1 \text{ tablet} \qquad \frac{\overset{2}{\cancel{60 \text{ mg}}}}{\underset{1}{\cancel{30 \text{ mg}}}} \times 1 \text{ tablet} = 2 \text{ tablets, not 20 tablets}$$

PRACTICE PROBLEMS—CHAPTER 9

Calculate one dose of the following drug orders. The tablets are scored in half.

1. Order: *Orinase 250 mg p.o. b.i.d.*

   Supply: Orinase 0.5 g tablets

   Give: _____ tablet(s)

2. Order: *codeine gr ss p.o. q.4h p.r.n., pain*

   Supply: codeine 15 mg tablets

   Give: _____ tablet(s)

3. Order: *Synthroid 0.075 mg p.o. q.d.*

   Supply: Synthroid 150 mcg tablets

   Give: _____ tablet(s)

4. Order: *phenobarbital gr $\frac{1}{6}$ p.o. t.i.d.*

   Supply: phenobarbital elixir 20 mg per 5 mL

   Give: _____ mL

5. Order: *Keflex 500 mg p.o. q.i.d.*

   Supply: Keflex 250 mg per 5 mL

   Give: _____ mL

6. Order: *Inderal 20 mg p.o. q.i.d.*

   Supply: Inderal 10 mg tablets

   Give: _____ tablet(s)

7. Order: *Amoxil 400 mg p.o. q.6h*

   Supply: Amoxil 250 mg per 5 mL

   Give: _____ mL

8. Order: *Diabenese 150 mg p.o. b.i.d.*

   Supply: Diabenese 0.1 g tablets

   Give: _____ tablet(s)

9. Order: *Aspirin gr v p.o. q.d.*

   Supply: Aspirin 325 mg tablets

   Give: _____ tablet(s)

10. Order: *codeine gr $\frac{1}{4}$ p.o. q.d.*

    Supply: codeine 30 mg tablets

    Give: _____ tablet(s)

11. Order: *Inderal 30 mg p.o. q.i.d.*

    Supply: Inderal 20 mg tablets

    Give: _____ tablet(s)

12. Order: *Synthroid 300 mcg p.o. q.d.*

    Supply: Synthroid 0.3 mg tablets

    Give: _____ tablet(s)

13. Order: *Lasix 60 mg p.o. q.d.*

    Supply: Lasix 40 mg tablets

    Give: _____ tablet(s)

14. Order: *Tylenol c̄ codeine gr $\frac{1}{8}$ p.o. q.d.*

    Supply: Tylenol with 7.5 mg codeine tablets

    Give: _____ tablet(s)

15. Order: *penicillin G 400,000 U p.o. q.i.d.*

    Supply: Pentids (penicillin G) 250 mg (400,000 U) tablets

    Give: _____ tablet(s)

16. Order: *Vasotec 7.5 mg p.o. q.d.*

    Supply: Vasotec 5 mg and 10 mg tablets

    Select: _____ mg tablets

    and give _____ tablet(s)

17. Order: *V-Cillin K 300,000 U p.o. q.i.d.*

    Supply: V-Cillin K 200,000 U/5 mL

    Give: _____ mL

18. Order: *Neomycin 0.75 g p.o. b.i.d.*

    Supply: Neomycin 500 mg tablets

    Give: _____ tablet(s)

19. Order: *Halcion 0.25 mg p.o. h.s.*

    Supply: Halcion 0.125 mg tablets

    Give: _____ tablet(s)

20. Order: *Roxanol gr $\frac{1}{10}$ p.o. q.3–4h p.r.n. pain*

    Supply: Roxanol 10 mg/5 mL

    Give: _____ mL

21. Order: *Decadron 750 mcg p.o. b.i.d.*

    Supply: Decadron 0.75 mg and 1.5 mg tablets

    Select: _____ mg tablets

    Give: _____ tablet(s)

22. Order: *Edecrin 12.5 mg p.o. b.i.d.*

    Supply: Edecrin 25 mg tablets

    Give: _____ tablet(s)

23. Order: *Urecholine 50 mg p.o. t.i.d.*

    Supply: Urecholine 25 mg tablets

    Give: _____ tablet(s)

24. Order: *erythromycin 0.5 g p.o. q.12h*

    Supply: erythromycin 250 mg tablets

    Give: _____ tablet(s)

25. Order: *glyburide 2.5 mg p.o. q.d.*

    Supply: glyburide 1.25 mg tablets

    Give: _____ tablet(s)

26. Order: *Tranxene 7.5 mg p.o. q.AM*

    Supply: Tranxene 3.75 mg capsules

    Give: _____ capsules

27. Order: *phenobarbital gr $\frac{3}{4}$ p.o. q.d.*

    Supply: phenobarbital 15 mg, 30 mg, and 60 mg scored tablets

    Which strength of tablet(s) would you select, and how much would you give?

    Select: _____ mg tablets

    Give: _____ tablet(s)

28. Order: *acetaminophen 240 mg p.o. q.4–6h p.r.n., pain or T > 102°F*

    Supply: acetaminophen drops 80 mg per 0.8 mL

    Give: _____ mL

29. Order: *acetaminophen 160 mg p.o. q.4–6h p.r.n., pain or T > 102°F*

    Supply: acetaminophen liquid 80 mg per $\frac{1}{2}$ t

    Give: _____ mL

30. Order: *Coumadin 7.5 mg p.o. q.d.*

    Supply: Coumadin 2.5 mg tablets

    Give: _____ tablet(s)

See the three medication administration records and accompanying labels on the following pages for questions 31 through 45.

Calculate one dose of each of the drugs prescribed. Labels A–O provided on pages 183–185 are the drugs you have available. Indicate the letter corresponding to the label you select.

	ORIGINAL ORDER DATE	DATE STARTED/RENEWED	MEDICATION - DOSAGE	ROUTE	11-7	7-3	3-11	11-7	7-3	3-11
					SCHEDULE			DATE 1/5/xx		
31.	1/5/xx	1/5	Tegretol 200 mg b.i.d.	PO		9	9		9 GP	9 MS
32.	1/5/xx	1/5	Allegra 60 mg b.i.d.	PO		9	9		9 GP	9 MS
33.	1/5/xx	1/5	sucralfate 1000 mg b.i.d.	PO		9	9		9 GP	9 MS
34.	1/5/xx	1/5	Naprosyn 0.5 g q.i.d.	PO		9 1			9 GP 1 GP	5 MS 9 MS

MEDICATION ADMINISTRATION RECORD

PAGE _____ of _____

PRN

INJECTION SITES
B - RIGHT ARM
C - RIGHT ABDOMEN
D - RIGHT ANTERIOR THIGH
G - LEFT ARM
H - LEFT ABDOMEN
J - LEFT ANTERIOR THIGH
L - LEFT BUTTOCKS
M - RIGHT BUTTOCKS

SIGNATURE OF NURSE ADMINISTERING MEDICATIONS

11-7 GP G. Pickar, R.N.

7-3 MS M. Smith, R.N.

3-11

Patient, Mary Q.

RECOPIED BY:

CHECKED BY:

ALLERGIES: NKA

① ORIGINAL COPY

31. Select: _____

    Give: _____

32. Select: _____

    Give: _____

33. Select: _____

    Give: _____

34. Select: _____

    Give: _____

PAGE _____ of _____

MEDICATION ADMINISTRATION RECORD

	ORIGINAL ORDER DATE	DATE STARTED / RENEWED	MEDICATION - DOSAGE	ROUTE	SCHEDULE 11-7	7-3	3-11	DATE 1/5/xx 11-7	7-3	3-11	DATE 11-7	7-3	3-11	DATE 11-7	7-3	3-11	DATE 11-7	7-3	3-11
35.	1/5/xx	1/5	Synthroid 0.2 mg q.d.	PO		9		GP 9											
36.	1/5/xx	1/5	Diabeta 5 mg q.d.	PO		9		GP 9											
37.	1/5/xx	1/5	erythromycin 0.8 g q.12h	PO	12 6	12	6	GP 12	MS 6										
38.	1/5/xx	1/5	Klonopin 500 mcg t.i.d.	PO		9	9	GP 9	MS 9										
39.	1/5/xx	1/5	Aldactone 0.1g q.d.	PO		9	9	GP 9	MS 9										

PRN

INJECTION SITES		B - RIGHT ARM	D - RIGHT ANTERIOR THIGH	H - LEFT ABDOMEN	L - LEFT BUTTOCKS
		C - RIGHT ABDOMEN	G - LEFT ARM	J - LEFT ANTERIOR THIGH	M - RIGHT BUTTOCKS

DATE GIVEN	TIME	INT.	ONE - TIME MEDICATION - DOSAGE	RT.	11-7	7-3	3-11	11-7	7-3	3-11	11-7	7-3	3-11	11-7	7-3	3-11	11-7	7-3	3-11
					SCHEDULE			DATE 1/5/xx			DATE			DATE			DATE		

SIGNATURE OF NURSE ADMINISTERING MEDICATIONS

11-7	
7-3	GP G. Pickar, R.N.
3-11	MS M. Smith, R.N.

DATE GIVEN | TIME | INT. | MEDICATION-DOSAGE-CONT. | RT.

LITHO IN U.S.A. R6506 (7-92) D395538

Patient, John Q.

RECOPIED BY:

CHECKED BY:

ALLERGIES:

602-31 (7-XX) (MPC# 1355)

(1)

ORIGINAL COPY

35. Select: _____

    Give: _____

36. Select: _____

    Give: _____

37. Select: _____

    Give: _____

38. Select: _____

    Give: _____

39. Select: _____

    Give: _____

ORIGINAL ORDER DATE	DATE STARTED / RENEWED	MEDICATION - DOSAGE	ROUTE	SCHEDULE 11-7	7-3	3-11	DATE 1/5/xx 11-7	7-3	3-11	DATE 11-7	7-3	3-11	DATE 11-7	7-3	3-11	DATE 11-7	7-3	3-11
40. 1/5/xx	1/5	digoxin 0.5 mg q.d.	PO		9			9 GP										
41. 1/5/xx	1/5	potassium chloride 40 mEq c̄ Ʒiv juice b.i.d.	PO		8 9	9		9 GP	9 MS									
42. 1/5/xx	1/5	Lopid 0.6 g b.i.d. ac	PO		7³⁰	4³⁰		7³⁰ GP	4³⁰ MS									
43. 1/5/xx	1/5	Furosemide 40 mg q.d.	PO		9			9 GP										
44. 1/5/xx	1/5	Lopressor 100 mg b.i.d.	PO		9	9		9 GP	9 MS									

PRN

45. 1/5/xx	1/5	Percocet 1 tab q.4h p.r.n. headache	PO					7³⁰ GP 11³⁰ GP										

INJECTION SITES

B - RIGHT ARM   D - RIGHT ANTERIOR THIGH   H - LEFT ABDOMEN   L - LEFT BUTTOCKS
C - RIGHT ABDOMEN   G - LEFT ARM   J - LEFT ANTERIOR THIGH   M - RIGHT BUTTOCKS

DATE GIVEN	TIME	INT.	ONE - TIME MEDICATION - DOSAGE	RT.	SCHEDULE 11-7	7-3	3-11	DATE 1/5/xx			DATE			DATE			DATE		

SIGNATURE OF NURSE ADMINISTERING MEDICATIONS

11-7

7-3   GP G. Pickar R.N.

3-11   MS M. Smith, R.N.

DATE GIVEN	TIME	INT.	MEDICATION-DOSAGE-CONT.	RT.

Doe, Jane Q.

RECOPIED BY:

CHECKED BY:

LITHO IN U.S.A. K6508 (7-92) D395538

ALLERGIES: **NKA**

602-31 (7-XX) (MPC# 1355)

(1)

ORIGINAL COPY

PAGE _____ of _____

MEDICATION ADMINISTRATION RECORD

40. Select: _____   43. Select: _____

    Give: _____   Give: _____

41. Select: _____   44. Select: _____

    Give: _____   Give: _____

42. Select: _____   45. Select: _____

    Give: _____   Give: _____

A

NDC 0088-1102-47

60 mg Hoechst Marion Roussel

ALLEGRA™
(fexofenadine hydrochloride)

60 mg

100 Capsules

50013685

Each capsule contains: fexofenadine hydrochloride........ 60 mg
Dosage and Administration: Read package insert for prescribing
information. **CAUTION:** Federal law prohibits dispensing without prescription. **Warning:** Keep out of reach of children. **Pharmacist:** Dispense in light, light-resistant container as
defined in USP. **Important:** This package is
not child resistant. Store at controlled room
temperature 68–77°F (20–25°C).

© 1997, Hoechst Marion Roussel, Inc.
US Patents 4,254,129; 5,375,693; 5,578,610

Mfd jointly by:
Hoechst Marion Roussel, Inc.
Kansas City, MO 64137 USA
and
Marion & Company
Mandi, Puerto Rico 00674

Exp

B

TAMPER-EVIDENT CONTAINER. DO NOT USE IF SEAL IS BROKEN !

STORE AT
ROOM TEMPERATURE.
DISPENSE IN
LIGHT-RESISTANT CONTAINERS.

NDC 18393-272-62
NAPROSYN®
[NAPROXEN] TABLETS
250 mg

CAUTION: Federal law prohibits
dispensing without prescription.
PACKAGE NOT CHILD-RESISTANT
500 TABLETS

6505-01-046-0126
USUAL DOSE: SEE ACCOMPANYING
PRESCRIBING INFORMATION.

SYNTEX
SYNTEX PUERTO RICO, INC.
HUMACAO, P.R. 00661

07-0272-62-07

18393-272-62

U. S. Patent Nos. 3,904,682; 3,998,906 and others.

C

NDC 0088-1712-53

**Carafate®
Tablets**
sucralfate

1 gram

120 Tablets

❧ **Aventis**

Rx ONLY
Each CARAFATE® Tablet contains 1g sucralfate.
Dosage and Administration: See package insert for
dosage information.
WARNING: Keep out of reach of children.
Pharmacist: Dispense in light-resistant, tight
container with child-resistant closure.
Important: This package is not
child-resistant.
**Store at controlled room tem-
perature 59–86°F (15–30°C).**
Aventis Pharmaceuticals Inc.
Kansas City, MO 64137
USA   ©2000
www.aventispharma-us.com

0088-1712-53

Exp   50059224

D

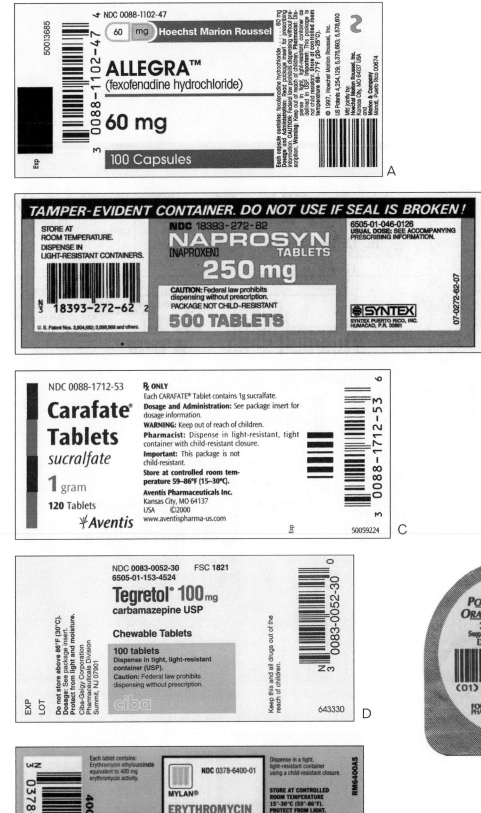

NDC 0083-0052-30   FSC **1821**
6505-01-153-4524

Tegretol® 100 mg
carbamazepine USP

Chewable Tablets

100 tablets
Dispense in tight, light-resistant
container (USP).
Caution: Federal law prohibits
dispensing without prescription.

ciba

Do not store above 86°F (30°C).
Dosage: See package insert.
Protect from light and moisture.
Ciba-Geigy Corporation
Pharmaceuticals Division
Summit, NJ 07901

EXP
LOT

Keep this and all drugs out of the
reach of children.

0083-0052-30

643330

E

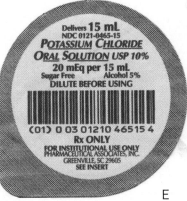

Delivers **15 mL**
NDC 0121-0465-15
**POTASSIUM CHLORIDE
ORAL SOLUTION** USP 10%
20 mEq per 15 mL
Sugar Free   Alcohol 5%
DILUTE BEFORE USING

(01) 0 03 01210 46515 4
Rx ONLY
FOR INSTITUTIONAL USE ONLY
PHARMACEUTICAL ASSOCIATES, INC.
GREENVILLE, SC 29605
SEE INSERT

F

Each tablet contains:
Erythromycin ethylsuccinate
equivalent to 400 mg
erythromycin activity.

NDC 0378-6400-01

MYLAN®

**ERYTHROMYCIN
ETHYLSUCCINATE
TABLETS, USP
400 mg**
Erythromycin Activity

100 TABLETS   **Rx only**

Dispense in a tight,
light-resistant container
using a child-resistant closure.

**STORE AT CONTROLLED
ROOM TEMPERATURE
15°-30°C (59°-86°F).
PROTECT FROM LIGHT.**

Usual Adult Dose: One
tablet every six hours.
See insert.

**DOSAGE MAY BE GIVEN
WITHOUT REGARD TO MEALS.**

Mylan Pharmaceuticals Inc.
Morgantown, WV 26505

RM6400A5

400 mg

0378-6400-01

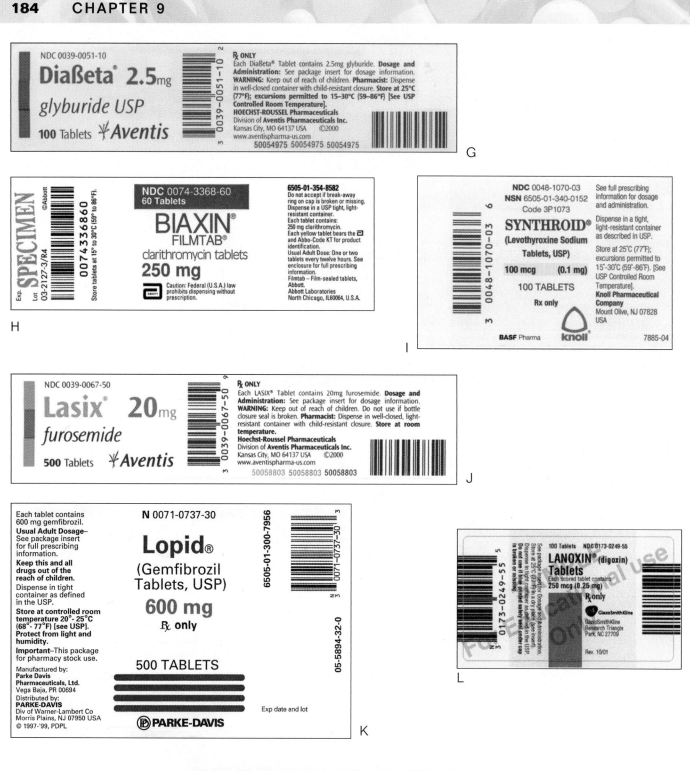

NDC 0039-0051-10

Diaßeta® 2.5mg

glyburide USP

100 Tablets ⚕ *Aventis*

Rx ONLY
Each DiaBeta® Tablet contains 2.5mg glyburide. **Dosage and Administration:** See package insert for dosage information. **WARNING:** Keep out of reach of children. **Pharmacist:** Dispense in well-closed container with child-resistant closure. Store at 25°C (77°F); excursions permitted to 15–30°C (59–86°F) [See USP Controlled Room Temperature].
HOECHST-ROUSSEL Pharmaceuticals
Division of **Aventis** Pharmaceuticals Inc.
Kansas City, MO 64137 USA   ©2000
www.aventispharma-us.com
50054975 50054975 50054975

G

SPECIMEN ©Abbott
Exp. Lot 03-2127-3/R4
Store tablets at 15° to 30°C (59° to 86°F).
00743368860

NDC 0074-3368-60
60 Tablets

BIAXIN®
FILMTAB®
clarithromycin tablets
250 mg

Caution: Federal (U.S.A.) law prohibits dispensing without prescription.

6505-01-354-8582
Do not accept if break-away ring on cap is broken or missing.
Dispense in a USP tight, light-resistant container.
Each tablet contains: 250 mg clarithromycin.
Each yellow tablet bears the 🄰 and Abbo-Code KT for product identification.
Usual Adult Dose: One or two tablets every twelve hours. See enclosure for full prescribing information.
Filmtab – Film-sealed tablets, Abbott.
Abbott Laboratories
North Chicago, IL 60064, U.S.A.

H

NDC 0048-1070-03
NSN 6505-01-340-0152
Code 3P1073

SYNTHROID®
(Levothyroxine Sodium Tablets, USP)

100 mcg   (0.1 mg)

100 TABLETS

Rx only

BASF Pharma   knoll

See full prescribing information for dosage and administration.
Dispense in a tight, light-resistant container as described in USP.
Store at 25°C (77°F); excursions permitted to 15°-30°C (59°-86°F). [See USP Controlled Room Temperature].
Knoll Pharmaceutical Company
Mount Olive, NJ 07828 USA

7885-04

I

NDC 0039-0067-50

Lasix® 20mg

furosemide

500 Tablets ⚕ *Aventis*

Rx ONLY
Each LASIX® Tablet contains 20mg furosemide. **Dosage and Administration:** See package insert for dosage information. **WARNING:** Keep out of reach of children. Do not use if bottle closure seal is broken. **Pharmacist:** Dispense in well-closed, light-resistant container with child-resistant closure. **Store at room temperature.**
Hoechst-Roussel Pharmaceuticals
Division of **Aventis** Pharmaceuticals Inc.
Kansas City, MO 64137 USA   ©2000
www.aventispharma-us.com
50058803 50058803 50058803

J

Each tablet contains 600 mg gemfibrozil.
Usual Adult Dosage– See package insert for full prescribing information.
Keep this and all drugs out of the reach of children.
Dispense in tight container as defined in the USP.
Store at controlled room temperature 20°- 25°C (68°- 77°F) [see USP].
Protect from light and humidity.
Important–This package for pharmacy stock use.
Manufactured by:
Parke Davis Pharmaceuticals, Ltd.
Vega Baja, PR 00694
Distributed by:
PARKE-DAVIS
Div of Warner-Lambert Co
Morris Plains, NJ 07950 USA
© 1997-'99, PDPL

N 0071-0737-30

Lopid®
(Gemfibrozil Tablets, USP)
600 mg
Rx only

500 TABLETS

6505-01-300-7956
0071-0737-30
05-5894-32-0
Exp date and lot

Ⓟ **PARKE-DAVIS**

K

100 Tablets   NDC 0173-0249-55

LANOXIN® (digoxin)
Tablets
Each scored tablet contains 250 mcg (0.25 mg)

Rx only

GlaxoSmithKline
Research Triangle Park, NC 27709

See package insert for Dosage and Administration. Store at 25°C (77°F) in a dry place (see insert). Dispense in tight container as defined in the USP. Do not use if blue printed safety seal under cap is broken or missing.

0173-0249-55

Rev. 10/01

For educational use only

L

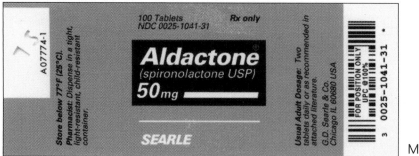

100 Tablets   Rx only
NDC 0025-1041-31

Aldactone®
(spironolactone USP)
50mg

SEARLE

A07774-1
Store below 77°F (25°C).
Pharmacist: Dispense in a tight, light-resistant, child-resistant container.

Usual Adult Dosage: Two tablets daily or as recommended in attached literature.
G.D. Searle & Co.
Chicago IL 60680 USA

FOR POSITION ONLY
UPC @100%
0025-1041-31

M

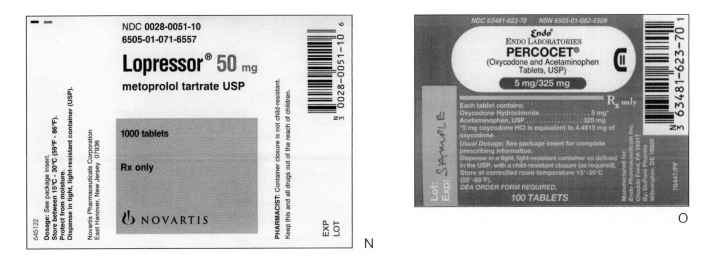

Calculate one dose of the medications indicated on the MAR. Labels P–S provided on the following page are the drugs available. Indicate the letter corresponding to the label you select.

46. Select: _____   48. Select: _____

    Give: _____   Give: _____

47. Select: _____   49. Select: _____

    Give: _____   Give: _____

	ORIGINAL ORDER DATE	DATE STARTED / RENEWED	MEDICATION - DOSAGE	ROUTE	SCHEDULE 11-7	7-3	3-11	DATE 3/8/xx 11-7	7-3	3-11	DATE 11-7	7-3	3-11	DATE 11-7	7-3	3-11	DATE 11-7	7-3	3-11
46.	3/8/xx	3/8	Zantac 300 mg h.s.	PO			10			10 MS										
47.	3/8/xx	3/8	Inderal 80 mg b.i.d.	PO		9	9		9 GP	9 MS										
48.	3/8/xx	3/8	Lasix 20 mg b.i.d.	PO		9	9		9 GP	9 MS										
49.	3/8/xx	3/8	Slow-K 600 mg q.d.	PO		9			9 GP											

MEDICATION ADMINISTRATION RECORD

PAGE _____ of _____

PRN

INJECTION SITES

B - RIGHT ARM
C - RIGHT ABDOMEN
D - RIGHT ANTERIOR THIGH
G - LEFT ARM
H - LEFT ABDOMEN
J - LEFT ANTERIOR THIGH
L - LEFT BUTTOCKS
M - RIGHT BUTTOCKS

DATE GIVEN	TIME	INT.	ONE - TIME MEDICATION - DOSAGE	RT.	11-7	7-3	3-11	...

SCHEDULE

SIGNATURE OF NURSE ADMINISTERING MEDICATIONS

11-7   GP G. Pickar R.N.

7-3

MS M. Smith, R.N.

3-11

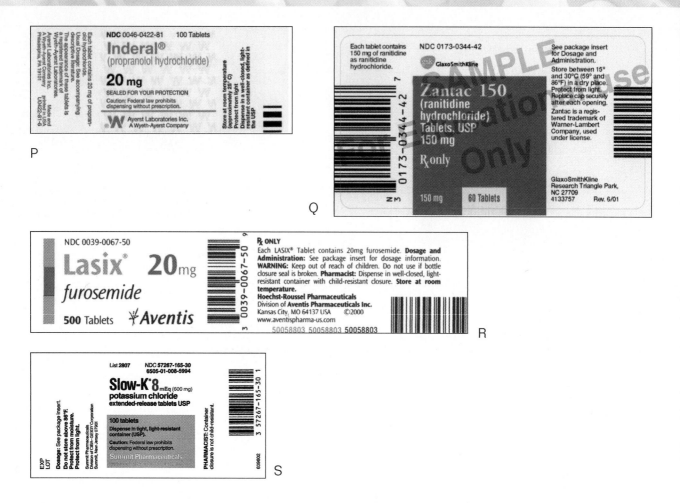

P

Q

R

S

50. Critical Thinking Skill: Describe the strategy to prevent this medication error.

possible scenario

Suppose the physician ordered *Betapen VK 5 mL (250 mg) p.o. q.i.d.* for a patient with an upper respiratory tract infection. The pharmacy supplied *Betapen VK 125 mg per 5 mL*. In a rush to administer the medication on time, the nurse read the order as "Betapen VK 5 mL," checked the label for Betapen VK and poured that amount and administered the drug. In a hurry, the nurse failed to recognize that 5 mL of the supply dosage of 125 mg per 5 mL did not provide the ordered dosage of 250 mg and underdosed the patient.

potential outcome

The patient received one-half of the ordered dosage of antibiotic needed to treat the respiratory infection. If this error was not caught, the patient's infection would not be halted. This would add to the patient's illness time and might lead to a more severe infection. Additional tests might be required to determine why the patient was not responding to the medication.

prevention

_____

_____

After completing these problems, see page 484 to check your answers.

CHAPTER

10

Parenteral Dosage of Drugs

OBJECTIVES

Upon mastery of Chapter 10, you will be able to calculate the parenteral dosages of drugs. To accomplish this you will also be able to:

- Apply the three steps for dosage calculations: convert, think, and calculate.
- Use the formula $\frac{D}{H} \times Q = X$ to calculate the amount to give.
- Measure insulin in a matching insulin syringe.
- Compare the calibration of U-100 insulin syringe units to milliliters (100 U = 1 mL).

The term *parenteral* is used to designate routes of administration other than gastrointestinal, such as the injection routes of IM, SC, ID, and IV. In this chapter intramuscular (IM), subcutaneous (SC), and intravenous (IV) injections will be emphasized. Intravenous flow-rate calculations are discussed in Chapters 14–16.

Intramuscular indicates an injection given into a muscle, such as Demerol given IM for pain. *Subcutaneous* means an injection given into the subcutaneous tissue, such as an insulin injection for the management of diabetes given SC. *Intravenous* refers to an injection given directly into a vein, either by direct injection (IV push) or diluted in a larger volume of intravenous fluid and administered as part of an intravenous infusion. When a patient has an IV site or IV infusing, the IV injection route is frequently used to administer parenteral drugs rather than the IM route. *Intradermal* (ID) means an injection given under the skin, such as an allergy test or tuberculin skin test.

INJECTABLE SOLUTIONS

Most parenteral medications are prepared in liquid or solution form, and packaged in dosage vials, ampules, or prefilled syringes (Figure 10-1). Injectable drugs are measured in syringes.

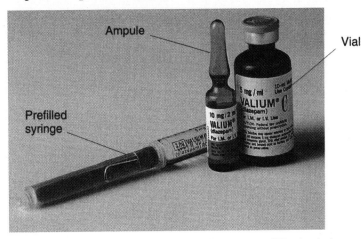

FIGURE 10-1 Parenteral Solutions (Courtesy of Roche Laboratories)

> **RULE**
>
> The maximum dosage volume to be administered per intramuscular injection site for:
> 1. An average 150 lb adult = 3 mL
> 2. Children age 6 to 12 years = 2 mL
> 3. Children birth to age 5 years = 1 mL

For example, if you must give an adult patient 4 milliliters of a drug, divide the dose into two injections of 2 milliliters each. The condition of the patient must be considered when applying this rule. *Adults or children who have decreased muscle or subcutaneous tissue mass or poor circulation may not be able to tolerate the maximum dosage volumes.*

To solve parenteral dosage problems, apply the same steps used for the calculation of oral dosages.

> **REMEMBER**
>
> | Step 1 | Convert | All units of measurement to the same system, and all units to the same size. |
> | Step 2 | Think | Estimate the logical amount. |
> | Step 3 | Calculate | $\dfrac{\text{D (desired)}}{\text{H (have)}} \times \text{Q (quantity)} = \text{X (amount)}$ |

Use the following rules to help you decide which size syringe to select to administer parenteral dosages.

> **RULE**
>
> As you calculate parenteral dosages:
> 1. Round the amount to be administered (X) to tenths if the amount is greater than 1 mL, and measure it in a 3 mL syringe.
> 2. Measure amounts of less than 1 mL rounded to hundredths, and all amounts less than 0.5 mL, in a 1 mL syringe.
> 3. Amounts of 0.5 to 1 mL, calculated in tenths, can be accurately measured in either a 1 mL or 3 mL syringe.

Let's look at some examples of appropriate syringe selections for the dosages to be measured and review how to read the calibrations. Refer to Chapter 6, *Equipment Used in Dosage Measurement*, regarding how to measure medication in a syringe. To review, the top black ring should align with the desired calibration, not the raised midsection and not the bottom ring. Look carefully at the illustrations that follow.

Example 1:

Measure 0.33 mL in a 1 mL syringe.

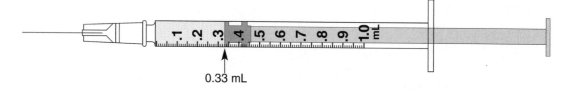

0.33 mL

Example 2:

Round 1.33 mL to 1.3 mL, and measure in a 3 mL syringe.

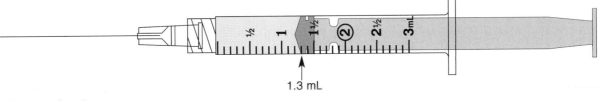

1.3 mL

Example 3:

Measure 0.6 mL in either a 1 mL or 3 mL syringe. (Notice that the amount is measured in tenths so the 3 mL syringe would be preferable.)

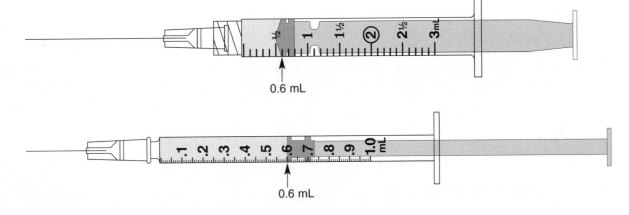

0.6 mL

0.6 mL

Example 4:

Measure 0.65 mL in a 1 mL syringe. (Notice that the amount is measured in hundredths and is less than 1 mL.)

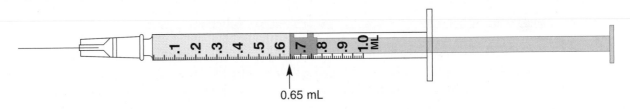

0.65 mL

An amber color has been added to selected syringe drawings throughout the text *to simulate a specific amount of medication,* as indicated in the example or problem. Because the color used may not correspond to the actual color of the medications named, **it must not be used as a reference for identifying medications.**

Let's look at some examples of parenteral dosage calculations.

Example 1:

The drug order reads *Vistaril 100 mg IM stat.* Available is *Vistaril Intramuscular Solution 50 mg/mL* in a 10 mL multiple-dose vial. How many milliliters should be administered to the patient?

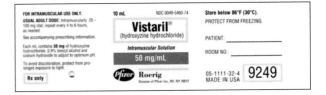

| Step 1 | Convert | No conversion is necessary. |
| Step 2 | Think | You want to give more than 1 mL. In fact, you want to give twice as much, because 100 mg is twice as much as 50 mg. |

Step 3   Calculate $\dfrac{D}{H} \times Q = \dfrac{\overset{2}{\cancel{20}\ \cancel{mg}}}{\underset{1}{\cancel{10}\ \cancel{mg}}} \times 1\,mL = 2\,mL$

given intramuscularly immediately

Select a *3 mL syringe and measure 2 mL* of Vistaril 50 mg/mL. Look carefully at the illustration to clearly identify the part of the black rubber stopper that measures the exact dosage.

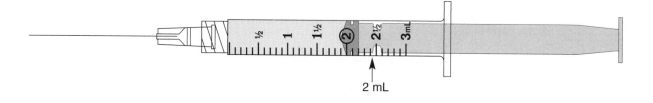

2 mL

Example 2:

The drug order reads *Nubain 5 mg SC q.3–6h p.r.n., pain*. The 10 mL multiple dose vial is labeled *Nubain 20 mg per mL injection*.

Step 1   Convert   No conversion necessary.

Step 2   Think   You want to give less than 1 mL. Actually you want to give $\dfrac{1}{4}$ or 0.25 of a mL.

Step 3   Calculate $\dfrac{D}{H} \times Q = \dfrac{\overset{1}{\cancel{5}\ \cancel{mg}}}{\underset{4}{\cancel{20}\ \cancel{mg}}} \times 1\,mL = \dfrac{1}{4}\,mL = 0.25\,mL$

given subcutaneously as needed for pain every 3 to 6 hours

NDC 63481-509-05

NUBAIN®
(Nalbuphine HCl) R_x only
20 mg/mL injection
10 mL Multiple Dose Vial

Each mL contains: 20 mg nalbuphine HCl, 0.94% sodium citrate hydrous, 1.26% citric acid anhydrous, and 0.2% of a 9:1 mixture of methyl and propylparaben, as preservatives. pH is adjusted, if necessary, to 3.5 to 3.7 with hydrochloric acid.

FOR IM, SC OR IV USE
Usual Dosage: See package insert for complete prescribing information.
Store at 25°C (77°F); excursions permitted to 15°-30°C (59°-86°F).
PROTECT FROM EXCESSIVE LIGHT.

Manufactured for:
Endo Pharmaceuticals Inc.
Chadds Ford, PA 19317
                          70361/OK

Lot: SAMPLE

Exp:

> **REMEMBER**
>
> Dosages measured in hundredths (such as 0.25 mL) and all amounts less than 0.5 mL should be prepared in a 1 mL syringe, which is calibrated in hundredths. However, if the route is IM, you may need to change needles to a more appropriate length.

Select a *1 mL syringe and measure 0.25 mL* of Nubain 20 mg/mL. Look carefully at the illustration to clearly identify the part of the black rubber stopper that measures the exact dosage.

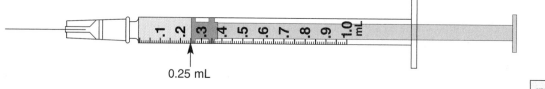

0.25 mL

Example 3:

Drug order: *meperidine hydrochloride 60 mg IM q.3–4h p.r.n., pain*

Available: *meperidine HCl injection 75 mg/mL*

Step 1   Convert   No conversion is necessary.

Step 2   Think   You want to give less than 1 mL but more than 0.5 mL.

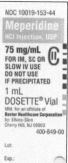

NDC 10019-153-44
Meperidine
HCl Injection, USP
75 mg/mL
FOR IM, SC OR
SLOW IV USE
DO NOT USE
IF PRECIPITATED
1 mL
DOSETTE® Vial
Mfd. for an affiliate of
Baxter Healthcare Corporation
by: Elkins-Sinn
Cherry Hill, NJ 08003
                    400-849-00

Lot:

Exp.:

Step 3 Calculate $\dfrac{D}{H} \times Q = \dfrac{\overset{4}{\cancel{60}\,\text{mg}}}{\underset{5}{\cancel{75}\,\text{mg}}} \times 1\ \text{mL} = \dfrac{4}{5}\ \text{mL} = 0.8\ \text{mL}$

given intramuscularly every 3 to 4 hours as needed for pain

Select a 1 mL or 3 mL syringe and draw up all of the contents of the 1 mL dosette vial. Then *discard 0.2 mL to administer 0.8 mL* of meperidine 75 mg/mL. You must discard the 0.2 mL in the presence of another nurse because meperidine is a controlled substance. As a controlled substance, you cannot just leave 0.2 mL in the single dosette vial.

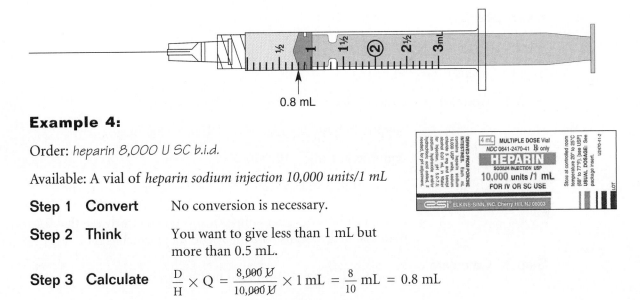

0.8 mL

Example 4:

Order: *heparin 8,000 U SC b.i.d.*

Available: A vial of *heparin sodium injection 10,000 units/1 mL*

Step 1 Convert   No conversion is necessary.

Step 2 Think   You want to give less than 1 mL but more than 0.5 mL.

Step 3 Calculate $\dfrac{D}{H} \times Q = \dfrac{8,000\ \cancel{U}}{10,000\ \cancel{U}} \times 1\ \text{mL} = \dfrac{8}{10}\ \text{mL} = 0.8\ \text{mL}$

given subcutaneously twice daily

Select a *1 mL* or a *3 mL syringe and measure 0.8 mL* of heparin 10,000 U/mL. Heparin is a very potent anticoagulant drug. It is safest to measure it in a 1 mL syringe.

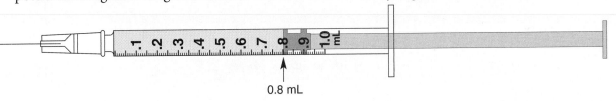

0.8 mL

Example 5:

Order: *Cleocin Phosphate 150 mg IM q.12h*

Available: *Cleocin Phosphate (clindamycin injection) 300 mg/2 mL*

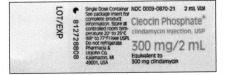

Step 1 Convert   No conversion is necessary.

Step 2 Think   You want to give less than 2 mL. Actually, you want to give 150 mg, which is $\frac{1}{2}$ of 300 mg and $\frac{1}{2}$ of 2 mL, or 1 mL. Calculate to double-check your estimate.

Step 3 Calculate $\dfrac{D}{H} \times Q = \dfrac{\overset{1}{\cancel{150}\,\text{mg}}}{\underset{2}{\cancel{300}\,\text{mg}}} \times 2\ \text{mL} = \dfrac{\overset{1}{\cancel{2}}}{\underset{1}{\cancel{2}}}\ \text{mL} = 1\ \text{mL}$

given intramuscularly every 12 hours

Select a *3 mL syringe, and measure 1 mL* of Cleocin 300 mg/2 mL.

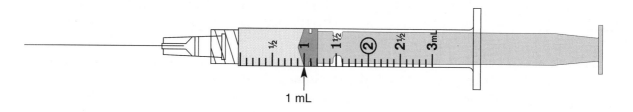

1 mL

Example 6:

Order: *Robinul 150 mcg IM stat*

Supply: *Robinul 0.2 mg/mL*

Step 1	Convert	Order: *Robinul 150 mcg*
		Supply: Robinul 0.2 mg = 0.2 × 1000 = 200 mcg
		Equivalent: 1 mg = 1000 mcg

Step 2   Think   You want to give less than 1 mL but more than 0.5 mL. Be careful with the units and decimals. Don't be fooled into thinking 0.2 mg is less than 150 mcg. After conversion you can clearly see that 0.2 mg is more than 150 mcg; because 0.2 mg = 200 mcg, which is more than 150 mcg.

Step 3   Calculate $\dfrac{D}{H} \times Q = \dfrac{\overset{3}{\cancel{150 \text{ mcg}}}}{\underset{4}{\cancel{200 \text{ mcg}}}} \times 1 \text{ mL} = \dfrac{3}{4} \text{ mL} = 0.75 \text{ mL}$

given intramuscularly immediately

Select a *1 mL syringe, and measure 0.75 mL* of Robinul 0.2 mg/mL. You may have to change needles, as this is an IM injection.

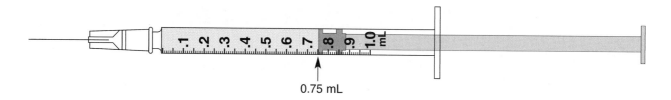

0.75 mL

Example 7:

The drug order reads *morphine sulfate gr $\frac{1}{6}$ IM q.3–4h p.r.n., pain,* and the label on the dosette vial states *morphine sulfate 10 mg/mL.*

Step 1   Convert   Order: *morphine sulfate* $gr\dfrac{1}{6} = \dfrac{1}{\cancel{6}_{1}} \times \dfrac{\overset{10}{\cancel{60}}}{1} = 10 \text{ mg}$

Equivalent: gr i = 60 mg

Supply: morphine sulfate 10 mg/mL

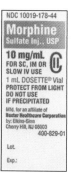

Step 2   Think   Now it is obvious that you want to give 1 mL.

Step 3   Calculate $\dfrac{D}{H} \times Q = \dfrac{\cancel{10}^{\,1}\ \cancel{mg}}{\underset{1}{\cancel{10}}\ \cancel{mg}} \times 1\ mL = 1\ mL$

given intramuscularly every 3 to 4 hours as needed for pain

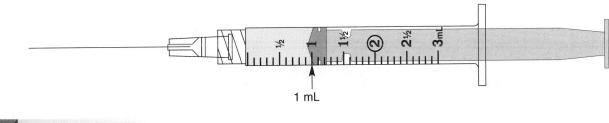

1 mL

QUICK REVIEW

- To solve parenteral dosage problems, apply the three steps to dosage calculations:

  STEP 1   CONVERT

  STEP 2   THINK

  STEP 3   CALCULATE $\dfrac{\mathbf{D}\ (desired)}{\mathbf{H}\ (have)} \times \mathbf{Q}$ (quantity) $= \mathbf{X}$ (amount)

- Prepare a maximum of 3 mL per intramuscular injection site for an average-size adult, 2 mL per site for children ages 6 through 12, and 0.5 to 1 mL for children under age 6.
- Calculate dose volumes and prepare injectable fractional doses in a syringe using these guidelines:
  - Standard doses more than 1 mL: Round to *tenths* and measure in a 3 mL syringe. The 3 mL syringe is calibrated to 0.1 mL increments. Example: 1.53 mL is rounded to 1.5 mL and drawn up in a 3 mL syringe.
  - Small (less than 0.5 mL) doses: Round to *hundredths* and measure in a 1 mL syringe. Critical care and children's doses less than 1 mL calculated in hundredths should also be measured in a 1 mL syringe. The 1 mL syringe is calibrated in 0.01 mL increments. Example: 0.257 mL is rounded to 0.26 mL and drawn up in a 1 mL syringe.
  - Amounts of 0.5–1 mL calculated in tenths, can be accurately measured in either a 1 mL or 3 mL syringe.

REVIEW SET 27

Calculate the amount you will prepare for each dose. The labels provided represent the drugs available. Draw an arrow to the syringe calibration that corresponds to the amount you will administer. Indicate doses that have to be divided.

1. Order: *Depo-Provera 1 g IM stat*

    Give: _____ mL

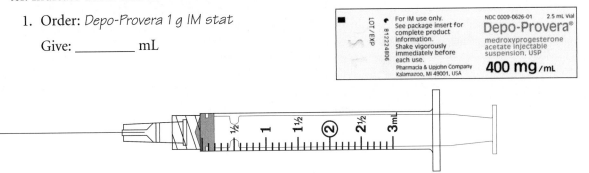

2. Order: *Bicillin CR 900/300 2,400,000 U IM stat*

   Give: _____ mL

BICILLIN® C-R 900/300
1,200,000 UNITS per 2 mL
(900,000 UNITS PENICILLIN G BENZATHINE
AND 300,000 UNITS PENICILLIN G PROCAINE
INJECTABLE SUSPENSION)
FOR DEEP IM INJECTION ONLY

Dist. By: Monarch Pharm., Inc.
Bristol, TN
TUBEX®
TL 128-4
EXP

0.5 mL   1 mL   1.5 mL   2 mL

0.5 mL   1 mL   1.5 mL   2 mL

3. Order: *digoxin 600 mcg IV stat*

   Give: _____ mL

LANOXIN®   2 mL
(digoxin) Injection   R only
500 mcg (0.5 mg) in 2 mL
(250 mcg [0.25 mg] per mL)
Store at 25°C (77°F) [see insert].
PROTECT FROM LIGHT.
Dist.: GlaxoSmithKline
Research Triangle Park, NC 27709
Made in Canada
4144627
Rev. 3/02   **220201**

LOT

EXP

½   1   1½   ②   2½   3mL

4. Order: *dexamethasone sodium phosphate 1.5 mg IM q.12h*

   Give: _____ mL

NDC 63323-165-01   16501
DEXAMETHASONE
SODIUM PHOSPHATE
INJECTION, USP
equivalent to
4 mg/mL
Dexamethasone Phosphate
For IM or IV Use, See Insert
For Other Routes
1 mL
Sterile, Nonpyrogenic
Usual Dosage: See Insert.
Rx only
American Pharmaceutical
Partners, Inc.
Los Angeles, CA 90024
401779A

.1   .2   .3   .4   .5   .6   .7   .8   .9   1.0
                                              mL

5. Order: *Tigan 200 mg IM stat, then 100 mg q.6h p.r.n., nausea*

   Give: _____ mL stat and _____ mL q.6h

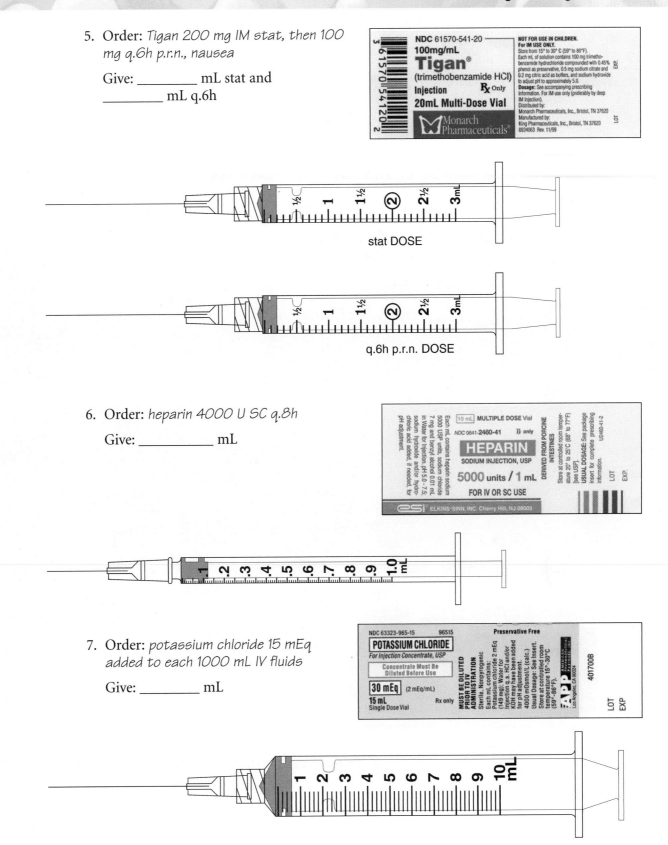

NDC 61570-541-20
100mg/mL
Tigan®
(trimethobenzamide HCl)
Injection ℞ Only
20mL Multi-Dose Vial
Monarch Pharmaceuticals®

NOT FOR USE IN CHILDREN.
For IM USE ONLY.
Store from 15° to 30° C (59° to 86°F).
Each mL of solution contains 100 mg trimethobenzamide hydrochloride compounded with 0.45% phenol as preservative, 0.5 mg sodium citrate and 0.2 mg citric acid as buffers, and sodium hydroxide to adjust pH to approximately 5.0.
Dosage: See accompanying prescribing information. For IM use only (preferably by deep IM injection).
Distributed by:
Monarch Pharmaceuticals, Inc., Bristol, TN 37620
Manufactured by:
King Pharmaceuticals, Inc., Bristol, TN 37620
0934063 Rev. 11/99

stat DOSE

q.6h p.r.n. DOSE

6. Order: *heparin 4000 U SC q.8h*

   Give: _____ mL

10 mL MULTIPLE DOSE Vial
NDC 0641-2460-41   ℞ only
HEPARIN
SODIUM INJECTION, USP
5000 units / 1 mL
FOR IV OR SC USE
esi ELKINS-SINN, INC. Cherry Hill, NJ 08003

DERIVED FROM PORCINE INTESTINES

Store at controlled room temperature 20° to 25°C (68° to 77°F) [see USP].
USUAL DOSAGE: See package insert for complete prescribing information. U2460-41-2

Each mL contains heparin sodium 5000 USP units, sodium chloride 7 mg and benzyl alcohol 0.01 mL in Water for Injection. pH 5.0 - 7.5; sodium hydroxide and/or hydrochloric acid added, if needed, for pH adjustment.

7. Order: *potassium chloride 15 mEq added to each 1000 mL IV fluids*

   Give: _____ mL

NDC 63323-965-15   96515
POTASSIUM CHLORIDE
For Injection Concentrate, USP
Concentrate Must Be Diluted Before Use
30 mEq (2 mEq/mL)
15 mL
Single Dose Vial   Rx only

Preservative Free

MUST BE DILUTED PRIOR TO IV ADMINISTRATION
Sterile, Nonpyrogenic.
Each mL contains:
Potassium chloride 2 mEq (149 mg); Water for Injection q.s. HCl and/or KOH may have been added for pH adjustment.
4000 mOsmol/L (calc.)
Usual Dosage: See insert.
Store at controlled room temperature 15°-30°C (59°-86°F).

401700B
LOT
EXP

8. Order: *meperidine hydrochloride 35 mg IM q.4h p.r.n., pain*

   Give: _____ mL

9. Order: *Bumex 500 mcg IV bolus stat*

   Give: _____ mL

10. Order: *Morphine sulfate gr $\frac{1}{4}$ IM q.3–4h p.r.n., pain*

    Give: _____ mL

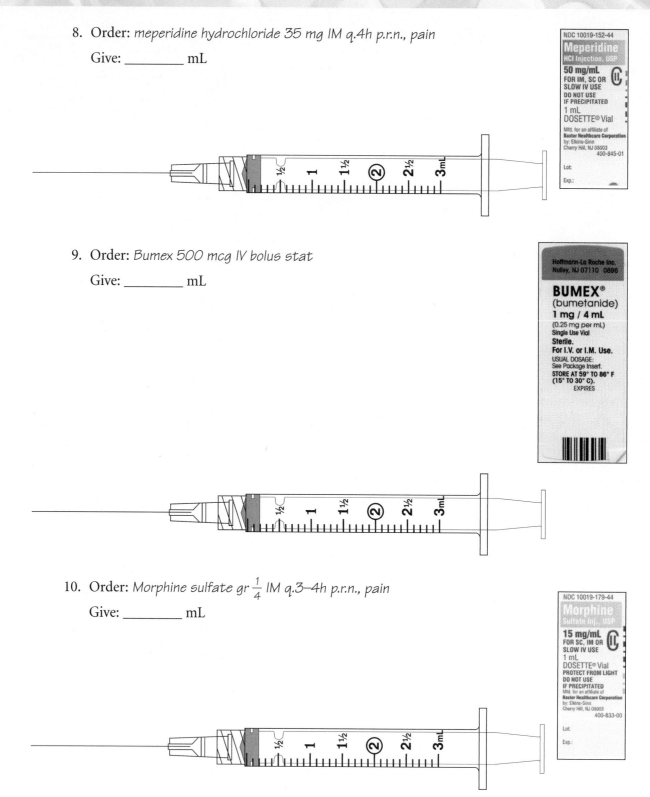

11. Order: *methotrexate 30 mg IM q.d. ×
5 days*

    Give: _____ mL

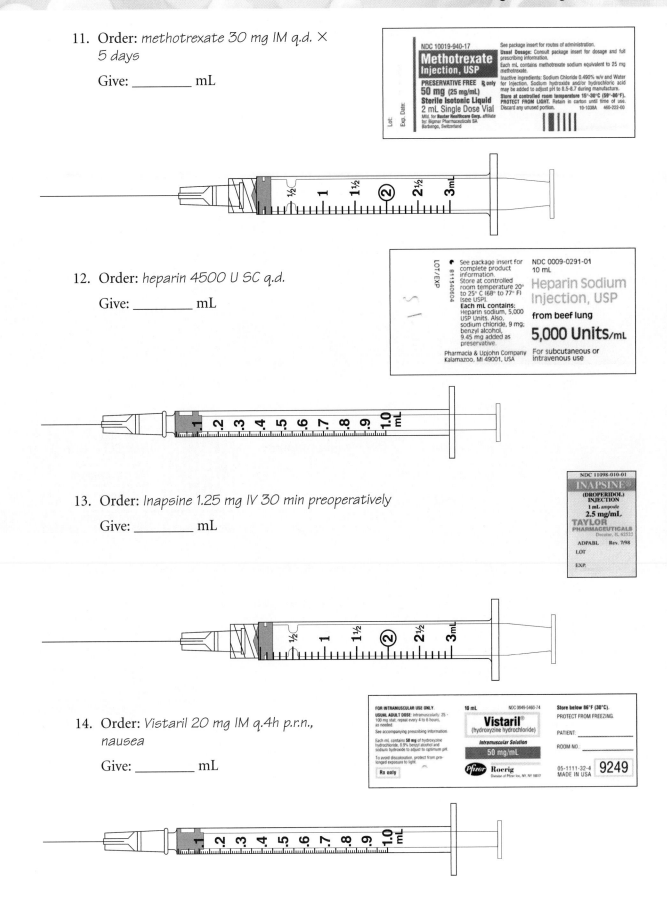

NDC 10019-940-17

**Methotrexate
Injection, USP**

PRESERVATIVE FREE ℞ only
50 mg (25 mg/mL)
**Sterile Isotonic Liquid
2 mL Single Dose Vial**
Mfd. for **Baxter Healthcare Corp.** affiliate
by: Bigmar Pharmaceuticals SA
Barbengo, Switzerland

See package insert for routes of administration.
Usual Dosage: Consult package insert for dosage and full
prescribing information.
Each mL contains methotrexate sodium equivalent to 25 mg
methotrexate.
Inactive ingredients: Sodium Chloride 0.490% w/v and Water
for Injection. Sodium hydroxide and/or hydrochloric acid
may be added to adjust pH to 8.5-8.7 during manufacture.
**Store at controlled room temperature 15°-30°C (59°-86°F).
PROTECT FROM LIGHT.** Retain in carton until time of use.
Discard any unused portion.   10-1038A   460-222-00

Lot:
Exp. Date:

12. Order: *heparin 4500 U SC q.d.*

    Give: _____ mL

LOT/EXP
811540604

• See package insert for
complete product
information.
Store at controlled
room temperature 20°
to 25° C (68° to 77° F)
(see USPI).
Each mL contains:
Heparin sodium, 5,000
USP Units. Also,
sodium chloride, 9 mg;
benzyl alcohol,
9.45 mg added as
preservative.

Pharmacia & Upjohn Company
Kalamazoo, MI 49001, USA

NDC 0009-0291-01
10 mL

**Heparin Sodium
Injection, USP**

from beef lung

5,000 Units/mL

For subcutaneous or
intravenous use

13. Order: *Inapsine 1.25 mg IV 30 min preoperatively*

    Give: _____ mL

NDC 11098-010-01

INAPSINE®
**(DROPERIDOL)
INJECTION**
1 mL ampoule
2.5 mg/mL
**TAYLOR
PHARMACEUTICALS**
Decatur, IL 62522

ADPABL   Rev. 7/98

LOT

EXP.

14. Order: *Vistaril 20 mg IM q.4h p.r.n.,
nausea*

    Give: _____ mL

FOR INTRAMUSCULAR USE ONLY
USUAL ADULT DOSE: Intramuscularly: 25 -
100 mg stat, repeat every 4 to 6 hours,
as needed.
See accompanying prescribing information.

Each mL contains **50 mg** of hydroxyzine
hydrochloride, 0.9% benzyl alcohol and
sodium hydroxide to adjust to optimum pH.

To avoid discoloration, protect from prolonged exposure to light.

Rx only

10 mL   NDC 0049-5460-74

Vistaril®
(hydroxyzine hydrochloride)

Intramuscular Solution

50 mg/mL

Pfizer Roerig
Division of Pfizer Inc. NY, NY 10017

Store below 86°F (30°C).
PROTECT FROM FREEZING.

PATIENT: _____

ROOM NO.: _____

05-1111-32-4   **9249**
MADE IN USA

15. Order: *Terramycin 150 mg IM q.12h*

    Give: _____ mL

16. Order: *Calcijex 1.5 mcg IV 3 times/wk q.o.d. M-W-F*

    Give: _____ mL

17. Order: *vitamin B$_{12}$ 0.5 mg IM once/week*

    Give: _____ mL

18. Order: *Zantac 20 mg IM q.6h*

    Give: _____ mL

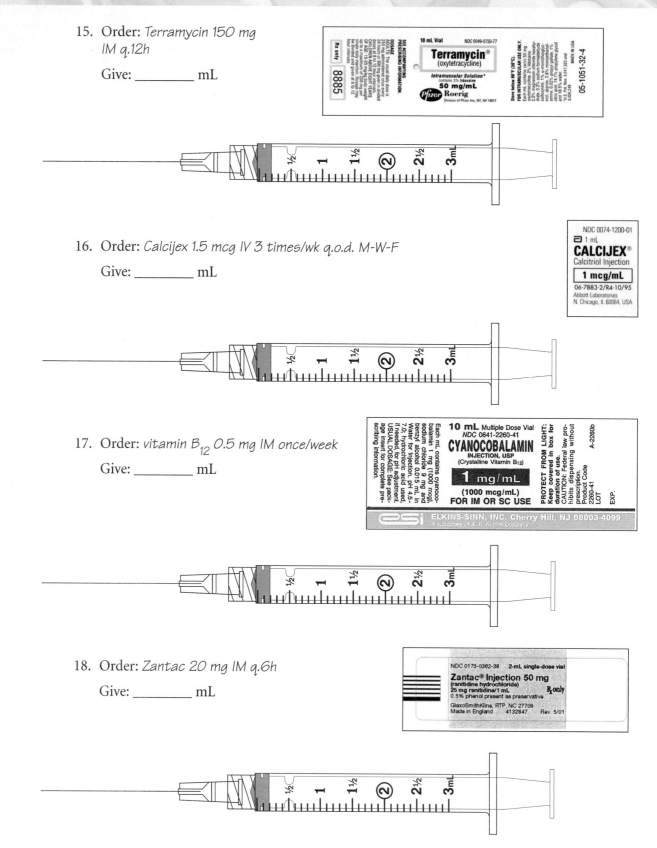

19. Order: *Phenergan 12.5 mg IM stat*

    Give: _____ mL

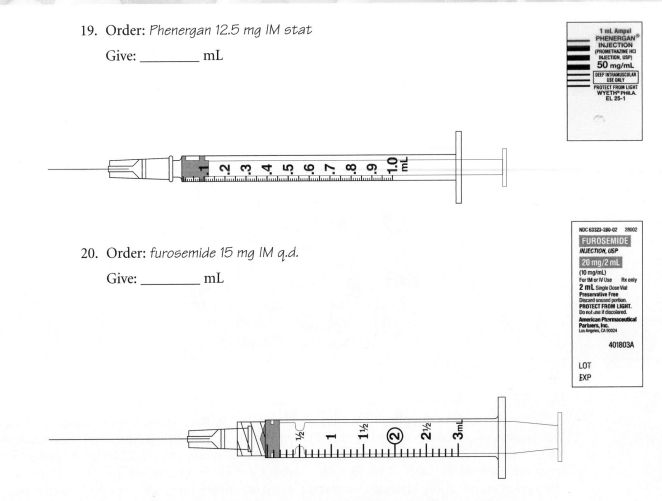

20. Order: *furosemide 15 mg IM q.d.*

    Give: _____ mL

After completing these problems, see pages 485–488 to check your answers.

INSULIN

Insulin, a hormone made in the pancreas, is necessary for the metabolism of glucose, proteins, and fats. Patients who are deficient in insulin (insulin-dependent diabetics) are required to take insulin by injection daily. Insulin is a ready-to-use solution that is measured in units (U). The most common supply dosage is *100 U per mL.*

MATH TIP

The supply dosage of insulin is **100 U per mL**, which is abbreviated on the label as **U-100**. Think: U-100 = 100 U per mL.

Insulin is also available as 500 U per mL (or U-500). This supply dosage is used only under special circumstances and is not commercially dispensed.

CAUTION

Accuracy in insulin preparation and administration is critical. Inaccuracy is potentially life-threatening. It is essential for nurses to *understand the information on the insulin label*, to correctly *interpret the insulin order*, and to *select the correct syringe* to measure insulin for administration.

Insulin Label

Figure 10-2 identifies the essential components of insulin labels. The insulin label includes important information. For example, the *brand and generic names,* the *supply dosage* or *concentration,* and the *storage* instructions are details commonly found on most parenteral drug labels. Chapter 8 explains these and other typical drug label components. Let's look closely at different insulin types classified by the insulin *action times* and insulin *species,* which are critical identifiers of this important hormone supplement.

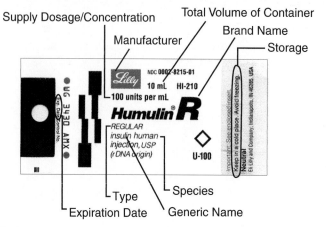

FIGURE 10-2 Insulin Label

Insulin Action Times

Figure 10-3 shows a sampling of insulin labels arranged by the three action times: rapid-acting (Regular, Lispro), intermediate-acting (Lente, NPH or *Neutral Protamine Hagedorn*), and long-acting (Ultralente). Regular and NPH insulin are the two types of insulin used most often. Notice the uppercase, bold letters on each insulin label: **R** for Regular insulin; **L** for Lente insulin; **N** for NPH insulin; and **U** for Ultralente insulin. These letters are important visual identifiers when selecting the insulin type.

Species of Insulin

Insulin comes from various sources:
- human insulin (the most common species)
  a. biosynthetic—bacteria genetically altered to create human insulin
  b. semisynthetic—pork insulin chemically altered to produce human insulin
- beef insulin—from the pancreas of cattle
- pork insulin—from the pancreas of pigs
- beef–pork mixture—a combination of beef and pork insulin
  Note: Beef–pork insulins are being phased out.

> **CAUTION**
>
> Avoid a potentially life-threatening medication error. Carefully read the label, and compare it to the drug order to ensure that you select the correct action time and species of insulin.

Premixed, Combination Insulin

Two premixed insulin combinations that are commercially available are 70/30 U-100 insulin and 50/50 U-100 insulin (Figure 10-4, page 202). The 70/30 insulin concentration means there is 70% NPH insulin and 30% Regular insulin in each unit. Therefore, if the physician orders 10 units of 70/30 insulin, the patient would receive 7 units of NPH insulin (70% or 0.7 × 10 U = 7 U) and 3 units of Regular insulin (30% or 0.3 × 10 U = 3 U) in the 70/30 concentration. If the physician orders 20 units of 70/30 insulin, the patient would receive 14 units (0.7 × 20 = 14) of NPH and 6 units (0.3 × 20 = 6) of Regular insulin.

The 50/50 insulin concentration means there is 50% NPH insulin and 50% Regular insulin in each unit. Therefore, if the physician orders 12 units of 50/50 insulin, the patient would receive 6 units of NPH insulin (50% or 0.5 × 12 U = 6 U) and 6 units of Regular insulin (50% or 0.5 × 12 U = 6 U).

Rapid-Acting

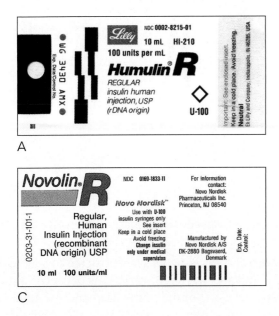

A

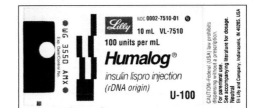

B

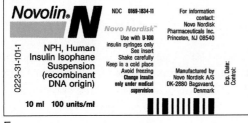

C

Intermediate-Acting

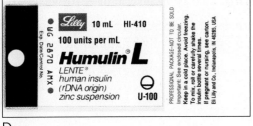

D

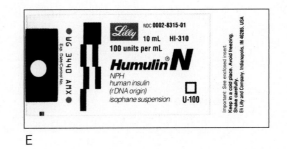

E

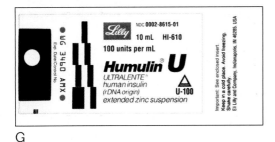

F

Long-Acting

G

FIGURE 10-3 Labels for Insulin Types Grouped by Action Times

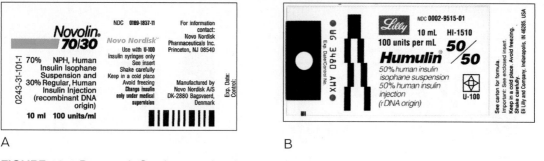

A   B

FIGURE 10-4 Premixed, Combination Insulins

Interpreting the Insulin Order

Insulin orders must be written clearly and contain specific information to ensure correct administration and prevent errors. An insulin order should contain:

1. The *brand name, including the species and action time.* Patients are instructed to stay with the same manufacturer's brand-name insulin and species. Slight variations between brands can affect an individual's response. Verify both the usual brand name used and the actual insulin supplied with the patient before administration. Different species of insulin may cause allergy-like symptoms in some patients, so check carefully. Look for one of the three action times: rapid-acting (*Regular*), intermediate-acting (*Lente, NPH*), and long-acting (*Ultralente*).

2. The *supply dosage (concentration) and number of units* to be given; for example, U-100 insulin 40U

3. The *route* of administration and *time or frequency.* All insulin may be administered subcutaneously (SC), and Regular insulin may additionally be administered intravenously (IV).

Examples:

Humulin R Regular U-100 insulin 14 U SC stat

Novolin N NPH U-100 insulin 24 U SC $\frac{1}{2}$ hour $\overline{a}$ breakfast

Insulin Coverage—The "Sliding Scale"

A special insulin order is sometimes needed to "cover" a patient's increasing blood sugar level that is not yet regulated. *Only* Regular insulin will be used, because of its rapid action. The physician will specify the amount of insulin in units, which "slide" up or down based on a specific blood sugar level range. Sliding scales are individualized for each patient. Here's an example of a sliding-scale order:

Example:

Order: *Humulin R Regular U-100 insulin SC based on glucose reading at 1600*

If the patient's blood glucose is 290, you would administer 6 U of Humulin R Regular U-100 insulin.

Insulin Dose	Glucose Reading*
No coverage	Glucose < 160
2 U	160–220
4 U	221–280
6 U	281–340
8 U	341–400

*Glucose > 400: Hold insulin; call MD stat.

Measuring Insulin in an Insulin Syringe

The insulin syringe and measurement of insulin were introduced in Chapter 6. This critical skill warrants your attention again. Once you understand how insulin is packaged and how to use the insulin syringe, you will find insulin dosage simple.

RULE

- Measure insulin in an insulin syringe only. Do not use a 3 mL or 1 mL syringe to measure insulin.
- Use U-100 insulin syringes to measure U-100 insulin only. Do not measure other drugs supplied in units in an insulin syringe.

Measuring insulin with the insulin syringe is very simple. The insulin syringe makes it possible to obtain a correct dosage without mathematical calculation. Let's look at three different insulin syringes. They are the *standard* (100 unit) capacity and the *lo-dose* (50 unit and 30 unit) capacity.

Standard U-100 Insulin Syringe

Example 1:

The Standard U-100 insulin syringe in Figure 10-5 is a dual-scale syringe with 100 U/mL capacity. It is calibrated on one side in *even*-numbered, 2-unit increments (2, 4, 6, ...) with every 10 units labeled (10, 20, 30, ...). It is calibrated on the reverse side in odd-numbered, 2 unit increments (1, 3, 5, ...) with every 10 units labeled (5, 15, 25, ...). The measurement of 73 units of U-100 insulin is illustrated in Figure 10-5.

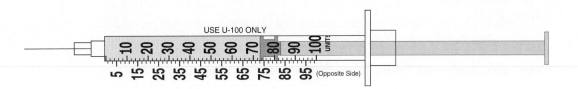

FIGURE 10-5 Standard U-100 Insulin Syringe Measuring 73 U

CAUTION

Look carefully at the increments on the dual scale. The volume from one mark to the next (on either side) is 2 units. You are probably comfortable counting by 2s for even numbers. Pay close attention when counting by 2s with odd numbers.

Lo-Dose U-100 Insulin Syringes

Example 1:

The Lo-Dose U-100 insulin syringe in Figure 10-6 is a single-scale syringe with 50 U/0.5 mL capacity. It is calibrated in 1 unit increments with every five units (5, 10, 15, ...) labeled up to 50 units. The enlarged 50 unit calibration of this syringe makes it easy to read and use to measure low dosages of insulin. To measure 32 units, withdraw U-100 insulin to the 32 unit mark (Figure 10-6).

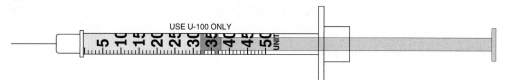

FIGURE 10-6 50-U Lo-Dose U-100 Insulin Syringe Measuring 32 U

Example 2:

The Lo-Dose U-100 insulin syringe in Figure 10-7 is a single-scale syringe with 30 U/0.3 mL capacity. It is calibrated in 1 unit increments with every five units (5, 10, 15, …) labeled up to 30 units. The enlarged 30 unit calibration accurately measures very small amounts of insulin, such as for children. To measure 12 units, withdraw U-100 insulin to the 12 unit mark (Figure 10-7).

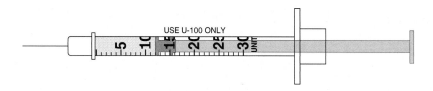

FIGURE 10-7 30-U Lo-Dose U-100 Insulin Syringe Measuring 12 U

> **CAUTION**
>
> Always choose the *smallest* capacity insulin syringe available for accurate insulin measurement. Use Standard and Lo-Dose U-100 syringes to measure U-100 insulin *only*. Although the Lo-Dose U-100 insulin syringes only measure a maximum of 30 or 50 units, they are still intended for the measurement of U-100 insulin only.

Be cautious when measuring. The Lo-Dose U-100 syringe is calibrated in 1 unit increments; the Standard U-100 insulin syringe is calibrated in 2 unit increments on the even and odd scales.

Combination Insulin Dosage

The patient may have two types of insulin prescribed to be administered at the same time. To avoid injecting the patient twice, it is common practice to draw up both insulins in the same syringe.

> **RULE**
>
> Draw up *clear insulin first*, then draw up cloudy insulin.
> Regular insulin is clear. NPH insulin is cloudy.
> **Think:** *First clear, then cloudy.* **Think:** *First Regular, then NPH.*

Example 1:

Order: *Novolin R Regular U-100 insulin 12 U with Novolin N NPH U-100 insulin 40 U SC ā breakfast.*

To accurately draw up both insulins into the same syringe, you will need to know the total units of both insulins: 12 + 40 = 52 units. Withdraw 12 units of the Regular U-100 insulin (clear) and then withdraw 40 more units of the NPH U-100 insulin (cloudy) up to the 52 unit mark (Figure 10-8). In this case, the smallest capacity syringe you can use is the Standard U-100 insulin syringe. Notice

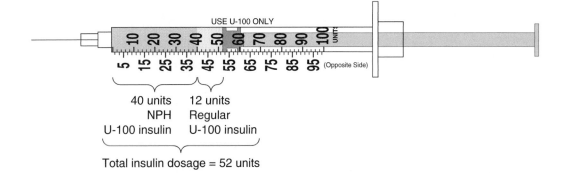

FIGURE 10-8 Combination Insulin Dosage

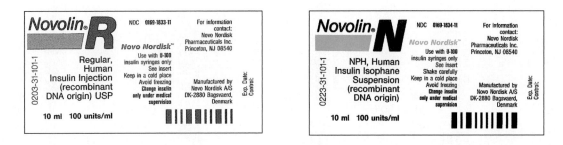

that the NPH insulin is drawn up last and is closest to the needle in the diagram. In reality, the drugs mix right away.

The second example gives step-by-step directions for this procedure. Look closely at Figures 10-9 and 10-10 to demonstrate the procedure as you study Example 2. Notice that to withdraw Regular insulin (clear) first and then NPH insulin (cloudy), you must inject the dose amount of air into the NPH insulin *before* you inject the dose amount of air into the Regular insulin.

Example 2:

The physician orders *Novolin R Regular U-100 insulin 10 U with Novolin N NPH U-100 insulin 30 U SC $\frac{1}{2}$ hour $\overline{a}$ dinner.*

1. Draw back and inject 30 units of air into the NPH insulin vial (cloudy liquid). Remove needle.

2. Draw back and inject 10 units of air into the Regular insulin vial (clear liquid) and leave the needle in the vial.

3. Turn the vial of Regular insulin upside down, and draw out the insulin to the 10 unit mark on the syringe. Make sure all air bubbles are removed.

4. Roll the vial of the NPH insulin in your hands to mix; do not shake it. Insert the needle into the NPH insulin vial, turn the vial upside down and slowly draw back to the 40 unit mark, being careful not to exceed the 40 unit calibration. 10 units of Regular + 30 units of NPH = 40 units of insulin total, Figure 10-10.

CAUTION

If you withdraw too much of the second insulin (NPH), you must discard the entire medication and start over.

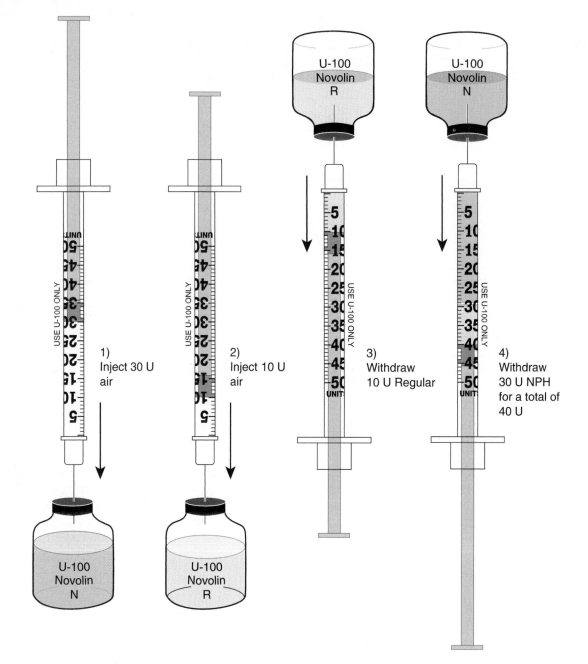

FIGURE 10-9 Procedure for Drawing Up Combination Insulin Dosage: 10 U Regular U-100 Insulin with 30 U NPH U-100 Insulin

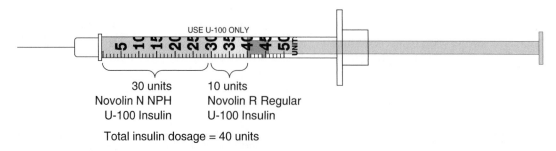

FIGURE 10-10 Combination Insulin Dosage

Avoiding Insulin Dosage Errors

Insulin dosage errors are very costly and, unfortunately, too common. They can be avoided by following two important rules.

RULE

1. Insulin dosages must be checked by two nurses.
2. When combination dosages are prepared, two nurses must verify each step of the process.

QUICK REVIEW

- Carefully read the physician's order, and match the supply dosage for type and species of insulin.
- Always measure insulin in an insulin syringe.
- An insulin syringe is used to measure insulin *only*. Insulin syringes must not be used to measure other medications measured in units.
- Use the smallest capacity insulin syringe possible to most accurately measure insulin doses.
- When drawing up combination insulin doses, think *clear first, then cloudy*.
- Avoid insulin dosage errors. The insulin dosage should be checked by two nurses.
- There are 100 units per mL for U-100 insulin.

REVIEW SET 28

Read the following labels. Identify the insulin brand name and its action time (rapid-acting, intermediate-acting, or long-acting).

1. Insulin brand name _____

   Action time _____

   NDC 0002-8215-01
   Lilly
   10 mL   HI-210
   100 units per mL
   Humulin® R
   REGULAR
   insulin human
   injection, USP
   (rDNA origin)
   U-100
   Important: See enclosed insert.
   Keep in a cold place. Avoid freezing.
   Neutral
   Eli Lilly and Company, Indianapolis, IN 46285, USA

2. Insulin brand name _____

   Action time _____

   Novolin. N
   Novo Nordisk™
   NDC 0169-1834-11
   NPH, Human
   Insulin Isophane
   Suspension
   (recombinant
   DNA origin)
   Use with U-100
   insulin syringes only
   See insert
   Shake carefully
   Keep in a cold place
   Avoid freezing
   Change insulin
   only under medical
   supervision
   For information
   contact:
   Novo Nordisk
   Pharmaceuticals Inc.
   Princeton, NJ 08540
   Manufactured by
   Novo Nordisk A/S
   DK-2880 Bagsvaerd,
   Denmark
   10 ml   100 units/ml

3. Insulin brand name _____

   Action time _____

   NDC 0002-8615-01
   Lilly
   10 mL   HI-610
   100 units per mL
   Humulin® U
   ULTRALENTE®
   human insulin
   (rDNA origin)
   extended zinc suspension
   U-100
   Important: See enclosed insert.
   Keep in a cold place. Avoid freezing.
   Shake carefully.
   Eli Lilly and Company, Indianapolis, IN 46285, USA

4. Insulin brand name   _____

   Action time   _____

5. Insulin brand name   _____

   Action time   _____

6. Describe the three syringes available to measure U-100 insulin. _____

   _____

7. What would be your preferred syringe choice to measure 24 units of U-100 insulin?

   _____

8. What would be your preferred syringe choice to measure 35 units of U-100 insulin?

   _____

9. There are 60 units of U-100 insulin per _____ mL.

10. There are 25 units of U-100 insulin per _____ mL.

11. 65 units of U-100 insulin should be measured in a(n) _____ syringe.

12. The 50 unit Lo-Dose U-100 insulin syringe is intended to measure U-50 insulin only. _____ (True) (False)

Identify the U-100 insulin dosage indicated by the colored area of the syringe.

13. _____ U

14. _____ U

15. _____ U

16. _____ U

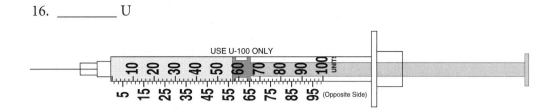

Draw an arrow on the syringe to identify the given dosages.

17. 80 units U-100 insulin

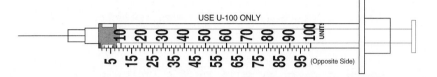

18. 15 units U-100 insulin

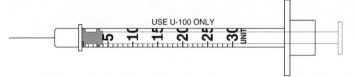

19. 66 units U-100 insulin

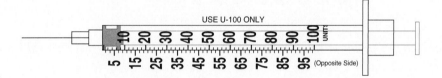

20. 16 units U-100 insulin

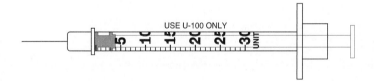

21. 32 units of U-100 insulin

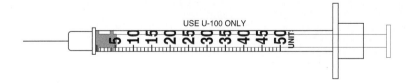

Draw arrows, and label the dosage for each of the combination insulin orders to be measured in the same syringe. Label and measure the insulins in the correct order, indicating which insulin will be drawn up first.

22. *Novolin R Regular U-100 insulin 21 U with Novolin N NPH U-100 insulin 15 U SC stat*

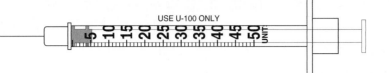

23. *Humulin R Regular U-100 insulin 16 U with Humulin N NPH U-100 insulin 42 U SC stat*

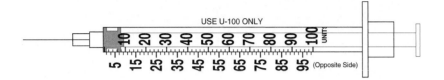

24. *Humulin R Regular U-100 insulin 32 U with Humulin N NPH U-100 insulin 40 U SC ā dinner*

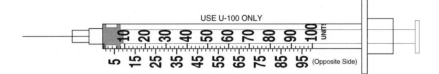

25. *Humulin R Regular U-100 insulin 8 U with Humulin N NPH U-100 insulin 12 U SC stat*

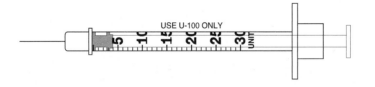

Use the following insulin sliding scale and medication order to answer questions 26 through 30.

Insulin Sliding Scale

Insulin Dose	Glucose Reading*
No coverage	Glucose < 160
2 U	160–220
4 U	221–280
6 U	281–340
8 U	341–400

*Glucose > 400: Hold insulin; call MD stat.

Order: *Humulin R Regular U-100 insulin SC ac per sliding scale.*

26. When will you check the patient's blood glucose level to determine the amount of insulin to give? _____

27. At what range of blood glucose levels will you administer insulin? _____

28. The patient's blood glucose level before breakfast is 250. What should you do? _____
    _____

29. The patient's blood glucose level before lunch is 150. How much insulin should you give now? _____

30. The patient's blood glucose level before dinner is 410. What should you do now?
    _____

After completing these problems, see pages 488–490 to check your answers.

CRITICAL THINKING SKILLS

Many insulin errors occur when the nurse fails to clarify an incomplete order. Let's look at an example of an insulin error when the order did not include the type of insulin to be given.

error

Failing to clarify an insulin order when the type of insulin is not specified.

possible scenario

Suppose the physician wrote an insulin order this way:

Humulin U-100 insulin 50 U a̅ breakfast

Because the physician did not specify the type of insulin, the nurse assumed it was Regular insulin and noted that on the medication administration record. Suppose the patient was given the Regular insulin for three days. On the morning of the third day, the patient developed signs of hypoglycemia (low blood glucose), including shakiness, tremors, confusion, and sweating.

potential outcome

A stat blood glucose would likely reveal a dangerously low glucose level. The patient would be given a glucose infusion to increase the blood sugar. The nurse may not realize the error until she and the doctor check the original order and find that the incomplete order was filled in by the nurse. When the doctor did not specify the type of insulin, the nurse assumed the physician meant Regular, which is short-acting, when in fact intermediate-acting NPH insulin was desired.

prevention

This error could have been avoided by remembering all the essential components of an insulin order: species, type of insulin (such as Regular or NPH), supply dosage, the amount to give in units, and the frequency. When you fill in an incomplete order, you are essentially practicing medicine without a license. This would be a clear malpractice incident. It does not make sense to put you and your patient in such jeopardy. A simple phone call would clarify the situation for everyone involved. Further, the nurse should have double-checked the dosage with another licensed practitioner. Had the nurse done so, the error could have been discovered prior to administration.

> ### SUMMARY
>
> You are now prepared to solve many of the dosage calculations you will encounter in your health care career. Oral and parenteral drug orders, written in the forms presented thus far, account for a large percentage of prescriptions. You have learned to think through the process from order to supply to amount administered, and to apply the formula $\frac{D}{H} \times Q = X$.
>
> Work the practice problems for Chapter 10. After completing the practice problems, you should feel comfortable and confident working dosage calculations. If not, seek additional instruction. Concentrate on accuracy. Remember, one error in dosage calculation can be a serious mistake for your patient.

PRACTICE PROBLEMS—CHAPTER 10

Calculate the amount you will prepare for one dose. Indicate the syringe you will select to measure the medication.

1. Order: *Demerol 20 mg IM q.3–4h p.r.n., pain*

    Supply: Demerol 50 mg/mL

    Give: _____ mL   Select _____ syringe

2. Order: *morphine sulfate gr $\frac{1}{4}$ IM stat*

    Supply: morphine sulfate 10 mg/mL

    Give: _____ mL   Select _____ syringe

3. Order: *Lanoxin 0.6 mg IV stat*

    Supply: Lanoxin 500 mcg/2 mL

    Give: _____ mL   Select _____ syringe

4. Order: *Vistaril 15 mg IM stat*

    Supply: Vistaril 25 mg/mL

    Give: _____ mL   Select _____ syringe

5. Order: *Cleocin 300 mg IM q.i.d.*

    Supply: Cleocin 0.6 g/4 mL

    Give: _____ mL   Select _____ syringe

6. Order: *potassium chloride 30 mEq added to each 1000 mL IV fluids*

    Supply: 30 mL multiple-dose vial potassium chloride 2 mEq/mL

    Give: _____ mL   Select _____ syringe

7. Order: *Atarax 40 mg IM q.4–6h p.r.n., agitation*

    Supply: Atarax 50 mg/mL

    Give: _____ mL   Select _____ syringe

8. Order: *Valium 5 mg IM q.4–6h p.r.n., agitation*

    Supply: Valium 10 mg/2 mL

    Give: _____ mL   Select _____ syringe

9. Order: *Tigan 100 mg IM q.6h p.r.n., nausea and vomiting*

   Supply: Tigan 200 mg/2 mL

   Give: _____ mL   Select _____ syringe

10. Order: *Dilantin 25 mg IV q.8h*

    Supply: Dilantin 100 mg/2 mL ampule

    Give: _____ mL   Select _____ syringe

11. Order: *atropine gr $\frac{1}{100}$ IM on call to O.R.*

    Supply: atropine 0.4 mg/mL

    Give: _____ mL   Select _____ syringe

12. Order: *Valium 3 mg IV stat*

    Supply: Valium 10 mg/2 mL

    Give: _____ mL   Select _____ syringe

13. Order: *heparin 6000 U SC q.12h*

    Supply: heparin 10,000 U/mL vial

    Give: _____ mL   Select _____ syringe

14. Order: *tobramycin sulfate 75 mg IM q.8h*

    Supply: Nebcin (tobramycin sulfate) 80 mg/2 mL

    Give: _____ mL   Select _____ syringe

15. Order: *morphine sulfate gr $\frac{1}{10}$ IM q.3h p.r.n., pain*

    Supply: morphine sulfate 10 mg/mL ampule

    Give: _____ mL   Select _____ syringe

16. Order: *atropine gr $\frac{1}{150}$ IM on call to O.R.*

    Supply: atropine 0.4 mg/mL

    Give: _____ mL   Select _____ syringe

17. Order: *ketorolac 20 mg IM q.6h p.r.n., severe pain*

    Supply: ketorolac 30 mg/mL

    Give: _____ mL   Select _____ syringe

18. Order: *Garamycin 40 mg IM q.8h*

    Supply: Garamycin 80 mg/2 mL

    Give: _____ mL   Select _____ syringe

19. Order: *Demerol 60 mg IM q.3h p.r.n., pain*

    Supply: Demerol 75 mg/1.5 mL

    Give: _____ mL   Select _____ syringe

20. Order: *Demerol 35 mg IM q.4h p.r.n., pain*

    Supply: Demerol 50 mg/1 mL

    Give: _____ mL   Select: _____ syringe

21. Order: *vitamin B₁₂ 0.75 mg IM q.d.*

    Supply: vitamin B$_{12}$ 1000 mcg/mL

    Give: _____ mL   Select _____ syringe

22. Order: *Aquamephyton 15 mg IM stat*

    Supply: Aquamephyton 10 mg per mL

    Give: _____ mL   Select _____ syringe

23. Order: *Phenergan 35 mg IM q.4h p.r.n., nausea and vomiting*

    Supply: Phenergan 50 mg/1 mL

    Give: _____ mL   Select _____ syringe

24. Order: *heparin 8000 U SC stat*

    Supply: heparin 10,000 U/1 mL

    Give: _____ mL   Select _____ syringe

25. Order: *morphine sulfate gr $\frac{1}{6}$ SC q.4h p.r.n., pain*

    Supply: morphine sulfate 8 mg/mL

    Give: _____ mL   Select _____ syringe

26. Order: *Lanoxin 0.4 mg IV stat*

    Supply: Lanoxin 500 mcg/2 mL

    Give: _____ mL   Select _____ syringe

27. Order: *Lasix 60 mg IV stat*

    Supply: Lasix 20 mg per 2 mL ampule

    Give: _____ mL   Select _____ syringe

28. Order: *heparin 4000 U SC q.6h*

    Supply: heparin 5000 U/1 mL

    Give: _____ mL   Select _____ syringe

29. Order: *Apresoline 30 mg IV q.6h*

    Supply: hydralazine (Apresoline) 20 mg per mL

    Give: _____ mL   Select _____ syringe

30. Order: *lidocaine 50 mg IV stat*

    Supply: lidocaine 2%

    Give: _____ mL   Select _____ syringe

31. Order: *Calan 2.5 mg IV push stat*

    Supply: Calan 10 mg/4 mL

    Give: _____ mL   Select _____ syringe

32. Order: *heparin 3500 U SC q.12h*

    Supply: heparin 5000 U/mL

    Give: _____ mL   Select _____ syringe

33. Order: *neostigmine 0.5 mg IM t.i.d.*

    Supply: neostigmine 1:2000

    Give: _____ mL   Select _____ syringe

34. Order: *KCl 60 mEq added to each 1000 mL IV fluid*

    Supply: KCl 2 mEq/1 mL

    Give: _____ mL   Select _____ syringe

35. Order: *Novolin R Regular U-100 insulin 16 U SC a.c.*

    Supply: Novolin R Regular U-100 insulin, with Standard 100 U and Lo-Dose 30 U U-100 insulin syringes

    Give: _____ U   Select _____ syringe

36. Order: *Novolin N NPH U-100 insulin 25 U SC ā breakfast*

    Supply: Novolin N NPH U-100 insulin with Standard 100 U and Lo-Dose 50 U U-100 insulin syringes

    Give: _____ U   Select _____ syringe

Calculate one dose of each of the drug orders numbered 37 through 48. Draw an arrow on the syringe indicating the calibration line that corresponds to the dose to be administered. The labels provided on pages 217–218 are the medications you have available. Indicate dosages that must be divided.

37. *Haldol 1.5 mg IM q.8h*

    Give: _____ mL

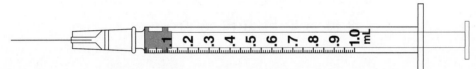

38. *Thorazine 40 mg IM q.6h*

    Give: _____ mL

39. *Inapsine 1 mg IV stat*

    Give: _____ mL

40. *Nebcin 100 mg IM q.8h*

    Give: _____ mL

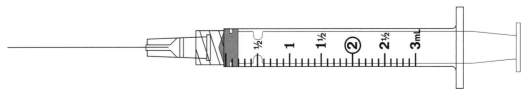

41. *epoetin alpha 12,000 U SC q.d. × 10 days*

    Give: _____ mL

42. *Humulin R Regular U-100 insulin 22 U SC stat*

    Give: _____ U

43. *meperidine 60 mg IM q.3–4h p.r.n., pain*

    Give: _____ mL

44. *Phenergan 15 mg IM q.3–4h p.r.n., nausea & vomiting*

    Give: _____ mL

45. *Reglan 7 mg IM stat*

    Give: _____ mL

46. *Neupogen 225 mcg SC q.d. × 2 weeks*

    Give: _____ mL

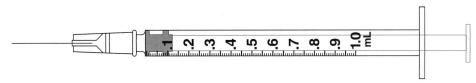

47. *Novolin R Regular U-100 insulin 32 U with Novolin N NPH U-100 insulin 54 U SC ā breakfast*

    Give: _____ total U

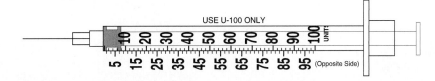

48. *Novolin 70/30 U-100 insulin 46 U SC ā dinner*

    Give: _____ U

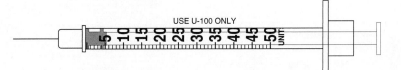

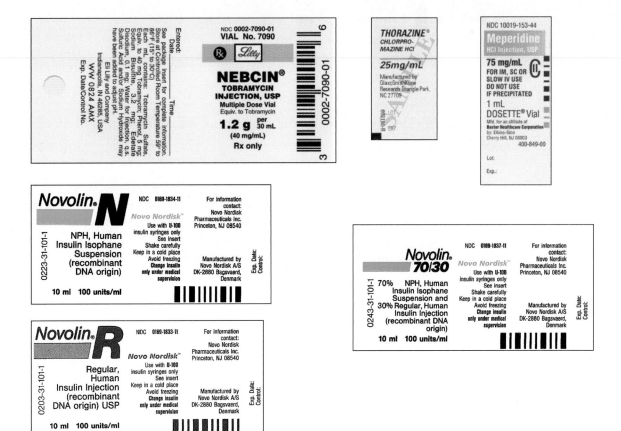

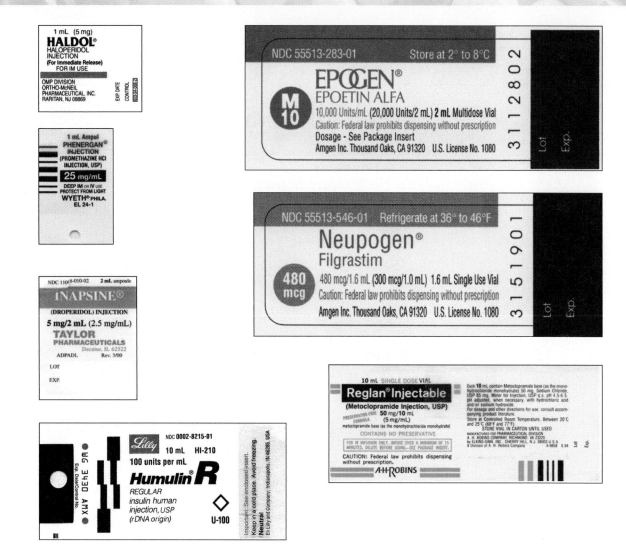

49. Critical Thinking Skill: Describe the strategy you would implement to prevent this medication error.

possible scenario

Suppose the physician ordered Humulin R U-100 insulin 20 units mixed with Humulin N U-100 insulin 40 units to be administered SC before breakfast. The nurse selected the vials of Humulin R and Humulin N U-100 insulin from the medication drawer and injected 20 units of air in the Humulin N vial and 40 units of air in the Humulin R vial, drew up 40 units of Humulin R and then drew up 20 units of Humulin N.

potential outcome

The patient received the incorrect dosage of insulin because the nurse drew up 40 units of Humulin R and 20 units of Humulin N instead of the dosage that was ordered: 20 units of Humulin R and 40 units of Humulin N. Because the patient received too much short-acting insulin (twice the amount ordered), the patient would likely show signs of hypoglycemia, such as shakiness, confusion, and diaphoresis.

prevention

50. Critical Thinking Skill: Describe the strategy you would implement to prevent this medication error.

possible scenario

Suppose the physician ordered 10 units of Novolin R U-100 insulin SC stat for a patient with a blood glucose of 300. The nurse selected the Novolin R U-100 insulin from the patient's medication drawer and selected a 1 mL syringe to administer the dose. The nurse looked at the syringe for the 10 unit mark and was confused as to how much should have been drawn up. The nurse finally decided to draw up 1 mL of insulin into the syringe, administered the dose, and then began to question whether the correct dosage was administered. The nurse called the supervisor for advice.

potential outcome

The patient would have received 10 times the correct dosage of insulin. Because this was a short-acting insulin, the patient would likely show signs of severe hypoglycemia, such as loss of consciousness and seizures. The likelihood of a successful outcome is questionable.

prevention

_____

_____

After completing these problems, see pages 490–493 to check your answers.

Reconstitution of Solutions

Upon mastery of Chapter 11, you will be prepared to reconstitute injectable and noninjectable solutions. To accomplish this you will also be able to:
- Define and apply the terms *solvent, solute,* and *solution.*
- Reconstitute and label medications supplied in powder or dry form.
- Differentiate between varying directions for reconstitution and select the correct set to prepare the dosage ordered.
- Calculate the amount of solute and solvent needed to prepare a desired strength and quantity of an irrigating solution or enteral feeding.

Some parenteral medications are supplied in powder form and must be mixed with water or some other liquid before administration. As more health care is provided in the home setting, nurses and other health care workers must dilute topical irrigants, soaks, and nutritional feedings. This process of mixing and diluting solutions is referred to as *reconstitution.*

The process of reconstitution is comparable to the preparation of hot chocolate from a powdered mix. By adding the correct amount of hot water (referred to as the *solvent* or *diluent*) to the package of powdered, hot chocolate drink mix (referred to as the *solute*), you prepare a tasty, hot beverage (the resulting *solution*).

The properties of solutions are important concepts to understand. Learn them well now, as we will apply them again when we examine intravenous solutions.

SOLUTION PROPERTIES

As you look at Figures 11-1 and 11-2, let's define the terms of reconstitution.
- *Solute*—a substance to be dissolved or diluted. It can be in solid or liquid form.
- *Solvent*—a substance (liquid) that dissolves another substance to prepare a solution. *Diluent* is a synonymous term.
- *Solution*—the resulting mixture of a solute plus a solvent.

To prepare a therapeutic *solution*, you will *add a solvent or diluent* (usually normal saline or water) *to a solute* (solid substance or concentrated stock solution) to obtain the required strength of a stated volume of a solution. This means that the solid substance or concentrate, called a *solute*, is diluted with a *solvent* to obtain a reconstituted *solution* of a weaker strength. However, the amount of the drug that was in the pure solute or concentrated stock solution still equals the amount of pure drug in the diluted solution. Only the solvent has been added to the solute, expanding the total volume.

Figure 11-1 shows that the amount of pure drug (solute) remains the same in the concentrated form and in the resulting solution. However, in solution, notice the solute particles are dispersed or suspended throughout the resulting weaker solution. The particles evident in Figure 11-1 are for illustration purposes only. In a solution, the solute would be dissolved.

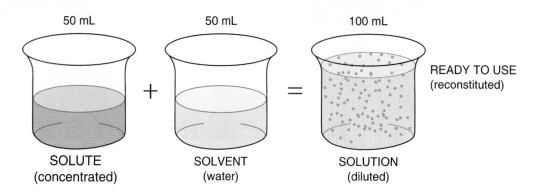

FIGURE 11-1 Concentrated Liquid Solute: 50 milliliters of concentrated solute diluted with 50 milliliters of solvent make 100 milliliters of diluted solution

The *strength of a solution* or *concentration* was briefly discussed in Chapters 8 and 9. Solution strength indicates the ratio of solute to solvent. Consider how each of these substances—solute and solvent—contributes a certain number of parts to the total solution.

Look at the Zithromax 500 mg label (Figure 11-2). The label directions indicate that 4.8 mL of sterile water (*solvent*) should be added to the powder (*solid solute*) to prepare the reconstituted *solution*. As the label indicates, the resulting supply dosage would be 100 mg of Zithromax per 1 mL of solution.

Let's thoroughly examine the reconstitution of powdered injectable medications.

RECONSTITUTION OF INJECTABLE MEDICATIONS IN POWDER FORM

Some medications are unstable when stored in solution or liquid form. Thus they are packaged in powdered form and must be dissolved or *reconstituted* by a liquid *solvent or diluent* and mixed thoroughly. Reconstitution is a necessary step in medication preparation to create a measurable and usable dosage form. The pharmacist often does this before dispensing liquid medications, for oral as well as parenteral routes. However, nurses need to understand reconstitution and know how to accomplish it. Some medications must be prepared by the nurse just prior to administration, as they become unstable when stored.

> **CAUTION**
>
> Before reconstituting injectable drugs, read and follow the label or package insert directions carefully. Consult a pharmacist with *any* questions.

Let's look at the rules for reconstituting injectable medications from powder to liquid form. Follow these rules carefully to ensure that the patient receives the intended solution.

> **RULE**
>
> When reconstituting injectable medications, you must determine both the *type* and *amount* of diluent to be used.

Some powdered medications are packaged by the manufacturer with special diluents for reconstitution. Sterile water and 0.9% sodium chloride (normal saline) are most commonly used as diluents in parenteral medications. Both sterile water (Figure 11-3) and normal saline are available *preservative-free* when intended for a single use only, as well as in *bacteriostatic* form with preservative when intended for more than one use. Carefully check the instructions and vial label for the appropriate diluent.

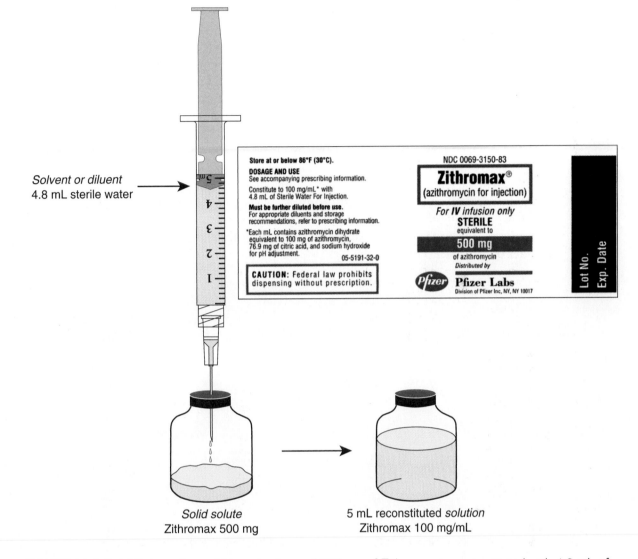

Solvent or diluent
4.8 mL sterile water

Store at or below 86°F (30°C).

DOSAGE AND USE
See accompanying prescribing information.

Constitute to 100 mg/mL* with
4.8 mL of Sterile Water For Injection.

Must be further diluted before use.
For appropriate diluents and storage
recommendations, refer to prescribing information.

*Each mL contains azithromycin dihydrate
equivalent to 100 mg of azithromycin,
76.9 mg of citric acid, and sodium hydroxide
for pH adjustment.
05-5191-32-0

CAUTION: Federal law prohibits
dispensing without prescription.

NDC 0069-3150-83

Zithromax®
(azithromycin for injection)

*For **IV** infusion only*
STERILE
equivalent to

500 mg
of azithromycin
Distributed by

Pfizer **Pfizer Labs**
Division of Pfizer Inc, NY, NY 10017

Lot No.
Exp. Date

Solid solute
Zithromax 500 mg

5 mL reconstituted *solution*
Zithromax 100 mg/mL

FIGURE 11-2 Solid Solute: the solid powder form of 500 mg of Zithromax is reconstituted with 4.8 mL of sterile water as the diluent to make 5 mL of Zithromax IV solution with the supply dosage of 100 mg/mL

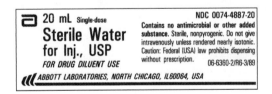

20 mL Single-dose
Sterile Water
for Inj., USP
FOR DRUG DILUENT USE
ABBOTT LABORATORIES, NORTH CHICAGO, IL 60064, USA

NDC 0074-4887-20
**Contains no antimicrobial or other added
substance.** Sterile, nonpyrogenic. Do not give
intravenously unless rendered nearly isotonic.
Caution: Federal (USA) law prohibits dispensing
without prescription.   06-6360-2/R6-3/89

FIGURE 11-3 Reconstitution Diluent for Parenteral Powdered Drugs

RULE

When reconstituting injectable medications, you must determine the *volume in mL* of diluent to be used for the route as ordered, then reconstitute the drug and *note the resulting supply dosage* on the vial.

Because many reconstituted parenteral medications can be administered either intramuscularly (IM) or intravenously (IV), it is essential to verify the route of administration before reconstituting the medication. Remember that the intramuscular volume of 3 mL or less per injection site is determined by the patient's age and condition and the intramuscular site selected. The directions take this into account by stating the minimum volume or quantity of diluent that should be added to the powdered drug for IM use. Often the powdered drug itself *adds* volume to the solution. The powder displaces the liquid as it dissolves and increases the total resulting volume. The resulting volume of the reconstituted drug is usually given on the label. This resulting volume determines the liquid's concentration or *supply dosage.*

Look at the directions on the Kefzol label, Figure 11-4. They state, "To prepare solution add 2 mL Sterile Water for Injection or 0.9% Sodium Chloride Injection. Provides a total volume of 2.2 mL (225 mg per mL)." Notice that when 2 mL of diluent is added and the powder is dissolved, the weight

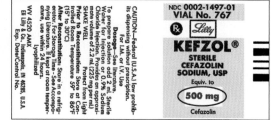

of the powder adds an additional 0.2 mL for a total solution volume of 2.2 mL. (The amount of diluent added will vary with each medication.) Thus, the supply dosage available after reconstitution is *225 mg of Kefzol per mL of solution.* Figure 11-4 demonstrates the reconstitution procedure for Kefzol 500 mg, to fill the order of *Kefzol 225 mg IM q.6h.*

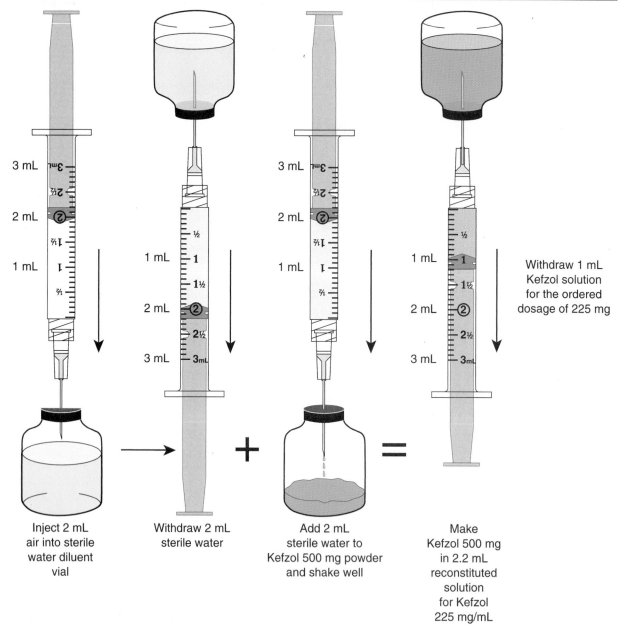

Inject 2 mL air into sterile water diluent vial

Withdraw 2 mL sterile water

Add 2 mL sterile water to Kefzol 500 mg powder and shake well

Make Kefzol 500 mg in 2.2 mL reconstituted solution for Kefzol 225 mg/mL

Withdraw 1 mL Kefzol solution for the ordered dosage of 225 mg

FIGURE 11-4 Kefzol Reconstitution Procedure to Fill the Order *Kefzol 225 mg IM q.6h*

Single-dose vials contain only enough medication for one dose, and the resulting contents are administered after the powder is diluted. But in some cases the nurse also may dilute a powdered medication in a multiple-dose vial that will yield more than one dose. When this is the case, it is important to clearly label the vial after reconstitution. Labeling is discussed in the next section.

TYPES OF RECONSTITUTED PARENTERAL SOLUTIONS

There are two types of reconstituted parenteral solutions: single strength and multiple strength. The simplest type to dilute is a *single-strength* solution. This type usually has the recommended dilution directions and resulting supply dosage printed on the label, such as the Kefzol 500 mg label in Figure 11-4 (page 224) and the Zithromax label in Figure 11-5.

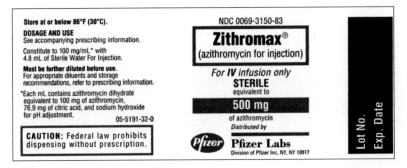

FIGURE 11-5 Zithromax Label

Some medications have several directions for dilution that allow the nurse to select the best supply dosage. This is called a *multiple-strength* solution and requires even more careful reading of the instructions, such as the Pfizerpen label shown in Figure 11-7 (page 227). Sometimes these directions for reconstitution will not fit on the vial label. You must consult the package insert or other printed instructions to ensure accurate dilution of the parenteral medication.

Let's look at some examples to clarify what the health care professional needs to do to correctly reconstitute and calculate dosages of parenteral medications supplied in powder form.

Single-Strength Solution/Single-Dose Vial

Example:

Order: *Zithromax 400 mg IV q.d. × 2 days*

Supply: 500 mg vial of powdered Zithromax with directions on the left side of the label as follows: "Constitute to 100 mg/mL with 4.8 mL of Sterile Water for injection" (Figure 11-5).

Carefully sort through and analyze the information provided on the label.

- First, how much and what type of diluent must you add? The directions state to *add 4.8 mL of Sterile Water.*
- Second, what is the resulting supply dosage or concentration? When reconstituted, the *supply dosage is Zithromax 100 mg/mL.*
- Third, what is the resulting total volume of the reconstituted solution? The *total volume is 5 mL.* The powder added 0.2 mL to the solution. You know this because the supply dosage is 100 mg/mL and you added 4.8 mL of diluent. Therefore, it is only logical that the total volume is 5 mL.
- Finally, to fill the order as prescribed, how many full doses are available in this vial? The order is for 400 mg and the single-dose vial contains 500 mg. This is enough for one full dose, but not enough for two full doses. Two doses would require 800 mg.

Now, let's put it all together.

This means you have available a vial of 500 mg of Zithromax to which you will add 4.8 mL of sterile water as the diluent. The powdered drug displaces 0.2 mL. The resulting 5 mL of the solution contains 500 mg of the drug, and there are 100 mg of Zithromax in each 1 mL of solution.

After reconstitution, you are ready to apply the same three steps of dosage calculation that you learned in Chapters 9 and 10.

Step 1 Convert   No conversion necessary

Order: *Zithromax 400 mg IV q.d. × 2 days*

Supply: 100 mg/mL

Step 2 Think   You want to give more than 1 mL. In fact, you want to give four times 1 mL.

Step 3 Calculate $\dfrac{D}{H} \times Q = \dfrac{\overset{4}{\cancel{400 \text{ mg}}}}{\underset{1}{\cancel{100 \text{ mg}}}} \times 1 \text{ mL} = \dfrac{4}{1} \text{ mL} = 4 \text{ mL}$

Give 4 mL Zithromax reconstituted to 100 mg/mL, intravenously each day for 2 days.

This vial of Zithromax 500 mg contains only one full ordered dose of reconstituted drug. Any remaining medication is usually discarded. Because this vial provides only one dose, you will not have to label and store any of the reconstituted drug.

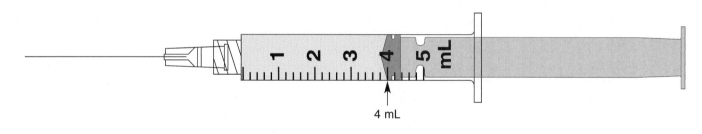

4 mL

Single-Strength Solution/Multiple-Dose Vial

Example

Suppose the drug order reads *Zithromax 250 mg IV q.d.* Using the same size vial of Zithromax and the same dilution instructions as in the previous example, you would now have 2 full doses of Zithromax, making this a multiple-dose vial.

$$\frac{D}{H} \times Q = \frac{250 \text{ mg}}{100 \text{ mg}} \times 1 \text{ mL} = 2.5 \text{ mL}$$

Select a 3 mL syringe and measure 2.5 mL of Zithromax reconstituted to 100 mg/mL.

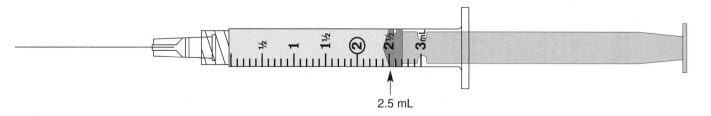

2.5 mL

> ## RULE
>
> When reconstituting multiple-dose injectable medications, verify the length of drug potency. Store the reconstituted drug appropriately with a reconstitution label attached.

If multiple doses result from the reconstitution of a powdered drug, the solution must be used in a timely manner. Because the drug potency (or stability) may be several hours to several days, check the drug label, package information sheet, or *Hospital Formulary* for how long the drug may be used after reconstitution. Store the drug appropriately at room temperature or refrigerate per the manufacturer's instructions. The package insert for Zithromax states, "Reconstituted solution is stable for 24 hours at or below room temperature (86° F) and 7 days when refrigerated."

> ## CAUTION
>
> The length of potency is different from the expiration date. The expiration date is provided by the manufacturer on the label. It indicates the *last* date the drug may be reconstituted and used.

When you reconstitute or mix a multiple-dose vial of medication in powdered form, it is important that the vial be *clearly labeled* with the *date* and *time* of preparation, the strength or *supply dosage* you prepared, *length of potency, storage directions,* and your *initials.* Because the medication becomes unstable after storage for long periods, the date and time are especially important. Figure 11-6 shows the proper label for the Zithromax reconstituted to 100 mg/mL. Because there are 2 doses of reconstituted drug in this vial, and 2 doses will be administered 24 hours apart (now at 0800, then again the next day at 0800), this drug should be refrigerated. Refrigeration will protect the potency of the drug in case the second dose is administered slightly later than 0800. Indicate the need for refrigeration on the label.

> 1/10/xx, 0800, reconstituted
> as 100 mg/mL. Expires 1/17/xx,
> 0800. Keep refrigerated. G.D.P.

FIGURE 11-6 Reconstitution Label for Zithromax

Multiple-Strength Solution/Multiple-Dose Vial

Some parenteral powdered medications have directions for preparing several different solution strengths, to allow you to select a particular dosage strength (Figure 11-7). This results in a reasonable amount to be given to a particular patient.

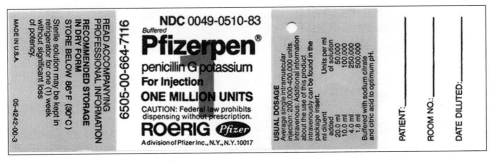

FIGURE 11-7 Pfizerpen Label

Example

Order: *penicillin G potassium 300,000 U IM q.i.d.*

Supply: Pfizerpen (penicillin G potassium) 1,000,000 U vial

This vial contains a total of 1,000,000 U of penicillin. The reconstitution instructions are shown on the right side of the label. The instructions detail four different parenteral solution supply dosages or concentrations that are determined by the added diluent volume. Let's look at each of the four instructions. Notice how these reconstituted concentrations differ and when each might be selected.

Add 20 mL Diluent

Refer to the first set of directions, which indicates to add 20 mL diluent to prepare 50,000 units per milliliter of solution. Is this a good choice for preparing the medication to fill the order?
What do we know?

- First, to follow the first set of directions, how much and what type of diluent must you add? The directions state to add 20 mL of diluent. (You must check the package insert to determine the type of diluent, as this information is not stated on the label. The package insert recommends 1–2% lidocaine for intramuscular injection to lessen the pain at the injection site.)
- Second, what is the concentration of the reconstituted penicillin? When adding 20 mL of diluent, the supply dosage or concentration is 50,000 U/mL.
- Third, what is the resulting total volume of this reconstituted solution? The total volume is 20 mL. You know this because the supply dosage is 50,000 U/mL or 1,000,000 U/20 mL. The volume of diluent is large enough that the powder dissolves without adding any significant additional volume.
- Finally, how many full doses of penicillin as ordered are available in this vial? The vial contains 1,000,000 U and the order is for 300,000 U. There are 3 full doses (plus some extra) in this vial. If you choose this concentration, a reconstitution label would be required. This means that when you add 20 mL of sterile diluent to this vial of powdered penicillin, the result is 1,000,000 units of penicillin in 20 mL of solution, with a concentration of 50,000 units per mL.
Apply the three steps of dosage calculation:

Step 1   Convert   No conversion necessary

Order: *penicillin G potassium 300,000 U IM q.i.d.*

Supply: 50,000 U/mL

Step 2   Think   You want to give more than 1 mL. In fact, you want to give six times 1 mL.

Step 3   Calculate $\dfrac{D}{H} \times Q = \dfrac{\overset{6}{\cancel{300,000}\ \cancel{U}}}{\underset{1}{\cancel{50,000}\ \cancel{U}}} \times 1\ \text{mL} = \dfrac{6}{1}\ \text{mL} = 6\ \text{mL}$

Because each dose is 6 mL and the total volume is 20 mL, you would have enough for 2 additional full doses. However, this is an IM dose, and 3 mL is the maximum volume for a large, adult muscle. To administer this order using this concentration, you would need to inject the patient with two 3 mL syringes filled with 3 mL of penicillin each. Therefore, this is a poor choice of reconstitution instructions to prepare this order.

Add 10 mL Diluent

Refer to the second set of directions on the penicillin label, which indicates to add 10 mL of diluent for 100,000 units per mL of solution. Would this prepare an appropriate concentration to fill the order?

What do we know?

- First, to correctly follow the second set of directions, how much and what type of diluent must you add? The directions state to add 10 mL of diluent. (You must check the package insert to determine the type of diluent, as this information is not stated on the label. The package insert recommends 1–2% lidocaine for IM injection.)
- Second, what is the concentration of the reconstituted penicillin? When adding 10 mL of diluent, the supply dosage or concentration is 100,000 U/mL.
- Third, what is the resulting total volume of this reconstituted solution? The total volume is 10 mL. You know this because the supply dosage is 100,000 U/mL or 1,000,000 U/10 mL. The solution volume is large enough that the powder does not add volume to the solution.
- Finally, how many full doses of penicillin as ordered are available in this vial? The vial contains 1,000,000 U and the order is for 300,000 U. There are 3 full doses (plus some extra) in this vial. If you select this set of instructions, you will need to add a reconstitution label to the vial after mixing.

This means when you add 10 mL of sterile diluent to this vial of powdered penicillin, the result is 1,000,000 units of penicillin in 10 mL of solution with a concentration of 100,000 units per mL.

Apply the three steps of dosage calculation:

Step 1 Convert   No conversion necessary

Order: *penicillin G potassium 300,000 U IM q.i.d.*

Supply: 100,000 U/mL

Step 2 Think   You want to give more than 1 mL. In fact, you want to give three times 1 mL.

Step 3 Calculate $\dfrac{D}{H} \times Q = \dfrac{\overset{3}{\cancel{300,000}\ \cancel{U}}}{\underset{1}{\cancel{100,000}\ \cancel{U}}} \times 1\,mL = \dfrac{3}{1}\,mL = 3\,mL$

Because each dose is 3 mL and the total volume is 10 mL, you would have enough for 2 additional full doses. As an IM dose, 3 mL is the maximum volume for a large, adult muscle. Although this is a safe volume and would require only one injection, perhaps another concentration would result in a lesser volume that would be more readily absorbed.

Add 4 mL Diluent

Refer to the third set of directions on the penicillin label, which indicates to add 4 mL of diluent for 250,000 units per mL of solution. Would this prepare an appropriate concentration to fill the order?

What is different about this set of directions? Let's analyze the information provided on the label.

- First, to follow the third set of directions, how much and what type of diluent must you add? The directions state to add 4 mL of diluent. (Remember, you must check the package insert to determine the type of diluent, as this information is not stated on the label. The recommendation is for 1–2% lidocaine.)
- Second, what is the supply dosage of the reconstituted penicillin? When adding 4 mL of diluent, the supply dosage is 250,000 U/mL.
- Third, what is the resulting total volume of this reconstituted solution? The total volume is 4 mL. You know this because the supply dosage is 250,000 U/mL or 1,000,000 U/4 mL. The powder does not add volume to the solution.
- Finally, how many full doses of penicillin are available in this vial? The vial contains 1,000,000 U and the order is for 300,000 U. Regardless of the concentration, there are still 3 full doses (plus some extra) in this vial. A reconstitution label would be needed.

This means that when you add 4 mL of sterile diluent to the vial of powdered penicillin, the result is 4 mL of solution with 250,000 U of penicillin per mL.

Calculate one dose.

Step 1 Convert   No conversion necessary

Order: *penicillin G potassium 300,000 U IM q.i.d.*

Supply: 250,000 U/mL

Step 2 Think   You want to give more than 1 mL but less than 2 mL.

Step 3 Calculate $\dfrac{D}{H} \times Q = \dfrac{\overset{6}{\cancel{300,000}\ \cancel{U}}}{\underset{5}{\cancel{250,000}\ \cancel{U}}} \times 1\,\text{mL} = \dfrac{6}{5}\,\text{mL} = 1.2\,\text{mL}$

given intramuscularly four times a day

Because each dose is 1.2 mL and the total volume is 4 mL, you would have enough for 2 additional full doses. As an IM dose, 3 mL is the maximum volume for a large, adult muscle. This concentration would result in a reasonable volume that would be readily absorbed. This is a good choice of concentration instructions to use to prepare this order.

Select a 3 mL syringe, and measure 1.2 mL of Pfizerpen reconstituted to 250,000 U/mL.

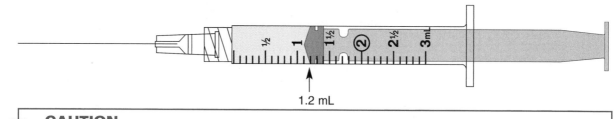

1.2 mL

CAUTION

The supply dosage of a reconstituted drug is an essential detail that the preparer must write on the multiple-dose vial label. Once a powdered drug is reconstituted, there is no way to verify how much diluent was actually added, unless it is properly labeled.

Be sure to add a label to the reconstituted Pfizerpen 250,000 U/mL vial, Figure 11-8.

1/30/xx, 0800, reconstituted as 250,000 U/mL. Expires 2/06/xx, 0800, keep refrigerated. G.D.P.

FIGURE 11-8 Reconstitution Label for Pfizerpen 1,000,000 U with 4 mL Diluent

Add 1.8 mL Diluent

The fourth set of directions instructs you to add 1.8 mL diluent for a solution concentration of 500,000 U/mL. Let's examine this information.
- First, to fulfill the fourth set of directions, how much and what type of diluent must you add? The directions state to add 1.8 mL of diluent. (You must check the package insert to determine the type of diluent, as this information is not stated on the label. Use 1–2% lidocaine.)
- Second, what is the supply dosage of the reconstituted penicillin? When adding 1.8 mL of diluent, the supply dosage is 500,000 U/mL.
- Third, what is the resulting total volume of this reconstituted solution? The total volume is 2 mL. You know this because the supply dosage is 500,000 U/mL or 1,000,000 U/2 mL. The powder

displaces 0.2 mL of the solution. (Notice that this is the most concentrated, or the strongest, of the four concentrations.)

- Finally, how many full doses of penicillin are available in this vial? The vial contains 1,000,000 U and the order is for 300,000 U. Notice that regardless of the concentration, there are 3 full doses (plus some extra) in this vial. You must prepare a different reconstitution label, as this is a different concentration.

Following the fourth set of directions, you add 1.8 mL of diluent to prepare 2 mL of solution with a resulting concentration of 500,000 U of penicillin in each 1 mL.

Calculate one dose.

Step 1	**Convert**	No conversion necessary
		Order: *penicillin G potassium 300,000 U IM q.i.d.*
		Supply: 500,000 U/mL
Step 2	**Think**	You want to give less than 1 mL.

Step 3 Calculate $\dfrac{D}{H} \times Q = \dfrac{\overset{3}{\cancel{300,000}}\ \cancel{U}}{\underset{5}{\cancel{500,000}}\ \cancel{U}} \times 1\,\text{mL} = \dfrac{3}{5}\,\text{mL} = 0.6\,\text{mL}$

given intramuscularly four times a day

Because each dose is 0.6 mL and the total volume is 2 mL, you would have enough for 2 additional full doses. This supply dosage would result in a reasonable volume for an IM injection for an infant, small child, or anyone with wasted muscle mass.

Select a *3 mL syringe, and measure 0.6 mL* of penicillin reconstituted to 500,000 units/mL.

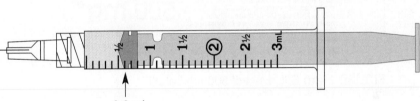

0.6 mL

Finally, add the label to the reconstituted penicillin G 500,000 U/mL vial, Figure 11-9.

1/30/xx, 0800, reconstituted as 500,000 U/mL. Expires 2/06/xx, 0800, keep refrigerated. G.D.P.

FIGURE 11-9 Reconstitution Label for Pfizerpen 1,000,000 U with 1.8 mL Diluent

As you can see from these four possible reconstituted strengths, three full doses are available from this multiple-dose vial in each case. The added diluent volume is the key factor that determines the resulting concentration. The *supply dosage* ultimately determines the *injectable volume per dose.*

MATH TIP

When multiple directions for diluting are given, the *smaller* the amount of diluent added, the *greater* or *stronger* the resulting solution concentration will be.

RECONSTITUTED PARENTERAL SOLUTIONS WITH VARIOUS ROUTES

A variety of drugs are labeled and packaged with reconstitution instructions. Some drugs are for IM use only and some are for IV use only, whereas others may be used for either. Some are even suitable for SC, IM, or IV administration. Carefully check the route and related reconstitution directions. The following material gives examples of several types of directions you will encounter.

Drugs with Injection Reconstitution Instructions—Either IM or IV

Example:

Order: *Solu-Medrol 200 mg IV q.6h*

Supply: 500 mg vial of powdered Solu-Medrol for IM or IV injection (Figure 11-10) with directions on the left side of the label that state, "Reconstitute with 8 mL Bacteriostatic Water for Injection with Benzyl Alcohol. When reconstituted as directed each 8 mL contains: Methylprednisolone sodium succinate equivalent to 500 mg methylprednisolone (62.5 mg per mL)."

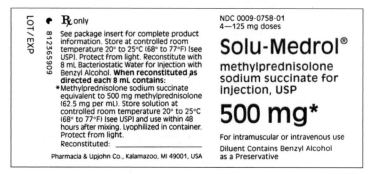

FIGURE 11-10 Solu-Medrol 500 mg Label

What do we know?
- First, to fill the order, how much and what type of diluent must you add? The directions state to add 8 mL of bacteriostatic water for injection with benzyl alcohol.
- Second, what is the supply dosage of the reconstituted Solu-Medrol? When adding 8 mL of diluent, the supply dosage is 62.5 mg/mL.
- Third, what is the resulting total volume of this reconstituted solution? The total volume is 8 mL. You know this because 62.5 mg/mL × 8 mL = 500 mg.
- Finally, how many full doses of Solu-Medrol are available in this vial? The vial contains 500 mg and the order is for 200 mg. There are two full doses in the vial. A reconstitution label is needed.

This means that you have available a vial of 500 mg of Solu-Medrol to which you will add 8 mL of diluent. The final yield of the solution is 62.5 mg per mL, which is your supply dosage.
Calculate one dose.

Step 1   Convert   No conversion necessary

Order: *Solu-Medrol 200 mg IV q.6h*

Supply: 62.5 mg/mL

Step 2   Think   You want to give more than 1 mL. In fact, you want to give more than three times 1 mL.

Step 3 **Calculate**

$$\frac{D}{H} \times Q = \frac{200 \text{ mg}}{62.5 \text{ mg}} \times 1 \text{ mL} = 3.2 \text{ mL}$$

given intravenously every 6 hours

1/30/xx, 0800, reconstituted as 62.5 mg/mL. Expires 2/01/xx, 0800, store at room temperature 68–77°F. G.D.P.

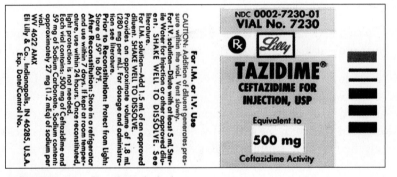

3.2 mL

Drugs with Different IM and IV Reconstitution Instructions

Notice that the Tazidime label (Figure 11-11) has one set of instructions for IM use and another set for IV administration. The nurse must carefully check the route ordered, and then follow the directions that correspond to that route. In such cases, it is important not to interchange the dilution instructions for IM and IV administrations.

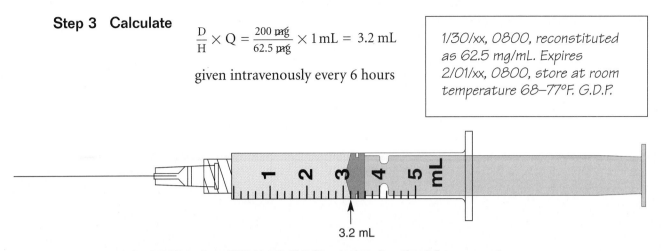

FIGURE 11-11 Tazidime Label

Example 1:

Order: *Tazidime 250 mg IM q.12h*

Supply: 500 mg vial of powdered Tazidime (Figure 11-11) with IM reconstitution directions that state, "For IM solution—Add 1.5 mL of an approved diluent. Provides an approximate volume of 1.8 mL (280 mg per mL)."

- First, to fill the order, how much and what type of diluent must you add? The directions state to add 1.5 mL of diluent. The label does not indicate what diluent you should use. You would refer to the package insert, which recommends sterile water, bacteriostatic water, or 0.5–1% lidocaine for injection.
- Second, what is the supply dosage of the reconstituted Tazidime? When adding 1.5 mL of diluent, the resulting supply dosage is 280 mg/mL.
- Third, how many full doses of Tazidime are available in this vial? The vial contains 500 mg and the order is for 250 mg. There are two full doses in the vial. A reconstitution label is needed.
- Finally, what is the resulting total volume of this reconstituted solution? The total volume is 1.8 mL, as indicated on the label for IM reconstitution.

This means that you have available a vial of 500 mg of Tazidime to which you will add 1.5 mL of diluent. The final yield of the solution is 1.8 mL with a supply dosage of 280 mg/mL.

Calculate one dose.

Step 1	Convert	No conversion necessary
		Order: *Tazidime 250 mg IM q.12h*
		Supply: 280 mg/mL
Step 2	Think	You want to give less than 1 mL.
Step 3	Calculate	$\dfrac{D}{H} \times Q = \dfrac{250\ \cancel{mg}}{280\ \cancel{mg}} \times 1\ mL = 0.89\ mL$
		given intramuscularly every 12 hours

> 1/30/xx, 0800, reconstituted
> as 280 mg/mL for IM use.
> Expires 1/31/xx, 0800, store at
> room temperature. G.D.P.

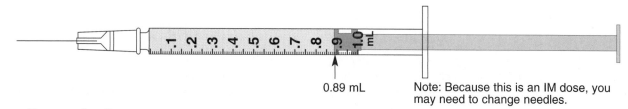

0.89 mL

Note: Because this is an IM dose, you
may need to change needles.

Example 2:

Order: *Tazidime 400 mg IV q.8h*

Supply: 500 mg vial of powdered Tazidime with IV reconstitution directions that state, "For IV solution—Dilute with at least 5 mL Sterile Water for injection or other approved diluent."

- First, to prepare the order, how much and what type of diluent must you add? The directions state to add 5 mL of sterile water.
- Second, what is the supply dosage of the reconstituted Tazidime? Notice that the insert does not give a final supply dosage. In this case, the diluent will be used in the supply dosage. When adding 5 mL of diluent, the resulting supply dosage is 500 mg/5 mL or 100 mg/mL.
- Third, what is the resulting total volume of this reconstituted solution? The total volume is 5 mL. Unless indicated otherwise, the solution volume is sufficient to dilute the powder without adding additional volume.
- Finally, how many full doses of Tazidime are available in this vial? The vial contains 500 mg and the order is for 400 mg. There is one full dose in the vial. No reconstitution label is needed.

This means that you have available a vial of 500 mg of Tazidime to which you will add 5 mL of diluent. The final yield of the solution is 5 mL with a supply dosage of 100 mg/mL. Most IV antibiotics are then further diluted in an approved IV solution and infused over a specified time period. You will learn more about this in the next section and in Chapter 16.

Calculate one dose.

Step 1	Convert	No conversion necessary
		Order: *Tazidime 400 mg IV q.8h*
		Supply: 100 mg/mL
Step 2	Think	You want to give more than 1 mL.
Step 3	Calculate	$\dfrac{D}{H} \times Q = \dfrac{\overset{4}{\cancel{400}}\ \cancel{mg}}{\underset{1}{\cancel{100}}\ \cancel{mg}} \times 1\ mL = 4\ mL$
		given intravenously every 8 hours

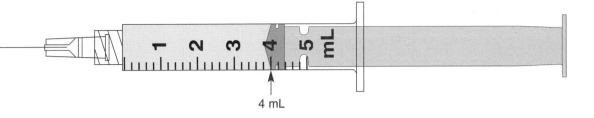

4 mL

Drugs with Instructions to "See Package Insert" for Dilution and Administration

Some labels only give the dosage strength contained in the vial and other minimal information that is insufficient to properly reconstitute or safely store the drug. To prepare the powdered medication, you must see the package insert. Look at the Amphocin label and the accompanying package insert (Figure 11-12). The label instructs you to "See insert for reconstitution and dosage information." The following example demonstrates the use of the package insert for calculating the dosage.

AVOID ERRORS
READ CAREFULLY

STOP Verify the product name and dosage if dose exceeds 1.5 mg/kg.

See insert for reconstitution and dosage information.

Store under refrigeration 2° to 8°C (36° to 46°F).

Protect from light during administration.

SEE BOTTOM OF CARTON FOR EXP. DATE AND LOT NO.

Each vial contains a sterile, lyophilized cake providing 50 mg amphotericin B and 41 mg sodium desoxycholate buffered with 20.2 mg sodium phosphates (consisting of mono and dibasic sodium phosphate, phosphoric acid and sodium hydroxide).

PHARMACIA

Patient

Room No.

Dose

Manufactured for:
Pharmacia & Upjohn Co.
A subsidiary of
Pharmacia Corporation
Kalamazoo, MI 49001, USA

By:
SP Pharmaceuticals
Albuquerque, NM 87109, USA

817 170 002

1 Vial   NDC 0013-1405-44

Amphocin®
amphotericin B
for injection, USP

50 mg
FOR INTRAVENOUS INFUSION ONLY

STOP Verify the product name and dosage if dose exceeds 1.5 mg/kg.

℞ only   ***PHARMACIA***

Manufactured for:
Pharmacia & Upjohn Co.
A subsidiary of
Pharmacia Corporation
Kalamazoo, MI 49001, USA

By:
SP Pharmaceuticals
Albuquerque, NM 87109, USA

PREPARATION OF SOLUTIONS

Reconstitute as follows: An initial concentrate of 5 mg amphacericin B per mL is first prepared by rapidly expressing 10 mL Sterile Water for injection, USP *without a bacteriostatic agent* directly into the lyephilized cake, using a sterile needle (minimum diameter: 20 gague) and syringe. Shake the vial immediately until the colloidal solution is clear. The infusion solution, providing 0.1 mg amphocericim B per mL, is then obtained by further dilution (1:50) with 5% Dextrose injection, USP *of pH above 4.2.* The pH of each container of Dextrose injection should be ascertained before use. Commercial Dextrose Injection usually has a pH above 4.2, however, if it is below 4.2, then 1 or 2 mL of buffer should be added to the Dextrose injection before it is used to dilute the concentrated solution of amphotericin B. The recommended buffer has the following composition

Dibasic sodium phosphate (anhydrous)	1.59 g
Monobasic sodium phosphate (anhydrous)	0.96 g
Water for injection, USP	qs 100.0 mL

The buffer should be sterilized before it is added to the Dextrose injection, either by filtration through a bacterial retentive stone mat or membrane, or by autoclaving for 30 minutes at 15 lb pressure (121°C). **CAUTION: Aseptic technique must be strictly observed in all handling,** since no preservative or bacteriostatic agent is present in the anobiotic or in the materials used to prepare it for administration. **All entries into the vial or into the diluents must be made with a sterile needle. Do not reconstitute with saline solutions. The use of any diluent other than the ones recommended or the presence of a bacteriostatic agent** (e.g. benzyl alcohol) **in the diluent may cause precipitation of the antibiotic. Do not use the initial concentrate or the infusion solution if there is any evidence of precipitation or foreign matter in either one.**

An in-line membrane filter may be used for intraveneous infusion of amphocericin B; **however, the mean pore diameter of the filter should not be less than 1.0 micron in order to assure passage of the antibiotic dispersion.**

FIGURE 11-12 Amphocin Label and Portion of Package Insert

Example:

Order: *Amphocin 37.5 mg IV q.d.*

Supply: Amphocin 50 mg

Look at the preparation instructions given in the package insert (Figure 11-12).
- First, to fill the order, how much and what type of diluent must you add? The directions advise the preparer, for initial concentration, to add 10 mL of sterile water for injection without a bacteriostatic agent and then to further dilute the solution containing 5 mg/mL to 0.1 mg/mL by adding 1 mL (5 mg) of solution to 49 mL of 5% Dextrose and Water Injection for a 1:50 dilution. (We will use the latter information after we calculate the dosage.)
- Second, what is the supply dosage of the reconstituted Amphocin? When adding 10 mL of diluent, the supply dosage is 5 mg/mL.
- Third, what is the resulting total volume of this reconstituted solution? The total volume is 10 mL. You know this because the supply dosage is 5 mg/mL or 50 mg/10 mL. The powder does not add significant volume to this solution.
- Finally, how many full doses of Amphocin are available in this vial? The vial contains 50 mg and the order is for 37.5 mg. There is enough for one full dose in the vial, but not enough for two full doses. No reconstitution label is needed.

This means that you have available a vial of 50 mg of Amphocin to which you will add 10 mL of diluent. The final yield of the solution is 5 mg/mL, which is your supply dosage. Each 1 mL (5 mg) must be further diluted with 49 mL of IV solution for administration.

Calculate one dose of the initial concentration (before further dilution).

Step 1	Convert	No conversion necessary

Order: *Amphocin 37.5 mg IV q.d.*

Supply: Amphocin 5 mg/mL

Step 2	Think	You want to give more than 1 mL, but less than 10 mL.

Step 3   Calculate $\dfrac{D}{H} \times Q = \dfrac{37.5 \text{ mg}}{5 \text{ mg}} \times 1\,\text{mL} = 7.5\,\text{mL}$

given intravenously daily

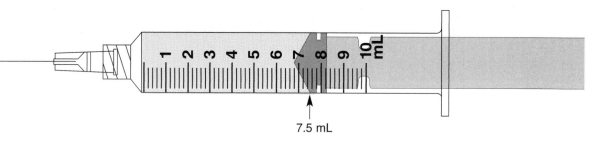

7.5 mL

Recall that the instructions indicate that further dilution of the initial concentration is required before administration: *further dilute the solution containing 5 mg/mL to 0.1 mg/mL by adding 1 mL (5 mg) of solution to 49 mL of 5% Dextrose and Water Injection.* We have 7.5 mL of concentrated solution; therefore, we need to add it to *7.5 × 49 = 367.5 or 368 mL* of IV solution before administering this drug intravenously. You can also use ratio-proportion to calculate this.

$$\frac{49}{1} \times \frac{X}{7.5}$$

X = 367.5 mL = 368 mL

QUICK REVIEW

It is important that you remember the following points when reconstituting drugs:

- If any medicine remains for future use after reconstitution, clearly label:
  1. date and time of preparation
  2. strength or concentration per volume
  3. potency expiration
  4. recommended storage
  5. your initials
- Read all instructions carefully. If no instructions accompany the vial, confer with the pharmacist before proceeding.
- When reconstituting multiple-strength parenteral powders, select the dosage strength that is appropriate for the patient's age, size, and condition.
- Carefully select the correct reconstitution directions for IM or IV administration.

REVIEW SET 29

Calculate the amount you will prepare for each dose. The labels provided are the drugs available. Draw an arrow to the syringe calibration that corresponds with the amount you will draw up and prepare a reconstitution label, if neded.

1. Order: *Ceftazidime 200 mg IM q.i.d.*

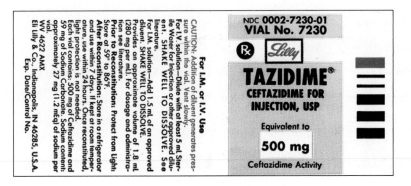

Reconstitute with _____ mL diluent for a concentration of _____ mg/mL.

Give: _____ mL

How many full doses are available in this vial? _____ dose(s).

Prepare a reconstitution label for the remaining solution.

Reconstitution Label

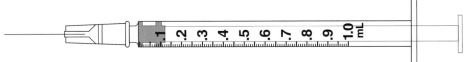

2. Order: *bacitracin 2500 U IM q.12h*

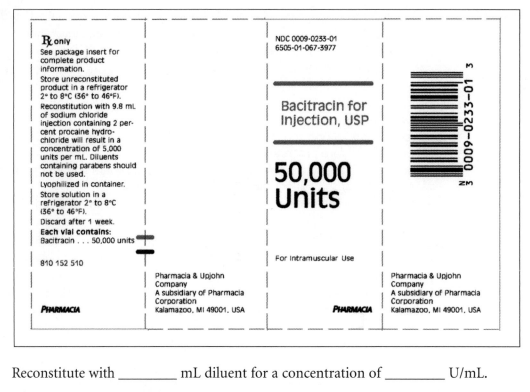

Reconstitute with _____ mL diluent for a concentration of _____ U/mL.

Give: _____ mL

How many full doses are available in this vial? _____ dose(s).

Prepare a reconstitution label for the remaining solution.

Reconstitution Label

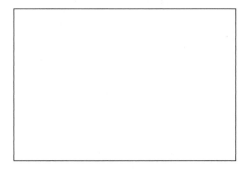

3. Order: *Librium 25 mg IM q.6h p.r.n., agitation*

Package insert states: "Add 2 mL Special Diluent to yield 100 mg per 2 mL."

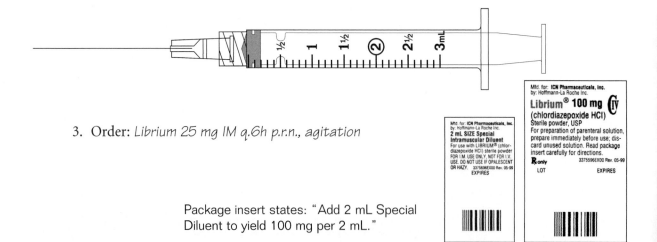

Reconstitute with _____ mL diluent for a concentration of _____ mg/_____ mL.

Give: _____ mL

How many full doses are available in this vial? _____ dose(s).

Does this reconstituted medication require a reconstitution label? _____
Explain: _____

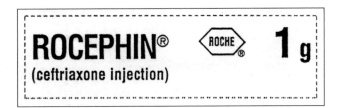

4. Order: *Zithromax 0.5 g IV q.d.*

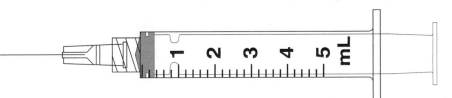

Store at or below 86°F (30°C).

DOSAGE AND USE
See accompanying prescribing information.
Constitute to 100 mg/mL* with
4.8 mL of Sterile Water For Injection.

Must be further diluted before use.
For appropriate diluents and storage
recommendations, refer to prescribing information.

*Each mL contains azithromycin dihydrate
equivalent to 100 mg of azithromycin,
76.9 mg of citric acid, and sodium hydroxide
for pH adjustment. 05-5191-32-0

CAUTION: Federal law prohibits
dispensing without prescription.

NDC 0069-3150-83

Zithromax®
(azithromycin for injection)

For **IV** infusion only
STERILE
equivalent to

500 mg
of azithromycin
Distributed by
Pfizer **Pfizer Labs**
Division of Pfizer Inc, NY, NY 10017

Lot No.
Exp. Date

Reconstitute with _____ mL diluent for a concentration of _____ mg/mL.

Give: _____ mL

How many full doses are available in this vial? _____ dose(s).

Does this reconstituted medication require a reconstitution label? _____

Explain: _____

5. Order: *Rocephin 750 mg IM q.d.*

ROCEPHIN® ⬡ROCHE⬡® **1 g**
(ceftriaxone injection)

See portion of package insert on next page.

DIRECTIONS FOR USE: Intramuscular Administration: Reconstitute Rocephin powder with the appropriate diluent (see COMPATIBILITY-STABILITY section).

Vial Dosage Size	Amount of Diluent to be Added
250 mg	0.9 mL
500 mg	1.8 mL
1 gm	3.6 mL
2 gm	7.2 mL

After reconstitution, each 1 mL of solution contains approximately 250 mg equivalent of ceftriaxone. If required, more dilute solutions could be utilized. As with all intramuscular preparations, Rocephin should be injected well within the body of a relatively large muscle; aspiration helps to avoid unintentional injection into a blood vessel.

Intravenous Administration: Rocephin should be administered intravenously by infusion over a period of 30 minutes. Concentrations between 10 mg/mL and 40 mg/mL are recommended; however, lower concentrations may be used if desired. Reconstitute vials or "piggyback" bottles with an appropriate I.V. diluent (see COMPATIBILITY-STABILITY section).

Vial Dosage Size	Amount of Diluent to be Added
250 mg	2.4 mL
500 mg	4.8 mL
1 gm	9.6 mL
2 gm	19.2 mL

After reconstitution, each 1 mL of solution contains approximately 100 mg equivalent of ceftriaxone. Withdraw entire contents and dilute to the desired concentration with the appropriate I.V. diluent.

Piggyback Bottle Dosage Size	Amount of Diluent to be Added
1 gm	10 mL
2 gm	20 mL

After reconstitution, further dilute to 50 mL or 100 mL volumes with the appropriate I.V. diluent.

10 gm Bulk Pharmacy Container: This dosage size is *NOT FOR DIRECT ADMINISTRATION.* Reconstitute powder with 95 mL of an appropriate I.V. diluent. Before parenteral administration, withdraw the required amount, then further dilute to the desired concentration.

COMPATIBILITY AND STABILITY: Rocephin sterile powder should be stored at room temperature—77°F (25°C)—or below and protected from light. After reconstitution, protection from normal light is not necessary. The color of solutions ranges from light yellow to amber, depending on the length of storage, concentration and diluent used.

ROCEPHIN® (ceftriaxone sodium injection)

Rocephin *intramuscular* solutions remain stable (loss of potency less than 10%) for the following time periods:

Diluent	Concentration mg/mL	Storage Room Temp. (25°C)	Storage Refrigerated (4°C)
Sterile Water for Injection	100	3 days	10 days
	250	24 hours	3 days
0.9% Sodium Chloride Solution	100	3 days	10 days
	250	24 hours	3 days
5% Dextrose Solution	100	3 days	10 days
	250	24 hours	3 days
Bacteriostatic Water + 0.9% Benzyl Alcohol	100	24 hours	10 days
	250	24 hours	3 days
1% Lidocaine Solution (without epinephrine)	100	24 hours	10 days
	250	24 hours	3 days

Rocephin *intravenous* solutions, at concentrations of 10, 20 and 40 mg/mL, remain stable (loss of potency less than 10%) for the following time periods stored in glass or PVC containers:

Diluent	Storage Room Temp. (25°C)	Storage Refrigerated (4°C)
Sterile Water	3 days	10 days
0.9% Sodium Chloride Solution	3 days	10 days
5% Dextrose Solution	3 days	10 days
10% Dextrose Solution	3 days	10 days
5% Dextrose + 0.9% Sodium Chloride Solution*	3 days	Incompatible
5% Dextrose + 0.45% Sodium Chloride Solution	3 days	Incompatible

*Data available for 10-40 mg/mL concentrations in this diluent in PVC containers only.

Similarly, Rocephin *intravenous* solutions, at concentrations of 100 mg/mL, remain stable in the I.V. piggyback glass containers for the above specified time periods.

The following *intravenous* Rocephin solutions are stable at room temperature (25°C) for 24 hours, at concentrations between 10 mg/mL and 40 mg/mL: Sodium Lactate (PVC container), 10% Invert Sugar (glass container), 5% Sodium Bicarbonate (glass container), Freamine III (glass container), Normosol-M in 5% Dextrose (glass and PVC containers), Ionosol-B in 5% Dextrose (glass container), 5% Mannitol (glass container), 10% Mannitol (glass container).

After the indicated stability time periods, unused portions of solutions should be discarded.

Rocephin reconstituted with 5% Dextrose or 0.9% Sodium Chloride solution at concentrations between 10 mg/mL and 40 mg/mL, and then stored in frozen state (−20°C) in PVC (Viaflex) or polyolefin containers, remains stable for 26 weeks.

Frozen solutions should be thawed at room temperature before use. After thawing, unused portions should be discarded. **DO NOT REFREEZE.**

Rocephin solutions should *not* be physically mixed with or piggybacked into solutions containing other antimicrobial drugs or into diluent solutions other than those listed above, due to possible incompatibility.

Reconstitute with _____ mL diluent for an initial concentration of _____ mg/mL.
Give: _____ mL

How many full doses are available in this vial? _____ dose(s)

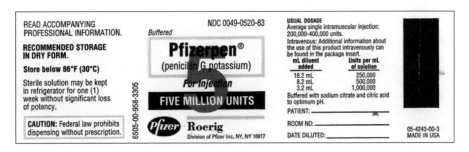

6. Order: *penicillin G potassium 1,000,000 U IM q.6h*

READ ACCOMPANYING PROFESSIONAL INFORMATION.		NDC 0049-0520-83	USUAL DOSAGE Average single intramuscular injection: 200,000-400,000 units.

Buffered

Pfizerpen®
(penicillin G potassium)
For Injection
FIVE MILLION UNITS

RECOMMENDED STORAGE IN DRY FORM.

Store below 86°F (30°C)

Sterile solution may be kept in refrigerator for one (1) week without significant loss of potency.

CAUTION: Federal law prohibits dispensing without prescription.

6505-00-958-3305

Pfizer Roerig
Division of Pfizer Inc, NY, NY 10017

USUAL DOSAGE
Average single intramuscular injection: 200,000-400,000 units.
Intravenous: Additional information about the use of this product intravenously can be found in the package insert.

mL diluent added	Units per mL of solution
18.2 mL	250,000
8.2 mL	500,000
3.2 mL	1,000,000

Buffered with sodium citrate and citric acid to optimum pH.

PATIENT: _____
ROOM NO: _____
DATE DILUTED: _____

05-4243-00-3
MADE IN USA

Describe the three concentrations and calculate the amount to give for each of the supply dosage concentrations.

Reconstitute with _____ mL diluent for a concentration of _____ U/mL, and give _____ mL.

Reconstitute with _____ mL diluent for a concentration of _____ U/mL, and give _____ mL.

Reconstitute with _____ mL diluent for a concentration of _____ U/mL, and give _____ mL.

Indicate the concentration you would choose and explain the rationale for your selection.

Select _____ U/mL and give _____ mL. Rationale: _____

_____

How many full doses are available in this vial? _____ dose(s)

Prepare a reconstitution label for the remaining solution.

Reconstitution Label

7. Order: *Solu-Medrol 175 mg IM q.d.*

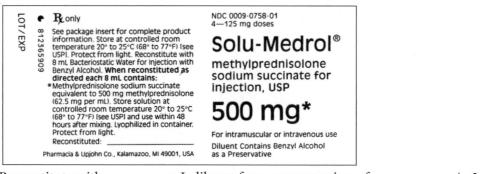

Reconstitute with _____ mL diluent for a concentration of _____ mg/mL.

Give: _____ mL

How many full doses are available in this vial? _____ dose(s).

Prepare a reconstitution label for the remaining solution.

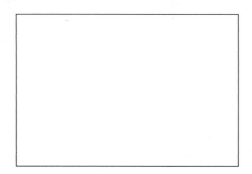

Reconstitution Label

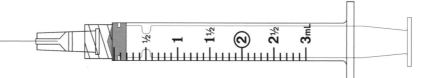

8. Order: *Pipracil 200 mg IM q.6h*

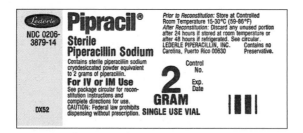

Package insert states, "Add 4 mL suitable diluent (sterile water or 0.9% NaCl) to yield 1 g/2.5 mL."

Reconstitute with _____ mL diluent for a concentration of _____ g/_____ mL. or _____ mg/_____ mL.

Give: _____ mL

How many full doses are available in this vial? _____ dose(s).

Prepare a reconstitution label for the remaining solution.

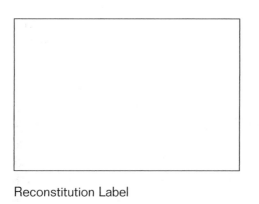

Reconstitution Label

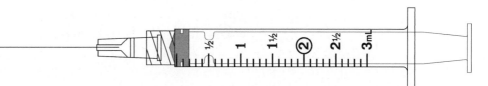

9. **Order:** *penicillin G potassium 500,000 U IM q.6h*

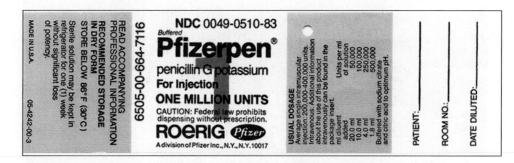

Describe the four concentrations and calculate the amount to give for each of the supply dosage concentrations.

Reconstitute with _____ mL diluent for a concentration of _____ U/mL, and give _____ mL.

Reconstitute with _____ mL diluent for a concentration of _____ U/mL, and give _____ mL.

Reconstitute with _____ mL diluent for a concentration of _____ U/mL, and give _____ mL.

Reconstitute with _____ mL diluent for a concentration of _____ U/mL, and give _____ mL.

Indicate the concentration you would choose and explain the rationale for your selection.

Select _____ U/mL and give _____ mL. Rationale: _____

_____

How many full doses are available in this vial? _____ dose(s)

Prepare a reconstitution label for the remaining solution.

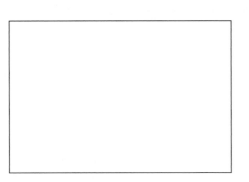

Reconstitution Label

10. Order: *Unasyn 1500 mg IM q.6h*

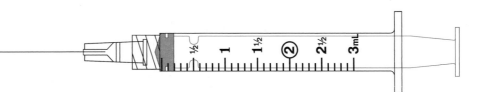

Package insert directions state:

Unasyn Vial Size	Volume Diluent to Be Added	Withdrawal Volume
1.5 g	3.2 mL	4.0 mL
3.0 g	6.4 mL	8.0 mL

Reconstitute with _____ mL diluent for a concentration of _____ g/_____ mL or _____ mg/mL.

Give: _____ mL

How many full doses are in this vial? _____ dose(s)

11. Order: *methylprednisolone succinate 24 mg IM q.d.*

Package insert with 40 mg Act-O-Vial system states,

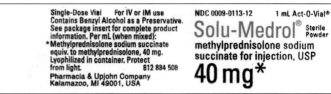

"Press down on plastic activator to force accompanying 1 mL diluent into the lower compartment."

The resulting concentration is _____ mg/mL.

Give _____ mL

How many full doses are available in this vial? _____ dose(s)

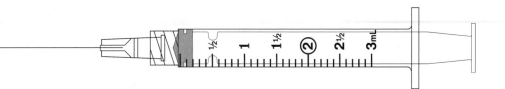

12. Order: *Fortaz 250 mg IV q.12h*

Lot _____	NDC 0173-0379-34	See package insert for Dosage and Administration. Before constitution, store between 15° and 30°C (59° and 86°F) and protect from light.
Exp. _____	**Fortaz®** (ceftazidime for injection)	**IMPORTANT:** The vial is under reduced pressure. Addition of diluent generates a positive pressure. Before constituting, see Instructions for Constitution. To prepare IV solution, add 10 mL of Sterile Water for Injection. After constitution, solutions maintain potency for 24 hours at room temperature (not exceeding 25°C [77°F]) or for 7 days under refrigeration. Constituted solutions in Sterile Water for Injection may be frozen. See package insert for details. Color changes do not affect potency. This vial contains 236 mg of sodium carbonate. The sodium content is approximately 108 mg (4.7 mEq).
	2 g R only Equivalent to 2 g of ceftazidime. For IV use.	GlaxoSmithKline, Research Triangle Park, NC 27709 Made in England Rev. 1/02

Reconstitute with _____ mL diluent for a concentration of _____ g/_____ mL or _____ mg/mL.

Give: _____ mL

How many full doses are available in this vial? _____ dose(s).

Will the drug remain potent to use all available doses? _____
Explain: _____

Prepare a reconstitution label for the remaining solution.

Reconstitution Label

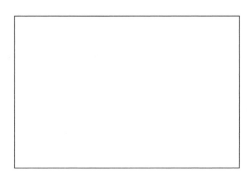

13. Order: *Rocephin 1500 mg IV q.6h in 50 mL D₅W (5% Dextrose & Water IV solution)*

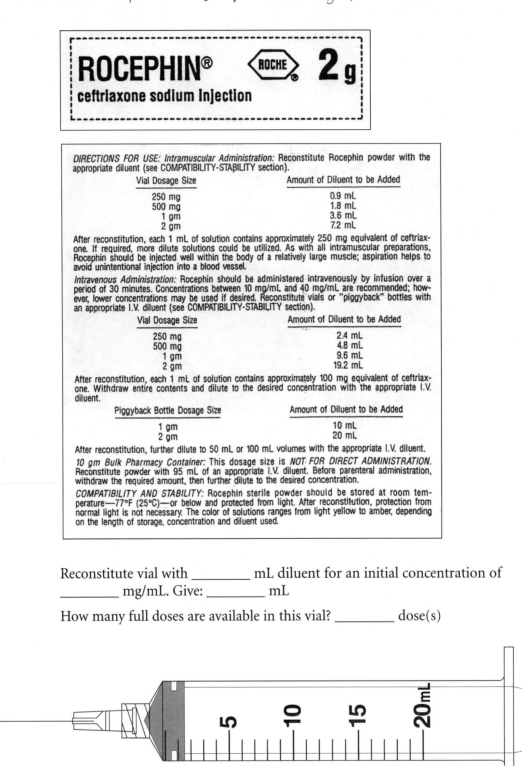

ROCEPHIN®   〈ROCHE〉 **2 g**
ceftriaxone sodium injection

DIRECTIONS FOR USE: *Intramuscular Administration:* Reconstitute Rocephin powder with the appropriate diluent (see COMPATIBILITY-STABILITY section).

Vial Dosage Size	Amount of Diluent to be Added
250 mg	0.9 mL
500 mg	1.8 mL
1 gm	3.6 mL
2 gm	7.2 mL

After reconstitution, each 1 mL of solution contains approximately 250 mg equivalent of ceftriaxone. If required, more dilute solutions could be utilized. As with all intramuscular preparations, Rocephin should be injected well within the body of a relatively large muscle; aspiration helps to avoid unintentional injection into a blood vessel.

Intravenous Administration: Rocephin should be administered intravenously by infusion over a period of 30 minutes. Concentrations between 10 mg/mL and 40 mg/mL are recommended; however, lower concentrations may be used if desired. Reconstitute vials or "piggyback" bottles with an appropriate I.V. diluent (see COMPATIBILITY-STABILITY section).

Vial Dosage Size	Amount of Diluent to be Added
250 mg	2.4 mL
500 mg	4.8 mL
1 gm	9.6 mL
2 gm	19.2 mL

After reconstitution, each 1 mL of solution contains approximately 100 mg equivalent of ceftriaxone. Withdraw entire contents and dilute to the desired concentration with the appropriate I.V. diluent.

Piggyback Bottle Dosage Size	Amount of Diluent to be Added
1 gm	10 mL
2 gm	20 mL

After reconstitution, further dilute to 50 mL or 100 mL volumes with the appropriate I.V. diluent.

10 gm Bulk Pharmacy Container: This dosage size is *NOT FOR DIRECT ADMINISTRATION.* Reconstitute powder with 95 mL of an appropriate I.V. diluent. Before parenteral administration, withdraw the required amount, then further dilute to the desired concentration.

COMPATIBILITY AND STABILITY: Rocephin sterile powder should be stored at room temperature—77°F (25°C)—or below and protected from light. After reconstitution, protection from normal light is not necessary. The color of solutions ranges from light yellow to amber, depending on the length of storage, concentration and diluent used.

Reconstitute vial with _____ mL diluent for an initial concentration of _____ mg/mL. Give: _____ mL

How many full doses are available in this vial? _____ dose(s)

ROCEPHIN® (ceftriaxone sodium injection)

Rocephin *intramuscular* solutions remain stable (loss of potency less than 10%) for the following time periods:

Diluent	Concentration mg/mL	Storage Room Temp. (25°C)	Refrigerated (4°C)
Sterile Water for Injection	100	3 days	10 days
	250	24 hours	3 days
0.9% Sodium Chloride Solution	100	3 days	10 days
	250	24 hours	3 days
5% Dextrose Solution	100	3 days	10 days
	250	24 hours	3 days
Bacteriostatic Water + 0.9% Benzyl Alcohol	100	24 hours	10 days
	250	24 hours	3 days
1% Lidocaine Solution (without epinephrine)	100	24 hours	10 days
	250	24 hours	3 days

Rocephin *intravenous* solutions, at concentrations of 10, 20 and 40 mg/mL, remain stable (loss of potency less than 10%) for the following time periods stored in glass or PVC containers:

Diluent	Storage Room Temp. (25°C)	Refrigerated (4°C)
Sterile Water	3 days	10 days
0.9% Sodium Chloride Solution	3 days	10 days
5% Dextrose Solution	3 days	10 days
10% Dextrose Solution	3 days	10 days
5% Dextrose + 0.9% Sodium Chloride Solution*	3 days	Incompatible
5% Dextrose + 0.45% Sodium Chloride Solution	3 days	Incompatible

*Data available for 10-40 mg/mL concentrations in this diluent in PVC containers only.

Similarly, Rocephin *intravenous* solutions, at concentrations of 100 mg/mL, remain stable in the I.V. piggyback glass containers for the above specified time periods.

The following *intravenous* Rocephin solutions are stable at room temperature (25°C) for 24 hours, at concentrations between 10 mg/mL and 40 mg/mL: Sodium Lactate (PVC container), 10% Invert Sugar (glass container), 5% Sodium Bicarbonate (glass container), Freamine III (glass container), Normosol-M in 5% Dextrose (glass and PVC containers), Ionosol-B in 5% Dextrose (glass container), 5% Mannitol (glass container), 10% Mannitol (glass container).

After the indicated stability time periods, unused portions of solutions should be discarded.

Rocephin reconstituted with 5% Dextrose or 0.9% Sodium Chloride solution at concentrations between 10 mg/mL and 40 mg/mL, and then stored in frozen state (−20°C) in PVC (Viaflex) or polyolefin containers, remains stable for 26 weeks.

Frozen solutions should be thawed at room temperature before use. After thawing, unused portions should be discarded. **DO NOT REFREEZE.**

Rocephin solutions should *not* be physically mixed with or piggybacked into solutions containing other antimicrobial drugs or into diluent solutions other than those listed above, due to possible incompatibility.

14. Order: *Nebcin 200 mg IV q.8h*

Reconstitute with _____ mL diluent for a concentration of _____ mg/mL.

Give: _____ mL

How many full doses are available in this vial? _____ dose(s).

Prepare a reconstitution label for the remaining solution.

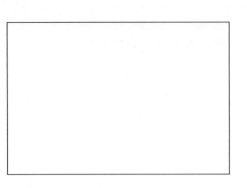

Reconstitution Label

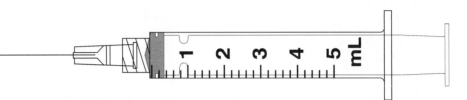

15. Order: *Kefzol 250 mg IM q.6h*

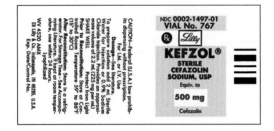

Reconstitute with _____ mL diluent for a concentration of _____ mg/mL.

Give: _____ mL

How many full doses are available in this vial? _____ dose(s).

Prepare a reconstitution label for the remaining solution.

Reconstitution Label

After completing these problems, see pages 493–498 to check your answers.

RECONSTITUTION OF NONINJECTABLE SOLUTIONS

Now let's look at reconstitution of noninjectable solutions, such as nutritional formulas and irrigating solutions. In most cases, the nurse or health care professional must dilute a liquid concentrate (*solute*) with water or saline (*solvent*) to make a weaker *solution*.

Solution Concentration

An important concept for understanding solution concentration or strength is that the amount of solvent used to decrease the total concentration is determined by the desired final strength of the solution. The *less* solvent added, the more concentrated the final solution strength; the *more* solvent added, the less concentrated the final solution strength. Think of orange juice concentrate as a way to illustrate this concept. The directions call for 3 cans of water to be added to 1 can of orange juice concentrate. The result is "reconstituted juice," a ready-to-drink beverage. If you like a stronger orange taste, you might add only 2 cans of water, making it a *more* concentrated juice, but you get *less total volume* to drink. If you have several people wanting to drink orange juice, you might choose to add 4 cans of water to the final total volume. You get *more* volume, but the orange juice is *less* concentrated; therefore, it is more dilute, because you have increased the water (solvent) content. Note that in either case, the amount of orange juice concentrate in the final solution is the same.

Medical notation to express the strength of a solution uses either a ratio, percent, or fraction. The fraction is the preferred form because it is easily applied in calculation and helps explain the ratio of solute to total solution. Recall that a ratio or percent can also be expressed as a fraction.

> ### RULE
>
> When a fraction expresses the strength of a solution, made from a liquid concentrate:
> - The *numerator* of the fraction is the number of parts of *solute*.
> - The *denominator* of the fraction is the total number of parts of total *solution*.
> - The *difference* between the denominator (final solution) and the numerator (parts of solute) is the number of parts of *solvent*.

Let's describe some solutions made from liquid concentrates.

Example 1:

$\frac{1}{4}$ *strength reconstituted orange juice* made from canned frozen concentrate

$\frac{1}{4}$ strength $= \frac{\text{1 part (can) of frozen orange juice concentrate}}{\text{4 parts (cans) of total reconstituted orange juice}}$

- 1 part (can) frozen orange juice concentrate (*solute*, numerator)
- 4 parts (cans) of total reconstituted orange juice (*solution*, denominator)
- $4 - 1 = 3$ parts (cans) of water (*solvent*)

Three cans of water added to one can frozen orange juice concentrate makes four cans of a final reconstituted orange juice solution. The resulting $\frac{1}{4}$ strength reconstituted orange juice is comparable to the strength of fresh juice.

Example 2:

$\frac{1}{3}$ *strength nutritional formula*

- 1 part concentrate formula as the solute
- 3 parts of total solution
- $3 - 1 = 2$ parts solvent (water)

Calculating Solutions

To prepare a prescribed solution of a certain strength from a solute, you can apply a similar formula to the one you learned for calculating dosages: $\frac{D}{H} \times Q = X$.

RULE

To prepare solutions,
1. D (Desired solution strength) × Q (Quantity of desired solution) = X (Amount of solute)
   or you can apply ratio-proportion to find the amount of solute:
   Ratio for desired solution strength = $\frac{\text{Amount of solute}}{\text{Quantity of desired solution}}$
2. Quantity of desired solution − Amount of solute = Amount of solvent

---

In this application, "D" is the strength of the desired solution, which is written as a fraction. "Q" is the amount of solution you desire to prepare, usually expressed as mL or ounces. The unknown "X" you are solving for is the quantity or amount of solute you will need to add to the solvent to prepare the desired solution. Let's look at how this rule and formula are applied in health care.

TOPICAL SOLUTIONS/IRRIGANTS

Topical or irrigating solutions may be mixed from powders, salts, or liquid concentrates. Asepsis in mixing, storage, and use is essential. Liquids can quickly harbor microorganisms. Our focus here is to review the essentials of reconstitution, but nurses and other health care professionals need to be alert at all times to the chain of infection.

Most often nurses and other health care professionals will further dilute ready-to-use solutions, which are called *full-strength* or stock solutions, to create a less concentrated liquid. Consider the desired solution strength as well as the final volume needed for the task.

Example 1:

Hydrogen peroxide, which is usually available full strength as a 3% solution, can be very drying to the skin and should not be directly applied undiluted. For use as a topical antiseptic, the therapeutic protocol is to reconstitute hydrogen peroxide to $\frac{1}{2}$ strength with normal saline used as the solvent. You decide to make 4 ounces that can be kept in a sterile container at the patient's bedside for traction pin care.

Step 1	**Convert**	No conversion is necessary.
Step 2	**Think**	The fraction represents the desired solution strength: $\frac{1}{2}$ strength means 1 part solute (hydrogen peroxide) to 2 total parts solution. The amount of solvent is 2 − 1 = 1 part saline. Because you need 4 oz of solution, you estimate that you will need $\frac{1}{2}$ of it as solute and $\frac{1}{2}$ of it as solvent, or 2 oz hydrogen peroxide and 2 oz saline to make a total of 4 oz of $\frac{1}{2}$ strength hydrogen peroxide.
Step 3	**Calculate**	$D \times Q = X$

$\frac{1}{2}$ (Strength of desired solution) × 4 oz (Quantity desired) = X (Amount of solute)

$\frac{1}{2} \times 4 \text{ oz} = 2 \text{ oz solute}$

You could also use ratio-proportion, if you prefer.

Remember that $\frac{1}{2}$ strength $= \frac{1 \text{ part solute}}{2 \text{ parts total solution}}$. Here, the desired solution strength is $\frac{1}{2}$. The quantity of solution desired is 4 oz. You want to know how much solute (X oz) you will need.

$$\frac{1}{2} \times \frac{X \text{ oz}}{4 \text{ oz}} \begin{array}{l} \text{(solute)} \\ \text{(solution)} \end{array}$$

$$2X = 4$$

$$\frac{2X}{2} = \frac{4}{2}$$

$$X = 2 \text{ oz of solute}$$

X (2 oz) is the quantity of solute (full-strength hydrogen peroxide) you will need to prepare the desired solution (4 oz of $\frac{1}{2}$ strength hydrogen peroxide). The amount of solvent is 4 oz − 2 oz = 2 oz. If you add 2 ounces of full-strength hydrogen peroxide (solute) to 2 ounces of normal saline (solvent) you will prepare 4 ounces of a $\frac{1}{2}$ strength hydrogen peroxide topical antiseptic.

Example 2:

Suppose a physician orders a patient's *wound irrigated with $\frac{2}{3}$ strength hydrogen peroxide and normal saline solution q.4h while awake.* You will need 60 mL per irrigation and will do 3 irrigations during your 12 hour shift. You will need to prepare 60 mL × 3 irrigations = 180 mL total solution. How much stock hydrogen peroxide and normal saline will you need?

Step 1 Convert   No conversion is necessary.

Step 2 Think   You want to make $\frac{2}{3}$ strength, which means 2 parts solute (concentrated hydrogen peroxide) to 3 total parts solution. The amount of solvent is 3 − 2 = 1 part saline. Because you need 180 mL of solution, you estimate that you will need $\frac{2}{3}$ of it as solute ($\frac{2}{3} \times 180 = 120$ mL) and $\frac{1}{3}$ of it as solvent ($\frac{1}{3} \times 180 = 60$ mL).

Step 3 Calculate $D \times Q = \frac{2}{3} \times 180$ mL = 120 mL of solute

Or, use ratio-proportion, if you prefer.

$$\frac{2}{3} \times \frac{X \text{ mL}}{180 \text{ mL}} \begin{array}{l} \text{(solute)} \\ \text{(solution)} \end{array}$$

$$3X = 360$$

$$\frac{3X}{3} = \frac{360}{3}$$

$$X = 120 \text{ mL of solute}$$

"X" (120 mL) is the quantity of solute (hydrogen peroxide) you will need to prepare the desired solution (180 mL of $\frac{2}{3}$ strength). Because you desire to make a total of 180 mL of solution for wound irrigation, the amount of solvent you need is 180 − 120 = 60 mL of normal saline. Therefore, to make 180 mL of $\frac{2}{3}$ strength hydrogen peroxide, mix 120 mL full-strength hydrogen peroxide and 60 mL normal saline.

ORAL AND ENTERAL FEEDINGS

The principles of reconstitution are frequently applied to nutritional liquids for children and adults with special needs. Premature infants require increased calories for growth yet cannot take large volumes of fluid. Children who suffer from intestinal malabsorption require incremental changes as their bodies adjust to more concentrated formulas. Adults, especially the elderly, also experience nutritional problems that can be remedied with liquid nutrition. Prepared solutions that are taken orally or through feeding tubes are usually available and ready to use from manufacturers. Nutritional solutions may also be mixed from powders or liquid concentrates. Figure 11-13 shows examples of the

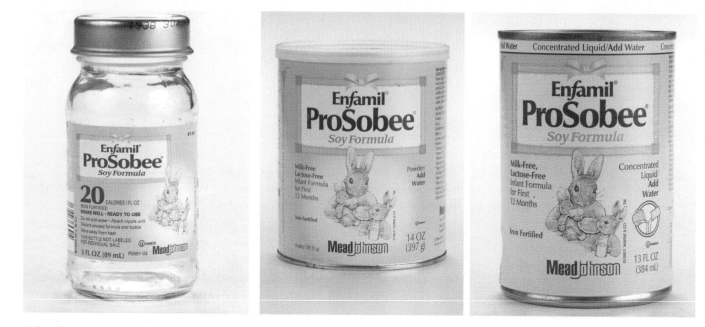

FIGURE 11-13 Nutritional Formulas

three forms of one nutritional formula. Directions on the label detail how much water should be added to the powdered form or liquid concentrate. Nutritionists provide further expertise in creating complex solutions for special patient needs.

As mentioned previously, health care professionals must be alert at all times to the chain of infection. Asepsis in mixing, storage, and use of nutritional liquids is essential. Because they contain sugars, such liquids have an increased risk for contamination during preparation and spoilage during storage and use. These are important concepts to teach a patient's family members.

Diluting Ready-to-Use Nutritional Liquids

Ready-to-use nutritional liquids are those solutions that are normally administered directly from the container without any further dilution. Most ready-to-use formulas contain 20 calories per ounce and are used for children and adults. The manufacturer balances the solute (nutrition) and solvent (water) to create a balanced, full-strength solution. However, some children and adults require less than full-strength formula for a short period to normalize intestinal absorption. Nutritional formulas are diluted with sterile water or tap water for oral use. Consult the facility policy regarding the use of tap water to reconstitute nutritional formulas. Let's look at a few typical examples.

Example 1:

A physician orders *Ensure $\frac{1}{4}$ strength 120 mL q.2h via NG tube × 3 feedings* for a patient who is recovering from gastric surgery. Available are 4 and 8 ounce cans of Ensure ready-to-use formula.

Step 1	**Convert**	Approximate equivalent: 1 oz = 30 mL; Larger → Smaller: (×) 4 oz = 4 × 30 = 120 mL and 8 oz = 8 × 30 = 240 mL
Step 2	**Think**	You need 120 mL total reconstituted formula for each of 3 feedings. This is a total of 120 × 3 = 360 mL. But you must dilute the full-strength formula to $\frac{1}{4}$ strength. You know that $\frac{1}{4}$ strength means 1 part formula to 4 parts solution. The solvent needed is 4 − 1 = 3 parts water. You will need $\frac{1}{4}$ of the solution as solute ($\frac{1}{4}$ × 360 mL = 90 mL) and $\frac{3}{4}$ of the solution as solvent ($\frac{3}{4}$ × 360 mL = 270 mL). Therefore, if you mix 90 mL of full-strength formula with 270 mL of water, you will have 360 mL of $\frac{1}{4}$ strength formula.

Step 3 Calculate $D \times Q = \frac{1}{4} \times 360 \text{ mL} = 90 \text{ mL full-strength Ensure}$

Or, use ratio-proportion.

$$\frac{1}{4} \diagdown\mkern-13mu\diagup \frac{X \text{ mL}}{360 \text{ mL}}$$

$$4X = 360$$

$$\frac{4X}{4} = \frac{360}{4}$$

$$X = 90 \text{ mL of full-strength Ensure}$$

You need 90 mL of the formula (solute). Use 90 mL from the 4 oz can because it contains 120 mL. (You will have 30 mL left over.) The amount of solvent needed is 360 − 90 = 270 mL water. Add 270 mL water to 90 mL of full-strength Ensure to make a total of 360 mL of $\frac{1}{4}$ strength Ensure. You now have enough for 3 full feedings. Administer 120 mL to the patient for each feeding.

Example 2:

The physician orders *800 mL of $\frac{3}{4}$ strength Sustacal through a gastrostomy tube over 8 hours* to supplement a patient while he sleeps. Sustacal ready-to-use formula comes in 10 ounce cans.

Step 1 Convert 1 oz = 30 mL; 10 oz = 10 × 30 = 300 mL

Step 2 Think The ordered solution strength is $\frac{3}{4}$. This means "3 parts solute to 4 total parts in solution." You know that $\frac{3}{4}$ of the 800 mL will be solute or full-strength Sustacal ($\frac{3}{4} \times 800 = 600$ mL) and $\frac{1}{4}$ of the solution will be solvent or water ($\frac{1}{4} \times 800 = 200$ mL). This proportion of solute to solvent will reconstitute the Sustacal to the required $\frac{3}{4}$ strength and total volume of 800 mL.

Step 3 Calculate $D \times Q = \frac{3}{4} \times 800 \text{ mL} = 600 \text{ mL of full-strength Sustacal}$

Or, use ratio-proportion.

$$\frac{3}{4} \diagdown\mkern-13mu\diagup \frac{X \text{ mL}}{800 \text{ mL}}$$

$$4X = 2400$$

$$\frac{4X}{4} = \frac{2400}{4}$$

$$X = 600 \text{ mL of full-strength Sustacal}$$

You need 600 mL of the formula (solute). Because the 10 ounce can contains 300 mL, you will need 2 cans (600 mL) to prepare the $\frac{3}{4}$ strength Sustacal as ordered. The amount of solvent needed is 800 mL − 600 mL = 200 mL water. Add 200 mL water to 600 mL (or 2 cans) of full-strength Ensure to make a total of 800 mL of $\frac{3}{4}$ strength Sustacal for the full feeding.

QUICK REVIEW

- *Solute*—a concentrated or solid substance to be dissolved or diluted.
- *Solvent*—or diluent, a liquid substance that dissolves another substance to prepare a solution.
- *Solution*—the resulting mixture of a solute plus a solvent.
- When a fraction expresses the strength of a desired solution to be made from a liquid concentrate:
  - The *numerator* of the fraction is the number of parts of *solute*.
  - The *denominator* of the fraction is the total number of parts of *solution*.
  - The *difference between the denominator and the numerator* is the number of parts of *solvent*.

- To prepare solutions:
  1. D (Desired solution strength) × Q (Quantity of desired solution) = X (Amount of solute)
     or, Ratio for desired solution strength = $\dfrac{\text{Amount of solute}}{\text{Quantity of desired solution}}$
  2. Quantity of desired solution − Amount of solute = Amount of solvent.

REVIEW SET 30

Explain how you would prepare each of the following solutions, using liquid stock hydrogen peroxide as the solute and saline as the solvent.

1. 480 mL of $\frac{1}{3}$ strength for wound irrigation. _____

2. 4 ounces of $\frac{1}{4}$ strength for skin cleansing. _____

3. 240 mL of $\frac{3}{4}$ strength for skeletal pin care. _____

4. 16 ounces of $\frac{1}{2}$ strength for wound care. _____

Explain how you would prepare each of the following from ready-to-use nutritional formulas for the specified time period. Note which supply would require the least discard of unused formula.

5. $\frac{1}{3}$ strength Ensure 900 mL via NG tube over 9 h. Supply: Ensure 4, 8, 12 ounce cans.

_____

6. $\frac{1}{4}$ strength Isomil 4 oz p.o. q.4 h for 24 h. Supply: Isomil 3, 6, 12 ounce cans. _____

_____

7. $\frac{2}{3}$ strength Sustacal 300 mL p.o. q.i.d. Supply: Sustacal 5 and 10 ounce cans. _____

_____

8. $\frac{1}{2}$ strength Ensure 26 oz via gastrostomy tube over 5 h. Supply: 4, 8, 12 ounce cans.

_____

9. $\frac{1}{2}$ strength Sustacal 250 mL p.o. q.i.d. Supply: Sustacal 5 and 10 ounce cans. _____

_____

10 $\frac{3}{4}$ strength Isomil 8 oz p.o. q.4 h for 24 h. Supply: Isomil 3, 6, 12 ounce cans. _____

_____

11. $\frac{2}{3}$ strength Ensure 6 oz via gastrostomy tube over 2 h. Supply: 4, 8, 12 ounce cans.

_____

12. $\frac{1}{4}$ strength Ensure 16 oz via NG tube over 6 h. Supply: Ensure 4, 8, 12 ounce cans.

_____

After completing these problems, see page 498 to check your answers.

CRITICAL THINKING SKILLS

Errors in formula dilution occur when the nurse fails to correctly calculate the amount of solute and solvent needed for the required solution strength.

error

Incorrect calculation of solute and solvent.

(continues)

(continued)

possible scenario

Suppose the physician ordered $\frac{1}{3}$ strength Isomil 90 mL p.o. q.3h for four feedings for an infant recovering from gastroenteritis. The concentration will be increased after these feedings. The nurse knows she will give all four feedings during her 12 hour shift, so she makes up 360 mL of formula. She takes a 3 ounce bottle of ready-to-use Isomil and adds three, 3 ounce bottles of water for oral use. She thinks, "One-third means 1 bottle of formula and 3 bottles of water. The amount I need even works out!"

potential outcome

What the nurse has actually mixed is a $\frac{1}{4}$ strength solution. Because the infant is getting a more dilute solution than intended, the amount of water to solute is increased and the incremental tolerance of more concentrated formula could be jeopardized. Thinking the child is tolerating $\frac{1}{3}$ strength, the physician might increase it to $\frac{2}{3}$ strength, and the infant may have problems digesting this more concentrated formula. His progress could be slowed or even set back.

prevention

The nurse should have thought through the meaning of the terms of a solution. If so, she would have recognized that $\frac{1}{3}$ strength meant 1 part solute (formula) to 3 total parts of solution with 2 parts water, not 1 part formula to 3 parts water. She should have applied the calculation formula or ratio-proportion to determine the amount of solute (full strength Isomil) needed and the amount of solvent (water) to add. If she did not know how to prepare the formula, she should have conferred with another nurse or called the pharmacy or dietary services for assistance. Never guess. Think and calculate with accuracy.

PRACTICE PROBLEMS—CHAPTER 11

Calculate the amount you will prepare for one dose. Indicate the syringe you will select to measure the medication.

1. Order: *Zosyn 2.5 g IV q.8h*

   Supply: 3.375 g vial of powdered Zosyn

   Directions: Reconstitute Zosyn with 5 mL of a diluent from the list for a total solution volume of 5 mL.

   The concentration is _____ g/_____ mL

   Give: _____ mL

   Select: _____ syringe

2. Order: *Ampicillin 500 mg IM q.4h*

   Supply: Ampicillin 500 mg

   Directions: Reconstitute with 1.8 mL diluent for a concentration of 250 mg/mL

   Give: _____ mL

   Select: _____ syringe

3. Order: *Ancef 500 mg IV q.6h*

   Supply: Ancef 1 g

   Directions: Reconstitute with 2.5 mL diluent to yield 3 mL with concentration of 330 mg/mL

   Give: _____ mL

   Select: _____ syringe

4. Order: *ceftriaxone sodium 750 mg IV q.6h in 50 mL 5% Dextrose & Water IV solution*

Supply: See label and package insert for Rocephin IV vial.

ROCEPHIN® ⬡ROCHE⬡ **2 g**
ceftriaxone sodium Injection

DIRECTIONS FOR USE: *Intramuscular Administration:* Reconstitute Rocephin powder with the appropriate diluent (see COMPATIBILITY-STABILITY section).

Vial Dosage Size	Amount of Diluent to be Added
250 mg	0.9 mL
500 mg	1.8 mL
1 gm	3.6 mL
2 gm	7.2 mL

After reconstitution, each 1 mL of solution contains approximately 250 mg equivalent of ceftriaxone. If required, more dilute solutions could be utilized. As with all intramuscular preparations, Rocephin should be injected well within the body of a relatively large muscle; aspiration helps to avoid unintentional injection into a blood vessel.

Intravenous Administration: Rocephin should be administered intravenously by infusion over a period of 30 minutes. Concentrations between 10 mg/mL and 40 mg/mL are recommended; however, lower concentrations may be used if desired. Reconstitute vials or "piggyback" bottles with an appropriate I.V. diluent (see COMPATIBILITY-STABILITY section).

Vial Dosage Size	Amount of Diluent to be Added
250 mg	2.4 mL
500 mg	4.8 mL
1 gm	9.6 mL
2 gm	19.2 mL

After reconstitution, each 1 mL of solution contains approximately 100 mg equivalent of ceftriaxone. Withdraw entire contents and dilute to the desired concentration with the appropriate I.V. diluent.

Piggyback Bottle Dosage Size	Amount of Diluent to be Added
1 gm	10 mL
2 gm	20 mL

After reconstitution, further dilute to 50 mL or 100 mL volumes with the appropriate I.V. diluent.

10 gm Bulk Pharmacy Container: This dosage size is *NOT FOR DIRECT ADMINISTRATION.* Reconstitute powder with 95 mL of an appropriate I.V. diluent. Before parenteral administration, withdraw the required amount, then further dilute to the desired concentration.

COMPATIBILITY AND STABILITY: Rocephin sterile powder should be stored at room temperature—77°F (25°C)—or below and protected from light. After reconstitution, protection from normal light is not necessary. The color of solutions ranges from light yellow to amber, depending on the length of storage, concentration and diluent used.

Add _____ mL diluent to the vial.

The concentration is _____ mg/mL

Give: _____ mL

How many full doses are available in this vial? _____

Select: _____ syringe

ROCEPHIN® (ceftriaxone sodium injection)

Rocephin *intramuscular* solutions remain stable (loss of potency less than 10%) for the following time periods:

Diluent	Concentration mg/mL	Storage Room Temp. (25°C)	Storage Refrigerated (4°C)
Sterile Water for Injection	100	3 days	10 days
	250	24 hours	3 days
0.9% Sodium Chloride Solution	100	3 days	10 days
	250	24 hours	3 days
5% Dextrose Solution	100	3 days	10 days
	250	24 hours	3 days
Bacteriostatic Water + 0.9% Benzyl Alcohol	100	24 hours	10 days
	250	24 hours	3 days
1% Lidocaine Solution (without epinephrine)	100	24 hours	10 days
	250	24 hours	3 days

Rocephin *intravenous* solutions, at concentrations of 10, 20 and 40 mg/mL, remain stable (loss of potency less than 10%) for the following time periods stored in glass or PVC containers:

Diluent	Storage Room Temp. (25°C)	Storage Refrigerated (4°C)
Sterile Water	3 days	10 days
0.9% Sodium Chloride Solution	3 days	10 days
5% Dextrose Solution	3 days	10 days
10% Dextrose Solution	3 days	10 days
5% Dextrose + 0.9% Sodium Chloride Solution*	3 days	Incompatible
5% Dextrose + 0.45% Sodium Chloride Solution	3 days	Incompatible

*Data available for 10-40 mg/mL concentrations in this diluent in PVC containers only.

Similarly, Rocephin *intravenous* solutions, at concentrations of 100 mg/mL, remain stable in the I.V. piggyback glass containers for the above specified time periods.

The following *intravenous* Rocephin solutions are stable at room temperature (25°C) for 24 hours, at concentrations between 10 mg/mL and 40 mg/mL: Sodium Lactate (PVC container), 10% Invert Sugar (glass container), 5% Sodium Bicarbonate (glass container), Freamine III (glass container), Normosol-M in 5% Dextrose (glass and PVC containers), Ionosol-B in 5% Dextrose (glass container), 5% Mannitol (glass container), 10% Mannitol (glass container).

After the indicated stability time periods, unused portions of solutions should be discarded.

Rocephin reconstituted with 5% Dextrose or 0.9% Sodium Chloride solution at concentrations between 10 mg/mL and 40 mg/mL, and then stored in frozen state (–20°C) in PVC (Viaflex) or polyolefin containers, remains stable for 26 weeks.

Frozen solutions should be thawed at room temperature before use. After thawing, unused portions should be discarded. **DO NOT REFREEZE.**

Rocephin solutions should *not* be physically mixed with or piggybacked into solutions containing other antimicrobial drugs or into diluent solutions other than those listed above, due to possible incompatibility.

5. Order: *cefepime 500 mg IM q.12h*

Supply: Maxipime (cefepime) 1 g

Directions: Reconstitute with 2.4 mL diluent for an approximate available volume of 3.6 mL and a concentration of 280 mg/mL.

Give: _____ mL

Select: _____ syringe

How many full doses are available in this vial? _____ dose(s).

Prepare a reconstitution label for the remaining solution. The drug is stable for up to 7 days refrigerated and 24 hours at controlled room temperature.

Reconstitution Label

6. Order: *Synercid 375 mg IV q.8h*

   Supply: Synercid 500 mg

   Directions: Reconstitute with 5 mL sterile water for a concentration of 100 mg/mL.

   Give: _____ mL

   Select: _____ syringe

   How many full doses are available in this vial? _____

Calculate one dose of each of the drug orders numbered 7 through 15. The labels shown on pages 259–260 are the medications you have available. Indicate which syringe you would select to measure the dose to be administered. Specify if a reconstitution label is required for multiple-dose vials.

7. Order: *Kefzol 300 mg IV q.8h*

   Reconstitute with _____ mL diluent for a concentration of _____ mg/mL and give _____ mL.

   Select: _____ syringe

   How many full doses are available in this vial? _____ dose(s)

   Is a reconstitution label required? _____

8. Order: *Solu-Medrol 200 mg IV q.6h*

   Reconstitute with _____ mL diluent for a concentration of _____ mg/mL and give _____ mL.

   Select: _____ syringe

   How many full doses are available in this vial? _____ dose(s)

   Is a reconstitution label required? _____

9. Order: *Tazidime 350 mg IM q.12h*

   Reconstitute with _____ mL diluent for a concentration of _____ mg/mL and give _____ mL.

   Select: _____ syringe

   How many full doses are available in this vial? _____ dose(s)

   Is a reconstitution label required? _____

10. Order: *Bacitracin 7500 U IM q.12h*

    Reconstitute with _____ mL diluent for a concentration of _____ U/mL and give _____ mL.

    Select: _____ syringe

    How many full doses are available in this vial? _____ dose(s)

    Is a reconstitution label required? _____

11. Order: *Fortaz 1.25 g IV q.12h*

    Reconstitute with _____ mL diluent for a concentration of _____ g/_____ mL and give _____ mL.

    Select: _____ syringe

    How many full doses are available in this vial? _____ dose(s)

    Is a reconstitution label required? _____

12. Order: *Nebcin 150 mg IV q.8h*

Reconstitute with _____ mL diluent for a concentration of _____ mg/mL and give _____ mL.

Select: _____ syringe

How many full doses are available in this vial? _____ dose(s)

Is a reconstitution label required? _____

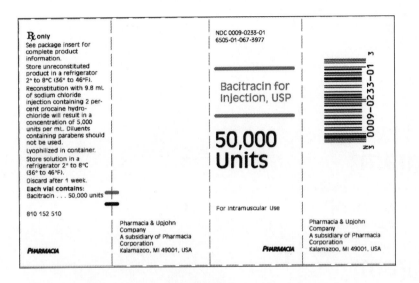

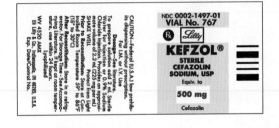

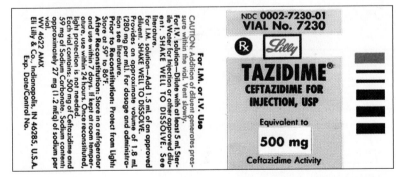

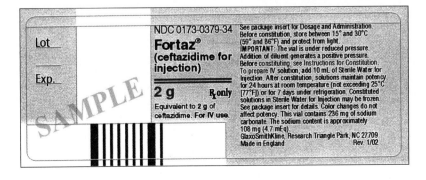

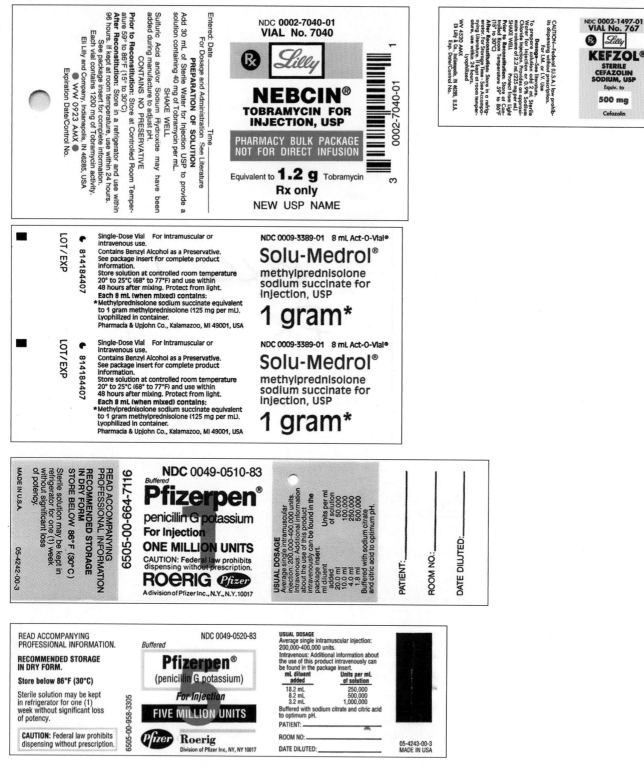

13. Order: *penicillin G potassium 2,000,000 U IM q.8h*

Reconstitute with _____ mL diluent for a concentration of _____ U/mL and give _____ mL.

Select: _____ syringe

How many full doses are available in this vial? _____ dose(s)

Is a reconstitution label required? _____

14. Order: *penicillin G potassium 1,000,000 U IM q.8h*

    Reconstitute with _____ mL diluent for a concentration of _____ U/mL and give _____ mL.

    Select: _____ syringe

    How many full doses are available in this vial? _____ dose(s)

    Is a reconstitution label required? _____

15. Order: *Kefzol 400 mg IV q.6h*

    Reconstitute with _____ mL diluent for a concentration of _____ mg/mL and give _____ mL.

    Select: _____ syringe

    How many full doses are available in this vial? _____ dose(s)

    Is a reconstitution label required? _____

Explain how you would prepare each of the following hydrogen peroxide (solute) and normal saline (solvent) irrigation orders:

16. 16 ounces of $\frac{1}{8}$ strength solution _____

17. 320 mL of $\frac{3}{8}$ strength solution _____

18. 80 mL of $\frac{5}{8}$ strength solution _____

19. 18 ounces of $\frac{2}{3}$ strength solution _____

20. 1 pt of $\frac{7}{8}$ strength solution _____

21. 1 L of $\frac{1}{4}$ strength solution _____

Explain how you would prepare each of the following from ready-to-use nutritional formulas for the specified time period. Note how many cans or bottles of supply are needed and how much unused formula would remain from the used supply.

22. Order: $\frac{1}{4}$ *strength Enfamil 12 mL via NG tube q.h. for 10 hours*

    Supply: Enfamil 3 ounce bottles.

    _____

23. Order: $\frac{3}{4}$ *strength Sustacal 360 mL over 4 hours via gastrostomy*

    Supply: Sustacal 10 ounce cans

    _____

24. Order: $\frac{2}{3}$ *strength Ensure. Give 90 mL q.h. for 5 hours via NG tube.*

    Supply: Ensure 8 ounce cans

    _____

25. Order: $\frac{3}{8}$ *strength Enfamil. Three patients need 32 ounces of the* $\frac{3}{8}$ *strength Enfamil for one feeding each.*

    Supply: Enfamil 6 ounce bottles

    _____

26. Order: $\frac{1}{8}$ *strength Ensure. Give 160 mL stat via NG tube*

    Supply: Ensure 4 ounce cans

    _____

27. Order: $\frac{1}{2}$ strength Ensure 55 mL hourly for 10 hours via gastrostomy tube

    Supply: Ensure 12 ounce cans

The nurse is making up $\frac{1}{4}$ strength Enfamil formula for several infants in the nursery.

28. If 8 ounce cans of ready-to-use Enfamil are available, how many cans of formula will be needed to make 48 ounces of reconstituted $\frac{1}{4}$ strength Enfamil? _____ can(s)

29. How many ounces of water will be added to the Enfamil in question 28 to correctly reconstitute the $\frac{1}{4}$ strength Enfamil? _____ ounce(s)

30. Critical Thinking Skill: Describe the strategy you would implement to prevent this medication error.

possible scenario

Suppose a physician ordered *penicillin G potassium 1,000,000 U IM stat* for a patient with a severe staph infection. Look at the label of the medication available on hand.

The nurse, in a hurry to give the stat medication, selected the first concentration given on the label: 250,000 Units/mL. Next the nurse calculated the dosage using the $\frac{D}{H} \times Q = X$ formula.

$$\frac{D}{H} \times Q = \frac{1,000,000 \text{ U}}{250,000 \text{ U}} \times 1 \text{ mL} = 4 \text{ mL}$$

The nurse added 18.2 mL diluent to the vial and drew up 4 mL of medication. It was not until the nurse drew up the 4 mL that the error was recognized. The nurse realized that 4 mL IM should not be administered in one injection site. The nurse called the pharmacy for another vial of penicillin G and prepared the dose again, using 3.2 mL of diluent for a concentration of 1,000,000 Units/mL. To give 1,000,000 U the nurse easily calculated to give 1 mL, which was a safe volume of medication for IM injection in adults.

potential outcome

Had the nurse given the 4 mL in one intramuscular injection, the patient would likely have developed an abcess at the site, due to the excessive volume of medication being given into the muscle. The patient's hospital stay would likely have been lengthened. Further, the nurse and the hospital may have faced a malpractice suit. The alternative would have been to divide the dose into two injections. Although the patient would have received the correct dosage, to give two injections when only one was necessary would have been poor nursing judgment.

prevention

After completing these problems, see pages 498–500 to check your answers.

Using Ratio-Proportion to Calculate Dosages

OBJECTIVES

Upon mastery of Chapter 12, you will be able to calculate the dosages of drugs using the ratio-proportion method. To accomplish this, you will also be able to:

- Convert all units of measurement to the same system and same size units.
- Consider the reasonable amount of the drug to be administered.
- Set up and solve the dosage calculation ratio-proportion: ratio for the dosage you have on hand equals the ratio for the desired dosage.

You may prefer to calculate drug dosages by the ratio-proportion method. It is presented here as an alternative to the formula method $\frac{D}{H} \times Q = X$ found in Chapters 9 to 11.

If you preferred to perform conversions by the ratio-proportion method presented in Chapter 4, then you will likely want to use ratio-proportion to solve dosage problems. Try both methods: $\frac{D}{H} \times Q = X$ and *ratio-proportion*. Choose the one that is easier and more logical to you.

RULE

Ratio for the dosage you have on hand equals ratio for the desired dosage.

Recall that a proportion is a relationship comparing two ratios. When setting up the first ratio to calculate a drug dosage, use the supply dosage or drug concentration information available on the drug label. This is the drug you *have on hand*. Set up the second ratio using the drug order or the *desired dosage* and the amount or volume you will give to the patient. (This is the unknown or "X".) Keep the *known* information on the left side of the proportion and the *unknown* on the right. Refer to Chapters 1, 2, and 4 to review information about ratios and proportions, if needed.

REMEMBER

$$\frac{\text{Dosage on hand}}{\text{Amount on hand}} = \frac{\text{Dosage desired}}{\text{X Amount desired}}$$

For example, the physician *orders* 500 milligrams of amoxicillin, and you *have on hand* a drug labeled Amoxil (amoxicillin) 250 mg per capsule. The proportion is:

$$\frac{250 \text{ mg}}{1 \text{ cap}} \bowtie \frac{500 \text{ mg}}{\text{X cap}} \quad \text{(Cross-multiply and solve for X)}$$

$250 \text{ X} = 500$

$\frac{250 \text{X}}{250} = \frac{500}{250}$ (Simplify)

$\text{X} = 2 \text{ capsules}$

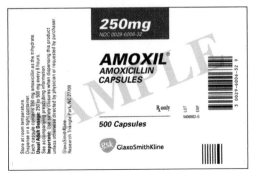

Use the same three steps to calculate dosages learned in Chapters 9 through 11. Substitute the ratio-proportion method for the formula $\frac{D}{H} \times Q = X$ in step 3. Remember that proportions compare like things. Therefore, you must first convert all units to the same system and to the same size. As pointed out in Chapter 4, notice that the ratio must follow the same sequence. The proportion is set up so that like units are across from each other. The numerators of each represent the weight of the dosage, and the denominators represent the amount. It is important to keep like units in order, such as mg as the numerators (on top) and capsules as the denominators (on the bottom). Labeling units helps you to recognize if you have set up the equation in the proper sequence. If you are careful to use the full three-step method and "think through" for the logical dosage, you will also minimize the potential for error.

REMEMBER

Step 1	Convert	All units to the same system, and all units to the same size.
Step 2	Think	Estimate the reasonable amount.
Step 3	Calculate	$\frac{\text{Dosage on hand}}{\text{Amount on hand}} = \frac{\text{Dosage desired}}{\text{X Amount desired}}$

Example 1:

Order: *Thorazine 15 mg IM stat*

Supply: Thorazine 25 mg per mL

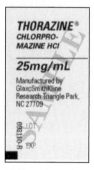

Step 1	Convert	No conversion is necessary.
Step 2	Think	You want to give less than 1 mL; in fact, you want to give $\frac{15}{25}$ of a mL or $\frac{3}{5}$ mL = 0.6 mL.
Step 3	Calculate	$\frac{\text{Dosage on hand}}{\text{Amount on hand}} = \frac{\text{Dosage desired}}{\text{X Amount desired}}$

$$\frac{25 \text{ mg}}{1 \text{ mL}} \diagup\!\!\!\!\diagdown \frac{15 \text{ mg}}{\text{X mL}} \quad \text{(Cross-multiply)}$$

$$25X = 15$$

$$\frac{25X}{25} = \frac{15}{25} \text{ (Simplify)}$$

$$X = \frac{3}{5} = 0.6 \text{ mL given intramuscularly now}$$

Example 2:

Order: *Ritalin 15 mg p.o. q.d.*

Supply: Ritalin 10 mg tablets

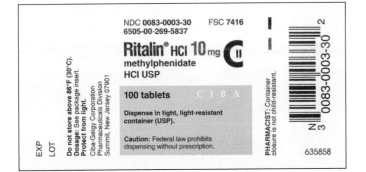

Step 1	Convert	No conversion is necessary.

Step 2 Think   You want to give more than one tablet. In fact, you want to give $1\frac{1}{2}$ times more or $1\frac{1}{2}$ tablets.

Step 3 Calculate

$$\frac{\text{Dosage on hand}}{\text{Amount on hand}} = \frac{\text{Dosage desired}}{\text{X Amount desired}}$$

$$\frac{10 \text{ mg}}{1 \text{ tab}} \diagdown\!\!\!\diagup \frac{15 \text{ mg}}{\text{X tab}} \quad \text{(Cross-multiply)}$$

$$10X = 15$$

$$\frac{10X}{10} = \frac{15}{10} \text{ (Simplify)}$$

$$X = 1\frac{1}{2} \text{ tablets given orally once daily}$$

Example 3:

Order: *Lopid 0.6 g p.o. b.i.d.*

Supply: Lopid 600 mg tablets

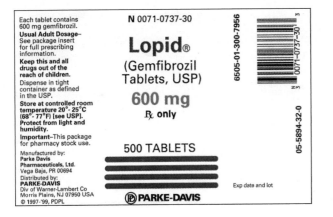

Step 1   Convert   Equivalent 1 g = 1000 mg

$$\frac{1\,g}{1000\,mg} \diagdown \diagup \frac{0.6\,g}{X\,mg}\ \text{(Cross-multiply)}$$

X = 600 mg

0.6 g = 600 mg

Step 2   Think   You want to give 600 mg and each tablet supplies 600 mg. It is obvious that you want to give 1 tablet.

Step 3   Calculate $\dfrac{\text{Dosage on hand}}{\text{Amount on hand}} = \dfrac{\text{Dosage desired}}{\text{X Amount desired}}$

$$\frac{600\,mg}{1\,tab} \diagdown \diagup \frac{600\,mg}{X\,tab}\ \text{(Cross-multiply)}$$

600X = 600

$$\frac{600X}{600} = \frac{600}{600}\ \text{(Simplify)}$$

X = 1 tablet given orally twice daily

Example 4:

Order: *codeine gr $\frac{1}{4}$ q.6h p.r.n., severe cough*

Supply: codeine 30 mg tablets

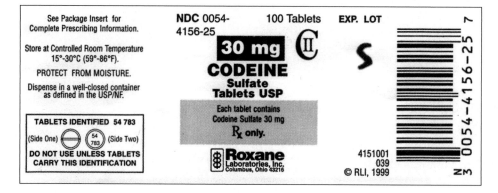

Step 1   Convert   Equivalent gr i = 60 mg

$$\frac{gr\,i}{60\,mg} \diagdown \diagup \frac{gr\,\frac{1}{4}}{X\,mg}\ \text{(Cross-multiply)}$$

$X = \frac{1}{4} \times 60 = \frac{60}{4} = 15\,mg$

$gr\,\frac{1}{4} = 15\,mg$

Step 2   Think   You want to give less than 1 tablet. Actually, you want to give $\frac{1}{2}$ tablet.

Step 3   Calculate $\dfrac{\text{Dosage on hand}}{\text{Amount on hand}} = \dfrac{\text{Dosage desired}}{\text{X Amount desired}}$

$$\frac{30 \text{ mg}}{1 \text{ tab}} \bowtie \frac{15 \text{ mg}}{X \text{ tab}} \text{ (Cross-multiply)}$$

$$30X = 15$$

$$\frac{30X}{30} = \frac{15}{30} \text{ (Simplify)}$$

$$X = \frac{1}{2} \text{ tablet given orally three times a day}$$

Example 5:

Order: *clindamycin 0.6 g IV q.12h*

Supply: Cleocin phosphate (clindamycin) 300 mg/2 mL

	Single Dose Container NDC 0009-0870-21 2 mL Vial

LOT/EXP   8127288808

Single Dose Container NDC 0009-0870-21   2 mL Vial
See package insert for complete product information. Store at controlled room temperature 20° to 25°C (68° to 77°F) [see USP]. Do not refrigerate. Pharmacia & Upjohn Co. Kalamazoo, MI 49001, USA

Cleocin Phosphate®
clindamycin injection, USP
300 mg/2 mL
Equivalent to
300 mg clindamycin

Step 1   Convert   Equivalent: 1 g = 1000 mg

$$\frac{1 \text{ g}}{1000 \text{ mg}} \bowtie \frac{0.6 \text{ g}}{X \text{ mg}} \text{ (Cross-multiply)}$$

$$X = 0.6X \times 1000 = 600 \text{ mg}$$

$$0.6 \text{ g} = 600 \text{ mg}$$

Step 2   Think   You want to give more than 2 mL. In fact, you want two times 2 mL or 4 mL.

Step 3   Calculate $\dfrac{\text{Dosage on hand}}{\text{Amount on hand}} = \dfrac{\text{Dosage desired}}{X \text{ Amount desired}}$

$$\frac{300 \text{ mg}}{2 \text{ mL}} \bowtie \frac{600 \text{ mg}}{X \text{ mL}} \text{ (Cross-multiply)}$$

$$300X = 1200$$

$$\frac{300X}{300} = \frac{1200}{300} \text{ (Simplify)}$$

$$X = \frac{1200}{300} = 4 \text{ mL given intravenously every 12 hours}$$

QUICK REVIEW

When calculating dosages using the ratio and proportion method:
- Ratio for dosage you have on hand equals ratio for desired dosage.
- $\dfrac{\text{Dosage on hand}}{\text{Amount on hand}} = \dfrac{\text{Dosage desired}}{X \text{ Amount desired}}$
- Drug dosages cannot be accurately calculated until all units of measurement are in the same system and the same size.
- Always **convert** first, then **think** or reason for the logical answer before you finally **calculate**.

REVIEW SET 31

Use the ratio-proportion method to calculate the amount you will prepare for each dose.

1. Order: *Premarin 1.25 mg p.o. q.d.*

   Supply: Premarin 0.625 mg tablets

   Give: _____ tablet(s)

2. Order: *Tagamet 150 mg p.o. q.i.d. c̄ meals & h.s.*

   Supply: Tagamet liquid 300 mg per 5 mL

   Give: _____ mL

3. Order: *Thiamine 80 mg IM stat*

   Supply: Thiamine 100 mg per 1 mL

   Give: _____ mL

4. Order: *Demerol 35 mg IM q.4h p.r.n., pain*

   Supply: Demerol 50 mg per 1 mL

   Give: _____ mL

5. Order: *lithium 12 mEq p.o. t.i.d.*

   Supply: lithium 8 mEq per 5 mL

   Give: _____ mL

6. Order: *Ativan 2.4 mg IM h.s. p.r.n., anxiety*

   Supply: Ativan 4 mg per 1 mL

   Give: _____ mL

7. Order: *Prednisone 7.5 mg p.o. q.d.*

   Supply: Prednisone 5 mg (scored) tablets

   Give: _____ tablet(s)

8. Order: *Hydrochlorothiazide 30 mg p.o. b.i.d.*

   Supply: Hydrochlorothiazide 50 mg/5 mL

   Give: _____ mL

9. Order: *Theophylline 160 mg p.o. q.6h*

   Supply: Theophylline 80 mg per 15 mL

   Give: _____ mL

10. Order: *Tofranil 20 mg IM h.s.*

    Supply: Tofranil 25 mg per 2 mL

    Give: _____ mL

11. Order: *Indocin 15 mg p.o. t.i.d.*

    Supply: Indocin Suspension 25 mg/5 mL

    Give: _____ mL

12. Order: *Ativan 2 mg IM 2 h pre-op*

    Supply: Ativan 4 mg per mL

    Give: _____ mL

13. Order: *Luminal gr ss p.o. t.i.d.*

    Supply: Luminal 15 mg tablets

    Give: _____ tablet(s)

14. Order: *Diabinese 125 mg p.o. q.d.*

    Supply: Diabinese 100 mg or 250 mg tablets

    Select: _____ mg

    Give: _____ tablet(s)

15. Order: *Thorazine 60 mg IM stat*

    Supply: Thorazine 25 mg per mL

    Give: _____ mL

16. Order: *Synthroid 0.15 mg p.o. q.d.*

    Supply: Synthroid 75 mcg tablets

    Give: _____ tablet(s)

17. Order: *Choledyl Elixir 160 mg p.o. q.6h*

    Supply: Choledyl Elixir 100 mg per 5 mL

    Give: _____ mL

18. Order: *Solu-Medrol 100 mg IV q.6h*

    Supply: Solu-Medrol 80 mg per mL

    Give: _____ mL

19. Order: *Prolixin Elixir 8 mg p.o. q.8h*

    Supply: Prolixin Elixir 2.5 mg per 5 mL

    Give: _____ mL

20. Order: *Trimox 350 mg p.o. q.8h*

    Supply: Trimox 250 mg per 5 mL

    Give: _____ mL

After completing these problems, see pages 500–501 to check your answers.

For more practice, recalculate the amount you will prepare for each dose in Review Sets 25 through 29 using the ratio-proportion method.

CRITICAL THINKING SKILLS

Medication errors are often caused by setting up ratio and proportion problems incorrectly. Let's look at an example to identify the nurse's error.

error

Using the ratio and proportion method of calculation incorrectly.

possible scenario

Suppose the physician ordered *Keflex 80 mg p.o. q.i.d.* for a child with an upper respiratory infection, and the Keflex is supplied in an oral suspension with 250 mg per 5 mL. The nurse decided to calculate the dosage using the ratio and proportion method and set up the problem this way:

$$\frac{80 \text{ mg}}{5 \text{ mL}} = \frac{250 \text{ mg}}{X \text{ mL}}$$

80X = 1250

$$\frac{80X}{80} = \frac{1250}{80}$$

X = 15.6 mL

The nurse gave the child 15 mL of Keflex for two doses. The next day as the nurse prepared the medication in the medication room, another nurse observed the nurse pour 15 mL in a medicine cup and asked about the dosage. At that point, the nurse realized the error.

potential outcome

The child would likely have developed complications from overdosage of Keflex, such as renal impairment and liver damage. When the physician was notified of the errors, he would likely have ordered the medication discontinued and the child's blood urea nitrogen (BUN) and liver enzymes monitored. An incident report would be filed and the family notified of the error.

prevention

This type of calculation error occurred because the nurse set up the ratio and proportion problem incorrectly. The dosage on hand and amount on hand were not both set up on the left (or same) side of the proportion. The problem should have been calculated this way:

$$\frac{250 \text{ mg}}{5 \text{ mL}} = \frac{80 \text{ mg}}{X \text{ mL}}$$

250X = 400

$$\frac{250X}{250} = \frac{400}{250}$$

X = 1.6 mL

In addition, had the nurse used step 2 in the calculation process, the nurse would have realized the dose required was less than 5 mL, not more. In calculating ratio and proportion problems, remember to keep the weight of medication and the amount of the *known* together on the left side of the proportion, and the weight and the amount of the *unknown* together on the right side. In this scenario the patient would have received almost 10 times the amount of medication ordered by the physician each time the nurse committed the error. You know this

(continues)

(continued)

because there are 250 mg in 5 mL, and the nurse gave 15 mL. You can use ratio and proportion to determine how many mg of Keflex the child received in the scenario.

$$\frac{250 \text{ mg}}{5 \text{ mL}} = \frac{X \text{ mg}}{15 \text{ mL}}$$

5X = 3750

X = 750 mg, not 80 mg as ordered

Obviously the nurse did not think through for the logical amount, and either miscalculated the dosage three times or did not bother to calculate the dosage again, preventing identification of the error.

PRACTICE PROBLEMS—CHAPTER 12

Use the ratio-proportion method to calculate the amount you prepare for each dose.

1. Order: *lactulose 30 g in 100 mL fluid p.r. t.i.d.*

   Supply: lactulose 3.33 g per 5 mL

   Give: _____ mL in 100 mL

2. Order: *penicillin G potassium 500,000 U IM q.i.d.*

   Supply: penicillin G potassium 5,000,000 U per 20 mL

   Give: _____ mL

3. Order: *Keflex 100 mg p.o. q.i.d.*

   Supply: Keflex oral suspension 250 mg per 5 mL

   Give: _____ mL

4. Order: *amoxicillin 125 mg p.o. q.i.d.*

   Supply: amoxicillin 250 mg per 5 mL

   NOTE: You are giving home-care instructions.

   Give: _____ t

5. Order: *Benadryl 25 mg IM stat*

   Supply: Benadryl 10 mg per 1 mL

   Give: _____ mL

6. Order: *Benadryl 40 mg p.o. stat*

   Supply: Benadryl 12.5 mg per 5 mL

   Give: _____ mL

7. Order: *penicillin G potassium 350,000 U IM b.i.d.*

   Supply: penicillin G potassium 500,000 U per 2 mL

   Give: _____ mL

8. Order: *Valium 3.5 mg IM q.6h p.r.n., anxiety*

   Supply: Valium 10 mg per 2 mL

   Give: _____ mL

9. Order: *tobramycin sulfate 90 mg IM q.8h*

   Supply: tobramycin sulfate 80 mg per 2 mL

   Give: _____ mL

10. Order: *heparin 2500 U SC b.i.d.*

    Supply: heparin 20,000 U per mL

    Give: _____ mL

11. Order: *Compazine 8 mg IM q.6h p.r.n., nausea*

    Supply: Compazine 10 mg per 2 mL

    Give: _____ mL

12. Order: *gentamycin 60 mg IM q.6h*

    Supply: gentamycin 80 mg per 2 mL

    Give: _____ mL

13. Order: *Pipracil 500 mg IM b.i.d.*

    Supply: Pipracil 1 g per 2.5 mL

    Give: _____ mL

14. Order: *Nilstat Oral Suspension 250,000 U p.o. q.i.d.*

    Supply: Nilstat Oral Suspension 100,000 U per mL

    Give: _____ mL

15. Order: *Ilosone 80 mg p.o. q.4h*

    Supply: Ilosone 250 mg per 5 mL

    Give: _____ mL

16. Order: *potassium chloride 10 mEq p.o. stat*

    Supply: potassium chloride 20 mEq per 15 mL

    Give: _____ mL

17. Order: *Unipen 400 mg IM q.6h*

    Supply: Unipen 1 g per 4 mL

    Give: _____ mL

18. Order: *Synthroid 150 mcg p.o. q.d.*

    Supply: Synthroid 0.075 mg tablets

    Give: _____ tablet(s)

19. Order: *amoxicillin 400 mg p.o. q.8h*

    Supply: amoxicillin 250 mg per 5 mL

    Give: _____ mL

20. Order: *Dilantin 225 mg IV stat*

    Supply: Dilantin 50 mg per mL

    Give: _____ mL

21. Order: *Elixophyllin 160 mg p.o. q.6h*

    Supply: Elixophyllin 80 mg per 15 mL

    Give: _____ mL

22. Order: *Thorazine 35 mg IM stat*

    Supply: chlorpromazine (Thorazine) 25 mg per mL

    Give: _____ mL

23. Order: *Add potassium chloride 30 mEq to 1000 mL D$_5$W IV*

    Supply: KCl (potassium chloride) 40 mEq per 20 mL

    Add: _____ mL

24. Order: *Phenergan 25 mg via NG tube h.s.*

    Supply: Phenergan 6.25 mg per 5 mL

    Give: _____ mL

25. Order: *Ceclor 300 mg p.o. t.i.d.*

    Supply: Ceclor 125 mg per 5 mL

    Give: _____ mL

26. Critical Thinking Skill: Describe the strategy you would implement to prevent this medication error.

    possible scenario

    The physician ordered *Amoxil 50 mg p.o. q.i.d.* for a child with an upper respiratory infection. Amoxil is supplied in an oral suspension with 125 mg/5 mL. The nurse calculated the dose this way:

    $$\frac{125 \text{ mg}}{50 \text{ mg}} = \frac{X \text{ mL}}{5 \text{ mL}}$$

    $$50X = 625$$

    $$\frac{50X}{50} = \frac{625}{50}$$

    $$X = 12.5 \text{ mL}$$

    potential outcome

    The patient received a large overdose and should have received only 2 mL. The child would likely develop complications from overdosage of amoxicillin. When the physician was notified of the error, she would likely have ordered the medication discontinued and had extra blood lab work done. An incident report would be filed and the family notified of the error.

    prevention

    _____

    _____

After completing these problems, see pages 501–502 to check your answers.

Pediatric and Adult Dosages Based on Body Weight

OBJECTIVES

Upon mastery of Chapter 13, you will be able to calculate drug dosages based on body weight and verify the safety of medication orders. To accomplish this you will also be able to:

- Convert pounds to kilograms.
- Consult a reputable drug resource to calculate the recommended safe dosage per kilogram of body weight.
- Compare the ordered dosage with the recommended safe dosage.
- Determine whether the ordered dosage is safe to administer.
- Apply body weight dosage calculations to patients across the life span.

Only a doctor, dentist, or nurse practitioner (in some states) may prescribe the dosage of medications. However, before administering a drug, the nurse should know if the ordered dosage is safe. This is important for adults and critical for infants, children, frail elderly, and critically ill adults.

> ### CAUTION
>
> Those who administer drugs to patients are legally responsible for recognizing incorrect and unsafe dosages and for alerting the prescribing practitioner.

The one who administers a drug is just as responsible for the patient's safety as the one who prescribes it. For the protection of the patient and yourself, you must familiarize yourself with the recommended dosage of drugs or consult a reputable drug reference, such as the *package insert* that accompanies the drug or the *Hospital Formulary*.

Standard adult dosage is determined by the drug manufacturer. Dosage is usually recommended based on the requirements of an average-weight adult. Frequently an adult range is given, listing a minimum and maximum safe dosage, allowing the nurse to simply compare what is ordered to what is recommended.

Dosages for infants and children are based on their unique and changing body differences. The prescribing practitioner must consider the weight, height, body surface, age, and condition of the child as contributing factors to safe and effective medication dosages. The two methods currently used for calculating safe pediatric dosages are *body weight* (such as mg/kg), and *body surface area* (BSA, measured in square meters, m^2). The body weight method is more common in pediatric situations and is emphasized in this chapter. The BSA method is based on both weight and height. It is used primarily in oncology and critical care situations. BSA is discussed in Chapter 15. Although used most frequently in pediatrics, both the body weight and BSA methods are also used for adults, especially in critical care situations. The calculations are the same.

ADMINISTERING MEDICATIONS TO CHILDREN

Numerically, the infant's or child's dosage appears smaller, but *proportionally* pediatric dosages are frequently much larger per kilogram of body weight than the usual adult dosage. Infants—birth to one year—have a greater percentage of body water and diminished ability to absorb water-soluble drugs, necessitating dosages of oral and some parenteral drugs that are higher than those given to persons of larger size. Children—age one to 12 years—metabolize drugs more readily than adults, which necessitates higher dosages. Both infants and children, however, are growing, and their organ systems are still maturing. Immature physiological processes related to absorption, distribution, metabolism, and excretion put them continuously at risk for overdose, toxic reactions, and even death. Adolescents—age 13 to 18 years—are often erroneously thought of as adults because of their body weight (greater than 110 pounds or 50 kilograms) and mature physical appearance. In fact, they should still be regarded as physiologically immature, with unpredictable growth spurts and hormonal surges. Drug therapy for the pediatric population is further complicated because very little detailed pharmacologic research has been done on children and adolescents. The infant or child, therefore, must be frequently evaluated for desired clinical responses to medications, and serum drug levels are needed to help adjust some drug dosages. It is important to remember that administration of an incorrect dosage to adult patients is dangerous, but with a child, the risk is even greater. Therefore, using a reputable drug reference to verify safe pediatric dosages is a critical health care skill.

Two well-written drug references written especially for pediatrics are *Pediatric Drugs and Nursing Implications* (2nd ed.), by Ruth McGillis Bindler and Linda Berner Howry, 1997, Upper Saddle River, NJ: Prentice Hall, and *Pediatric Medications: A Handbook for Nurses,* by Susan Miller and Joanne Fioravanti, 1997, St. Louis: Mosby-Year Book, Inc. There are also a variety of pocket-size pediatric drug handbooks. Two widely used handbooks are *Johns Hopkins Hospital: The Harriet Lane Handbook* (16th ed.), Johns Hopkins Hospital, 2002, St. Louis: Mosby-Year Book, Inc., and *Pediatric Dosage Handbook: Including Neonatal Dosing, Drug Administration, & Extemporaneous Preparations, 2001–2002* (8th ed.), by Carol K. Taketomo, et al., 2002, Cleveland: LEXI-COMP.

CONVERTING POUNDS TO KILOGRAMS

The body weight method uses calculations based on the person's weight in kilograms. Recall that the pounds to kilograms conversion was introduced in Chapter 4.

> **REMEMBER**
>
> **1 kg = 2.2 lb** and **1 lb = 16 oz**
> Simply stated, weight in pounds is approximately twice the metric weight in kg; or weight in kg is approximately $\frac{1}{2}$ of weight in pounds. You can estimate kg by halving the weight in lb.

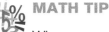

> **MATH TIP**
>
> When converting pounds to kilograms, round kilogram weight to one decimal place (tenths).

Example 1:

Convert 45 lb to kg

Approximate equivalent: 1 kg = 2.2 lb

Think: $\frac{1}{2}$ of 45 = approximately 23

Smaller → Larger: (÷)

45 lb = 45 ÷ 2.2 = 20.45 kg = 20.5 kg

Example 2:

Convert 10 lb 12 oz to kg

Approximate equivalents: 1 kg = 2.2 lb

$$1 \text{ lb} = 16 \text{ oz}$$

Smaller → Larger: ($\div$)

$$12 \text{ oz} = 12 \div 16 = \frac{\overset{3}{\cancel{12}}}{\underset{4}{\cancel{16}}} = \frac{3}{4} \text{ lb; so } 10 \text{ lb } 12 \text{ oz} = 10\frac{3}{4} \text{ lb}$$

Think: $\frac{1}{2}$ of $10\frac{3}{4}$ = approximately 5

Smaller → Larger: ($\div$)

$10\frac{3}{4}$ lb = 10.75 $\div$ 2.2 = 4.88 kg = 4.9 kg

BODY WEIGHT METHOD FOR CALCULATING SAFE PEDIATRIC DOSAGE

The most common method of prescribing and administering the therapeutic amount of medication for a child is to calculate the amount of drug according to the child's body weight in **kilograms**. The nurse then compares the child's *ordered dosage* to the recommended *safe dosage* from a reputable drug resource before administering the medication. The intent is to ensure that the ordered dosage is safe and effective *before* calculating the amount to give and administering the dose to the patient.

> ### RULE
>
> To verify safe pediatric dosage:
> 1. Convert the child's weight from pounds to kilograms (rounded to tenths).
> 2. Calculate the safe dosage in mg/kg or mcg/kg (rounded to tenths) for a child of this weight, as recommended by a reputable drug reference: **multiply mg/kg by child's weight in kg**.
> 3. Compare the *ordered dosage* to the *recommended dosage*, and decide if the dosage is safe.
> 4. If safe, calculate the amount to give and administer the dose; if the dosage seems unsafe, consult with the ordering practitioner before administering the drug.
> NOTE: The *dosage per kg* may be mg/kg, mcg/kg, g/kg, mEq/kg, U/kg, mU/kg, etc.

For each pediatric medication order, you must ask yourself, "Is this dosage safe?" Let's work through some examples.

Single-Dosage Drugs

Example:

Single-dosage drugs are intended to be given once or p.r.n. Dosage ordered by the body weight method is based on **mg/kg/dose, calculated by multiplying the recommended mg by the patient's kg weight for each dose.**

The physician orders *morphine sulfate 1.8 mg IM stat.* The child weighs 79 lb. Is this dosage safe?

1. **Convert lb to kg.** Approximate equivalent: 1 kg = 2.2 lb

   Think: $\frac{1}{2}$ of 79 = approximately 40

   Smaller → Larger: ($\div$)

   79 lb = 79 $\div$ 2.2 = 35.90 kg = 35.9 kg

2. **Calculate mg/kg as recommended by a reputable drug resource.** A reputable drug resource indicates that the usual IM/SC dosage may be initiated at 0.05 mg/kg/dose.

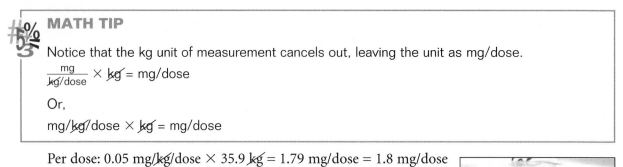

> **MATH TIP**
>
> Notice that the kg unit of measurement cancels out, leaving the unit as mg/dose.
>
> $\frac{mg}{kg/dose} \times kg = mg/dose$
>
> Or,
>
> $mg/kg/dose \times kg = mg/dose$

Per dose: $0.05 \text{ mg/kg/dose} \times 35.9 \text{ kg} = 1.79 \text{ mg/dose} = 1.8 \text{ mg/dose}$

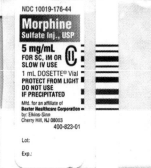

FIGURE 13-1
Morphine Label

3. **Decide if the dosage is safe by comparing ordered and recommended dosages.** For this child's weight, 1.8 mg is the recommended dosage and 1.8 mg is the ordered dosage. Yes, the dosage is safe.

4. **Calculate one dose.** Apply the three steps of dosage calculation.

   Order: *morphine sulfate 1.8 mg IM stat*

   Supply: morphine sulfate 5 mg/mL (Figure 13-1)

Step 1   Convert   No conversion is necessary.

Step 2   Think   You want to give less than 1 mL. Estimate that you want to give less than 0.5 mL.

Step 3   Calculate $\frac{D}{H} \times Q = \frac{1.8 \text{ mg}}{5 \text{ mg}} \times 1 \text{ mL} = 0.36 \text{ mL}$

Or, apply the ratio and proportion method.

$$\frac{5 \text{ mg}}{1 \text{ mL}} \times\!\!\!\times \frac{1.8 \text{ mg}}{X \text{ mL}}$$

$5X = 1.8$

$\frac{5X}{5} = \frac{1.8}{5}$

$X = 0.36 \text{ mL}$

This is a small, child's dose. Measure 0.36 mL in a 1 mL syringe. Route is IM. Needle may need to be changed.

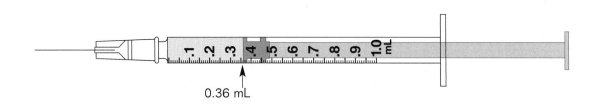

0.36 mL

Single-Dosage Range

Example:

Some single-dosage medications indicate a minimum and maximum range, or a safe dosage range.

The practitioner orders *Vistaril 20 mg IM q.4–6h, p.r.n., nausea.* The child weighs 44 lb. Is this a safe dosage?

1. **Convert lb to kg.** Approximate equivalent: 1 kg = 2.2 lb

   Think: $\frac{1}{2}$ of 44 = 22

   44 lb = 44 ÷ 2.2 = 20 kg

2. **Calculate recommended dosage.** A reputable drug resource indicates that the usual IM dosage is 0.5 mg to 1 mg/kg/dose every 4 to 6 hours as needed. Notice that the recommended dosage is represented as a range of "0.5–1 mg/kg/dose" for dosing flexibility. Calculate the minimum and maximum safe dosage range.

   Minimum per dose: 0.5 mg/kg/dose × 20 kg = 10 mg/dose

   Maximum per dose: 1 mg/kg/dose × 20 kg = 20 mg/dose

3. **Decide if the ordered dosage is safe.** The recommended dosage range is 10 mg to 20 mg, and the ordered dosage of 20 mg is within this range. Yes, the ordered dosage is safe.

4. **Calculate one dose.** Apply the three steps of dosage calculation.

   Order: *Vistaril 20 mg IM q.4–6h p.r.n., nausea*

   Supply: Vistaril 50 mg/mL (Figure 13-2)

FOR INTRAMUSCULAR USE ONLY.
USUAL ADULT DOSE: Intramuscularly: 25 - 100 mg stat; repeat every 4 to 6 hours, as needed.
See accompanying prescribing information.
Each mL contains **50 mg** of hydroxyzine hydrochloride, 0.9% benzyl alcohol and sodium hydroxide to adjust to optimum pH.
To avoid discoloration, protect from prolonged exposure to light.
Rx only

10 mL   NDC 0049-5460-74

Vistaril®
(hydroxyzine hydrochloride)
Intramuscular Solution
50 mg/mL

Pfizer **Roerig**
Division of Pfizer Inc, NY, NY 10017

Store below 86°F (30°C).
PROTECT FROM FREEZING.
PATIENT: _____
ROOM NO.: _____

05-1111-32-4   9249
MADE IN USA

FIGURE 13-2 Vistaril Label

Step 1	Convert	No conversion is necessary.
Step 2	Think	Estimate that you want to give less than 1 mL; in fact, you want to give less than 0.5 mL.

Step 3 **Calculate** $\dfrac{D}{H} \times Q = \dfrac{2\emptyset \text{ mg}}{5\emptyset \text{ mg}} \times 1\,\text{mL} = \dfrac{2}{5}\,\text{mL} = 0.4\,\text{mL}$

Or, apply the ratio-proportion method.

$$\dfrac{50 \text{ mg}}{1 \text{ mL}} \underset{\diagdown}{\overset{\diagup}{\times}} \dfrac{20 \text{ mg}}{X \text{ mL}}$$

$50X = 20$

$\dfrac{50X}{50} = \dfrac{20}{50}$

$X = 0.4\,\text{mL}$

This is a small, child's dose. Measure it in a 1 mL syringe. Route is IM. Needle may need to be changed.

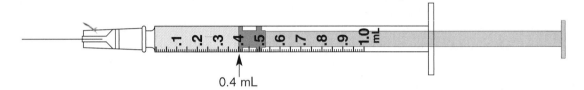

0.4 mL

Routine or Round-the-Clock Drugs

Example:

Routine or round-the-clock drugs are intended to produce a continuous effect on the body over 24 hours. They are recommended as a *total daily dosage:* **mg/kg/day to be divided into some number of individual doses,** such as "three divided doses," "four divided doses," "divided doses every 8 hours," and so on. "Three divided doses" means the drug total daily dosage is divided equally and is administered three times per day, either t.i.d. or q.8h. Likewise, "four divided doses" means the total daily drug dosage is divided equally and administered four times per day either q.i.d. or q.6h. Recommendations like "divided doses every 8 hours" specifies that the total daily drug dosage should be divided equally and administered q.8h.

The practitioner orders *Ceclor 100 mg p.o. t.i.d.* The child weighs $33\frac{1}{2}$ lb. Is this dosage safe?

1. **Convert lb to kg.** Approximate equivalent: 1 kg = 2.2 lb

   Think: $\frac{1}{2}$ of 33 = approximately 17

   $33\frac{1}{2}$ lb = 33.5 lb = 33.5 ÷ 2.2 = 15.22 lb = 15.2 lb

2. **Calculate recommended dosage.** Figure 13-3 shows the recommended dosage on the drug label, "Usual dose—Children, 20 mg per kg a day . . . in three divided doses." First, calculate the total daily dosage: 20 mg/kg/day × 15.2 kg = 304 mg/day. Then, divide this total daily dosage into 3 doses: 304 mg ÷ 3 doses = 101.3 mg/dose.

3. **Decide if the ordered dosage is safe.** Yes, the ordered dosage is safe, because this is an *oral* dose and 100 mg is a *reasonably safe* dosage for a 101.3 recommended single dosage. Think: To give 101.3 mg you would calculate $\dfrac{D}{H} \times Q = \dfrac{101.3 \text{ mg}}{125 \text{ mg}} \times 5\,\text{mL} = 4.05\,\text{mL}$, which would be rounded to 4 mL. Notice in step 4 that to administer 100 mg, the dose is also 4 mL because of rounding.

NDC 0002-5057-18
75 mL (When Mixed) M-5057

℞ *Lilly*

CECLOR®
CEFACLOR FOR
ORAL SUSPENSION
USP

125 mg
per 5 mL

CAUTION—Federal (U.S.A.)
law prohibits dispensing
without prescription.

FIGURE 13-3 Ceclor Label

4. **Calculate one dose.** Apply the three steps of dosage calculation.

   Order: *Ceclor 100 mg p.o. t.i.d.*

   Supply: *Ceclor 125 mg/5 mL*

Step 1	**Convert**	No conversion is necessary.
Step 2	**Think**	You want to give less than 5 mL. Estimate that you want to give between 2.5 mL and 5 mL.
Step 3	**Calculate**	

$$\frac{D}{H} \times Q = \frac{\overset{4}{\cancel{100}\text{ mg}}}{\underset{5}{\cancel{125}\text{ mg}}} \times 5 \text{ mL} = \frac{4}{\cancel{5}} \text{ mL} \times \cancel{5} \text{ mL} = 4 \text{ mL}$$

Or, apply the ratio-proportion method.

$$\frac{125 \text{ mg}}{5 \text{ mL}} \times\!\!\!\!\diagup\!\!\!\! \frac{100 \text{ mg}}{X \text{ mL}}$$

$$125X = 500$$

$$\frac{125X}{125} = \frac{500}{125}$$

$$X = 4 \text{ mL}$$

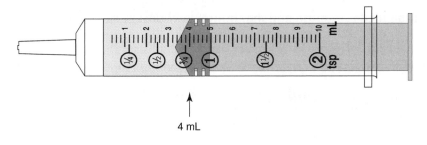

4 mL

Total Daily Dosage Range per Kilogram

Example:

Many medications are recommended by a minimum and maximum mg/kg range per day to be divided into some number of doses. Amoxicillin is an antibiotic that is used to treat a variety of infections in adults and children. It is often given in divided doses round-the-clock for a total daily dosage.

Suppose the physician orders *amoxicillin 200 mg p.o. q.8h* for a child who weighs 22 lb. Is this dosage safe?

1. **Convert lb to kg.** Approximate equivalent: 1 kg = 2.2 lb

   Think: $\frac{1}{2}$ of 22 = 11

   22 lb = 22 ÷ 2.2 = 10 kg

2. **Calculate recommended dosage.** Look at the label for Amoxil (amoxicillin), Figure 13-4. The label describes the recommended dosage as "20 to 40 mg/kg/day in divided doses every 8 hours . . . ."

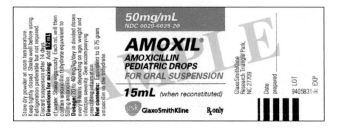

FIGURE 13-4 Amoxil Label

Calculate the minimum and maximum dosage for each single dose. The label recommends that the total daily dosage be divided and administered every 8 hours, resulting in 3 doses in 24 hours.

Minimum total daily dosage: 20 mg/kg/day × 10 kg = 200 mg/day

Minimum dosage for each single dose: 200 mg ÷ 3 doses = 66.7 mg/dose

Maximum total daily dosage: 40 mg/kg/day × 10 kg = 400 mg/day

Maximum dosage for each single dose: 400 mg ÷ 3 doses = 133.3 mg/dose

The single dosage range is 66.7 to 133.3 mg/dose.

3. **Decide if the ordered dosage is safe.** The ordered dosage is 200 mg, and the allowable, safe dosage is 66.7 to 133.3 mg/dose. No, this dosage is too high and is not safe.

4. **Contact the prescriber to discuss the order.**

You can save yourself a calculation step with the following shortcut, based on the total daily dosage.

Calculate recommended minimum and maximum daily dosage range for *this* child.

You know the total daily dosage is divided into 3 doses in 24 hours.

Minimum total daily dosage: 20 mg/kg/day × 10 kg = 200 mg/day

Maximum total daily dosage: 40 mg/kg/day × 10 kg = 400 mg/day

Daily dosage per this order: 200 mg/dose × 3 doses/day = 600 mg/day

Decide if the ordered daily dosage is safe. The ordered daily dosage is 600 mg, and the allowable safe daily dosage is 200 to 400 mg/day. No, the dosage ordered is too high and is not safe.

Total Daily Dosage Range per Kilogram with Maximum Daily Allowance

Example:

Some medications have a range of mg/kg/day recommended, with a maximum allowable total amount per day also specified.

The physician orders *cefazolin 2.1 g IV q.8h* for a child with a serious joint infection. The child weighs 95 lb. The drug reference indicates that the usual IM or IV dosage of cefazolin for infants and children is 50 to 100 mg/kg/day divided every 8 hours; maximum dosage is 6 g/day. This means that regardless of how much the child weighs, the maximum safe allowance of this drug is 6 g per 24 hours.

1. **Convert lb to kg.** Approximate equivalent: 1 kg = 2.2 lb

   Think: $\frac{1}{2}$ of 95 = approximately 48

   95 lb = 95 ÷ 2.2 = 43.18 kg = 43.2 kg

2. **Calculate recommended dosage.**

   Minimum mg/kg/day: 50 mg/kg/day × 43.2 kg = 2160 mg/day

   Minimum mg/dose: 2160 mg ÷ 3 doses = 720 mg/dose or 0.72 g/dose
   (720 mg/dose = 720 ÷ 1000 = 0.72 g/dose)

   Maximum mg/kg/day: 100 mg/kg/day × 43.2 kg = 4320 mg/day, which is still below the maximum allowable per day dosage of 6 g or 6000 mg.

   Maximum mg/dose: 4320 mg ÷ 3 doses = 1440 mg/dose or 1.44 g/dose
   (1440 mg/dose = 1440 ÷ 1000 = 1.44 g/dose)

3. **Decide if the dosage is safe.** No, the dosage is too high. It exceeds both the highest mg/kg/dose extreme of the range (1440 mg/dose), and it exceeds the maximum allowable dosage. At 6 g/day, no more than 2 g/dose would be allowed. The ordered dosage of 2.1 g is not safe, because 3 doses/day would deliver 6.3 g of the drug (2.1 g × 3 = 6.3 g). This example points out the importance of carefully reading all dosage recommendations.

4. **Contact the prescriber to discuss the order.**

Underdosage

Example:

Underdosage, as well as overdosage, can be a hazard. If the medication is necessary for the treatment or comfort of the patient, then giving too little can be just as hazardous as giving too much. Dosage that is less than the recommended therapeutic amount is also considered unsafe, because it may be ineffective.

The nurse notices a baby's fever has not come down below 102.6°F in spite of several doses of ibuprofen that the physician ordered as an antipyretic (fever reducer). The order reads *ibuprofen 40 mg p.o. q.6h p.r.n., temp > 101.6°F*. The 7-month-old baby weighs $17\frac{1}{2}$ lb.

1. **Convert lb to kg.** Approximate equivalent: 1 kg = 2.2 lb.

   Think: $\frac{1}{2}$ of $17\frac{1}{2}$ = approximately 9

   $17\frac{1}{2}$ lb = 17.5 lb = 17.5 ÷ 2.2 = 7.95 kg = 8 kg

2. **Calculate safe dosage.** The drug reference states "Usual dosage . . . oral: Children: . . . Antipyretic: 6 months–12 years: Temperature < 102.5°F (39°C) 5 mg/kg/dose; temperature > 102.5°F: 10 mg/kg/dose; given every 6–8 hr; Maximum daily dose: 40 mg/kg/day."

   The recommended safe mg/kg dosage to treat this child's fever of 102.6°F is based on 10 mg/kg/dose. For the 8 kg child, per dose, 10 mg/kg/dose × 8 kg = 80 mg/dose.

3. **Decide if the dosage is safe.** The nurse realizes that the dosage as ordered is insufficient to lower the child's fever. Because it is below the recommended therapeutic dosage, it is unsafe.

4. **Contact the physician.** Upon discussion with the physician, the doctor agrees and revises the order to *ibuprofen 80 mg p.o. q.6h p.r.n., Temp > 102.5°F* and *ibuprophen 40 mg p.o. q.6h p.r.n., fever < 102.5°F*. Underdosage with an antipyretic may result in serious complications of hyperthermia. Likewise, consider how underdosage with an antibiotic may lead to a superinfection and underdosage of a pain reliever may be inadequate to effectively treat the patient's pain, delaying recovery. Remember, the information in the drug reference provides important details related to specific use of medications and appropriate dosages for certain age groups to provide safe, therapeutic dosing. Both the physician and nurse must work together to ensure accurate and safe dosages that are within the recommended parameters as stated by the manufacturer on the label, in a drug insert, or in a reputable drug reference.

CAUTION

Once an adolescent attains a weight of 50 kg (110 lb) or greater, the standard adult dosage is frequently prescribed instead of a calculated dosage by weight. The health care professional must carefully verify that the order for a child's dosage *does not exceed* the maximum adult dosage recommended by the manufacturer.

CAUTION

Many over-the-counter preparations, such as fever reducers and cold preparations, have printed dosing instructions that show the recommended child dose *per pound*, Figure 13-5. Manufacturers understand that most parents in the United States measure their child's weight in pounds and are most familiar with household measurement. The recommended dosage is measured in teaspoons. Recall that pounds and teaspoons are primarily used for measurement in the home setting. In the clinical setting, you should measure body weight in kg and calculate dosage by the body weight method, using recommended dosage in mg/kg, not mg/lb.

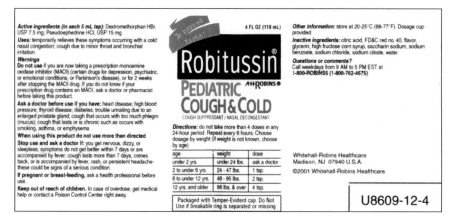

FIGURE 13-5 Label with Dosage-Per-Lb Instructions

COMBINATION DRUGS

Some medications contain two drugs combined into one solution or suspension. To calculate the safe dosage of these medications, the nurse should consult a pediatric drug reference. Often the nurse will need to calculate the *safe* dosage for each of the medications combined in the solution or suspension. Combination drugs are usually ordered by the amount to give or dose volume.

Example 1:

The physician orders *Pediazole 6 mL p.o. q.6h* for a child weighing 44 lb. The pediatric drug reference states that Pediazole is a combination drug containing 200 mg of erythromycin ethylsuccinate with 600 mg of sulfisoxazole acetyl in every 5 mL oral suspension. The usual dosage for Pediazole is 50 mg erythromycin and 150 mg sulfisoxazole/kg/day in equally divided doses administered every 6 hours. Is the dose volume ordered safe?

Because this is a combination drug, notice that the order is for the dose volume (6 mL). To verify that the dose is safe, you must calculate the recommended dosage and the recommended quantity to give to supply that dosage for each drug component.

1. **Convert lb to kg.** Approximate equivalent: 1 kg = 2.2 lb

   Think: $\frac{1}{2}$ of 44 = 22

   44 lb = 44 ÷ 2.2 = 20 kg

2. **Calculate the safe dosage for each drug component.**

   erythromycin per day: 50 mg/kg/day × 20 kg = 1000 mg/day; divided into 4 doses/day
   1000 mg ÷ 4 doses = 250 mg/dose

   sulfisoxazole per day: 150 mg/kg/day × 20 kg = 3000 mg/day; divided into 4 doses/day
   3000 mg ÷ 4 doses = 750 mg/dose

3. **Calculate the volume of medication recommended for one dose for each drug component.**

   erythromycin: 250 mg is the recommended dosage; the supply has 200 mg/5 mL.

$$\frac{D}{H} \times Q = \frac{\overset{5}{\cancel{250}} \text{ mg}}{\underset{4}{\cancel{200}} \text{ mg}} \times 5 \text{ mL} = \frac{25}{4} \text{ mL} = 6.25 \text{ mL} = 6 \text{ mL recommended to deliver 250 mg erythromycin}$$

   As this is an oral dosage, it is safely and reasonably rounded to 6 mL.

   Or, use ratio-proportion.

$$\frac{200 \text{ mg}}{5 \text{ mL}} \diagdown\!\!\!\!\diagup \frac{250 \text{ mg}}{X \text{ mL}}$$

   200X = 1250

   $$\frac{200X}{200} = \frac{1250}{200}$$

   X = 6.25 mL = 6 mL recommended to deliver 250 mg erythromycin sulfisoxazole: 750 mg is the recommended dosage; 600 mg/5 mL is the supply.

$$\frac{D}{H} \times Q = \frac{\overset{5}{\cancel{750}} \text{ mg}}{\underset{4}{\cancel{600}} \text{ mg}} \times 5\,\text{mL} = \frac{25}{4}\,\text{mL} = 6.25\,\text{mL} = 6\,\text{mL recommended to}$$
$$\text{deliver 750 mg sulfisoxazole}$$

Or, use ratio-proportion.

$$\frac{600\text{ mg}}{5\text{ mL}} \underset{\displaystyle\times}{} \frac{750\text{ mg}}{X\text{ mL}}$$

$$600X = 3750$$

$$\frac{600X}{600} = \frac{3750}{600}$$

X = 6.25 mL = 6 mL recommended to deliver 750 mg sulfisoxazole

4. **Decide if the dose ordered is safe.** The ordered dose is 6 mL, and the appropriate dose based on the recommended dosage for each component is 6 mL. The dose is safe. **Realize that because this is a combination product; 6 mL contains *both* medications delivered in this suspension.** Therefore, 6 mL is given, not 6 mL plus 6 mL.

Example 2:

The physician orders *Septra suspension (co-trimoxazole) 7.5 cc (1½ t) p.o. q.12h* for a child who weighs 22 lb. The drug reference states that Septra is a combination drug containing trimethoprim (TMP) 40 mg and sulfamethoxazole 200 mg in 5 mL oral suspension. It further states that the usual dosage of Septra is based on the TMP component, which is 6 to 12 mg/kg/day p.o. in divided doses q.12h for a mild to moderate infection. Is this dose volume safe?

1. **Convert lb to kg.** Approximate equivalent: 1 kg = 2.2 lb

   Think: $\frac{1}{2}$ of 22 = 11

   22 lb = 22 ÷ 2.2 = 10 kg

2. **Calculate the safe dose for the TMP range.**

   TMP minimum daily dosage: 6 mg/kg/day × 10 kg = 60 mg/day

   Divided into 2 doses/day: 60 mg ÷ 2 doses = 30 mg/dose

   TMP maximum daily dosage: 12 mg/kg/day × 10 kg = 120 mg/day

   Divided into 2 doses/day: 120 mg ÷ 2 doses = 60 mg/dose

3. **Calculate the volume of medication for the dosage range.**

   Minimum dose volume: $\dfrac{D}{H} \times Q = \dfrac{\overset{3}{\cancel{30}} \text{ mg}}{\underset{4}{\cancel{40}} \text{ mg}} \times 5\,\text{mL} = \dfrac{15}{4}\,\text{mL} = 3.75\,\text{mL, minimum per dose}$

   Or, use ratio-proportion.

   $$\frac{40\text{ mg}}{5\text{ mL}} \underset{\displaystyle\times}{} \frac{30\text{ mg}}{X\text{ mL}}$$

   $$40X = 150$$

   $$\frac{40X}{40} = \frac{150}{40}$$

   X = 3.75 mL, minimum per dose

Maximum dose volume: $\dfrac{D}{H} \times Q = \dfrac{\overset{3}{\cancel{60}\text{ mg}}}{\underset{2}{\cancel{40}\text{ mg}}} \times 5\,\text{mL} = \dfrac{15}{2}\,\text{mL} = 7.5\,\text{mL}$, maximum per dose

Or, use ratio-proportion.

$$\dfrac{40\text{ mg}}{5\text{ mL}} \bowtie \dfrac{60\text{ mg}}{X\text{ mL}}$$

$40X = 300$

$\dfrac{40X}{40} = \dfrac{300}{40}$

$X = 7.5$ mL, maximum per dose

4. **Decide if the dose volume is safe.** Because the physician ordered 7.5 mL, the dose falls within the safe range and is a safe dose.

What dosage of TMP did the physician actually order per dose for this child?

Using the formula, $\dfrac{D}{H} \times Q = X$, write in the quantities you already know.

$\dfrac{D\text{ mg}}{40\text{ mg}} \times 5\text{ mL} = 7.5\text{ mL}$ Solve for the unknown "D," desired dosage.

$\dfrac{5D}{40} \bowtie \dfrac{7.5}{1}$ Notice you now have a ratio-proportion.

$5D = 300$

$\dfrac{5D}{5} = \dfrac{300}{5}$

$D = 60$ mg   This is the dosage of TMP you would give in one 7.5 mL dose, which matches the upper limit of the safe dosage range.

Or, you could have started with a ratio-proportion: ratio for dosage on hand equals ratio for desired dosage.

$\dfrac{40\text{ mg}}{5\text{ mL}} \bowtie \dfrac{D\text{ mg}}{7.5\text{ mL}}$ The unknown "D" is the desired dosage.

$5D = 300$

$\dfrac{5D}{5} = \dfrac{300}{5}$

$D = 60$ mg

Example 3:

The pediatric oral surgeon orders *Tylenol and codeine (acetaminophen and codeine phosphate) suspension 10 mL p.o. q.4–6h p.r.n., pain* for a child weighing 42 lb, who had two teeth repaired. The drug reference states that Tylenol and codeine is a combination drug containing 120 mg of acetaminophen and 12 mg of codeine phosphate per 5 mL. Safe dosage is based on the codeine component, which is 0.5–1 mg/kg/dose every 4 to 6 hours as needed. Is this dose volume safe?

1. **Convert lb to kg.** Approximate equivalent: 1 kg = 2.2 lb

Think: $\dfrac{1}{2}$ of 42 = 21

42 lb = 42 ÷ 2.2 = 19.09 kg = 19.1 kg

2. **Calculate the safe dosage range for the codeine.**

    codeine minimum per dose: 0.5 mg/kg/dose $\times$ 19.1 kg = 9.55 mg/dose = 9.6 mg/dose

    codeine maximum per dose: 1 mg/kg/dose $\times$ 19.1 kg = 19.1 mg/dose

3. **Calculate the volume of medication for the minimum and maximum dose.**

    Minimum dose volume:　　　$\dfrac{D}{H} \times Q = \dfrac{9.6 \text{ mg}}{12 \text{ mg}} \times 5\,\text{mL} = 4\,\text{mL}$, minimum per dose

    Or, use ratio-proportion.

    $\dfrac{12 \text{ mg}}{5 \text{ mL}} \diagdown\!\!\!\!\diagup \dfrac{9.6 \text{ mg}}{X \text{ mL}}$

    $12X = 48$

    $\dfrac{12X}{12} = \dfrac{48}{12}$

    $X = 4\,\text{mL}$, minimum per dose

    Maximum dose volume:　　　$\dfrac{D}{H} \times Q = \dfrac{19.1 \text{ mg}}{12 \text{ mg}} \times 5\,\text{mL} = 7.95\,\text{mL} = 8\,\text{mL}$, maximum per dose

    Or, use ratio-proportion.

    $\dfrac{12 \text{ mg}}{5 \text{ mL}} \diagdown\!\!\!\!\diagup \dfrac{19.1 \text{ mg}}{X \text{ mL}}$

    $12X = 95.5$

    $\dfrac{12X}{12} = \dfrac{95.5}{12}$

    $X = 7.95\,\text{mL} = 8\,\text{mL}$, maximum per dose

4. **Decide if the dose volume is safe.** The ordered dose of 10 mL exceeds the maximum safe dose range; the dose is not safe. Contact the physician to discuss the order.

Be sure to take the time to double-check pediatric dosage. The health care provider who administers the medication has the last opportunity to ensure safe drug therapy.

ADULT DOSAGES BASED ON BODY WEIGHT

Some adult dosage recommendations are based on body weight, too, although less frequently than for children. The information you learned about calculating and verifying children's body weight dosages can be applied to adults. It is important that you become familiar and comfortable with reading labels, drug inserts, and drug reference books to check any order that appears questionable.

Let's look at information found in a drug insert about the adult dosage recommendations for the drug Ticar (ticaricillin) (Figure 13-6). Notice that the adult dosage is recommended by body weight.

BODY WEIGHT DOSAGE CALCULATION WORKSHEET

Some students find the following worksheet helpful when calculating dosage ranges based on body weight for either adults or children. First convert the weight in lb to kg.

TICAR®

Adults:

Bacterial septicemia Respiratory tract infections Skin and soft-tissue infections Intra-abdominal infections Infections of the female pelvis and genital tract	200 to 300 mg/kg/day by I.V. infusion in divided doses every 4 or 6 hours. (The usual dose is 3 grams given every 4 hours [18 grams/day] or 4 grams given every 6 hours [16 grams/day] depending on weight and the severity of the infection.)

Urinary tract infections
  Complicated:
 	
  Uncomplicated:
	150 to 200·mg/kg/day by I.V. infusion in divided doses every 4 or 6 hours.
	(Usual recommended dosage for average [70 kg] adults: 3 grams q.i.d.)
	1 gram I.M. or direct I.V. every 6 hours.

FIGURE 13-6 Section of Ticar Package Insert

Example:

Order: *Ticar 4g IV q.6h* for a patient with bacterial septicemia

Supply: Ticar 200 mg/mL

Recommended adult dosage from package insert: 200–300 mg/kg/day q.4–6h

Patient's weight: 150 lb

Convert lb to kg.

Think: $\frac{1}{2}$ of 150 = 75

150 lb = 150 ÷ 2.2 = 68.2 kg

	Minimum Dosage	Maximum Dosage
Body Weight (kg)	68.2 kg	68.2 kg
× Recommended Dosage	× 200 mg/kg/day	× 300 mg/kg/day
Total Daily Dosage	13,640 mg/kg/day	20,460 mg/kg/day
÷ # Doses/Day	÷ 4 doses/day	÷ 4 doses/day
Dosage Range/Dose	3410 mg/dose q.6h to	5115 mg/dose q.6h

The ordered dosage of Ticar 4 g (or 4000 mg) is within the recommended range and is safe.

Calculate the amount to give for 1 dose.

Step 1 Convert 4 g = 4 × 1000 = 4000 mg

Step 2 Think 4000 mg is 20 times 200 mg, so you want to give 20 mL.

Step 3 Calculate $\dfrac{D}{H} \times Q = \dfrac{\overset{20}{\cancel{4000}}\,mg}{\underset{1}{\cancel{200}}\,mg} \times 1\ mL = 20\ mL$ given intravenously every 6 hours

---

QUICK REVIEW

To use the body weight method to verify the safety of pediatric and adult dosages:
- Convert body weight from pounds and ounces to kilograms: 1 kg = 2.2 lb; 1 lb = 16 oz.
- Calculate the recommended safe dosage in mg/kg.
- Compare the ordered dosage with the recommended dosage to decide if the dosage is safe.
- If the dosage is safe, calculate the amount to give for 1 dose; if not, notify the prescriber.
- Combination drugs are ordered by dose volume. Check a reputable drug reference to be sure the dose ordered contains the safe amount of each drug as recommended.

REVIEW SET 32

Calculate one dose of safe pediatric dosages.

1. Order: *Pathocil 125 mg p.o. q.6h* for a child who weighs 55 lb. The recommended dosage of Pathocil (dicloxacillin sodium) for children weighing less than 40 kg is 12.5–25 mg/kg/day p.o. in equally divided doses q.6h for moderate to severe infections.

   Child's weight: _____25_____ kg   *12.5 mg/kg/day × 25 kg =*

   Recommended minimum daily dosage for this child: __312.5__ mg/day

   Recommended minimum single dosage for this child: __78.1__ mg/dose

   Recommended maximum daily dosage for this child: __625__ mg/day

   Recommended maximum single dosage for this child: __156.3__ mg/dose

   Is the dosage ordered safe? __yes__

2. Dicloxacillin sodium is available as an oral suspension of 62.5 mg per 5 mL. If the dosage ordered in question 1 is safe, give ____10____ mL. If not safe, explain why not and describe what you should do. _____

   _____

3. Order: *Chloromycetin 55 mg IV q.12h* for an 8-day-old infant who weighs 2200 g. The recommended dosage of Chloromycetin (chloramphenicol) for neonates less than 2 kg is 25 mg/kg once daily; and for neonates more than 2 kg and over 7 days of age is ✗50 mg/kg/day divided q.12h.

   Child's weight: __2.2__ kg

   Recommended daily dosage for this child: __110__ mg/day

   Recommended single dosage for this child: __55__ mg/dose

   Is the dosage ordered safe? __yes__

4. Chloramphenicol is available as a solution for injection of 1 g per 10 mL. If the dosage ordered in question 3 is safe, give _____ mL. If not safe, explain why not and describe what you should do. _____

   _____

5. Order: *Suprax 120 mg p.o. q.d.* for a child who weighs 33 lb. The recommended dosage of Suprax (cefixime) for children under 50 kg is 8 mg/kg p.o. once daily or 4 mg/kg q.12h.

   Child's weight: _____ kg

   Recommended single dosage for this child: _____ mg/dose

   Is the dosage ordered safe? _____

6. Suprax is available as a suspension of 100 mg per 5 mL in a 50 mL bottle. If the dosage ordered in question 5 is safe, give _____ mL. If not safe, explain why not and describe what you should do. _____

   _____

   How many doses are available in the bottle of Suprax? _____ dose(s)

7. Order: *Panadol 480 mg p.o. q.4–6h p.r.n. for temperature ≥ 101.6°F.* The child's weight is 32 kg. The recommended child's dosage of Panadol (acetaminophen) is 10–15 mg/kg/dose p.o. q.4–6h p.r.n. for fever.

   Child's weight: _____ kg

   Recommended minimum single dosage for this child: _____ mg/dose

   Recommended maximum single dosage for this child: _____ mg/dose

   Is the dosage ordered safe? _____

8. Panadol is available as a suspension of 160 mg per 5 mL. If the dosage ordered in question 7 is safe, give _____ mL. If not safe, explain why not and describe what you should do. _____

   _____

9. Order: *Keflex 125 mg p.o. q.6h* for a child who weighs 44 lb. The recommended pediatric dosage of Keflex (cephalexin) is 25–50 mg/kg/day in 4 equally divided doses.

   Child's weight: _____ kg

   Recommended minimum daily dosage for this child: _____ mg/day

   Recommended minimum single dosage for this child: _____ mg/dose

   Recommended maximum daily dosage for this child: _____ mg/day

   Recommended maximum single dosage for this child: _____ mg/dose

   Is the dosage ordered safe? _____

10. Keflex is available in a suspension of 125 mg per 5 mL. If the dosage ordered in question 9 is safe, give _____ mL. If not safe, explain why not and describe what you should do.

    _____

    _____

The labels provided represent the drugs available to answer questions 11 through 25. Verify safe dosages, indicate the amount to give, and draw an arrow on the accompanying measuring device. Explain unsafe dosages and describe the appropriate action to take.

11. Order: *Nebcin 8 mg IM q.6h* for an infant who weighs 5000 g. The recommended pediatric dosage of Nebcin (tobramycin) is 2–2.5 mg/kg q.8h or 1.5–1.9 mg/kg q.6h.

    Infant's weight: _____ kg

    Recommended minimum single dosage for this infant: _____ mg/dose

    Recommended maximum singe dosage for this infant: _____ mg/dose

    Is the dosage ordered safe? _____

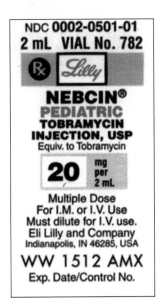

12. If the dosage ordered in question 11 is safe, give _____ mL. If not safe, explain why not and describe what you should do. _____

_____

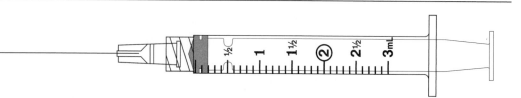

13. Order: *Kantrex 34 mg IV q.8h* for an infant who weighs 7 lb 8 oz. The recommended dosage of Kantrex (kanamycin sulfate) for adults and children is 15 mg/kg/day in 2 or 3 equal doses, not to exceed 1.5 g/day.

Child's weight: ___3.4___ kg

Recommended daily dosage for this child: ___51___ mg/day

Recommended single dosage for this child: ___17___ mg/dose

Is the dosage ordered safe? ___Yes___

NDC 0015-3512-20
EQUIVALENT TO   NSN 6505-00-926-9202
75 mg KANAMYCIN per 2 mL
KANTREX®
Kanamycin Sulfate Injection, USP
Pediatric Injection
FOR I.M. OR I.V. USE
CAUTION: Federal law prohibits dispensing without prescription.
MAXIMUM DOSE: 15 MG/KG/DAY

14. If the dosage ordered in question 13 is safe, give ___0.7___ mL. If not safe, explain why not and describe what you should do. ___17 mg/dose exceeds___

_____

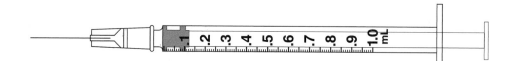

15. Order: *Bactrim pediatric suspension 7.5 mL p.o. q.12h* for a child who weighs 15 kg and has an urinary tract infection. The recommended dosage of Bactrim (trimethoprim and sulfamethoxazole) for such infections in children is based on the trimethoprim at 8 mg/kg/day in 2 equal doses.

Recommended daily trimethoprim dosage for this child: ___320___ mg/day

Recommended single trimethoprim dosage for this child: ___160___ mg/dose

Recommended single dose for this child: ___21.3___ mL/dose

Is the dose ordered safe? _____

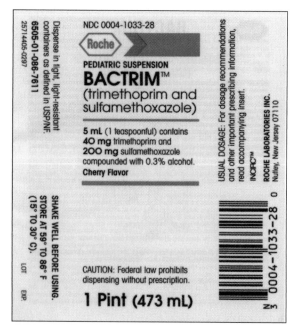

NDC 0004-1033-28
Roche
PEDIATRIC SUSPENSION
BACTRIM™
(trimethoprim and sulfamethoxazole)
5 mL (1 teaspoonful) contains
40 mg trimethoprim and
200 mg sulfamethoxazole
compounded with 0.3% alcohol.
Cherry Flavor
CAUTION: Federal law prohibits dispensing without prescription.
1 Pint (473 mL)

Dispense in tight, light-resistant containers as defined in USP/NF.
6505-01-086-7611
2571405-0297
SHAKE WELL BEFORE USING.
STORE AT 59° TO 86° F
(15° TO 30° C).
LOT   EXP.

USUAL DOSAGE: For dosage recommendations and other important prescribing information, read accompanying insert.
INCIRC™
ROCHE LABORATORIES INC.
Nutley, New Jersey 07110

16. If the dose ordered in question 15 is safe, give _____ mL. If not safe, explain why not and describe what you should do. _____

_____

The dose ordered is equivalent to _____ teaspoons.

17. Order: *gentamicin 40 mg IV q.8h* for a premature neonate who is 5 days old and weighs 1800 g. The recommended dosage of gentamicin for children is 2–2.5 mg/kg q.8h; for neonates, it is 2.5 mg/kg q.8h; and for premature neonates less than 1 week of age, it is 2.5 mg/kg q.12h.

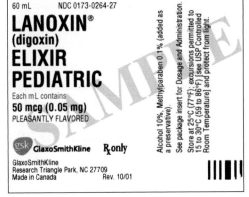

Neonate's weight: _____ kg

Recommended single dosage for this neonate: _____ mg/dose

Is the ordered dosage safe? _____

18. If the dosage ordered in question 17 is safe, give _____ mL. If not safe, explain why not and describe what you should do. _____

_____

19. Order: *Lanoxin 0.15 mg p.o. q.12h* for a maintenance dose for a 9-year-old child who weighs 70 lb. The recommended maintenance pediatric dosage of Lanoxin (digoxin) tablets and elixir is 7–10 mcg/kg/day divided and given in 2 to 3 equal doses per day.

Child's weight: _____ kg

Recommended minimum daily dosage for this child: _____ mg/day

Recommended minimum single dosage for this child: _____ mg/dose

Recommended maximum daily dosage for this child: _____ mg/day

Recommended maximum single dosage for this child: _____ mg/dose

Is the dosage ordered safe? _____

20. If the dosage ordered in question 19 is safe, give _____ mL. If not safe, explain why not and describe what you should do. _____

_____

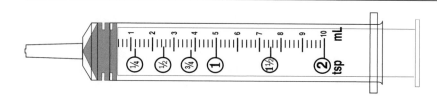

21. Order: *Amoxil oral suspension 100 mg p.o. q.8h* for a child who weighs 39 lb. Recommended dosage: See label.

Child's weight: _____ kg

Recommended minimum daily dosage for this child: _____ mg/day

Recommended minimum single dosage for this child: _____ mg/dose

Recommended maximum daily dosage for this child: _____ mg/day

Recommended maximum single dosage for this child: _____ mg/dose

AMOXIL®
125mg/5mL

125mg/5mL
NDC 0029-6008-22

AMOXIL®
AMOXICILLIN
FOR ORAL
SUSPENSION

Directions for mixing: Tap bottle until all powder flows freely. Add approximately 1/3 total amount of water for reconstitution (total=116 mL); shake vigorously to wet powder. Add remaining water; again shake vigorously. Each 5 mL (1 teaspoonful) will contain amoxicillin trihydrate equivalent to 125 mg amoxicillin.
Usual Adult Dosage: 250 to 500 mg every 8 hours.
Usual Child Dosage: 20 to 40 mg/kg/day in divided doses every 8 hours, depending on age, weight and infection severity. See accompanying prescribing information.
Keep tightly closed.
Shake well before using.
Refrigeration preferable but not required.
Discard suspension after 14 days.

℞ only

150mL
(when reconstituted)

LOT
EXP.

gsk **GlaxoSmithKline**

Net contents: Equivalent to 3.75 grams amoxicillin. Store dry powder at room temperature.

GlaxoSmithKline
Research Triangle Park, NC 27709

3 0029-6008-22 4

9405813-G

Is the dosage ordered safe? _____

22. If the dosage ordered in question 21 is safe, give _____ mL. If not safe, explain why not and describe what you should do. _____

_____

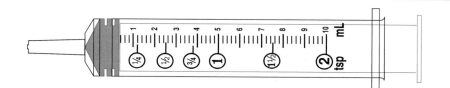

23. Order: *Terramycin 100 mg IM q.8h* for a 9-year-old child who weighs 55 lb. Recommended pediatric dosage: See label.

Child's weight: _____ kg

Recommended minimum daily dosage for this child: _____ mg/day

Recommended minimum single dosage for this child: _____ mg/dose

Recommended maximum daily dosage for this child: _____ mg/day

Recommended maximum single dosage for this child: _____ mg/dose

Is the dosage ordered safe? _____

10 mL Vial   NDC 0049-0750-77

℞ only
8885

SEE ACCOMPANYING
PRESCRIBING INFORMATION

DOSAGE
ADULTS: The usual daily dose is 250 mg administered once every 24 hours or 300 mg given in divided doses at 8 to 12 hour intervals. **CHILDREN ABOVE EIGHT YEARS OF AGE:** 15-25 mg/kg body weight up to a maximum of 250 mg per single dose every 24 hours. This may be divided and given at 8 to 12 hour intervals.

Terramycin®
(oxytetracycline)

*Intramuscular Solution**
contains 2% lidocaine
50 mg/mL

Pfizer **Roerig**
Division of Pfizer Inc, NY, NY 10017

Store below 86°F (30°C).
FOR INTRAMUSCULAR USE ONLY.
Each mL contains (w/v) 50 mg oxytetracycline, 2% lidocaine, 2.5% magnesium chloride hexahydrate, 0.3% sodium formaldehyde sulfoxylate, 1% α-monoethanolamine, approx. 2.6% monoethanolamine, 0.02% propyl gallate, 1% citric acid, 74.1% propylene glycol and 18.5% water.
*U.S. Pat. Nos. 3,017,323 and 3,026,248

05-1051-32-4

MADE IN USA

24. If the dosage ordered in question 23 is safe, give _____ mL. If not safe, explain why not and describe what you should do. _____

_____

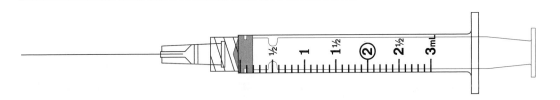

25. Order: *Terramycin 275 mg IM q.d.* for a 7-year-old child who weighs 21 kg. Recommended pediatric dosage: See label for question 23.

    Is the ordered dosage safe? _____ Explain: _____

_____

Refer to the following information from the package insert for Ticar to answer questions 26 through 30.

TICAR ®	
Adults:	
Bacterial septicemia	200 to 300 mg/kg/day by I.V. infusion in divided doses every 4 or 6 hours.
Respiratory tract infections	(The usual dose is 3 grams given every 4 hours [18 grams/day] or 4 grams given every 6 hours
Skin and soft-tissue infections	[16 grams/day] depending on weight and the severity of the infection.)
Intra-abdominal infections	
Infections of the female pelvis and genital tract	
Urinary tract infections	
Complicated:	150 to 200 mg/kg/day by I.V. infusion in divided doses every 4 or 6 hours.
	(Usual recommended dosage for average [70 kg] adults: 3 grams q.i.d.)
Uncomplicated:	1 gram I.M. or direct I.V. every 6 hours.

26. What is the recommended adult dosage of Ticar (ticaricillin) for bacterial septicemia?

_____

27. What is the recommended adult dosage of Ticar for a complicated urinary tract infection?

_____

28. What daily dosage range of Ticar should you expect for an adult with a complicated urinary tract infection who weighs 130 lb? _____ g to _____ g/day

29. What single dosage range of Ticar administered q.4h should you expect for the adult described in question 28? _____ g to _____ g/dose

30. What single dosage range of Ticar administered q.6h should you expect for the adult described in question 28? _____ g to _____ g/dose

After completing these problems, see pages 502–504 to check your answers.

CRITICAL THINKING SKILLS

Medication errors in pediatrics often occur when the nurse fails to properly identify the child before administering the dose.

(continues)

(continued)

error

Failing to identify the child before administering a medication.

possible scenario

Suppose the physician ordered *ampicillin 500 mg IV q.6h* for a child with pneumonia. The nurse calculated the dosage to be safe, checked to be sure the child had no allergies, and prepared the medication. The child had been assigned to a semiprivate room. The nurse entered the room and noted only one child in the room and administered the IV ampicillin to that child, without checking the identification of the child. Within an hour of the administered ampicillin the child began to break out in hives and had signs of respiratory distress. The nurse asked the child's mother, "Does Johnny have any known allergies?" The mother replied, "This is James, not Johnny, and yes, James is allergic to penicillin. His roommate, Johnny, is in the playroom." At this point the nurse realized the ampicillin was given to the wrong child, who was allergic to penicillin.

potential outcome

James's physician would have been notified and he would likely have ordered epinephrine SC stat (given for anaphylactic reactions), followed by close monitoring of the child. Anaphylactic reactions can range from mild to severe. Ampicillin is a derivative of penicillin and would not have been prescribed for a child such as James.

prevention

This error could easily have been avoided had the nurse remembered the cardinal rule of *identifying the child* before administering *any* medication. Children are very mobile, and you cannot assume the identity of a child simply because he is in a particular room. The correct method of identifying the child is to check the wrist or ankle band and compare it to the medication administration record with the child's name, room number, physician, and account number. Finally, remember that the first of the *six rights* of medication administration is the *right patient*.

PRACTICE PROBLEMS—CHAPTER 13

Convert the following weights to kilograms. Round to one decimal place.

1. 12 lb =   _____ kg   6. 6 lb 10 oz =   _____ kg

2. 8 lb 4 oz =   _____ kg   7. 52 lb =   _____ kg

3. 1570 g =   _____ kg   8. 890 g =   _____ kg

4. 2300 g =   _____ kg

5. 34 lb =   _____ kg

9. The recommended dosage of Nebcin (tobramycin) for adults with serious, non-life-threatening infections is 3 mg/kg/day in 3 equally divided doses q.8h. What should you expect the total daily dosage of Nebcin to be for an adult with a serious infection who weighs 80 kg? _____ mg/day

10. What should you expect the single dosage of Nebcin to be for the adult described in question 9? _____ mg/dose

The labels provided represent the drugs available to answer questions 11 through 42. Verify safe dosages and indicate the amount to give and draw an arrow on the accompanying measuring device. Explain unsafe dosages and describe the appropriate action to take.

11. Order: *gentamicin 40 mg IV q.8h* for a child who weighs 43 lb. The recommended dosage for children is 2–2.5 mg/kg q.8h.

    Child's weight: _____ kg

    Recommended minimum single dosage for this child: _____ mg/dose

    Recommended maximum single dosage for this child: _____ mg/dose

    Is the ordered dosage safe? _____

    NDC 63323-010-02   1002

    GENTAMICIN

    INJECTION, USP

    equivalent to 40 mg/mL
    Gentamicin

    80 mg/2 mL

    For IM or IV Use.
    Must be diluted for IV use.

    2 mL Multiple Dose Vial

    Sterile
    Usual Dosage: See insert.

    APP AMERICAN PHARMACEUTICAL PARTNERS

    Los Angeles, CA 90024

    401896A

    SAMPLE

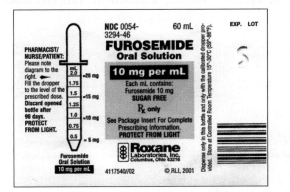

12. If the dosage ordered in question 11 is safe, give _____ mL. If not safe, explain why not and describe what you should do. _____

    _____

13. Order: *furosemide oral solution 10 mg p.o. b.i.d.* for a child who weighs 16 lb. The recommended pediatric dosage is 0.5–2 mg/kg b.i.d.

    Child's weight: _____ kg

    Recommended minimum single dosage for this child: _____ mg/dose

    Recommended maximum single dosage for this child: _____ mg/dose

    Is the ordered dosage safe? _____

    NDC 0054-3294-46   60 mL   EXP. LOT

    PHARMACIST/NURSE/PATIENT: Please note diagram to the right. Fill the dropper to the level of the prescribed dose. Discard opened bottle after 90 days. PROTECT FROM LIGHT.

    FUROSEMIDE Oral Solution

    10 mg per mL

    Each mL contains:
    Furosemide 10 mg
    SUGAR FREE

    Rx only

    See Package Insert For Complete Prescribing Information.
    PROTECT FROM LIGHT

    Roxane Laboratories, Inc.
    Columbus, Ohio 43216

    Furosemide Oral Solution 10 mg per mL

    4117540//02   © RLI, 2001

    Dispense only in this bottle and only with the calibrated dropper provided. Store at Controlled Room Temperature 15°–30°C (59°–86°F).

14. If the dosage ordered in question 13 is safe, give _____ mL. If not safe, explain why not and describe what you should do. _____

    _____

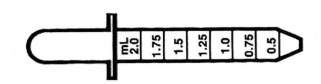

15. Order: *carbamazepine 150 mg p.o. b.i.d.* for a child who is 5 years old and weighs 40 lb. The recommended dosage for children under 6 years of age is 10–20 mg/kg/day in 2–4 divided doses per day, not to exceed 400 mg/day.

    Child's weight: _____ kg

    Recommended minimum daily dosage for this child: _____ mg/day

    Recommended minimum single dosage for this child: _____ mg/dose

    Recommended maximum daily dosage for this child: _____ mg/day

    Recommended maximum single dosage for this child: _____ mg/dose

    Is the dosage ordered safe? _____

NDC 0083-0019-76   FSC 1841
6505-01-302-4467

Tegretol®

carbamazepine USP

Suspension

100 mg/5 mL

IMPORTANT: Shake well before using.

Each 5 mL contains 100 mg carbamazepine USP.

450 mL

Dispense in tight, light-resistant container (USP).

Caution: Federal law prohibits dispensing without prescription.

Keep this and all drugs out of the reach of children.
Dosage: See package insert.
Do not store above 86°F (30°C).

Mfd. by:
Ciba-Geigy Canada, Ltd.
Dorval, Quebec, Canada

Dist. by:
Ciba-Geigy Corporation
Pharmaceuticals Division
Summit, NJ 07901

ciba

893972

0083-0019-76

P550631

16. If the dosage ordered in question 15 is safe, give _____ mL. If not safe, explain why not and describe what you should do. _____

    _____

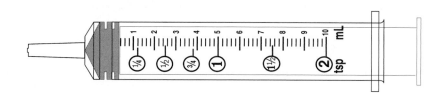

17. Order: *Depakene 150 mg p.o. b.i.d.* for a child who is 10 years old and weighs 64 lb. The recommended dosage for adults and children 10 years and older is 10–15 mg/kg/day up to a maximum of 60 mg/kg/day. If the total daily dosage exceeds 250 mg, divide the dose.

    Child's weight: _____ kg

    Recommended minimum daily dosage for this child: _____ mg/day

    Recommended minimum single dosage for this child: _____ mg/dose

    Recommended maximum daily dosage for this child: _____ mg/day

    Recommended maximum single dosage for this child: _____ mg/dose

    Is the dosage ordered safe? _____

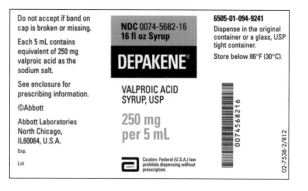

Do not accept if band on cap is broken or missing.

Each 5 mL contains equivalent of 250 mg valproic acid as the sodium salt.

See enclosure for prescribing information.

©Abbott

Abbott Laboratories
North Chicago,
IL60064, U.S.A.

Exp.

Lot

NDC 0074-5682-16
16 fl oz Syrup

DEPAKENE®

VALPROIC ACID
SYRUP, USP

250 mg
per 5 mL

Caution: Federal (U.S.A.) law prohibits dispensing without prescription.

6505-01-094-9241

Dispense in the original container or a glass, USP tight container.

Store below 86°F (30°C).

0074568216

02-7538-2/R12

18. If the dosage ordered in question 17 is safe, give _____ mL. If not safe, explain why not and describe what you should do. _____

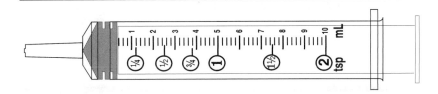

19. Order: *bacitracin 750 U I.M. q.8h* for an infant who weighs 2500 g. The recommended dosage for infants 2.5 kg and below: 900 units/kg/day in 2–3 divided doses; infants over 2.5 kg: 1000 units/kg/day in 2–3 divided doses.

Child's weight: _____ kg

Recommended daily dosage for this child: _____ U/day

Recommended single dosage for this child: _____ U/dose

Is the ordered dosage safe? _____

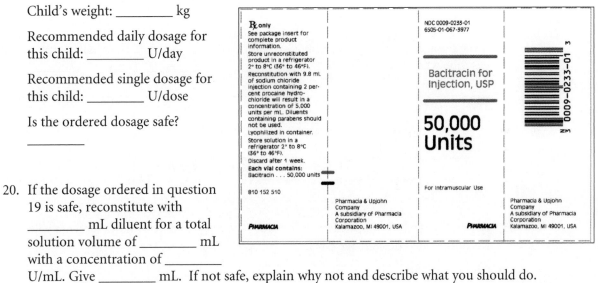

Rx only
See package insert for complete product information.
Store unreconstituted product in a refrigerator 2° to 8°C (36° to 46°F).
Reconstitution with 9.8 mL of sodium chloride injection containing 2 percent procaine hydrochloride will result in a concentration of 5,000 units per mL. Diluents containing parabens should not be used.
Lyophilized in container.
Store solution in a refrigerator 2° to 8°C (36° to 46°F).
Discard after 1 week.
Each vial contains:
Bacitracin . . . 50,000 units

810 152 510

NDC 0009-0233-01
6505-01-067-3977

Bacitracin for Injection, USP

50,000 Units

For Intramuscular Use

0009-0233-01

Pharmacia & Upjohn Company
A subsidiary of Pharmacia Corporation
Kalamazoo, MI 49001, USA

PHARMACIA

Pharmacia & Upjohn Company
A subsidiary of Pharmacia Corporation
Kalamazoo, MI 49001, USA

PHARMACIA

20. If the dosage ordered in question 19 is safe, reconstitute with _____ mL diluent for a total solution volume of _____ mL with a concentration of _____ U/mL. Give _____ mL. If not safe, explain why not and describe what you should do.

_____

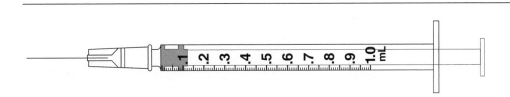

21. Order: *Amoxil oral suspension 150 mg p.o. q.8h* for a child who weighs 41 lb. Recommended dosage: See label on next page.

Child's weight: _____ kg

Recommended minimum daily dosage for this child: _____ mg/day

Recommended minimum single dosage for this child: _____ mg/dose

Recommended maximum daily dosage for this child: _____ mg/day

Recommended maximum single dosage for this child: _____ mg/dose

Is the dosage ordered safe? _____

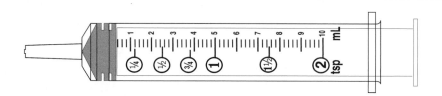

22. If the dosage ordered in question 21 is safe, give _____ mL. If not safe, explain why not and describe what you should do. _____

_____

23. Order: *Ceclor oral suspension 187 mg p.o. b.i.d.* for a child with otitis media who weighs $20\frac{1}{2}$ lb. Recommended dosage: See label.

   Child's weight: _____ kg

   Recommended daily dosage for this child: _____ mg/day

   Recommended single dosage for this child: _____ mg/dose

   Is the dosage ordered safe? _____

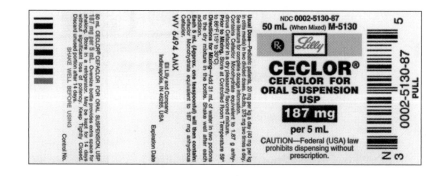

24. If the dosage ordered in question 23 is safe, give _____ mL. If not safe, explain why not and describe what you should do. _____

_____

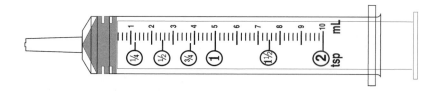

25. Order: *Narcan 100 mcg SC stat* for a child who weighs 22 lb. Recommended pediatric dosage: 0.01 mg/kg/dose.

    Child's weight: _____ kg

    Recommended single dosage for this child: _____ mg/dose

    Is the dosage ordered safe? _____

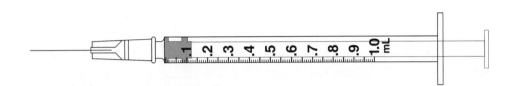

26. If the dosage ordered in question 25 is safe, give _____ mL. If not safe, explain why not and describe what you should do. _____

    _____

27. Order: *Nebcin 35 mg IV q.8h* for a child who weighs 14 kg. The recommended pediatric dosage of Nebcin (tobramycin) is 2–2.5 mg/kg q.8h or 1.5–1.9 mg/kg q.6h.

    Recommended minimum single dosage for this child: _____ mg/dose

    Recommended maximum single dosage for this child: _____ mg/dose

    Is the dosage ordered safe? _____

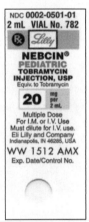

28. If the dosage ordered in question 27 is safe, give _____ mL. If not safe, explain why not and describe what you should do. _____

    _____

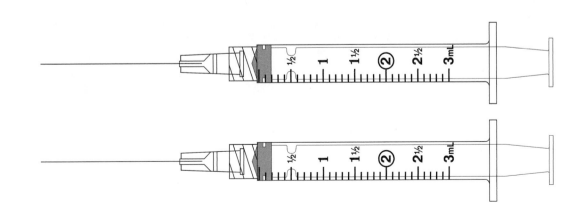

29. Order: *Rocephin 1 g IV q.12h* for a child with a serious infection who weighs 20 lb. The recommended pediatric dosage of Rocephin (ceftriaxone sodium) is a total daily dosage of 50–75 mg/kg, given once a day (or in equally divided doses twice a day), not to exceed 2 g/day.

Child's weight: _____ kg

Recommended minimum daily dosage for this child: _____ mg/day

Recommended minimum single dosage for this child: _____ mg/dose

Recommended maximum daily dosage for this child: _____ mg/day

Recommended maximum single dosage for this child: _____ mg/dose

Is the dosage ordered safe? _____

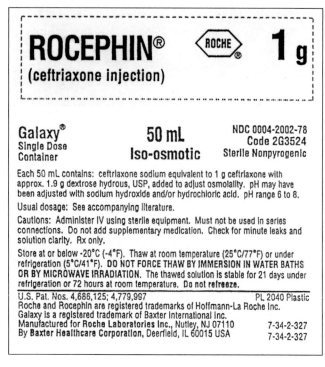

ROCEPHIN® ◇ROCHE◇ **1 g**
(ceftriaxone injection)

Galaxy®   **50 mL**   NDC 0004-2002-78
Single Dose   **Iso-osmotic**   Code 2G3524
Container   Sterile Nonpyrogenic

Each 50 mL contains: ceftriaxone sodium equivalent to 1 g ceftriaxone with approx. 1.9 g dextrose hydrous, USP, added to adjust osmolality. pH may have been adjusted with sodium hydroxide and/or hydrochloric acid. pH range 6 to 8.

Usual dosage: See accompanying literature.

Cautions: Administer IV using sterile equipment. Must not be used in series connections. Do not add supplementary medication. Check for minute leaks and solution clarity. Rx only.

Store at or below -20°C (-4°F). Thaw at room temperature (25°C/77°F) or under refrigeration (5°C/41°F). DO NOT FORCE THAW BY IMMERSION IN WATER BATHS OR BY MICROWAVE IRRADIATION. The thawed solution is stable for 21 days under refrigeration or 72 hours at room temperature. Do not refreeze.

U.S. Pat. Nos. 4,686,125; 4,779,997   PL 2040 Plastic
Roche and Rocephin are registered trademarks of Hoffmann-La Roche Inc.
Galaxy is a registered trademark of Baxter International Inc.
Manufactured for Roche Laboratories Inc., Nutley, NJ 07110   7-34-2-327
By Baxter Healthcare Corporation, Deerfield, IL 60015 USA   7-34-2-327

30. If the dosage ordered in question 29 is safe, give _____ mL. If not safe, explain why not and describe what you should do. _____

_____

31. Order: *Robinul 50 mcg IM 60 minutes pre-op* for a child who weighs 11.4 kg. The recommended pediatric pre-anesthesia dosage of Robinul (glycopyrrolate) is 0.002 mg/lb of body weight given intramuscularly.

Child's weight: _____ lb

Recommended single dosage for this child: _____ mg/dose

Is the dosage ordered safe? _____

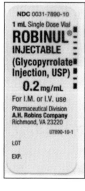

NDC 0031-7890-10
1 mL Single Dose Vial
ROBINUL®
INJECTABLE
(Glycopyrrolate
Injection, USP)
0.2 mg/mL
For I.M. or I.V. use
Pharmaceutical Division
A.H. Robins Company
Richmond, VA 23220
U7890-10-1
LOT
EXP.

32. If the dosage ordered in question 31 is safe, give _____ mL. If not safe, explain why not and describe what you should do. _____

_____

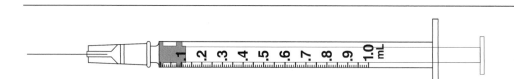

33. Order: *Tazidime 400 mg IV q.8h* for a 6-month-old infant with a serious infection who weighs 18 lb. The recommended dosage of Tazidime (ceftazidime) for infants and children 1 month–12 years is 30–50 mg/kg q.8h, not to exceed 6 g/day.

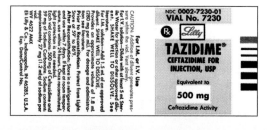

NDC 0002-7230-01
VIAL No. 7230
Ⓡ   *Lilly*
TAZIDIME®
CEFTAZIDIME FOR
INJECTION, USP
Equivalent to
500 mg
Ceftazidime Activity

Child's weight: _____ kg

The total daily dosage ordered for this infant: _____ mg/day or _____ g/day

Recommended minimum single dosage for this child: _____ mg/dose

Recommended maximum single dosage for this child: _____ mg/dose

Is the dosage ordered safe? _____

34. If the dosage ordered in question 33 is safe, reconstitute with _____ mL diluent for a total solution volume of _____ mL with a concentration of _____ mg/mL. Give _____ mL. If not safe, explain why not and describe what you should do. _____

_____

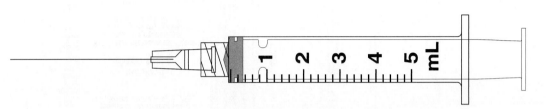

35. Order: *Augmentin 200 mg q.12h* for a 5-year-old child who weighs 45 lb. The recommended dosage of this combination drug is based on the amoxicillin at 25 mg/kg/day in divided doses q.12h or 20 mg/kg/day in divided doses q.8h.

Child's weight: _____ kg

Recommended daily dosage for this child: _____ mg/day

Recommended single dosage for this child: _____ mg/dose

Is the dosage ordered safe? _____

AUGMENTIN®
250mg/5mL

250mg/5mL
NDC 0029-6090-39

AUGMENTIN®
AMOXICILLIN/
CLAVULANATE POTASSIUM
FOR ORAL SUSPENSION
When reconstituted, each 5 mL contains:
AMOXICILLIN, 250 MG,
as the trihydrate
CLAVULANIC ACID, 62.5 MG,
as clavulanate potassium

Directions for mixing:
Tap bottle until all powder flows freely.
Add approximately 2/3 of total water
for reconstitution (total = 65 mL);
shake vigorously to wet powder. Add
remaining water; again shake vigorously.
Dosage: See accompanying prescribing
information.

Keep tightly closed.
Shake well before using.
Must be refrigerated.
Discard after 10 days.

75mL (when reconstituted)

Use only if inner seal is intact.
Net contents: Equivalent to
3.75 g amoxicillin and
0.938 g clavulanic acid
Store dry powder at room
temperature.
GlaxoSmithKline
Research Triangle Park,
NC 27709

3 0029-6090-39 7

LOT

EXP

gsk **GlaxoSmithKline**   **R only**   9405844-H

36. If the dosage ordered in question 35 is safe, give _____ mL. If not safe, explain why not and describe what you should do. _____

_____

37. Order: *Ceclor oral suspension 75 mg p.o. t.i.d.* for a child with an upper respiratory infection who weighs 18 lb. Recommended dosage: See label

    Child's weight: _____ kg

    Recommended daily dosage for this child: _____ mg/day

    Recommended single dosage for this child: _____ mg/dose

    Is the dosage ordered safe? _____

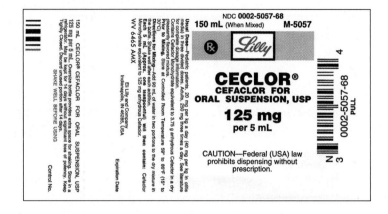

38. If the dosage ordered in question 37 is safe, give _____ mL. If not safe, explain why not and describe what you should do. _____

    _____

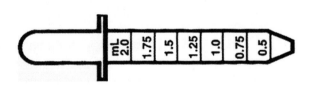

39. Order: *Vantin 100 mg p.o. q.i.d. × 10 days* for a 4-year-old child with tonsillitis who weighs 45 lb. Recommended dosage for children 5 months–12 years: 5 mg/kg (maximum of 100 mg/dose) q.12h (maximum daily dosage: 200 mg) for 5–10 days.

    Child's weight: _____ kg

    Recommended daily dosage for this child: _____ mg/day

    The total daily dosage ordered for this infant: _____ mg/day

    Is the dosage ordered safe? _____

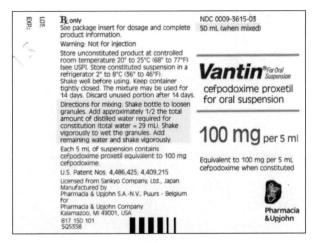

40. If the dosage ordered in question 39 is safe, give _____ mL. If not safe, explain why not and describe what you should do. _____

_____

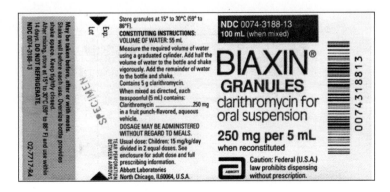

41. Order: *Biaxin 175 mg p.o. q.12h* for a child who weighs 51 lb. Recommended pediatric dosage: See label.

Child's weight: _____ kg

Recommended daily dosage for this child: _____ mg/day

Recommended single dosage for this child: _____ mg/dose

Is the dosage ordered safe? _____

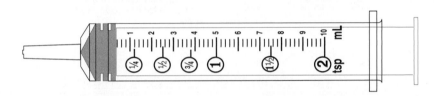

42. If the dosage ordered in question 41 is safe, give _____ mL. If not safe, explain why not and describe what you should do. _____

_____

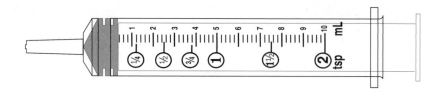

Questions 43 through 48 ask you to apply the steps on your own to determine safe dosages, just as you would do in the clinical setting. Calculate the amount to give and mark an arrow on the measuring device, or explain unsafe dosages and describe the appropriate action.

43. Order: *Solu-Medrol 10 mg IM q.6h* for a child who weighs 95 lb. Recommended pediatric dosage: Not less than 0.5 mg/kg/day

If the dosage ordered is safe, give _____ mL. If not safe, explain why not and describe what you should do. _____

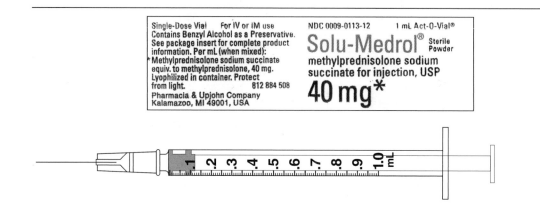

44. Order: *albuterol 1.4 mg p.o. t.i.d.* for a 2-year-old child who weighs 31 lb. Recommended pediatric dosage: 0.1 mg/kg, not to exceed 2 mg t.i.d.

If the dosage ordered is safe, give _____ mL. If not safe, explain why not and describe what you should do. _____

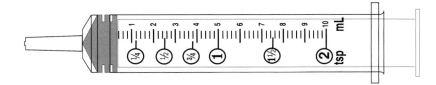

45. Order: *penicillin G potassium 450,000 U IM q.6h* for a child with a streptococcal infection who weighs 12 kg. Recommended pediatric dosage for streptococcal infections is 150,000 U/kg/day given in equal doses q.4–6h.

    If the dosage ordered is safe, reconstitute to a dosage supply of _____ U/mL and give _____ mL. If not safe, explain why not and describe what you should do. _____

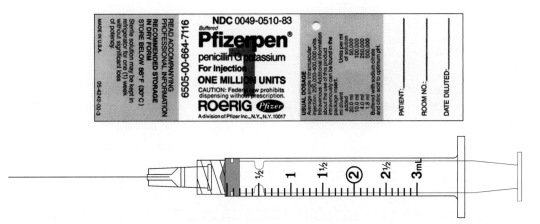

46. Order: *Klonopin 1 mg p.o. b.i.d.* for a 9-year-old child on initial therapy who weighs 56 lb. The recommended initial pediatric dosage of Klonopin (clonazepam) for children up to 10 years or 30 kg is 0.01–0.03 mg/kg/day in 2–3 divided doses up to a maximum of 0.05 mg/kg/day.

    If the dosage ordered is safe, give _____ tablet(s). If not safe, explain why not and describe what you should do. _____

    _____

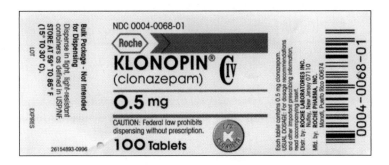

47. Order: *meperidine 20 mg SC q.3–4h p.r.n. pain* for a child who weighs 18 lb. Recommended pediatric dosage: 1.1–1.8 mg/kg q.3–4h p.r.n.; do not exceed adult dosage of 50–100 mg/dose.

    If the dosage ordered is safe, give _____ mL. If not safe, explain why not and describe what you should do. _____

    _____

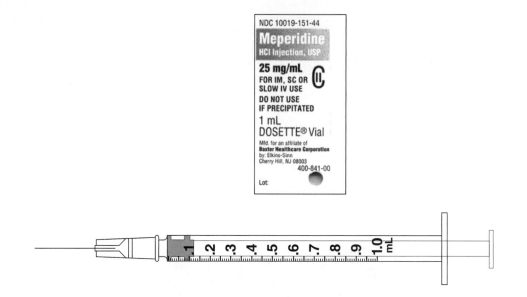

48. Order: *Kefzol 250 mg IM q.8h* for a 3-year-old child who weighs 35 lb. The recommended pediatric dosage of Kefzol (cefazolin sodium) for children over 1 month: 25–50 mg/kg/day in 3–4 divided doses.

    If the dosage ordered is safe, give _____ mL. If not safe, explain why not and describe what you should do. _____

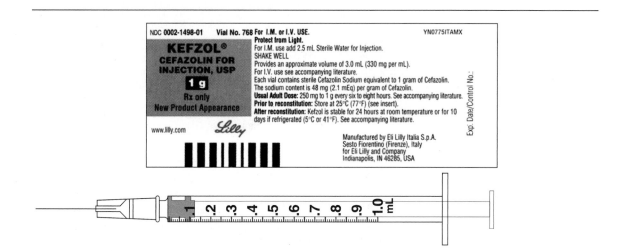

49. Refer back to questions 43 through 48. Identify which drugs require a reconstitution label.

    _____

    _____

50. Critical Thinking Skill: Describe the strategy or strategies you would implement to prevent this medication error.

    possible scenario

    Suppose the family practice resident ordered *tobramycin 110 mg IV q.8h* for a child with cystic fibrosis who weighs 10 kg. The pediatric reference guide states that the safe dosage of tobramycin for a child with severe infections is 7.5 mg/kg/day in 3 equally divided doses. The nurse received five admissions the evening of this order and thought, "I'm too busy to calculate the safe dosage this time." The pharmacist prepared and labeled the medication in a syringe and the nurse administered the first dose of the medication. An hour later the resident arrived on the pediatric unit and inquired if the nurse had given the first dose. When the nurse replied "yes," the resident became pale and stated, "I just realized that I ordered an adult dose of tobramycin. I had hoped you hadn't given the medication yet."

potential outcome

The resident's next step would likely have been to discontinue the tobramycin and order a stat tobramycin level. The level would most likely have been elevated, and the child would have required close monitoring for renal damage and hearing loss.

prevention

_____

_____

After completing these problems, see pages 504–509 to check your answers.

SECTION 3 SELF-EVALUATION

Chapter 9—Oral Dosage of Drugs

The following labels (A–N) represent the drugs you have available on your medication cart for the orders in questions 1 through 10. Select the correct label and identify the letter that corresponds to fill these medication orders. Calculate the amount to give.

1. Order: *Toprol-XL 0.2 g p.o. q.d.*

   Select label _____ and give _____ tab

2. Order: *Nexium 40 mg p.o. q.d.*

   Select label _____ and give _____ cap

3. Order: *Aricept 10 mg p.o. q.d.*

   Select label _____ and give _____ tab

4. Order: *ondansetron hydrochloride 6 mg p.o. b.i.d. × 2 days*

   Select label _____ and give _____ mL

5. Order: *potassium chloride 16 mEq p.o. q.d.*

   Select label _____ and give _____ mL

6. Order: *nitroglycerin 13 mg p.o. t.i.d.*

   Select label _____ and give _____ cap

7. Order: *Synthroid 0.05 mg p.o. q.d.*

   Select label _____ and give _____ tab

8. Order: *codeine gr $\frac{1}{4}$ p.o. q.4–6h p.r.n., cough*

   Select label _____ and give _____ tab

9. Order: *furosemide 12.5 mg p.o. b.i.d.*

   Select label _____ and give _____ mL

10. Order: *Proventil 3 mg p.o. t.i.d.*

    Select label _____ and give _____ mL

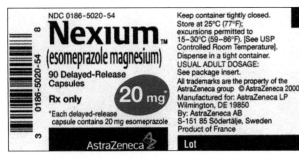

A

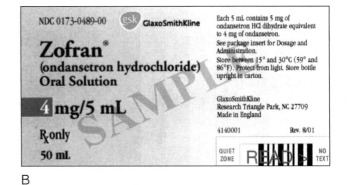

B

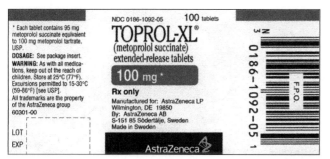

* Each tablet contains 95 mg metoprolol succinate equivalent to 100 mg metoprolol tartrate, USP.

DOSAGE: See package insert.
WARNING: As with all medications, keep out of the reach of children. Store at 25°C (77°F). Excursions permitted to 15-30°C (59-86°F) [see USP].
All trademarks are the property of the AstraZeneca group
60301-00

LOT
EXP

NDC 0186-1092-05   100 tablets

TOPROL-XL®
(metoprolol succinate)
extended-release tablets

100 mg*

Rx only

Manufactured for: AstraZeneca LP
Wilmington, DE 19850
By: AstraZeneca AB
S-151 85 Södertälje, Sweden
Made in Sweden

AstraZeneca

0186-1092-05

F.P.O.

C

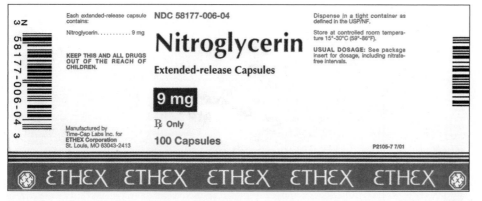

Each extended-release capsule contains:

Nitroglycerin . . . . 9 mg

KEEP THIS AND ALL DRUGS OUT OF THE REACH OF CHILDREN.

Manufactured by
Time-Cap Labs Inc. for
ETHEX Corporation
St. Louis, MO 63043-2413

NDC 58177-006-04

Nitroglycerin

Extended-release Capsules

9 mg

℞ Only
100 Capsules

Dispense in a tight container as defined in the USP/NF.

Store at controlled room temperature 15°-30°C (59°-86°F).

USUAL DOSAGE: See package insert for dosage, including nitrate-free intervals.

P2105-7 7/01

58177-006-04

ETHEX ETHEX ETHEX ETHEX ETHEX

D

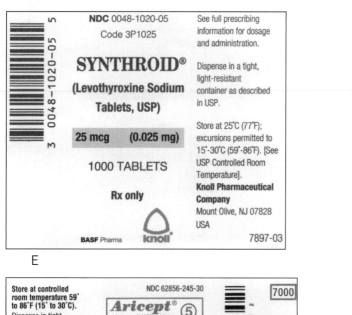

NDC 0048-1020-05
Code 3P1025

SYNTHROID®

(Levothyroxine Sodium Tablets, USP)

25 mcg   (0.025 mg)

1000 TABLETS

Rx only

BASF Pharma   knoll®

0048-1020-05

See full prescribing information for dosage and administration.

Dispense in a tight, light-resistant container as described in USP.

Store at 25°C (77°F); excursions permitted to 15°-30°C (59°-86°F). [See USP Controlled Room Temperature].

Knoll Pharmaceutical Company
Mount Olive, NJ 07828 USA

7897-03

E

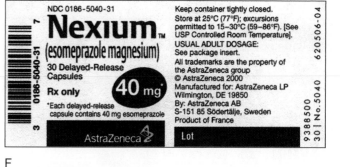

NDC 0186-5040-31

Nexium™
(esomeprazole magnesium)

30 Delayed-Release Capsules

Rx only

40 mg

*Each delayed-release capsule contains 40 mg esomeprazole

AstraZeneca

Keep container tightly closed.
Store at 25°C (77°F); excursions permitted to 15–30°C (59–86°F). [See USP Controlled Room Temperature].
USUAL ADULT DOSAGE: See package insert.
All trademarks are the property of the AstraZeneca group
© AstraZeneca 2000
Manufactured for: AstraZeneca LP
Wilmington, DE 19850
By: AstraZeneca AB
S-151 85 Södertälje, Sweden
Product of France

Lot

0186-5040-31

620506-04

9388500
30 | No.5040

F

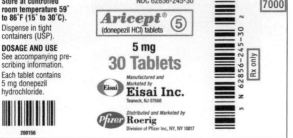

Store at controlled room temperature 59° to 86° F (15° to 30°C).
Dispense in tight containers (USP).

DOSAGE AND USE
See accompanying prescribing information.

Each tablet contains 5 mg donepezil hydrochloride.

NDC 62856-245-30

7000

Aricept® ⑤
(donepezil HCl) tablets

5 mg
30 Tablets

Manufactured and Marketed by
Eisai **Eisai Inc.**
Teaneck, NJ 07666

Distributed and Marketed by
Pfizer **Roerig**
Division of Pfizer Inc, NY, NY 10017

Rx only

62856-245-30

200156

G

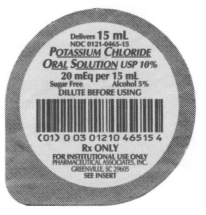

Delivers **15 mL**
NDC 0121-0465-15
POTASSIUM CHLORIDE ORAL SOLUTION USP 10%
20 mEq per 15 mL
Sugar Free   Alcohol 5%
DILUTE BEFORE USING

(01) 0 03 01210 46515 4

Rx ONLY
FOR INSTITUTIONAL USE ONLY
PHARMACEUTICAL ASSOCIATES, INC.
GREENVILLE, SC 29605
SEE INSERT

H

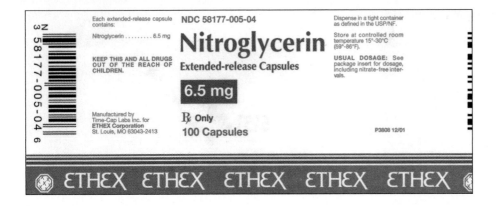

I

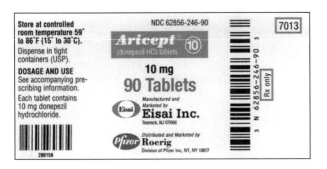

J

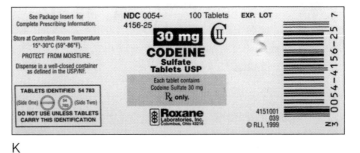

K

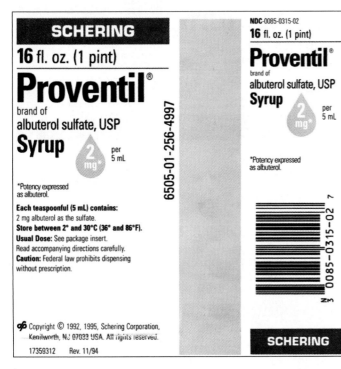

L

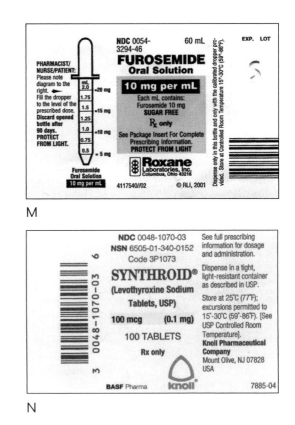

M

N

Chapter 10—Parenteral Dosage of Drugs

The following labels (A–H) represent the drugs you have available on your medication cart for the orders in questions 11 through 18. Select the correct label and identify the letter that corresponds to fill these parenteral medication orders. Calculate the amount to give.

11. Order: *vitamin B-12 0.2 mg SC q.d. × 10 days*

    Select label _____ and give _____ mL

12. Order: *Dilantin 175 mg IV stat*

    Select label _____ and give _____ mL

13. Order: *epinephrine 200 mcg SC stat*

    Select label _____ and give _____ mL

14. Order: *furosemide 8 mg IM q.d.*

    Select label _____ and give _____ mL

15. Order: *gentamicin 60 mg IV q.8h*

    Select label _____ and give _____ mL

16. Order: *heparin 750 U SC stat*

    Select label _____ and give _____ mL

17. Order: *morphine gr $\frac{1}{10}$ SC q.3–4h pr.n., pain*

    Select label _____ and give _____ mL

18. Order: *Narcan 0.3 mg IM stat*

    Select label _____ and give _____ mL

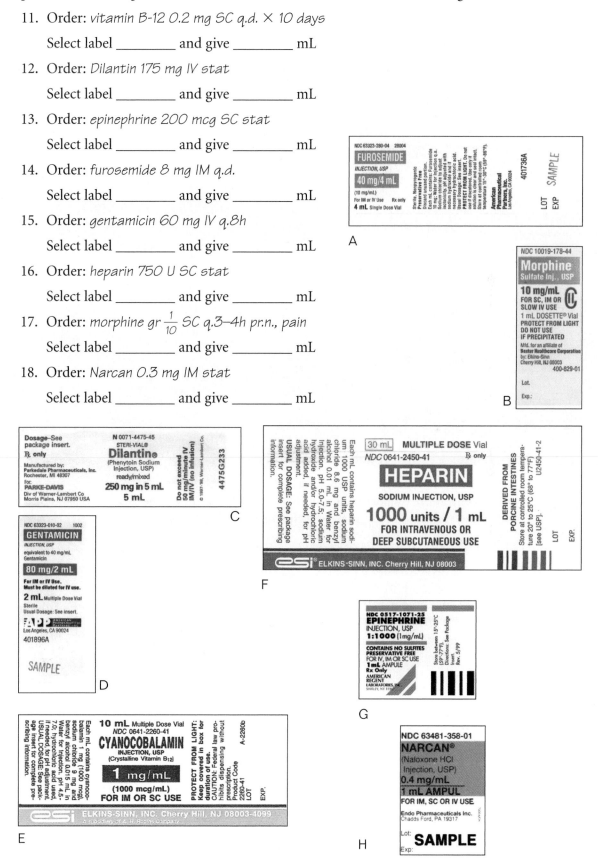

A

B

C

D

E

F

G

H

For questions 19 and 20, mark the amount to give on the correct syringe.

19. Order: *Humulin-N NPH U-100 insulin 48 U SC 30 min ā breakfast*

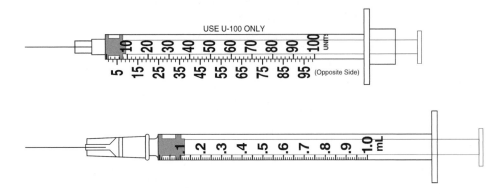

20. Order: *Novolin R Regular U-100 insulin 12 U c̄ Novolin N NPH U-100 insulin 28 U SC 30 min ā dinner*

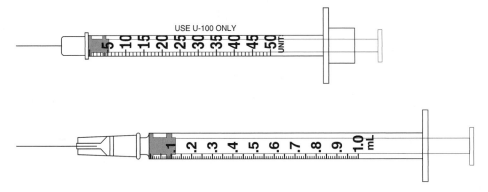

Chapter 11—Reconstitution of Solutions

For questions 21 through 26, specify the amount of diluent to add and the resulting solution concentration. Calculate the amount to give and indicate the dose with an arrow on the accompanying syringe. Finally, make a reconstitution label, if required.

21. Order: *Zithromax 500 mg IV q.d.*

Reconstitute with _____ mL diluent for a total solution volume of _____ mL with a concentration of _____ mg/mL.

Give: _____ mL

Store at or below 86°F (30°C).

DOSAGE AND USE
See accompanying prescribing information.
Constitute to 100 mg/mL* with
4.8 mL of Sterile Water For Injection.

Must be further diluted before use.
For appropriate diluents and storage
recommendations, refer to prescribing information.

*Each mL contains azithromycin dihydrate
equivalent to 100 mg of azithromycin,
76.9 mg of citric acid, and sodium hydroxide
for pH adjustment.
05-5191-32-0

CAUTION: Federal law prohibits
dispensing without prescription.

NDC 0069-3150-83

Zithromax®
(azithromycin for injection)

For **IV** infusion only
STERILE
equivalent to

500 mg

of azithromycin
Distributed by

Pfizer **Pfizer Labs**
Division of Pfizer Inc, NY, NY 10017

Lot No.
Exp. Date

22. Order: *vancomycin 500 mg IV q.6h*

    Package Insert Instructions: For IV use, dilute each 500 mg with 10 mL sterile water. Prior to administration, dilute further with 200 mL of dextrose or saline solution and infuse over 60 min. Aqueous solution is stable for 2 weeks.

    Reconstitute with _____ mL diluent for a total solution volume of _____ mL with a concentration of _____ g/_____ mL.

    Give: _____ mL

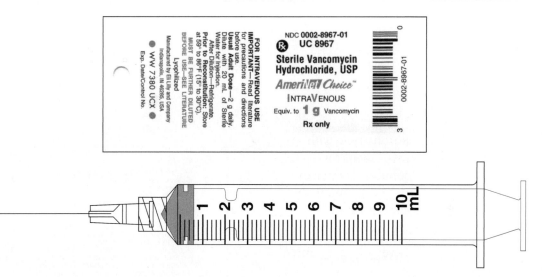

23. Order: *Tazidime 200 mg IM q.6h*

    Reconstitute with _____ mL diluent for a total solution volume of _____ mL with a concentration of _____ mg/mL.

    Give: _____ mL

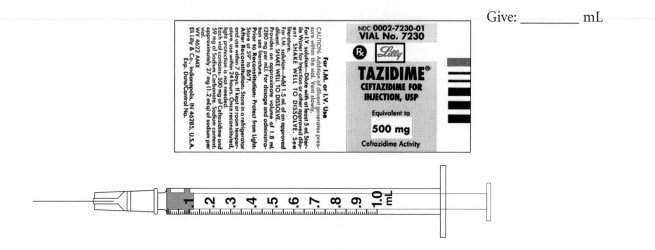

24. Order: *Kefzol 750 mg IM q.8h* (See label on next page.)

    Reconstitute with _____ mL diluent for a total solution volume of _____ mL with a concentration of _____ mg/mL.

    Give: _____ mL

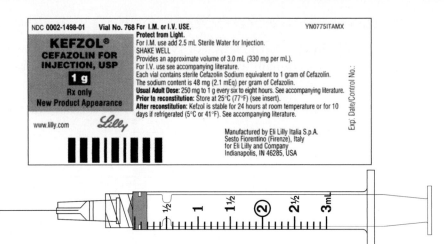

25. Order: *Solu-Medrol 250 mg IV q.6h*

    Reconstitute with _____
    mL diluent for a total
    solution volume of
    _____ mL with a
    concentration of _____
    mg/mL.

    Give: _____ mL

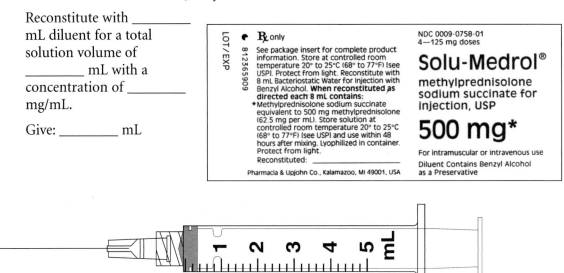

26. Order: *tobramycin 100 mg IV q.8h*

    Reconstitute with _____ mL diluent for a total solution volume of _____ mL with a concentration of _____ mg/mL.

    Give: _____ mL

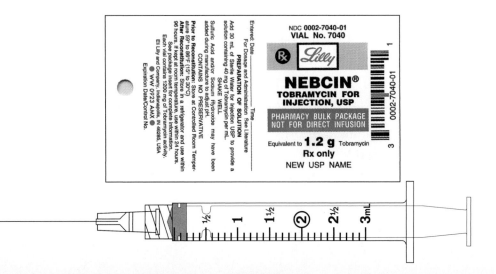

27. How many full doses are available of the medication supplied for question 26? _____ dose(s)

28. Will the medication supplied expire before it is used up for the order in question 26? _____ Explain: _____

Prepare the following therapeutic solutions.

29. 360 mL of $\frac{1}{3}$ strength hydrogen peroxide diluted with normal saline

    Supply: 60 mL stock hydrogen peroxide solution

    Add _____ mL solute and _____ mL solvent

30. 240 mL $\frac{3}{4}$ strength Ensure

    Supply: 8 ounce can of Ensure

    Add _____ mL Ensure and _____ mL water

Refer to the following order for questions 31 and 32.

Order: *Give $\frac{2}{3}$ strength Ensure 240 mL via NG tube q.3h.*

Supply: Ready-to-use Ensure 8 ounce can and sterile water.

31. How much sterile water would you add to the 8 ounce can of Ensure? _____ mL

32. How many feedings would this make? _____ feedings

Use the following information to answer questions 33 and 34.

You will prepare formula to feed 9 infants in the nursery. Each infant has an order for *4 ounces of $\frac{1}{2}$ strength Isomil formula q.3h.* You have 8 ounce cans of ready-to-use Isomil and sterile water.

33. How many cans of formula will you need to open to prepare the reconstituted formula for all 9 infants for one feeding each? _____ can(s)

34. How many mL of sterile water will you add to the Isomil to reconstitute the formula for one feeding for all 9 infants? _____ mL

Chapter 12—Using Ratio-Proportion to Calculate Dosages

Use ratio-proportion to calculate the dosages for questions 35 through 44. The following labels represent the drugs you have available.

35. Order: *meperidine 60 mg IM q.4h p.r.n., pain*

    Give: _____ mL

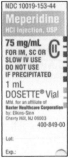

NDC 10019-153-44
Meperidine
HCl Injection, USP
75 mg/mL
FOR IM, SC OR
SLOW IV USE
DO NOT USE
IF PRECIPITATED
1 mL
DOSETTE® Vial
Mfd. for an affiliate of
Baxter Healthcare Corporation
by: Elkins-Sinn
Cherry Hill, NJ 08003
400-849-00
Lot:
Exp.:

36. Order: *methotrexate 175 mg IV stat*

    Give: _____ mL

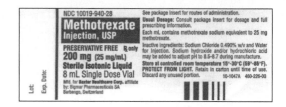

37. Order: *Phenergan 15 mg IM q.4–6h p.r.n., nausea*

    Give: _____ mL

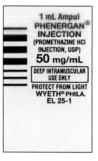

38. Order: *Nebcin 60 mg IV q.8h*

    Give: _____ mL

39. Order: *Thorazine 15 mg IM stat*

    Give: _____ mL

40. Order: *vancomycin 350 mg IV q.6h*

    Give: _____ mL

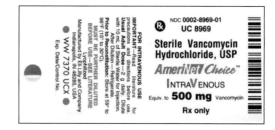

41. Order: *Nitrostat gr $\frac{1}{100}$ SL p.r.n., angina*

    Give: _____ tab

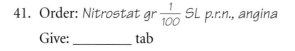

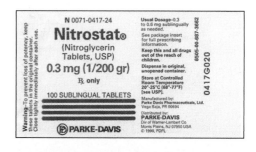

42. Order: *Procanbid 1 g p.o. b.i.d.*

    Give: _____ tab

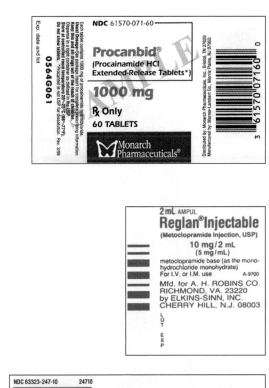

43. Order: *Reglan 15 mg IV q.3h × 3 doses*

    Give: _____ mL

44. Order: *levothyroxine 0.15 mg IV q.d.*

    Give: _____ mL

Chapter 13—Pediatric and Adult Dosages Based on Body Weight

Calculate and assess the safety of the following dosages. Mark safe dosages on the measuring device supplied.

45. Order: *morphine gr $\frac{1}{10}$ SC q.4h p.r.n. severe pain* for a child who weighs 67 lb. Recommended pediatric dosage: 100–200 mcg/kg q.4h, up to a maximum of 15 mg/dose.

    If the dosage ordered is safe, give _____ mL. If not safe, explain why not and describe what you should do. _____

    _____

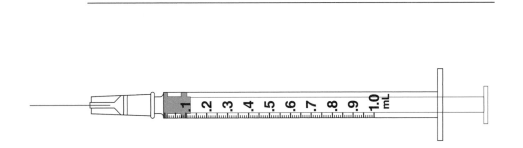

46. Order: *Amoxil pediatric drops 75 mg p.o. q.8h* for a 15 lb baby. Recommended dosage: See label.

    If the dosage ordered is safe, reconstitute with _____ mL diluent for a total solution volume of _____ mL and a concentration of _____ mg/mL and give _____ mL. If not safe, explain why not and describe what you should do. _____

    _____

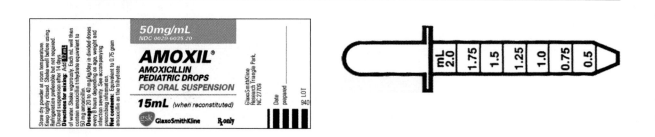

47. Order: *Dilantin 100 mg IV t.i.d.* for a child who weighs 20 kg. Recommended pediatric dosage: 5 mg/kg/day in 2–3 divided doses. If the dosage ordered is safe, give _____ mL. If not safe, explain why not and describe what you should do. _____

    _____

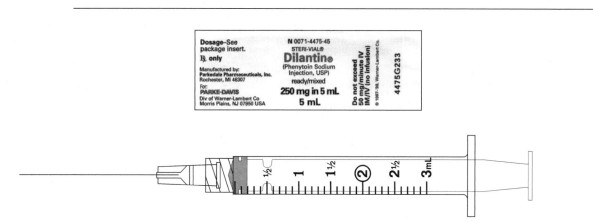

48. Order: *Ceclor 187 mg p.o. q.i.d.* for a child with otitis media who weighs 16 lb. Recommended dosage: See label.

    If the dosage ordered is safe, reconstitute with _____ mL diluent for a total solution volume of _____ mL and a concentration of _____ mg/mL. Give _____ mL. If not safe, explain why not and describe what you should do. _____

    _____

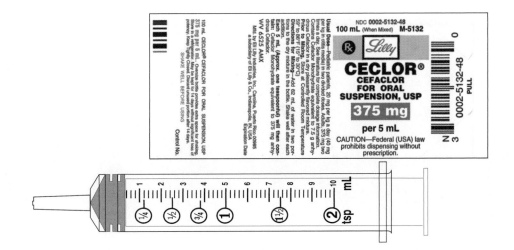

49. Order: *Kantrex 60 mg IM q.8h* for a child who weighs 16 lb. The recommended dosage of Kantrex for adults and children is 15 mg/kg/day in 2–3 divided doses, not to exceed 1.5 g/day.

    If the ordered dosage is safe, give _____ mL. If not safe, explain why not and describe what you should do. _____

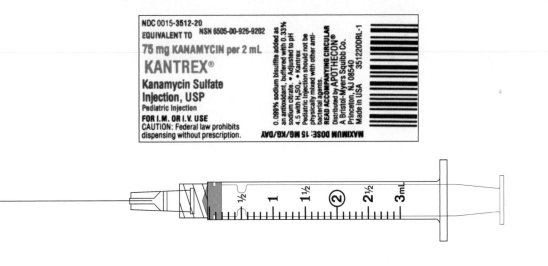

    _____

50. Refer to the recommended dosage of Kantrex in question 49. What would you expect the single q.8h dosage of Kantrex to be for an adult who weighs 275 lb?

    _____ mg/dose

After completing these problems, see pages 509–513 to check your answers. Give yourself two points for each correct answer.

Perfect score = 100   My score = _____

Minimum mastery score = 86 or higher (43 correct)

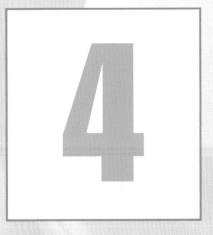

Advanced Calculations

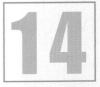
Intravenous Solutions, Equipment, and Calculations

OBJECTIVES

Upon mastery of Chapter 14, you will be able to calculate intravenous (IV) solution flow rate for electronic or manual infusion systems. To accomplish this you will also be able to:

- Identify common IV solutions and equipment.
- Calculate the amount of specific components in common IV fluids.
- Define the following terms: IV, peripheral line, central line, primary IV, secondary IV, saline/heparin locks, IV PB, and IV push.
- Calculate milliliters per hour: mL/h.
- Recognize the calibration or drop factor in gtt/mL as stated on the IV tubing package.
- Apply the formula method to calculate IV flow rate in gtt/min:

$$\frac{V \text{ (volume)}}{T \text{ (time in min)}} \times C \text{ (drop factor calibration)} = R \text{ (rate of flow)}$$

- Apply the shortcut method to calculate IV flow rate in gtt/min:

$$\frac{mL/h}{\text{drop factor constant}} = gtt/min$$

- Recalculate the flow rate when the IV is off schedule.
- Calculate small-volume piggyback IVs (IV PB).
- Calculate rate for IV push medications.
- Calculate IV infusion time.
- Calculate IV infusion volume.

Intravenous (IV) means the administration of fluids or medication through a vein. IV fluids are ordered for a variety of reasons. They may be ordered for replacement of lost fluids, to maintain fluid and electrolyte balance, or to administer IV medications. *Replacement fluids* are often ordered due to losses that may occur from hemorrhage, vomiting, or diarrhea. *Maintenance fluids* sustain normal fluid and electrolyte balance. They may be used for the patient who is not yet depleted but is beginning to show symptoms of depletion. They may also be ordered for the patient who has the potential to become depleted, such as the patient who is allowed nothing by mouth (NPO) for surgery.

IV fluids and drugs may be administered by two methods: *continuous* and *intermittent* infusion. Continuous IV infusions replace or maintain fluid and electrolytes and serve as a vehicle for drug administration. Intermittent, such as IV piggyback and IV push, infusions are used for IV administration of drugs and supplemental fluids. Intermittent peripheral infusion devices, also known as saline or heparin locks, are used to maintain venous access without continuous fluid infusion.

IV therapy is an important and challenging nursing role. This chapter covers the essential information and presents step-by-step calculations to help you gain a thorough understanding and mastery of this subject. Let's begin by analyzing IV solutions.

IV SOLUTIONS

IV solutions are ordered by a physician or prescribing practitioner; however, they are administered and monitored by the nurse. It is the responsibility of the nurse to ensure that the correct IV fluid is administered to the correct patient at the prescribed rate. IV fluids can be supplied in plastic solution bags or glass bottles with the volume of the IV fluid container typically varying from 50 mL to 1000 mL. Some IV bags may even contain more then 1000 mL. Solutions used for total parenteral nutrition usually contain 2000 mL or more in a single bag. The IV solution bag or bottle will be labeled with the exact components and amount of the IV solution. Health care practitioners often use abbreviations when communicating about the IV solution. Therefore, it is important for the nurse to know the common IV solution components and the solution concentration strengths represented by such abbreviations.

Solution Components

Glucose (dextrose), water, saline (sodium chloride or NaCl), and selected electrolytes and salts are found in IV fluids. Dextrose and sodium chloride are the two most common solute components. Learn these common IV component abbreviations.

REMEMBER

Common IV Component Abbreviations

Abbreviation	Solution Component
D	Dextrose
W	Water
S	Saline
NS	Normal Saline
NaCl	Sodium Chloride
RL	Ringer's Lactate
LR	Lactated Ringer's

Solution Strength

The abbreviation letters indicate the solution components, and the numbers indicate the solution strength or concentration of the components. The numbers may be written as subscripts in the medical order.

Example 1:

Suppose an order includes D_5W. This abbreviation means "Dextrose 5% in Water" and is supplied as 5% Dextrose Injection, Figure 14-1. This means that the solution strength of the solute (dextrose) is 5%. The solvent is water. Recall from Chapter 8 that parenteral solutions expressed in a percent indicate X g per 100 mL. Read the IV bag label and notice that "each 100 mL contains 5 g dextrose. . . ." For every 100 mL of solution, there are 5 g of dextrose.

Example 2:

Suppose a nurse writes D_5LR in the nurse's notes. This abbreviation means "Dextrose 5% in Lactated Ringer's" and is supplied as Lactated Ringer's and 5% Dextrose Injection, Figure 14-2.

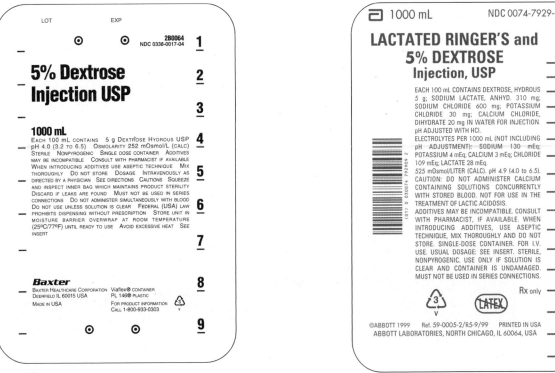

FIGURE 14-1 IV Solution Label: D₅W (Courtesy of Baxter Healthcare Corporation)

FIGURE 14-2 IV Solution Label: D₅LR (Courtesy of Abbott Laboratories, Inc.)

Example 3:

An order states, *D₅NS 1000 mL IV q.8h.* This order means "administer 1000 mL 5% dextrose in normal saline intravenously every 8 hours" and is supplied as 5% Dextrose and 0.9% Sodium Chloride, Figure 14-3. *Normal saline is the common term for 0.9% Sodium Chloride.* Another name is *physiologic saline.* The concentration of sodium chloride in normal saline is 0.9 g (or 900 mg) per 100 mL of solution.

Another common saline IV concentration is 0.45% Sodium Chloride (NaCl), Figure 14-4. Notice that 0.45% NaCl is $\frac{1}{2}$ the strength of 0.9% NaCl, which is normal saline. Thus, it is typically written as "$\frac{1}{2}$ NS" for $\frac{1}{2}$ normal saline. Other saline solution strengths include 0.33% NaCl (also abbreviated as $\frac{1}{3}$ NS) and 0.225% NaCl (also abbreviated as $\frac{1}{4}$ NS).

The goal of intravenous therapy, achieved through fluid infusion, is to maintain or regain fluid and electrolyte balance. When dextrose or saline (*solute*) is diluted in water for injection (*solvent*), the result is a *solution* that can be administered to maintain or approximate the normal blood plasma. Blood or serum concentration is called *tonicity* or *osmolarity* and is measured in milliOsmols per liter or mOsm/L. IV fluids are concentrated and classified as *isotonic* (the same tonicity or osmolarity as blood and other body serums), *hypotonic* (lower tonicity or osmolarity than blood and other body serums), or *hypertonic* (higher tonicity or osmolarity than blood and other body serums). Normal saline (0.9% NaCl or physiologic saline) is an isotonic solution. The osmolarity of a manufactured solution is detailed on the printed label. Look for the mOsm/L in the fine print under the solution name in Figures 14-1 through 14-4.

Figure 14-5 compares the three solution concentrations to normal serum osmolarity. Parenteral therapy is determined by unique patient needs, and these basic factors must be considered when ordering and infusing IV solutions.

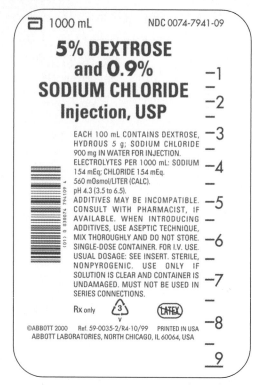

FIGURE 14-3 IV Solution Label: D₅NS (Courtesy of Abbott Laboratories, Inc.)

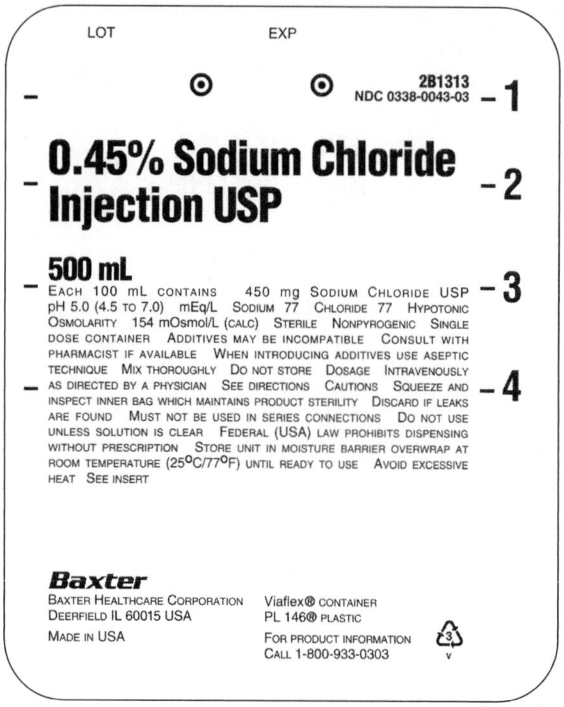

FIGURE 14-4 IV Solution Label: 0.45% NaCl (Courtesy of Baxter Healthcare Corporation)

Normal Serum Osmolarity
(Normal Average Tonicity—All Ages)
280–320 mOsm/L

Hypotonic (< 250 mOsm/L)	**Isotonic** (250–375 mOsm/L)	**Hypertonic** (> 375 mOsm/L)
Solvent exceeds solute—used to dilute excess serum electrolytes, as in hyperglycemia	*Solvent and solutes are balanced*—used to expand volume and maintain normal tonicity	*Solutes exceed solvent*—used to correct electrolyte imbalances, as in loss from excess vomiting and diarrhea
Example of IV solution: *0.45% Saline* (154 mOsm/L)	Examples of IV solution: *0.9% Saline* (308 mOsm/L) *Lactated Ringer's* (273 mOsm/L) *5% Dextrose in Water* (252 mOsm/L)	Example of IV solution: *5% Dextrose and 0.9% NaCl* (560 mOsm/L) *5% Dextrose and Lactated Ringer's* (525 mOsm/L)

FIGURE 14-5 Comparison of IV Solution Concentrations by Osmolarity

Solution Additives

Electrolytes also may be added to the basic IV fluid. Potassium chloride (KCl) is a common IV additive and is measured in *milliequivalents* (mEq). The order is usually written to indicate the amount of milliequivalents *per liter* (1000 mL) to be added to the IV fluid.

Example:

The physician orders $D_5NS \bar{c}$ *20 mEq KCl/L*. This means to add 20 milliequivalents potassium chloride per liter of 5% dextrose and 0.9% sodium chloride IV solution.

QUICK REVIEW

- Pay close attention to IV abbreviations: *letters* indicate the solution components and *numbers* indicate the concentration or solution strength.
- Dextrose and sodium chloride (NaCl) are common IV solutes.
- Solution strength expressed as a percent (%) indicates X g per 100 mL.
- Normal Saline is 0.9% sodium chloride: 0.9 g NaCl/100 mL solution.
- IV solution tonicity or osmolarity is measured in mOsm/L.
- D_5W and Normal Saline are common isotonic solutions.

REVIEW SET 33

For each of the following IV solutions labeled A through H:

a. Specify the *letter* of the illustration corresponding to the fluid abbreviation.

b. List the *solute(s)* of each solution, and identify the *strength (g/mL)* of each solute.

c. Identify the *osmolarity (mOsm/L)* of each solution.

d. Identify the *tonicity (isotonic, hypotonic, or hypertonic)* of each solution.

	a. Letter of Matching Illustration	b. Components and Strength	c. Osmolarity (mOsm/L)	d. Tonicity
1. NS	C	.99o	308	isotonic
2. D_5W	E	59o	252	
3. D_5NS	G			
4. $D_5\frac{1}{2}NS$	D			
5. $D_5\frac{1}{4}NS$	A			
6. D_5LR	H			
7. $D_5\frac{1}{2}NS \bar{c}$ 20 mEq KCl/L	B			
8. $\frac{1}{2}NS$	F			

After completing these problems, see page 513 to check your answers.

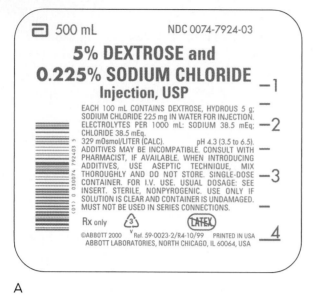

500 mL   NDC 0074-7924-03

5% DEXTROSE and 0.225% SODIUM CHLORIDE
Injection, USP

EACH 100 mL CONTAINS DEXTROSE, HYDROUS 5 g; SODIUM CHLORIDE 225 mg IN WATER FOR INJECTION. ELECTROLYTES PER 1000 mL: SODIUM 38.5 mEq; CHLORIDE 38.5 mEq.
329 mOsmol/LITER (CALC).   pH 4.3 (3.5 to 6.5). ADDITIVES MAY BE INCOMPATIBLE. CONSULT WITH PHARMACIST, IF AVAILABLE. WHEN INTRODUCING ADDITIVES, USE ASEPTIC TECHNIQUE, MIX THOROUGHLY AND DO NOT STORE. SINGLE-DOSE CONTAINER. FOR I.V. USE. USUAL DOSAGE: SEE INSERT. STERILE, NONPYROGENIC. USE ONLY IF SOLUTION IS CLEAR AND CONTAINER IS UNDAMAGED. MUST NOT BE USED IN SERIES CONNECTIONS.

Rx only   LATEX

©ABBOTT 2000   Ref. 59-0023-2/R4-10/99   PRINTED IN USA
ABBOTT LABORATORIES, NORTH CHICAGO, IL 60064, USA

—1
—2
—3
—4

A

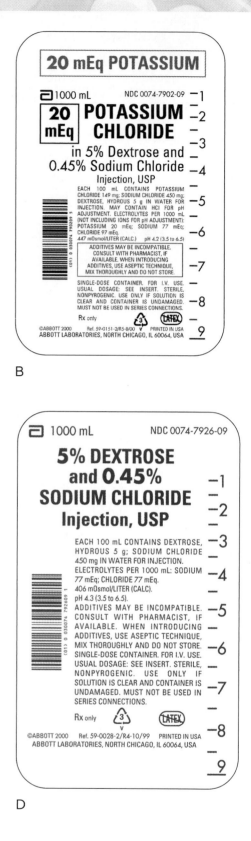

20 mEq POTASSIUM

1000 mL   NDC 0074-7902-09

20 mEq **POTASSIUM CHLORIDE**
in 5% Dextrose and 0.45% Sodium Chloride
Injection, USP

EACH 100 mL CONTAINS POTASSIUM CHLORIDE 149 mg; SODIUM CHLORIDE 450 mg; DEXTROSE, HYDROUS 5 g IN WATER FOR INJECTION. MAY CONTAIN HCl FOR pH ADJUSTMENT. ELECTROLYTES PER 1000 mL (NOT INCLUDING IONS FOR pH ADJUSTMENT): POTASSIUM 20 mEq; SODIUM 77 mEq; CHLORIDE 97 mEq.
447 mOsmol/LITER (CALC).   pH 4.2 (3.5 to 6.5)

ADDITIVES MAY BE INCOMPATIBLE. CONSULT WITH PHARMACIST, IF AVAILABLE. WHEN INTRODUCING ADDITIVES, USE ASEPTIC TECHNIQUE, MIX THOROUGHLY AND DO NOT STORE.

SINGLE-DOSE CONTAINER. FOR I.V. USE. USUAL DOSAGE: SEE INSERT. STERILE, NONPYROGENIC. USE ONLY IF SOLUTION IS CLEAR AND CONTAINER IS UNDAMAGED. MUST NOT BE USED IN SERIES CONNECTIONS.

Rx only   LATEX

©ABBOTT 2000   Ref. 59-0151-2/R5-8/00   PRINTED IN USA
ABBOTT LABORATORIES, NORTH CHICAGO, IL 60064, USA

—1
—2
—3
—4
—5
—6
—7
—8
—9

B

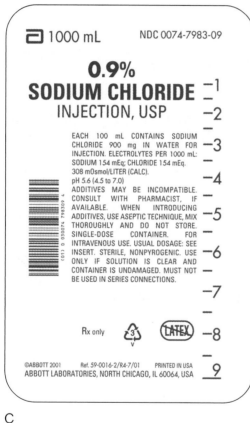

1000 mL   NDC 0074-7983-09

0.9% SODIUM CHLORIDE
INJECTION, USP

EACH 100 mL CONTAINS SODIUM CHLORIDE 900 mg IN WATER FOR INJECTION. ELECTROLYTES PER 1000 mL: SODIUM 154 mEq; CHLORIDE 154 mEq.
308 mOsmol/LITER (CALC).
pH 5.6 (4.5 to 7.0)
ADDITIVES MAY BE INCOMPATIBLE. CONSULT WITH PHARMACIST, IF AVAILABLE. WHEN INTRODUCING ADDITIVES, USE ASEPTIC TECHNIQUE, MIX THOROUGHLY AND DO NOT STORE. SINGLE-DOSE CONTAINER. FOR INTRAVENOUS USE. USUAL DOSAGE: SEE INSERT. STERILE, NONPYROGENIC. USE ONLY IF SOLUTION IS CLEAR AND CONTAINER IS UNDAMAGED. MUST NOT BE USED IN SERIES CONNECTIONS.

Rx only   LATEX

©ABBOTT 2001   Ref. 59-0016-2/R4-7/01   PRINTED IN USA
ABBOTT LABORATORIES, NORTH CHICAGO, IL 60064, USA

—1
—2
—3
—4
—5
—6
—7
—8
—9

C

1000 mL   NDC 0074-7926-09

5% DEXTROSE and 0.45% SODIUM CHLORIDE
Injection, USP

EACH 100 mL CONTAINS DEXTROSE, HYDROUS 5 g; SODIUM CHLORIDE 450 mg IN WATER FOR INJECTION. ELECTROLYTES PER 1000 mL: SODIUM 77 mEq; CHLORIDE 77 mEq.
406 mOsmol/LITER (CALC).
pH 4.3 (3.5 to 6.5).
ADDITIVES MAY BE INCOMPATIBLE. CONSULT WITH PHARMACIST, IF AVAILABLE. WHEN INTRODUCING ADDITIVES, USE ASEPTIC TECHNIQUE, MIX THOROUGHLY AND DO NOT STORE. SINGLE-DOSE CONTAINER. FOR I.V. USE. USUAL DOSAGE: SEE INSERT. STERILE, NONPYROGENIC. USE ONLY IF SOLUTION IS CLEAR AND CONTAINER IS UNDAMAGED. MUST NOT BE USED IN SERIES CONNECTIONS.

Rx only   LATEX

©ABBOTT 2000   Ref. 59-0028-2/R4-10/99   PRINTED IN USA
ABBOTT LABORATORIES, NORTH CHICAGO, IL 60064, USA

—1
—2
—3
—4
—5
—6
—7
—8
—9

D

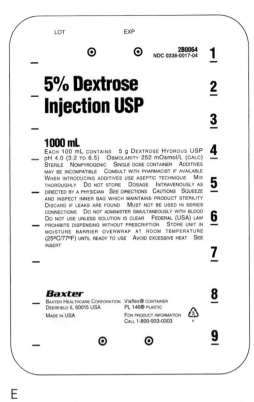

LOT   EXP

⊙   ⊙   2B0064
NDC 0338-0017-04   1

5% Dextrose
Injection USP   2

3

1000 mL   4
EACH 100 mL CONTAINS   5 g DEXTROSE HYDROUS USP
pH 4.0 (3.2 to 6.5) OSMOLARITY 252 mOsmol/L (CALC)
STERILE NONPYROGENIC SINGLE DOSE CONTAINER ADDITIVES
MAY BE INCOMPATIBLE CONSULT WITH PHARMACIST IF AVAILABLE
WHEN INTRODUCING ADDITIVES USE ASEPTIC TECHNIQUE   MIX   5
THOROUGHLY   DO NOT STORE   DOSAGE INTRAVENOUSLY AS
DIRECTED BY A PHYSICIAN SEE DIRECTIONS CAUTIONS SQUEEZE
AND INSPECT INNER BAG WHICH MAINTAINS PRODUCT STERILITY
DISCARD IF LEAKS ARE FOUND   MUST NOT BE USED IN SERIES   6
CONNECTIONS   DO NOT ADMINISTER SIMULTANEOUSLY WITH BLOOD
DO NOT USE UNLESS SOLUTION IS CLEAR   FEDERAL (USA) LAW
PROHIBITS DISPENSING WITHOUT PRESCRIPTION   STORE UNIT IN
MOISTURE BARRIER OVERWRAP AT ROOM TEMPERATURE   7
(25ºC/77ºF) UNTIL READY TO USE   AVOID EXCESSIVE HEAT SEE
INSERT

Baxter   8
BAXTER HEALTHCARE CORPORATION   VIAFLEX® CONTAINER
DEERFIELD IL 60015 USA   PL 146® PLASTIC
MADE IN USA   FOR PRODUCT INFORMATION
CALL 1-800-933-0303

⊙   9

E

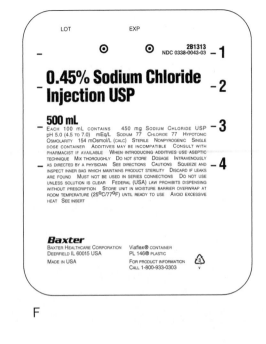

LOT   EXP

⊙   ⊙   2B1313
NDC 0338-0043-03   1

0.45% Sodium Chloride
Injection USP   2

500 mL   CONTAINS   450 mg SODIUM CHLORIDE USP   3
EACH 100 mL CONTAINS   450 mg SODIUM CHLORIDE USP
pH 5.0 (4.5 TO 7.0) mEq/L SODIUM 77 CHLORIDE 77 HYPOTONIC
OSMOLARITY   154 mOsmol/L (CALC) STERILE NONPYROGENIC SINGLE
DOSE CONTAINER ADDITIVES MAY BE INCOMPATIBLE CONSULT WITH
PHARMACIST IF AVAILABLE WHEN INTRODUCING ADDITIVES USE ASEPTIC
TECHNIQUE MIX THOROUGHLY DO NOT STORE DOSAGE INTRAVENOUSLY
AS DIRECTED BY A PHYSICIAN SEE DIRECTIONS CAUTIONS SQUEEZE AND   4
INSPECT INNER BAG WHICH MAINTAINS PRODUCT STERILITY DISCARD IF LEAKS
ARE FOUND   MUST NOT BE USED IN SERIES CONNECTIONS DO NOT USE
UNLESS SOLUTION IS CLEAR FEDERAL (USA) LAW PROHIBITS DISPENSING
WITHOUT PRESCRIPTION   STORE UNIT IN MOISTURE BARRIER OVERWRAP AT
ROOM TEMPERATURE (25ºC/77ºF) UNTIL READY TO USE AVOID EXCESSIVE
HEAT SEE INSERT

Baxter
BAXTER HEALTHCARE CORPORATION   VIAFLEX® CONTAINER
DEERFIELD IL 60015 USA   PL 146® PLASTIC
MADE IN USA   FOR PRODUCT INFORMATION
CALL 1-800-933-0303

F

ⓐ 1000 mL   NDC 0074-7941-09

5% DEXTROSE
and 0.9%   —1
SODIUM CHLORIDE   —2
Injection, USP

—3
EACH 100 mL CONTAINS DEXTROSE,
HYDROUS 5 g; SODIUM CHLORIDE
900 mg IN WATER FOR INJECTION.
ELECTROLYTES PER 1000 mL: SODIUM   —4
154 mEq; CHLORIDE 154 mEq.
560 mOsmol/LITER (CALC).
pH 4.3 (3.5 to 6.5).
ADDITIVES MAY BE INCOMPATIBLE.   —5
CONSULT WITH PHARMACIST, IF
AVAILABLE. WHEN INTRODUCING
ADDITIVES, USE ASEPTIC TECHNIQUE,
MIX THOROUGHLY AND DO NOT STORE.   —6
SINGLE-DOSE CONTAINER. FOR I.V. USE.
USUAL DOSAGE: SEE INSERT. STERILE,
NONPYROGENIC. USE ONLY IF
SOLUTION IS CLEAR AND CONTAINER IS   —7
UNDAMAGED. MUST NOT BE USED IN
SERIES CONNECTIONS.

Rx only △3 LATEX   —8

©ABBOTT 2000   Ref. 59-0035-2/R4-10/99   PRINTED IN USA
ABBOTT LABORATORIES, NORTH CHICAGO, IL 60064, USA

—9

G

ⓐ 500 mL   NDC 0074-7929-03

LACTATED RINGER'S and
5% DEXTROSE
Injection, USP   —1

EACH 100 mL CONTAINS DEXTROSE, HYDROUS 5 g; SODIUM
LACTATE, ANHYD. 310 mg; SODIUM CHLORIDE 600 mg;
POTASSIUM CHLORIDE 30 mg; CALCIUM CHLORIDE, DIHYDRATE
20 mg IN WATER FOR INJECTION. pH ADJUSTED WITH HCl.   —2
ELECTROLYTES PER 1000 mL (NOT INCLUDING pH ADJUSTMENT):
SODIUM 130 mEq; POTASSIUM 4 mEq; CALCIUM 3 mEq; CHLORIDE
109 mEq; LACTATE 28 mEq. 525 mOsmol/LITER (CALC). pH 4.9 (4.0
to 6.5). CAUTION: DO NOT ADMINISTER CALCIUM CONTAINING
SOLUTIONS CONCURRENTLY WITH STORED BLOOD. NOT FOR USE
IN THE TREATMENT OF LACTIC ACIDOSIS. ADDITIVES MAY BE
INCOMPATIBLE. CONSULT WITH PHARMACIST, IF AVAILABLE.   —3
WHEN INTRODUCING ADDITIVES, USE ASEPTIC TECHNIQUE, MIX
THOROUGHLY AND DO NOT STORE. SINGLE-DOSE CONTAINER.
FOR I.V. USE. USUAL DOSAGE: SEE INSERT. STERILE,
NONPYROGENIC. USE ONLY IF SOLUTION IS CLEAR AND
CONTAINER IS UNDAMAGED. MUST NOT BE USED IN SERIES
CONNECTIONS.

Rx only △3   LATEX   —4

©ABBOTT 1999 ᵛ Ref. 59-0001-2/R5-9/99   PRINTED IN USA
ABBOTT LABORATORIES, NORTH CHICAGO, IL 60064, USA

H

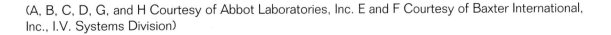

(A, B, C, D, G, and H Courtesy of Abbot Laboratories, Inc. E and F Courtesy of Baxter International, Inc., I.V. Systems Division)

CALCULATING COMPONENTS OF IV SOLUTIONS WHEN EXPRESSED AS A PERCENT

Recall from Chapter 8 that solution strength expressed as a percent (%) indicates X g per 100 mL. Understanding this concept allows you to calculate the total amount of solute per IV order.

Example 1:

Order: D_5W 1000 mL

Calculate the amount of dextrose in 1000 mL D_5W.

This can be calculated using ratio-proportion.

Recall that % indicates g per 100 mL; therefore, 5% dextrose is 5 g dextrose per 100 mL of solution.

$$\frac{5\text{ g}}{100\text{ mL}} \times \frac{X\text{ g}}{1000\text{ mL}}$$

100X = 5000

$$\frac{100X}{100} = \frac{5000}{100}$$

X = 50 g

1000 mL of D_5W contains 50 g of dextrose.

Example 2:

Order: $D_5\frac{1}{4}NS$ 500 mL

Calculate the amount of dextrose and sodium chloride in 500 mL.

D_5 = Dextrose 5% = 5 g dextrose per 100 mL

$$\frac{5\text{ g}}{100\text{ mL}} \times \frac{X\text{ g}}{500\text{ mL}}$$

100X = 2500

$$\frac{100X}{100} = \frac{2500}{100}$$

X = 25 g dextrose

$\frac{1}{4}$NS = 0.225% NaCl = 0.225 g NaCl per 100 mL

(Recall that NS or Normal Saline is 0.9% NaCl; therefore, $\frac{1}{4}$ NS is $\frac{1}{4} \times 0.9\%$ = 0.225% NaCl.)

$$\frac{0.225\text{ g}}{100\text{ mL}} \times \frac{X\text{ g}}{500\text{ mL}}$$

100X = 112.5

$$\frac{100X}{100} = \frac{112.5}{100}$$

X = 1.125 g NaCl

500 mL $D_5\frac{1}{4}$ NS contains 25 g dextrose and 1.125 g sodium chloride.

This concept is important because it helps you understand that IV solutions provide much more than fluid. They also provide other components. For example, now you know what you are administering to your patient when the IV order prescribes D_5W. Think, "I am hanging D_5W intravenous solution. Do I know what that this fluid contains? Yes, it contains dextrose as the solute and water as the solvent in the concentration of 5 g of dextrose in every 100 mL of solution." Regular monitoring and careful understanding of intravenous infusions cannot be stressed enough.

QUICK REVIEW

- Solution concentration expressed as a percent is X g of solute per 100 mL solution.

REVIEW SET 34

Calculate the amount of dextrose and/or sodium chloride in each of the following IV solutions.

1. 1000 mL of D_5NS $\frac{5}{100} \times \frac{9}{100}$

    dextrose _____ g

    sodium chloride _____ g

2. 500 mL of $D_5 \frac{1}{2}NS$

    dextrose _____ g

    sodium chloride _____ g

3. 250 mL of $D_{10}W$

    dextrose _____ g

4. 750 mL of NS

    sodium chloride _____ g

5. 500 mL of D_5 0.33% NaCl

    dextrose _____ g

    sodium chloride _____ g

6. 3 L of D_5NS

    dextrose _____ g

    sodium chloride _____ g

7. 0.5 L of $D_{10} \frac{1}{4}NS$

    dextrose _____ g

    sodium chloride _____ g

8. 300 mL of D_{12} 0.9% NaCl

    dextrose _____ g

    sodium chloride _____ g

9. 2 L of D_5 0.225% NaCl

    dextrose _____ g

    sodium chloride _____ g

10. 0.75 L of 0.45% NaCl

    sodium chloride _____ g

After completing these problems, see pages 513–514 to check your answers.

IV SITES

IV fluids may be ordered via a *peripheral line,* such as a vein in the arm, leg, or sometimes a scalp vein for infants, if other sites are inaccessible. Blood flowing through these veins can usually dilute the components in IV fluids. Glucose or dextrose is usually concentrated between 5 and 10% for short-term IV therapy. Peripheral veins can accommodate a maximum glucose concentration of 12%. The rate of infusion in peripheral veins should not exceed 200 mL in one hour.

IV fluids that are transparent flow smoothly into relatively small peripheral veins. When blood transfusion or replacement is needed, a larger vein is preferred to facilitate ease of blood flow. Whole blood or its components, especially packed cells, can be viscous and must be infused within a short period of time.

IV fluids may also be ordered via a *central line,* in which a special catheter is inserted to access a large vein in the chest. The subclavian vein, for example, may be used for a central line. Central lines may be accessed either directly through the chest wall or indirectly via a neck vein or peripheral vein in the arm. If a peripheral vein is used to access a central vein, you may see the term *peripherally inserted central catheter* or *PICC line.* Larger veins can accommodate higher concentrations of glucose (up to 35%) and other nutrients, and faster rates of IV fluids (> 200 mL in one hour). They are often utilized if the patient is expected to need IV therapy for an extended period of time.

MONITORING IVs

The nurse is responsible for monitoring the patient regularly during an IV infusion.

> **CAUTION**
>
> Generally the IV site and infusion should be checked *at least every 30 minutes to one hour* (according to hospital policy) for volume of remaining fluids, correct infusion rate, and signs of complications.

The major complications associated with IV therapy are phlebitis and infiltration. *Phlebitis* occurs when the vein becomes irritated, red, or painful. (Think: *warm and cordlike vein.*) *Infiltration* is when the IV catheter becomes dislodged from the vein and IV fluid escapes into the subcutaneous tissue. (Think: *cool and puffy skin.*) Should phlebitis or infiltration occur, the IV is discontinued and another IV site is chosen to restart the IV. The patient should be instructed to notify the nurse of any pain or swelling.

PRIMARY AND SECONDARY IVs

Primary IV tubing packaging and set are shown in Figures 14-6 and 14-7(a). This IV set is used to set up a typical or *primary IV*. Primary IV tubing includes a drip chamber, one or more injection ports, and a roller clamp, and is long enough to be attached to the hub of the IV catheter positioned in the patient's vein. The drip chamber is squeezed until it is half full of IV fluid, and IV fluid is run through the tubing prior to attaching it to the IV catheter to ensure that no air is in the tubing. The nurse can either regulate the rate manually using the roller clamp (Figure 14-7a) or place the tubing in an electronic infusion pump (Figures 14-12 through 14-15).

IV bags are often labeled with an infusion label (Figure 14-7b) that gives the nurse a visual check to monitor if the IV infusion is infusing on time as prescribed. These labels are attached to the IV bag and indicate the start and stop times of the infusion, as well as how the IV should be progressing, such as at 25 gtt/min. Each hour from the start time to the stop time the nurse should mark the label at the level where the solution should be.

Secondary IV tubing is used when giving medications. Secondary tubing is "piggybacked" into the primary line (Figure 14-8). This type of tubing generally is shorter and also contains a drip chamber and roller clamp. This gives access to the primary IV catheter without having to start another IV. You will notice that in this type of setup, the *secondary IV* set or *piggyback* is hung higher than the primary IV, to allow the secondary set of medication to infuse first. When administering primary IV fluids, choose primary IV tubing; when hanging piggybacks, select secondary IV tubing. IV piggybacks are discussed further at the end of this chapter.

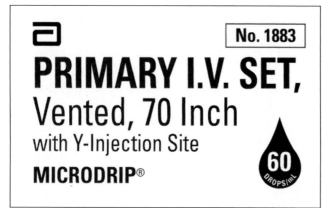

FIGURE 14-6 Primary Intravenous Infusion Set (Courtesy of Abbott Laboratories, Inc.)

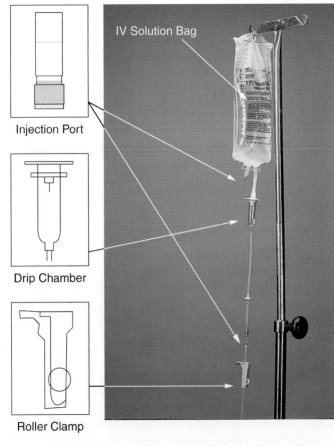

Injection Port

Drip Chamber

Roller Clamp

FIGURE 14-7 (a) Standard Straight Gravity Flow IV System

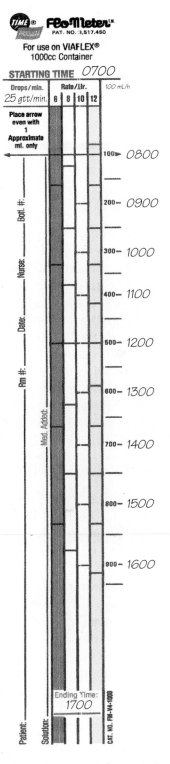

FIGURE 14-7 (b) Infusion Label

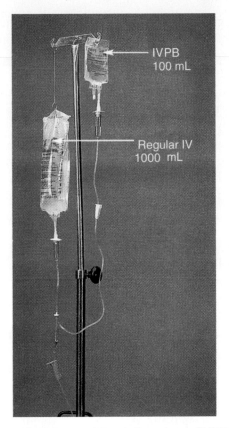

FIGURE 14-8 IV with Piggyback (IV PB)

BLOOD ADMINISTRATION TUBING

When blood is administered, a standard blood set (Figure 14-9) or a Y-type blood set (Figure 14-10) is commonly used. The "Y" refers to the two spikes that are attached above the drip chamber. One spike is attached to the blood container, and the other spike is attached to normal saline. Normal saline is used to dilute packed cells and to flush the IV tubing at the beginning and at the end of the transfusion. Blood is usually infused manually by gravity, and the roller clamp on the line is used to adjust the rate. Some electronic pumps may also be used for infusion of blood. In such cases, the nurse would program the pump in mL/h and then the pump would regulate the blood infusion. Blood infusion is calculated the same as any other IV fluid.

IV FLOW RATE

The *flow rate* of an IV infusion is ordered by the physician. It is the nurse's responsibility to regulate, monitor, and maintain this flow rate. Regulation of intravenous therapy is a critical skill in nursing. Because the fluids administered are infusing directly into the patient's circulatory system, careful monitoring is essential to be sure the patient does not receive too much or too little IV fluid and medication. It is also important for the nurse to accurately set and maintain the flow rate to administer the prescribed volume of the IV solution within the specified time period. The nurse records the IV fluids administered and IV flow rates on the IV administration record (IVAR) (Figure 14-11).

IV solutions are usually ordered for a certain volume to run for a stated period of time, such as *125 mL/h* or *1000 mL/8 h*. The nurse will use electronic or manual regulating equipment to monitor the flow rate. The calculations you must perform to set the flow rate will depend on the equipment used to administer the IV solutions.

ELECTRONICALLY REGULATED IVs

Frequently, IV solutions are regulated electronically by an infusion device, such as a controller or pump. The use of an electronic infusion device will be determined by the need to strictly regulate the IV. Manufacturers supply special volumetric tubing that must be used with their infusion devices. This special tubing ensures accurate, consistent IV infusions. Each device can be set for a specific flow rate and will set off an alarm if this rate is interrupted. Electronic units today are powered by direct (wall) current as well as an internal rechargeable battery. The battery takes over when the unit is unplugged, to allow for portability and patient ambulation.

Controllers (Figure 14-12) depend on gravity to maintain the desired flow rate by a compression/decompression mechanism that pinches the IV tubing, rather than forcing IV fluid into the system. They are often referred to as electronic flow clamps because they monitor the selected rate of infusion by either drop counting (drops per minute) or volumetric delivery (milliliters per hour).

Infusion pumps (Figure 14-13) do not rely on gravity but maintain the flow by displacing fluid at the prescribed rate. Resistance to flow within the system causes positive pressure in relation to the flow rate. The nurse or other user may preset a pressure alarm threshold. When the pressure sensed by the device reaches this threshold, the device stops pumping and sets off an alarm. The amount of change in pressure that results from infiltration or phlebitis may be insufficient to reach the alarm threshold. Therefore, users should not expect the device to stop infusing in the presence of these conditions.

A *syringe pump* (Figure 14-14) is a type of electronic infusion pump. It is used to infuse fluids or medications directly from a syringe. It is most often used in the neonatal and pediatric areas when small volumes of medication are delivered at very low rates. It is also used in anesthesia, labor and delivery, and in critical care when the drug cannot be mixed with other solutions or medications, or to reduce the volume of diluent fluid delivered to the patient. Syringe pumps can deliver in up to 16 different modes, including mL/h, volume/time, dose or body weight modes, mass modes such as U/h, and other specialty modes.

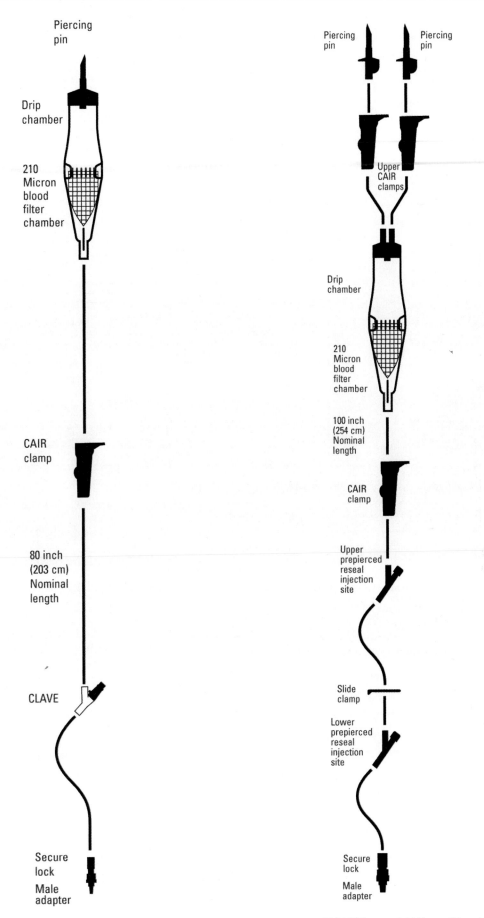

FIGURE 14-9 Standard Blood Set   **FIGURE 14-10** Y-Type Blood Set

Page: 1 of 1

DATE: 11/10/xx through

Correct	I.V. Order	Rate	Time	Initial	Site / Infusion Port	Pump / Other	Tubing Change
✓	D₅ ½ NS	100 ml/hr	0900	GP	LH / PIV	☐✓	✓

CIRCULATORY ACCESS SITE

Time	Gauge	Length	Type	Site	# Attempts	Dressing Change	Site Condition	IV Lock	Initial	Time D/C	Catheter Intact	Site Condition	Reason Code	Initial
0800	22	1½"	I	LH	1	✓	0	☐	GP					

Type:
I - Insyte
B - Butterfly
C - Cathlon
CVC - CVC
T - Tunnelled
IP - Implanted Port
PICC - PICC
A - Arterial Line
SG - Swan Ganz
DL - Dual Lumen Peripheral
UAC - UAC
UVC - UVC

Site:
L - Left
R - Right
H - Hand
FA - Forearm
UA - Upper Arm
SC - Subclavian
C - Chest
A - Antecubital
F - Femoral
J - Jugular
FT - Foot
S - Scalp
U - Umbilical
RA - Radial

Dressing Change:
T - Transparent
A - Air Occlusive
B - Bandaid
PR - Pressure Dressing

Reason Code:
1 - Infiltrate
2 - Physician Order
3 - Patient Removed
4 - Clotted
5 - Phlebitis
6 - Site Rotation
7 - Leaking
8 - Positional
9 - Not Patent
10 - Family Refused
Other:
D - Dial-a-flow

Infusion Port:
PIV - Peripheral IV
CVC - CVC
SG - Swan Ganz
D - Distal
M - Middle
P - Proximal
R - Red
BL - Blue
V - Venous
S - Sideport
AN - Access Needle
A - Arterial

Site Condition:
0
1+
2+
3+
4+
5+
Tubing Change:
P - Primary
S - Secondary
E - Extension
T - 3 Way Stopcock
H - Hemodynamic

ALLERGIES: NKA

Initial / Signature - Circulatory Access Site(s) checked hourly.

GP / G. Pickar, R.N. ___ / ___

___ / ___ ___ / ___

Reconciled by: ___

IV ADMINISTRATION RECORD

602-0203 (2-94)dlg)MPC#32258)

Smith, James 43y M

Dr. Jones Medical Service

Admitted 01-01-xx Rm 237-1

Adm. # 6634297

FIGURE 14-11 Intravenous Administration Record

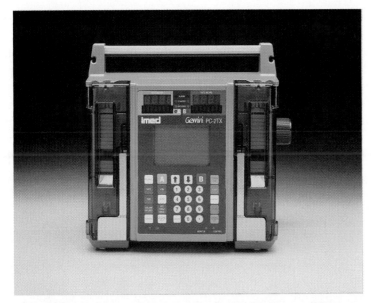

FIGURE 14-12 Volumetric Infusion Controller/Pump (Photo courtesy of Alaris Medical System)

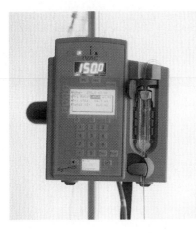

FIGURE 14-13 Infusion Pump (Photo courtesy of Alaris Medical System)

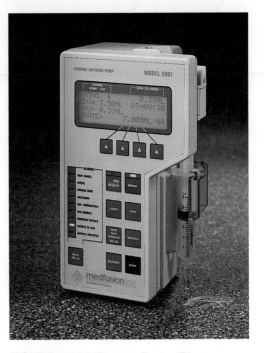

FIGURE 14-14 Syringe Pump (Photo courtesy of Medex, Inc.)

A *patient-controlled analgesia (PCA) pump* (Figure 14-15) is used to allow the patient to self-administer IV medication to control postoperative and other types of severe pain. The physician or other prescribing practitioner orders the pain medication, which is contained in a prefilled syringe locked securely in the IV pump. The patient presses the control button and receives the pain medication immediately rather than waiting for someone to bring it. The dose, frequency, and a safety "lock out" time are ordered and programmed into the pump, which delivers an individual therapeutic dose. The pump stores information about the frequency and dosage of the drug requested by and delivered to the patient. The nurse can display this information to document and evaluate pain management effectiveness. The nurse can also use such a pump to administer other IV push medications.

> **CAUTION**
>
> All electronic infusion devices must be monitored frequently (at least every 30 minutes to one hour) to ensure proper and safe functioning. Check the policy in your facility.

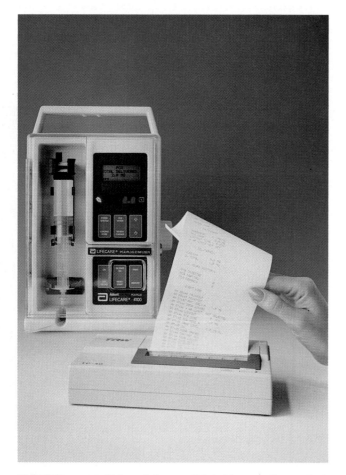

FIGURE 14-15 Abbott Lifecare PCA (Patient-Controlled Analgesia) Plus II Infusion System (Photo courtesy of Abbott Laboratories, Inc.)

CALCULATING FLOW RATES FOR ELECTRONIC REGULATORS IN mL/h

When an electronic infusion regulator is used, the IV volume is ordered by the physician and programmed into the device by the nurse. These devices are regulated in mL/h. Usually the physician orders the IV volume to be delivered in mL/h. If not, the nurse must calculate it.

> ### RULE
>
> To regulate an IV volume by electronic infusion pump or controller calibrated in mL/h, calculate:
>
> $\dfrac{\text{Total mL ordered}}{\text{Total h ordered}}$ = mL/h (rounded to a whole number)

Example:

Order reads: *D_5W 250 mL IV over the next 2 h by infusion pump*

Step 1 Think. The pump is set by the rate of mL per hour. So, if 250 mL is to be infused in two hours, how much will be infused in one hour? Yes, 125 mL will be infused in one hour. You would set the pump at 125 mL per hour.

Step 2 Use the formula:

$$\frac{\text{Total mL ordered}}{\text{Total h ordered}} = \text{mL/h}$$

$$\frac{250 \text{ mL}}{2 \text{ h}} = \frac{125 \text{ mL}}{1 \text{ h}}$$

Therefore, set the pump at 125 mL per hour (125 mL/h).

In most cases it is easy to calculate mL/h by dividing total mL by total h. However, an IV with medication added or a piggyback IV (IV PB) may be ordered to be administered in *less than one hour* by an electronic infusion device, but the pump or controller must still be set in mL/h.

> ### RULE
>
> $\dfrac{\text{Total mL ordered}}{\text{Total min ordered}}$ × 60 min/h = mL/h (rounded to a whole number)

Example:

Order: *Ampicillin 500 mg IV in 50 mL $D_5\frac{1}{2}NS$ in 30 min by controller*

Step 1 Think. The controller is set by the rate of mL per hour. If 50 mL is to be infused in 30 minutes, then 100 mL will be infused in 60 minutes, because 100 mL is twice as much as 50 mL and 60 minutes is twice as much as 30 minutes. Set the rate of the controller at 100 mL/h to infuse 50 mL/30 min.

Step 2 $\dfrac{\text{Total mL ordered}}{\text{Total min ordered}}$ × 60 min/h = mL/h

$$\frac{50 \text{ mL}}{\overset{}{\underset{1}{30 \text{ min}}}} \times \frac{\overset{2}{60 \text{ min}}}{1 \text{ h}} = 100 \text{ mL/h}$$

Or, you can use ratio-proportion.

$$\frac{50 \text{ mL}}{30 \text{ min}} \times \frac{X \text{ mL}}{60 \text{ min}}$$

$$30X = 3000$$

$$\frac{30X}{30} = \frac{3000}{30}$$

$$X = 100 \text{ mL/60 min or } 100 \text{ mL/h}$$

QUICK REVIEW

- $\frac{\text{Total mL ordered}}{\text{Total h ordered}} = \text{mL/h}$
- If the infusion time is less than one hour, then
  $\frac{\text{Total mL ordered}}{\text{Total min ordered}} \times 60 \text{ min/h} = \text{mL/h}$
- Round mL/h to a whole number.

REVIEW SET 35

Calculate the flow rate at which you will program the electronic infusion regulator for the following IV orders.

1. 1 L D_5W IV to infuse in 10 h by infusion pump

   Flow rate: _____ mL/h

2. 1800 mL Normal Saline IV to infuse in 15 h by controller

   Flow rate: _____ mL/h

3. 2000 mL D_5W IV in 24 h by controller

   Flow rate: _____ mL/h

4. 100 mL NS IV PB in 30 min by infusion pump

   Flow rate: _____ mL/h

5. 30 mL antibiotic in D_5W IV in 15 min by infusion pump

   Flow rate: _____ mL/h

6. 2.5 L NS IV in 20 h by controller

   Flow rate: _____ mL/h

7. 500 mL D_5LR IV in 4 h by controller

   Flow rate: _____ mL/h

8. 600 mL 0.45% NaCl IV in 3 h by infusion pump

   Flow rate: _____ mL/h

9. 150 mL antibiotic in D_5W IV in 2 h by infusion pump

   Flow rate: _____ mL/h

10. 3 L NS IV in 24 h by controller

    Flow rate: _____ mL/h

11. 1.5 L LR Injection IV in 24 h by infusion pump

    Flow rate: _____ mL/h

12. 240 mL D_{10}W IV in 10 h by controller

    Flow rate: _____ mL/h

13. 750 mL D_5W IV in 5 h by infusion pump

    Flow rate: _____ mL/h

14. 1.5 L D_5NS IV in 12 h by controller

    Flow rate: _____ mL/h

15. 380 mL D_5 0.45% NaCl in 9 h by infusion pump

    Flow rate: _____ mL/h

After completing these problems, see page 514 to check your answers.

MANUALLY REGULATED IVs

When an electronic infusion device is not used, the nurse manually regulates the IV rate. To do this, the nurse must calculate the ordered IV rate based on a certain *number of drops per minute (gtt/min)*. This actually represents the ordered milliliters per hour, as you will shortly see in the calculation.

The number of drops dripping per minute into the IV drip chamber (Figures 14-7a and 14-16) are counted and regulated by opening or closing the roller clamp. You actually place your watch at the level of the drip chamber and count the drops as they fall during a one-minute period (referred to as the *watch count*). This manual, gravity flow rate depends on the IV tubing calibration called the *drop factor*.

RULE

Drop factor = gtt/mL

The drop factor is the number of drops per milliliter (gtt/mL) a particular IV tubing set will deliver. It is stated on the IV tubing package (Figure 14-6) and varies according to the manufacturer of the IV equipment. Standard or *macrodrop* IV tubing sets have a drop factor of 10, 15, or 20 gtt/mL. All microdrip (or minidrip) IV tubing has a drop factor of 60 gtt/mL. Hospitals typically stock one macrodrop tubing for routine adult IV administration and the microdrip tubing for situations requiring more exact measurement.

Figure 14-16 compares macro- and microdrops. Figure 14-17 illustrates the size and number of drops in 1 mL for each drop factor. Notice that the fewer the number of drops per milliliter, the larger the actual drop size.

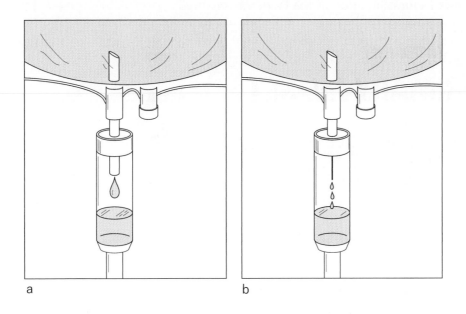

a   b

FIGURE 14-16 Intravenous Drip Chambers; Comparison of (a) Macrodrops and (b) Microdrops

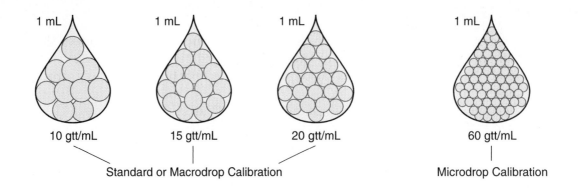

FIGURE 14-17 Comparison of Calibrated Drop Factors

REVIEW SET 36

Identify the drop factor calibration of the IV tubing pictured.

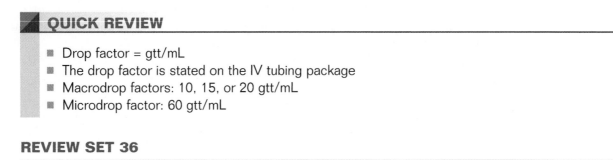

(Courtesy of Abbott Laboratories, Inc.)

1. _____ gtt/mL

(Courtesy of Abbott Laboratories, Inc.)

2. _____ gtt/mL

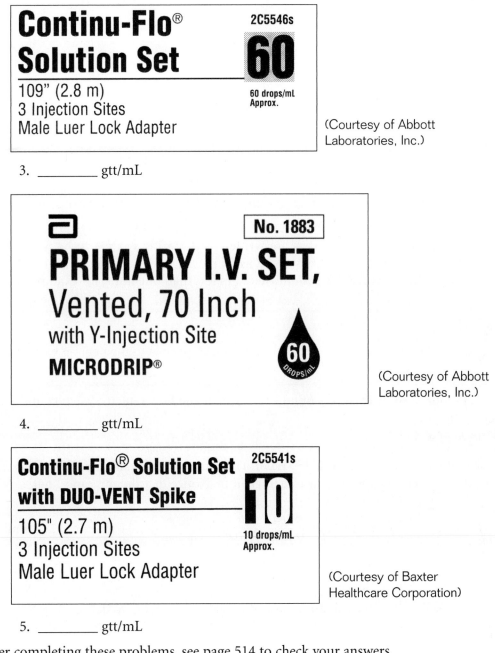

Continu-Flo® Solution Set

2C5546s

60

60 drops/mL
Approx.

109" (2.8 m)
3 Injection Sites
Male Luer Lock Adapter

(Courtesy of Abbott
Laboratories, Inc.)

3. _____ gtt/mL

No. 1883

PRIMARY I.V. SET,
Vented, 70 Inch
with Y-Injection Site
MICRODRIP®

60
DROPS/mL

(Courtesy of Abbott
Laboratories, Inc.)

4. _____ gtt/mL

Continu-Flo® Solution Set
with DUO-VENT Spike

2C5541s

10

10 drops/mL
Approx.

105" (2.7 m)
3 Injection Sites
Male Luer Lock Adapter

(Courtesy of Baxter
Healthcare Corporation)

5. _____ gtt/mL

After completing these problems, see page 514 to check your answers.

CALCULATING FLOW RATES FOR MANUALLY REGULATED IVs IN gtt/min

In this section you will learn two methods to calculate IV flow rate for manually regulated IVs: the formula method and the shortcut method.

Formula Method

The formula method can be used to determine the flow rate in drops per minute (*gtt/min*).

> ## RULE
>
> The formula method to calculate IV flow rate for manually regulated IVs ordered in mL/h or for a prescribed number of minutes is:
>
> $$\frac{V}{T} \times C = R$$
>
> $$\frac{\text{Volume (mL)}}{\text{Time (min)}} \times \text{Calibration or drop factor (gtt/mL)} = \text{Rate (gtt/min)}$$

In this formula:

> V = *volume* per hour to be infused in mL; ordered by the prescriber.
>
> C = *calibration* of tubing (drop factor) in gtt/mL.
>
> T = *time* converted to minutes; ordered by the prescriber or pharmacy .
>
> R = *rate* of flow in gtt/min. Think: The unknown is the "watch count."

IV fluid and medication orders are written as a specific volume to be infused in a certain time period. Most IV fluid orders are written as "X mL/h," which means X mL in 60 minutes. However, some IV medications are to be administered in less than one hour; for example, over 30 minutes.

> ## MATH TIP
>
> Carry calculations to one decimal place. Round gtt/min to the nearest whole number, because you can watch-count only whole drops.

Let's look at some examples of how to calculate the flow rate or "watch count" in gtt/min.

Example 1:

The physician orders D_5W IV @ 125 mL/h. The infusion set is calibrated for a drop factor of 10 gtt/mL. Calculate the IV flow rate in gtt/min. Notice that the mL cancel out, leaving *gtt/min*.

$$\frac{V}{T} \times C = \frac{125 \text{ mL}}{60 \text{ min}} \times 10 \text{ gtt/mL} = \frac{125 \text{ mL}}{\underset{6}{60} \text{ min}} \times \frac{\overset{1}{10} \text{ gtt}}{1 \text{ mL}} = \frac{125 \text{ gtt}}{6 \text{ min}} = 20.8 \text{ gtt/min} = 21 \text{ gtt/min}$$

Use your watch to count the drops and adjust the roller clamp to deliver 21 gtt/min.

Example 2:

Order: *Lactated Ringer's IV @ 150 mL/h.* The drop factor is 15 gtt/mL.

$$\frac{V}{T} \times C = \frac{150 \text{ mL}}{\underset{4}{60} \text{ min}} \times \overset{1}{15} \text{ gtt/mL} = \frac{150 \text{ gtt}}{4 \text{ min}} = 37.5 \text{ gtt/min} = 38 \text{ gtt/min}$$

Example 3:

Order: *Ampicillin 500 mg IV in 100 mL of NS, infuse over 45 min*

The drop factor is 20 gtt/mL. Notice that the time is less than one hour.

$$\frac{V}{T} \times C = \frac{100 \text{ mL}}{45 \text{ min}} \times 20 \text{ gtt/mL} = \frac{2000 \text{ gtt}}{45 \text{ min}} = 44.4 \text{ gtt/min} = 44 \text{ gtt/min}$$

> **MATH TIP**
>
> When the IV drop factor is 60 gtt/mL (microdrip sets), then the flow rate in gtt/min is the same as the volume ordered in mL/h.

Example 4:

Order: *D_5W NS IV @ 50 mL/h.* The drop factor is 60 gtt/mL. Notice that the order, 50 mL/h, is *the same as the flow rate* of 50 gtt/min when the drop factor is 60 gtt/mL.

$$\frac{V}{T} \times C = \frac{50 \cancel{mL}}{\cancel{60} \min} \times \cancel{60} \text{ gtt/}\cancel{mL} = 50 \text{ gtt/min}$$

Sometimes the prescriber will order a total IV volume to be infused over a total number of hours. In such cases, first calculate the mL/h, then calculate gtt/min.

RULE

The formula method to calculate IV flow rate for manually regulated IVs ordered in total volume and total hours is:

STEP 1 $\frac{\text{Total mL}}{\text{Total hours}} = \text{mL/h}$

STEP 2 $\frac{V}{T} \times C = R$

Example:

Order: *NS IV 3000 mL/24 h.* Drop factor is 15 gtt/min.

Step 1 $\frac{\text{Total mL}}{\text{Total h}} = \frac{3000 \text{ mL}}{24 \text{ h}} = 125 \text{ mL/h}$

Step 2 $\frac{V}{T} \times C = R$: $\frac{125 \text{ mL}}{60 \text{ min}} \times 15 \text{ gtt/mL} = \frac{125 \cancel{mL}}{\underset{4}{\cancel{60}} \min} \times \frac{\overset{1}{\cancel{15} \text{ gtt}}}{1 \cancel{mL}} = \frac{125 \text{ gtt}}{4 \text{ min}} = 31.2 \text{ gtt/min} = 31 \text{ gtt/min}$

QUICK REVIEW

- The formula method to calculate the flow rate, or watch count, in gtt/min for manually regulated IV rates ordered in mL/h or mL/minutes is:

  $\frac{\text{Volume (mL)}}{\text{Time (min)}} \times \text{Calibration or drop factor (gtt/mL)} = \text{Rate (gtt/min)}$

- When total volume and total hours are ordered, first calculate mL/h.
- When the drop factor calibration is 60 (microdrop sets), then the flow rate in gtt/min is the same as the ordered volume in mL/h.
- Round gtt/min to a whole number.

REVIEW SET 37

1. State the rule for the formula method to calculate IV flow rate in gtt/min when mL/h are known. _____

Calculate the flow rate or watch count in gtt/min.

2. Order: *3000 mL D5W IV @ 125 mL/h*

   Drop factor: 10 gtt/mL

   _____ gtt/min

3. Order: *250 mL LR IV @ 50 mL/h*

   Drop factor: 60 gtt/mL

   _____ gtt/min

4. Order: *100 mL NS bolus IV to infuse in 60 min*

   Drop factor: 20 gtt/mL

   _____ gtt/min

5. Order: $D_5 \frac{1}{2} NS$ *IV with 20 mEq KCl per liter to run at 25 mL/h*

   Drop factor: 60 gtt/mL

   _____ gtt/min

6. Order: *Two 500 mL units of whole blood IV to be infused in 4 h*

   Infusion set is calibrated to 20 drops per milliliter.

   _____ gtt/min

7. Hyperalimentation solution is ordered for 1240 mL to infuse in 12 h using an infusion set with tubing calibrated to 15 gtt/mL

   _____ gtt/min

8. Order: *D5NS IV @ 150 mL/h*

   Drop factor: 20 gtt/mL

   _____ gtt/min

9. Order: *150 mL NS bolus IV to infuse in 45 min*

   Drop factor: 15 gtt/mL

   _____ gtt/min

10. Order: *80 mL D5W antibiotic solution IV to infuse in 60 min*

    Drop factor: 60 gtt/mL

    _____ gtt/min

11. Order: *480 mL packed red blood cells IV to infuse in 4 h*

    Drop factor: 10 gtt/mL

    _____ gtt/min

12. Order: *D5W IV @ 120 mL/h*

    Drop factor: 15 gtt/mL

    _____ gtt/min

13. Order: *D5 0.33% NaCl IV @ 50 mL/h*

    Drop factor: 20 gtt/mL

    _____ gtt/min

14. Order: *2500 mL LR IV @ 165 mL/h*

    Drop factor: 20 gtt/mL

    _____ gtt/min

15. Order: *3500 mL D5LR IV to run at 160 mL/h*

    Drop factor: 15 gtt/mL

    _____ gtt/min

After completing these problems, see page 514 to check your answers.

Shortcut Method

By converting the volume and time in the formula method to mL/h (or mL/60 min), you can use a shortcut to calculate flow rate. This shortcut is derived from the drop factor (C), which cancels out each time and reduces the 60 minutes (T). You are left with the *drop factor constant*. Look at these examples.

Example 1:

Administer *Normal Saline 1000 mL IV at 125 mL/h* with a microdrop infusion set calibrated for *60 gtt/mL*. Use the formula $\frac{V}{T} \times C = R$.

$$\frac{V}{T} \times C = \frac{125 \ \cancel{mL}}{\underset{1}{\cancel{60} \ min}} \times \overset{1}{\cancel{60}} \ gtt/\cancel{mL} = \frac{125 \ gtt}{\textcircled{1} \ min} = 125 \ gtt/min$$

The drop factor constant for an infusion set with 60 gtt/mL is 1. Therefore, to administer 125 mL/h, set the flow rate at 125 gtt/min. Recall that when the drop factor is 60, then gtt/min = mL/h.

Example 2:

Administer *125 mL/h IV* with *20 gtt/mL* infusion set.

$$\frac{V}{T} \times C = \frac{125 \ \cancel{mL}}{\underset{3}{\cancel{60} \ min}} \times \overset{1}{\cancel{20}} \ gtt/\cancel{mL} = \frac{125 \ gtt}{\textcircled{3} \ min} = 41.6 \ gtt/min = 42 \ gtt/min$$

Drop factor constant = 3

Each drop factor constant is obtained by dividing 60 by the drop factor calibration from the infusion set.

REMEMBER

Drop Factor	Drop Factor Constant
10 gtt/mL	$\frac{60}{10} = 6$
15 gtt/mL	$\frac{60}{15} = 4$
20 gtt/mL	$\frac{60}{20} = 3$
60 gtt/mL	$\frac{60}{60} = 1$

Most hospitals consistently use infusion equipment manufactured by one company. Each manufacturer typically supplies one macrodrop and one microdrop system. You will become very familiar with the supplier used where you work; therefore, the shortcut method is very practical, quick, and simple to use.

RULE

The shortcut method to calculate IV flow rate is:

$$\frac{mL/h}{Drop \ factor \ constant} = gtt/min$$

Let's examine four examples using the shortcut method.

Example 1:

The IV order reads: *D_5W IV @ 125 mL/h*. The infusion set is calibrated for a drop factor of 10 gtt/mL. Drop factor constant: 6

$$\frac{mL/h}{Drop \ factor \ constant} = gtt/min$$

$$\frac{125 \ mL/h}{6} = 20.8 \ gtt/min = 21 \ gtt/min$$

Example 2:

Order reads *LR IV @ 150 mL/h.* The drop factor is 15 gtt/mL. Drop factor constant: 4

$$\frac{mL/h}{\text{Drop factor constant}} = gtt/min$$

$$\frac{150 \ mL/h}{4} = 37.5 \ gtt/min = 38 \ gtt/min$$

Example 3:

Order reads: *200 mL D$_5$$\frac{1}{2}$NS IV in 2 h*

Drop factor: 20 gtt/mL

Drop factor constant: 3

Step 1 $\dfrac{\text{Total mL}}{\text{Total h}} = mL/h$

$\dfrac{200}{2} = 100 \ mL/h$

Step 2 $\dfrac{mL/h}{\text{Drop factor constant}} = gtt/min$

$\dfrac{100 \ mL/h}{3} = 33.3 \ gtt/min = 33 \ gtt/min$

Example 4:

Order reads: *D$_5$W NS IV @ 50 mL/h.* The drop factor is 60 gtt/mL. Drop factor constant: 1

$$\frac{mL/h}{\text{Drop factor constant}} = gtt/min$$

$$\frac{50 \ mL/h}{1} = 50 \ gtt/min$$

Remember, when the drop factor is 60 (microdrop), set the flow rate at the same gtt/min as the mL/h.

CAUTION

For the shortcut method to work, the rate has to be written in mL/h. The shortcut method will not work if the time is less than one hour or is calculated in minutes, such as 15 or 75 minutes.

QUICK REVIEW

- The drop factor constant is 60 ÷ drop factor.

Drop Factor	Drop Factor Constant
10 gtt/mL	6
15 gtt/mL	4
20 gtt/mL	3
60 gtt/mL	1 → Set the flow rate at the same gtt/min as the mL/h.

- $\dfrac{mL/h}{\text{Drop factor constant}} = gtt/min$

REVIEW SET 38

1. The drop factor constant is derived by dividing _____ by the drop factor calibration.

Determine the drop factor constant for each of the following infusion sets.

2. 60 gtt/mL _____

3. 20 gtt/mL _____

4. 15 gtt/mL _____

5. 10 gtt/mL _____

6. State the rule for the shortcut method to calculate the IV flow rate in gtt/min. _____

_____

Calculate the IV flow rate in gtt/min using the shortcut method.

7. Order: _1000 mL D$_5$W IV to infuse @ 200 mL/h_

   Drop factor: 15 gtt/mL

   Flow rate: _____ gtt/min

8. Order: _750 mL D$_5$W to infuse @ 125 mL/h_

   Drop factor: 20 gtt/mL

   Flow rate: _____ gtt/min

9. Order: _500 mL D$_5$W 0.45% Saline IV to infuse @ 165 mL/h_

   Drop factor: 10 gtt/mL

   Flow rate: _____ gtt/min

10. Order: _2 L NS IV to infuse at 60 cc/h with microdrop infusion set of 60 gtt/mL_

    Flow rate: _____ gtt/min

11. Order: _400 cc D$_5$W IV to infuse @ 50 cc/h_

    Drop factor: 10 gtt/mL

    Flow rate: _____ gtt/min

12. Order: _3 L NS IV to infuse @ 125 mL/h_

    Drop factor: 15 gtt/mL

    Flow rate: _____ gtt/min

13. Order: _500 mL D$_5$LR to infuse in 6 h_

    Drop factor: 20 gtt/mL

    Flow rate: _____ gtt/min

14. Order: _0.5 L 0.45% NaCl IV to infuse in 20 h_

    Drop factor: 60 gtt/mL

    Flow rate: _____ gtt/min

15. Order: _650 mL D$_5$ 0.33% NaCl IV to infuse in 10 h_

    Drop factor: 10 gtt/mL

    Flow rate: _____ gtt/min

After completing these problems, see page 515 to check your answers.

SUMMARY

Calculating mL/h to program infusion devices and gtt/min to watch-count manually regulated IVs are two major IV calculations you need to know. Further, you have learned to calculate the supply dosage of certain IV solutes. These important topics warrant additional reinforcement and review.

QUICK REVIEW

- Solution strength expressed as a percent (%) indicates X g of solute per 100 mL of solution.
- When regulating IV flow rate for an electronic infusion device, calculate mL/h.
- When calculating IV flow rate to regulate an IV manually, calculate mL/h, find the drop factor, and calculate gtt/min by using the:

Formula Method: $\frac{V}{T} \times C = R$

or Shortcut Method: $\frac{mL/h}{\text{Drop factor constant}} = gtt/min$

- Carefully monitor patients receiving IV fluids at least hourly.
  - Check remaining IV fluids.
  - Check IV flow rate.
  - Observe IV site for complications.

REVIEW SET 39

Calculate the IV flow rate for these manually regulated IV administrations.

1. Order: *3000 mL 0.45% NaCl IV for 24 h*

   Drop factor: 15 gtt/mL

   Flow rate: _____ mL/h

   Flow rate: _____ gtt/min

2. Order: *200 mL D₅W IV to run @ 100 mL/h*

   Drop factor: Microdrop, 60 gtt/mL

   Flow rate: _____ gtt/min

3. Order: *800 cc D₅ ⅓ NS IV for 8 h*

   Drop factor: 20 gtt/mL

   Flow rate: _____ mL/h

   Flow rate: _____ gtt/min

4. Order: *1000 cc NS IV @ 50 cc/h*

   Drop factor: 60 gtt/mL

   Flow rate: _____ gtt/min

5. Order: *1500 mL D₅W IV for 12 h*

   Drop factor: 15 gtt/mL

   Flow rate: _____ mL/h

   Flow rate: _____ gtt/min

6. Order: *theophylline 0.5 g IV in 250 mL D₅W to run for 2 h by infusion pump*

   Drop factor: 60 gtt/mL

   Flow rate: _____ mL/h

   Flow rate: _____ gtt/min

7. Order: *2500 mL D₅ 0.45% NaCl IV @ 105 mL/h*

   Drop factor: 20 gtt/mL

   Flow rate: _____ gtt/min

8. Order: *500 mL D₅ 0.45% NaCl IV @ 100 mL/h*

   Drop factor: 10 gtt/mL

   Flow rate: _____ gtt/min

9. Order: *1200 mL NS IV @ 150 mL/h*

   Drop factor: 10 gtt/mL

   Flow rate: _____ gtt/min

Calculate the IV flow rate for these electronically regulated IV administrations.

10. Order: *1000 cc D₅ 0.45% NaCl to infuse over 8 h*

    Drop factor: On electronic infusion pump

    Flow rate: _____ mL/h

11. Order: *2000 cc D₅NS to infuse over 24 h*

    Drop factor: On electronic infusion controller

    Flow rate: _____ mL/h

12. Order: *500 cc LR to infuse over 4 h*

    Drop factor: On electronic infusion controller

    Flow rate: _____ mL/h

13. Order: *100 mL IV antibiotic to infuse in 30 min via electronic infusion pump*

    Flow rate: _____ mL/h

14. Order: *50 mL IV antibiotic to infuse in 20 min via electronic infusion pump*

    Flow rate: _____ mL/h

15. Order: *150 mL IV antibiotic to infuse in 45 min via electronic infusion pump*

    Flow rate: _____ mL/h

What is the total dosage of the solute(s) the patient will receive for each of the following orders?

16. *3000 mL $\frac{1}{2}$ NS IV*   NaCl: _____ g

17. *200 mL D₁₀ NS IV*   D: _____ g   NaCl: _____ g

18. *2500 mL NS IV*   NaCl: _____ g

19. *650 mL D₅ 0.33% NaCl IV*   D: _____ g   NaCl: _____ g

20. *1000 mL D₅ $\frac{1}{4}$ NS IV*   D: _____ g   NaCl: _____ g

After completing these problems, see pages 515–516 to check your answers.

ADJUSTING IV FLOW RATE

IV fluids, especially those with medicines added (called additives), are viewed as medications with specific dosages (rates of infusion, in this case). It is the responsibility of the nurse to maintain this rate of flow through careful calculations and close observation at regular intervals. Various circumstances, such as gravity, condition, and movement of the patient, can alter the set flow rate of an IV, causing the IV to run ahead of or behind schedule.

> **CAUTION**
>
> **It is not the discretion of the nurse to arbitrarily speed up or slow down the flow rate to catch up the IV.** This practice can result in serious conditions of over- or underhydration and electrolyte imbalance. Avoid off-schedule IV flow rates by regularly monitoring IVs at least every 30 minutes to one hour. Check your agency policy.

During your regular monitoring of the IV, if you find that the rate is not progressing as scheduled or is significantly ahead of or behind schedule, the physician may need to be notified as warranted by the patient's condition, hospital policy, or good nursing judgment. Some hospital policies allow the flow rate per minute to be adjusted a certain percentage of variation. A rule of thumb is that the flow rate per minute may be adjusted by *up to 25 percent more or less* than the original rate depending on the condition of the patient. In such cases, assess the patient. If the patient is stable, recalculate the flow rate to administer the total milliliters remaining over the number of hours remaining of the original order.

RULE

- Check for institutional policy regarding correcting off-schedule IV rates and the percentage of variation allowed. This variation should not exceed 25%.
- If adjustment is permitted, use the following formula to recalculate the mL/h and gtt/min for the time remaining and the percentage of variation.

Step 1 $\dfrac{\text{Remaining volume}}{\text{Remaining hours}}$ = Recalculated mL/h

Step 2 $\dfrac{V}{T} \times C$ = gtt/min

Step 3 $\dfrac{\text{Adjusted gtt/min} - \text{Ordered gtt/min}}{\text{Ordered gtt/min}}$ = % variation

The *% variation* will be positive (+) if the administration is slow and the rate has to be increased, and negative (–) if the administration is too fast and the rate has to be decreased.

Example 1:

The order reads *1000 mL D₅W @ 125 mL/h for 8 h.* The drop factor is 10 gtt/mL, and the IV is correctly set at 21 gtt/min. You would expect that after 4 hours, one-half of the total or 500 mL of the solution would be infused (125 mL/h × 4 h = 500 mL). However, when you check the IV bag the fourth hour after starting the IV, you find 600 milliliters remaining. The rate of flow is *behind schedule*, and the hospital allows a 25% IV flow variation with careful patient assessment and if the patient's condition is stable. The patient is stable, so you decide to compute a new flow rate for the remaining 600 milliliters to complete the IV fluid order in the remaining 4 hours.

Step 1 $\dfrac{\text{Remaining volume}}{\text{Remaining hours}}$ = Recalculated mL/h

$$\frac{600 \text{ mL}}{4\text{h}} = 150 \text{ mL/h}$$

Step 2 $\dfrac{V}{T} \times C = \dfrac{150 \text{ mL}}{\underset{6}{60 \text{ min}}} \times \overset{1}{10} \text{ gtt/mL} = \dfrac{150 \text{ gtt}}{6 \text{ min}} = 25 \text{ gtt/min}$ (Adjusted flow rate)

You could also use the shortcut method.

$$\frac{\text{mL/h}}{\text{Drop factor constant}} = \text{gtt/min}$$

$$\frac{150 \text{ mL/h}}{6} = 25 \text{ gtt/min}$$

Step 3 $\dfrac{\text{Adjusted gtt/min} - \text{Ordered gtt/min}}{\text{Ordered gtt/min}}$ = % of variation

$$\frac{25 - 21}{21} = \frac{4}{21} = 0.19 = 19\%;$$ within the acceptable 25% of variation depending on policy and patient's condition

Compare 25 gtt/min (in the last example) with the starting flow rate of 21 gtt/min. You can see that adjusting the total remaining volume over the total remaining hours changes the flow rate per minute very little. Most patients can tolerate this small amount of increase per minute over several hours. However, trying to catch up the lost 100 milliliters in one hour can be very dangerous. To infuse an extra 100 milliliters in one hour, with a drop factor of 10, you would need to speed up the IV to a much faster rate. Let's see what that rate would be.

$$\frac{V}{T} \times C = \frac{100 \text{ mL}}{\underset{6}{60 \text{ min}}} \times \overset{1}{10} \text{ gtt/mL} = \frac{100 \text{ gtt}}{6 \text{ min}} = 16.6 \text{ gtt/min} = 17 \text{ gtt/min more than the original rate}$$

To catch up the IV over the next hour, the flow rate would have to be 17 drops per minute faster than the original 21 drops per minute rate. The infusion would have to be set at 17 + 21 = 38 gtt/min for one hour and then slowed to the original rate. Such an increase would be $\frac{38 - 21}{21} = \frac{17}{21} = 81\%$ greater than the ordered rate. This could present a serious problem. **Do not do it! If permitted by hospital** policy, the flow rate for the remainder of the order must be recalculated when the IV is off sched-ule, and should never exceed a 25% adjustment.

Example 2:

The order reads: *500 mL LR to run over 10 h @ 50 mL/h.* The drop factor is 60 gtt/mL and the IV is correctly infusing at 50 gtt/min. After $2\frac{1}{2}$ hours, you find 300 mL remaining. Almost half of the total volume has already infused in about one-quarter the time. This IV infusion is *ahead of schedule.* You would compute a new flow rate of 300 mL to complete the IV fluid order in the remaining $7\frac{1}{2}$. hours. The patient would require close assessment for fluid overload.

Step 1 $\dfrac{\text{Remaining volume}}{\text{Remaining hours}} = \text{Recalculated mL/h}$

$\dfrac{300 \text{ mL}}{7.5 \text{ h}} = 40 \text{ mL/h}$

Step 2 $\dfrac{\text{V}}{\text{T}} \times \text{C} = \dfrac{40 \text{ mL}}{60 \text{ min}} \times \overset{1}{60} \text{ gtt/mL} = 40 \text{ gtt/min (Adjusted flow rate)}$

Or, you know when drop factor is 60, then mL/h = gtt/min.

Step 3 $\dfrac{\text{Adjusted gtt/min} - \text{Ordered gtt/min}}{\text{Ordered gtt/min}} = \% \text{ of variation}$

$\dfrac{40 - 50}{50} = \dfrac{-10}{50} = -0.2 = -20\% \text{ within the acceptable 25\% of variation}$

Remember, the negative percent of variation (−20%) indicates that the adjusted flow rate will be decreased.

A good rule of thumb is that the recalculated flow rate should not vary from the original rate by more than 25 percent. If the recalculated rate does vary from the original by more than 25 percent, contact your supervisor or the doctor for further instructions. The original order may have to be revised. Regular monitoring helps to prevent or minimize this problem.

Patients who require close monitoring for IV fluids will most likely have the IV regulated by an electronic infusion device. Because of the nature of their condition, "catching up" these IVs, if off schedule, is not recommended. If an IV regulated by an infusion pump or controller is off schedule or inaccurate, suspect that the infusion pump may need recalibration. Consult with your supervisor, as appropriate.

QUICK REVIEW

- Regular IV monitoring and patient assessment at least every 30 minutes to one hour is important to maintain prescribed IV flow rate.
- Do not arbitrarily speed up or slow down IV flow rates that are off schedule.
- Check hospital policy regarding adjustment of off-schedule IV flow rates and the percentage of variation allowed. If permitted, a rule of thumb is a maximum 25% variation for patients in stable condition.
- To recalculate off-schedule IV flow rate:

   Step 1 $\dfrac{\text{Remaining volume}}{\text{Remaining hours}} = \text{Recalculated mL/h}$

   Step 2 $\dfrac{\text{V}}{\text{T}} \times \text{C} = \text{gtt/min}$

   Step 3 $\dfrac{\text{Adjusted gtt/min} - \text{Ordered gtt/min}}{\text{Ordered gtt/min}} = \% \text{ variation}$

- Contact the prescribing health care professional for a new IV fluid order if the recalculated IV flow rate variation exceeds the allowed variation or if the patient's condition is unstable.

REVIEW SET 40

Compute the flow rate in drops per minute. Hospital policy permits recalculation of IVs when off schedule, with a maximum variation in rate of 25% for stable patients. Compute the % of variation.

1. Order: *1500 mL Lactated Ringer's IV for 12 h @ 125 mL/h*

   Drop factor: 20 gtt/mL

   Original flow rate: _____ gtt/min

   After 6 hours, there are 850 mL remaining; describe your action now.

   Time remaining: _____ h

   Recalculated flow rate: _____ mL/h

   Recalculated flow rate: _____ gtt/min

   Variation: _____ %

   Action: _____

2. Order: *1000 mL Lactated Ringer's IV for 6 h @ 167 mL/h*

   Drop factor: 15 gtt/mL

   Original flow rate: _____ gtt/min

   After 4 hours, there are 360 mL remaining; describe your action now.

   Time remaining: _____ h

   Recalculated flow rate: _____ mL/h

   Recalculated flow rate: _____ gtt/min

   Variation: _____ %

   Action: _____

3. Order: *1000 mL D$_5$W IV for 8 h @ 125 mL/h*

   Drop factor: 20 gtt/mL

   Original flow rate: _____ gtt/min

   After 4 hours, there are 800 mL remaining; describe your action now.

   Time remaining: _____ h

   Recalculated flow rate: _____ mL/h

   Recalculated flow rate: _____ gtt/min

   Variation: _____ %

   Action: _____

4. Order: *2000 mL NS IV for 12 h @ 167 mL/h*

   Drop factor: 10 gtt/mL

   Original flow rate: _____ gtt/min

   After 8 hours, there are 750 mL remaining; describe your action now.

   Time remaining: _____ h

   Recalculated flow rate: _____ mL/h

   Recalculated flow rate: _____ gtt/min

   Variation: _____ %

   Action: _____

5. Order: *1000 mL NS IV for 8 h @ 125 mL/h*

   Drop factor: 10 gtt/mL

   Original flow rate: _____ gtt/min

   After 4 hours, there are 750 mL remaining; describe your action now.

   Time remaining: _____ h

   Recalculated flow rate: _____ mL/h

   Recalculated flow rate: _____ gtt/min

   Variation: _____ %

   Action: _____

6. Order: *2000 mL NS IV for 16 h @ 125 mL/h*

   Drop factor: 15 gtt/mL

   Original flow rate: _____ gtt/min

   After 6 hours, 650 mL of fluid have infused; describe your action now.

   Solution remaining: _____ mL   Time remaining: _____ h

   Recalculated flow rate: _____ mL/h

   Recalculated flow rate: _____ gtt/min

   Variation: _____ %

   Action: _____

7. Order: *900 mL NS IV for 6 h @ 150 mL/h*

   Drop factor: 20 gtt/mL

   Original flow rate: _____ gtt/min

   After 3 hours, there are 700 mL remaining; describe your action now.

   Time remaining: _____ h

   Recalculated flow rate: _____ mL/h

   Recalculated flow rate: _____ gtt/min

   Variation: _____ %

   Action: _____

8. Order: *500 mL D₅NS IV for 5 h @ 100 mL/h*

   Drop factor: 20 gtt/mL

   Original flow rate: _____ gtt/min

   After 2 hours, there are 250 mL remaining; describe your action now.

   Time remaining: _____ h

   Recalculated flow rate: _____ mL/h

   Recalculated flow rate: _____ gtt/min

   Variation: _____ %

   Action: _____

9. Order: *1 L NS IV for 20 h @ 50 mL/h*

   Drop factor: 15 gtt/mL

   Original flow rate: _____ gtt/min

   After 10 hours, there are 600 mL remaining; describe your action now.

   Time remaining: _____ h

   Recalculated flow rate: _____ mL/h

   Recalculated flow rate: _____ gtt/min

   Variation: _____ %

   Action: _____

10. Order: *1000 mL D₅W IV for 10 h @ 100 mL/h*

    Drop factor: 60 gtt/mL

    Original flow rate: _____ gtt/min

    After 5 hours, there are 500 mL remaining; describe your action now.

    Time remaining: _____ h

    Recalculated flow rate: _____ mL/h

    Recalculated flow rate: _____ gtt/min

    Variation: _____ %

    Action: _____

After completing these problems, see pages 516–517 to check your answers.

INTERMITTENT IV INFUSIONS

Sometimes the patient needs to receive supplemental fluid therapy and/or IV medications but does not need continuous replacement or maintenance IV fluids. Several intermittent IV infusion systems are available to administer IV drugs. These include IV piggyback, IV locks for IV push drugs, the ADD-Vantage system, and volume control sets (such as Buretrol). Volume control sets are discussed in Chapter 15.

IV Piggybacks

A medication may be ordered to be dissolved in a small amount of IV fluid (usually 50 to 100 mL) and run "piggyback" to the regular IV fluids (Figure 14-8). Recall that the piggyback IV (or secondary IV) requires a secondary IV set.

The IV piggyback (IV PB) medication may come premixed by the manufacturer or pharmacy, or the nurse may need to properly prepare it. Whichever the case, it is always the responsibility of the nurse to accurately and safely administer the medication. The infusion time may be less than 60 minutes, so it is important to carefully read the order and recommended infusion time.

Sometimes the physician's order for the IV PB medication will not include an infusion time or rate. It is understood, when this is the case, that the nurse will follow the manufacturer's guidelines for infusion rates, keeping in mind the amount of fluid accompanying the medication and any standing orders that limit fluid amounts or rates. Appropriate infusion times are readily available in many drug reference books. Reference books are usually available on most nursing units, or you can consult with a hospital pharmacist.

Example 1:

Order: *Kefzol 0.5 g in 100 mL D$_5$W IV PB to run over 30 min*

Drop factor: 20 gtt/mL

What is the flow rate in gtt/min?

$$\frac{V}{T} \times C = \frac{100 \text{ mL}}{\overset{30 \text{ min}}{3}} \times \overset{2}{20} \text{ gtt/mL} = \frac{200 \text{ gtt}}{3 \text{ min}} = 66.6 \text{ gtt/min} = 67 \text{ gtt/min}$$

Example 2:

If an infusion pump or controller is used to administer the same order as in Example 1, remember that you would need to program the device in *mL/h*.

Step 1	**Think**	If 100 mL will be administered in 30 minutes or one-half hour, then 200 mL will be administered in 60 minutes or one hour.
Step 2	**Calculate**	Use ratio-proportion to calculate mL/h.

$$\frac{100 \text{ mL}}{30 \text{ min}} \bowtie \frac{X \text{ mL}}{60 \text{ min}} \quad (1 \text{ h} = 60 \text{ min})$$

$$30X = 6000$$

$$\frac{30X}{30} = \frac{6000}{30}$$

$$X = 200 \text{ mL/h}$$

Set the electronic IV PB regulator to 200 mL/h

Saline and Heparin IV Locks for IV Push Drugs

IV locks can be attached to the hub of the IV catheter that is positioned in the vein. The lock may be referred to as a *saline lock*, meaning that saline is used to flush or maintain the IV catheter patency, or a *heparin lock* if heparin is used to maintain the IV catheter patency. Sometimes a more general term, such as *intermittent peripheral infusion device*, may be used. Medications can be given *IV push*, meaning that a syringe is attached to the lock and medication is pushed in. An *IV bolus*, usually a quantity of IV fluid, can be run in over a specified period of time through an IV setup that is attached to the lock. Using either a saline or heparin lock allows for intermittent medication and fluid infusion. Heparin and saline locks are also being used for outpatient and home care medication therapy. Refer to the policy at your hospital or health care agency regarding the frequency, volume, and concentration of saline or heparin to be used to maintain the IV lock.

> **CAUTION**
>
> Heparin lock flush solution is usually concentrated to 10 units/mL or 100 units/mL. Much higher concentrations of heparin are given IV or SC, so carefully check the concentration.

Dosage calculations for IV push injections are the same as calculations for intramuscular (IM) injections. The IV push route of administration is often preferred when immediate onset of action is desired for persons with small or wasted muscle mass, poor circulation, or for drugs that have limited absorption from body tissues.

Drug literature and institutional guidelines recommend an acceptable rate (per minute or per incremental amount of time) for IV push drug administration. Most timed IV push administration recommendations are for 1–5 minutes or more. For smooth manual administration of IV push drugs, calculate the incremental volume to administer over 15-second intervals. You should time the administration with a digital or sweep second-hand watch or clock.

> **CAUTION**
>
> IV drugs are potent and rapid acting. Never infuse IV push drugs more rapidly than recommended by agency policy or pharmacology literature. Some drugs require further dilution after reconstitution for IV push administration. Carefully read package inserts and reputable drug resources for minimum dilution and minimum time for IV administration.

Example 1:

Order: *Ativan 3 mg IV Push 20 min preoperatively*

Supply: Ativan 4 mg/mL with drug literature guidelines of "IV infusion not to exceed 2 mg/min"

How much Ativan should you prepare?

Step 1 Convert   No conversion is necessary.

Step 2 Think   You want to give less than 1 mL.

Step 3 Calculate $\dfrac{D}{H} \times Q = \dfrac{3\ \text{mg}}{4\ \text{mg}} \times 1\,\text{mL} = 0.75\ \text{mL}$

What is a safe infusion time?

Use $\dfrac{D}{H} \times Q$ to calculate the time required to administer the drug as ordered. In this problem "Q" represents the quantity (or amount) of time for the supply rate: 1 min.

$$\frac{D}{H} \times Q = \frac{3\ \text{mg}}{2\ \text{mg}} \times 1\,\text{min} = \frac{3}{2}\ \text{min} = 1\frac{1}{2}\ \text{min}$$

Or use ratio-proportion to calculate the time required to administer the drug as ordered.

$$\frac{2\ \text{mg}}{1\ \text{min}} \diagdown\!\!\!\!\diagup \frac{3\ \text{mg}}{X\ \text{min}}$$

$$2X = 3$$

$$\frac{2X}{2} = \frac{3}{2}$$

$$X = 1\frac{1}{2}\ \text{min}$$

Administer 0.75 mL over $1\frac{1}{2}$ min.

How much should you infuse every 15 seconds?

Convert: 1 min = 60 sec; $1\frac{1}{2}$ min = $1\frac{1}{2} \times 60$ = 90 sec

$$\frac{0.75 \text{ mL}}{90 \text{ sec}} \times \frac{\text{X mL}}{15 \text{ sec}}$$

$90X = 11.25$

$$\frac{90X}{90} = \frac{11.25}{90}$$

X = 0.125 mL = 0.13 mL of Ativan 4 mg/mL infused IV push every 15 seconds will deliver 3 mg of Ativan.

This is a small amount. Use a 1 mL syringe to prepare 0.75 mL and slowly administer 0.13 mL every 15 seconds.

Example 2:

Order: *Cefizox 1500 mg IV push q.8h*

Supply: Cefizox 2 g powder with directions, "For direct IV administration, reconstitute each 1 g in 10 mL sterile water and give slowly over 3–5 minutes."

How much Cefizox should you prepare?

Step 1   Convert   2 g = 2 × 1000 = 2000 mg

Step 2   Think   If 1 g (or 1000 mg) requires 10 mL for dilution, then 2 g (or 2000 mg) requires 2 × 10 = 20 mL for dilution. Therefore, to administer 1500 mg, you will prepare more than 10 mL and less than 20 mL.

Step 3   Calculate $\dfrac{D}{H} \times Q = \dfrac{\overset{3}{\cancel{1500} \text{ mg}}}{\underset{1}{\cancel{2000} \text{ mg}}} \times \overset{5}{\cancel{20}} \text{ mL} = 15 \text{ mL}$

What is a safe infusion time?

This amount is larger than the Ativan dosage from Example 1, so you should use the longer infusion time recommendation (1 g per 5 min). Remember *Q* is the quantity of time to infuse the dosage you have on hand.

$$\frac{D}{H} \times Q = \frac{\overset{3}{\cancel{1500} \text{ mg}}}{\underset{2}{\cancel{1000} \text{ mg}}} \times 5 \text{ min} = \frac{15}{2} \text{ min} = 7.5 \text{ min}$$

Administer 15 mL over 7.5 min.

How much should you infuse every 15 seconds?

Convert: 1 min = 60 sec

7.5 min = 7.5 × 60 = 450 sec

$$\frac{15 \text{ mL}}{450 \text{ sec}} \bowtie \frac{X \text{ mL}}{15 \text{ sec}}$$

450 X = 225

$$\frac{450X}{450} = \frac{225}{450}$$

X = 0.5 mL of Cefizox 2 g/20 mL infused IV push every 15 seconds to deliver 1500 mg of Cefizox

Use a 20 mL syringe to prepare 15 mL and slowly infuse 0.5 mL every 15 seconds.

ADD-Vantage System

Another type of IV medication setup commonly used in hospitals is the ADD-Vantage system by Abbott Laboratories (Figure 14-18). This system uses a specially designed IV bag with a medication vial port. The medication vial comes with the ordered dosage and medication prepared in a powder form. The medication vial is attached to the special IV bag, and together they become the IV piggyback container. The powder is dissolved by the IV fluid and used within a specified time. This system maintains asepsis and eliminates the extra time and equipment (syringe and diluent vials) associated with reconstitution of powdered medications. Several drug manufacturers currently market many common IV antibiotics using products similar to the ADD-Vantage system.

QUICK REVIEW

- Intermittent IV infusions typically require more or less than 60 minutes of infusion time.
- Calculate IV PB flow rate in gtt/min: $\frac{V}{T} \times C = R$.
- Use a proportion to calculate IV PB flow rate in mL/h for an electronic infusion device.
- Use the three-step dosage calculation method to calculate the amount to give for IV push medications: convert, think, calculate ($\frac{D}{H} \times Q = X$).
- Use $\frac{D}{H} \times Q = X$ or ratio-proportion to calculate safe IV push time in minutes and seconds as recommended by reputable drug reference.

REVIEW SET 41

Calculate the IV PB or IV push flow rate.

1. Order: *Ancef 1 g in 100 cc D$_5$W IV PB to be infused over 45 min*

   Drop factor: 60 gtt/mL

   Flow rate: _____ gtt/min

2. Order: *Ancef 1 g in 100 cc D$_5$W IV PB to be administered by electronic infusion controller to infuse in 45 min*

   Flow rate: _____ mL/h

3. Order: *Kefzol 2 g IV PB diluted in 50 mL D$_5$W to infuse in 15 min*

   Drop factor: 15 gtt/mL

   Flow rate: _____ gtt/min

4. Order: *Kefzol 2 g IV PB diluted in 50 mL D$_5$W to infuse in 15 min by an electronic infusion pump*

   Flow rate: _____ mL/h

1 ASSEMBLE · USE ASEPTIC TECHNIQUE

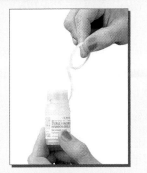

Swing the pull ring over the top of the vial and pull down far enough to start the opening. Then pull straight up to remove the cap. Avoid touching the rubber stopper and vial threads.

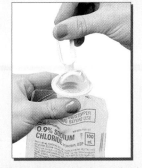

Hold diluent container and gently grasp the tab on the pull ring. Pull up to break the tie membrane. Pull back to remove the cover. Avoid touching the inside of the vial port.

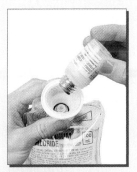

Screw the vial into the vial port until it will go no further. **Recheck the vial to assure that it is tight.** Label appropriately.

2 ACTIVATE · PULL PLUG/STOPPER TO MIX DRUG WITH DILUENT

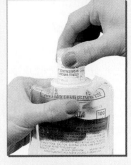

Hold the vial as shown. Push the drug vial down into container and grasp the inner cap of the vial through the walls of the container.

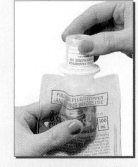

Pull the inner cap from the drug vial: allow drug to fall into diluent container for fast mixing. Do not force stopper by pushing on one side of inner cap at a time.

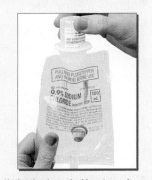

Verify that the plug and rubber stopper have been removed from the vial. The floating stopper is an indication that the system has been activated.

3 MIX AND ADMINISTER · WITHIN THE SPECIFIED TIME

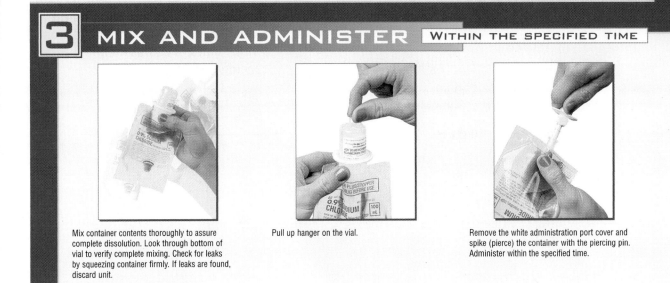

Mix container contents thoroughly to assure complete dissolution. Look through bottom of vial to verify complete mixing. Check for leaks by squeezing container firmly. If leaks are found, discard unit.

Pull up hanger on the vial.

Remove the white administration port cover and spike (pierce) the container with the piercing pin. Administer within the specified time.

FIGURE 14-18 ADD-Vantage System: Medications Can Be Added to Another Solution Being Infused (Reproduced with permission of Abbott Laboratories, Inc.)

5. Order: *50 mL IV PB antibiotic solution to infuse in 30 min*

   Drop factor: 60 gtt/mL

   Flow rate: _____ gtt/min

6. Order: *Zosyn 3 g in 100 mL D₅W IV PB to be infused over 40 min*

   Drop factor: 10 gtt/mL

   Flow rate: _____ gtt/min

7. Order: *Unasyn 1.5 g in 50 mL D₅W IV PB to be infused over 15 min*

   Drop factor: 15 gtt/mL

   Flow rate: _____ gtt/min

8. Order: *Merrem 1 g in 100 mL D₅W IV PB to be infused over 30 min*

   Use infusion pump.

   Flow rate: _____ mL/h

9. Order: *Keflin 750 mg in 50 mL NS IV PB to be infused over 20 min*

   Use infusion pump.

   Flow rate: _____ mL/h

10. Order: *oxacillin Sodium 900 mg in 125 mL D₅W IV PB to be infused over 45 min*

    Use infusion pump.

    Flow rate: _____ mL/h

11. Order: *Unasyn 0.5 g in 100 mL D₅W IV PB to be infused over 15 min*

    Drop factor: 20 gtt/mL

    Flow rate: _____ gtt/min

12. Order: *Keflin 500 mg in 50 mL NS IV PB to be infused over 20 min*

    Drop factor: 10 gtt/mL

    Flow rate: _____ gtt/min

13. Order: *Merrem 1 g in 100 mL D₅W IV PB to be infused over 50 min*

    Use infusion pump.

    Flow rate: _____ mL/h

14. Order: *oxacillin Sodium 900 mg in 125 mL D₅W IV PB to be infused over 45 min*

    Drop factor: 20 gtt/mL

    Flow rate: _____ gtt/min

15. Order: *Zosyn 1.3 g in 100 mL D₅W IV PB to be infused over 30 min*

    Drop factor: 60 gtt/mL

    Flow rate: _____ gtt/min

16. Order: *Lasix 120 mg IV push stat*

    Supply: Lasix 10 mg/mL with drug insert, which states, "IV injection not to exceed 40 mg/min."

    Give: _____ mL/_____ min or _____ mL/15 sec

17. Order: *Dilantin 150 mg IV push stat*

    Supply: Dilantin 250 mg/5 mL with drug insert, which states, "IV infusion not to exceed 50 mg/min."

    Give: _____ mL/_____ min or _____ mL/15 sec

18. Order: *morphine sulfate 6 mg IV push q.3h p.r.n., pain*

    Supply: Morphine sulfate 10 mg/mL with drug reference recommendation, which states, "IV infusion not to exceed 2.5 mg/min."

    Give: _____ mL/_____ min and _____ seconds or _____ mL/15 sec

19. Order: *cimetidine 300 mg IV push stat*

    Supply: Tagamet (cimetidine) 300 mg/2 mL

    Package insert instructions: "For direct IV injection, dilute 300 mg in 0.9% NaCl to a total volume of 20 mL. Inject over at least 2 minutes."

    Prepare _____ mL Tagamet

    Dilute with _____ mL 0.9% NaCl for a total of 20 mL of solution.

    Administer _____ mL/min or _____ mL/15 sec

20. Order: *Versed 1.5 mg IV push stat*

    Supply: Versed 1 mg/mL

    Instructions: "Slowly titrate to the desired effect using no more than 1.5 mg initially given over 2-min period."

    Prepare _____ mL Versed

    Give _____ mL/min or _____ mL/15 sec

After completing these problems, see pages 517–518 to check your answers.

CALCULATING IV INFUSION TIME

Intravenous solutions are usually ordered to be administered at a prescribed number of milliliters per hour, such as *1000 mL Lactated Ringer's IV to run at 125 mL per hour.* You may need to calculate the total infusion time so that you can anticipate when to add a new bag or bottle, or when to discontinue the IV.

RULE

To calculate IV infusion time:

- $\dfrac{\text{TOTAL volume}}{\text{mL/h}} = \text{TOTAL hours}$

Or use ratio-proportion: Ratio for prescribed flow rate in mL/h = Ratio for total mL per X total hours:

- $\dfrac{\text{mL}}{\text{h}} = \dfrac{\text{Total mL}}{\text{X Total h}}$

Example 1:

1000 mL LR IV to run at 125 mL/h. How long will this IV last?

$$\frac{1000 \text{ mL}}{125 \text{ mL/h}} = 8 \text{ h}$$

Or, use ratio-proportion.

$$\frac{125 \text{ mL}}{1 \text{ h}} \times \frac{1000 \text{ mL}}{X \text{ h}}$$

$$125X = 1000$$

$$\frac{125X}{125} = \frac{1000}{125}$$

$$X = 8 \text{ h}$$

Example 2:

1000 mL D₅W IV to infuse at 60 mL/h to being at 0600. At what time will this IV be complete?

$$\frac{1000 \ \text{mL}}{60 \ \text{mL/h}} = 16.6 \ \text{h} = 16 \frac{2}{3} \ \text{h}; \frac{2}{3} \ \text{h} = \frac{2}{3} \times 60 = 40 \ \text{min}; \ \text{Total time: 16 h and 40 min}$$

Or, use ratio-proportion:

$$\frac{60 \ \text{mL}}{1 \ \text{h}} \bowtie \frac{1000 \ \text{mL}}{\text{X h}}$$

$$60 \ \text{X} = 1000$$

$$\frac{60 \text{X}}{60} = \frac{1000}{60}$$

$$\text{X} = 16.6 \ \text{h} = 16\frac{2}{3} \ \text{h} = 16 \ \text{h and 40 min}$$

The IV will be complete at 0600 + 1640 = 2240 (or 10:40 PM).

You can also determine the infusion time if you know the volume, flow rate in gtt/min, and drop factor. Calculate the infusion time by using the $\frac{V}{T} \times C = R$ formula; T, time in minutes, is unknown.

> **RULE**
>
> Use the formula method to calculate time (T):
> $$\frac{V}{T} \times C = R$$

Example:

80 mL D₅W IV at 20 microdrops/min

The drop factor is 60 gtt/mL. Calculate the infusion time.

Step 1 $\frac{V}{T} \times C = R: \frac{80 \ \text{mL}}{\text{T min}} \times 60 \ \text{gtt/mL} = 20 \ \text{gtt/min}$

$$\frac{80 \ \text{mL}}{\text{T min}} \times \frac{60 \ \text{gtt}}{1 \ \text{mL}} = \frac{20 \ \text{gtt}}{1 \ \text{min}}$$

$$\frac{4800 \ \text{gtt}}{\text{T min}} = \frac{20 \ \text{gtt}}{1 \ \text{min}}$$

Then you apply ratio-proportion.

$$\frac{4800}{\text{T}} \bowtie \frac{20}{1}$$

$$20\text{T} = 4800$$

$$\frac{20\text{T}}{20} = \frac{4800}{20}$$

$$\text{T} = 240 \ \text{min}$$

Step 2   Convert: minutes to hours

$$240 \ \text{min} = \frac{240}{60} = 4 \ \text{h}$$

CALCULATING IV FLUID VOLUME

If you have an IV that is regulated at a particular flow rate (gtt/min) and you know the drop factor (gtt/mL) and the amount of time, you can determine the volume to be infused.

Apply the flow rate formula; V, volume, is unknown.

> **RULE**
>
> To calculate IV volume (V):
> $$\frac{V}{T} \times C = R$$

Example:

When you start your shift at 7 AM, there is an IV bag of D_5W *infusing at the rate of 25 gtt/min.* The infusion set is calibrated for a drop factor of *15 gtt/mL.* How much can you anticipate that the patient will receive during your 8-hour shift?

$$8\,h = 8 \times 60 = 480\ min$$

$$\frac{V}{T} \times C = R: \frac{V\ mL}{480\ min} \times 15\ gtt/mL = 25\ gtt/min$$

$$\frac{V\ mL}{480\ min} \times \frac{15\ gtt}{1\ mL} = \frac{25\ gtt}{1\ min}$$

$$\frac{15V\ gtt}{480\ min} = \frac{25\ gtt}{1\ min}$$

$$\frac{15V}{480} \bowtie \frac{25}{1}$$

$$15V = 12{,}000$$

$$\frac{15V}{15} = \frac{12{,}000}{15}$$

$$V = 800\ mL\ to\ be\ infused\ in\ 8\ h$$

If the IV is regulated in mL/h, you can also calculate the total volume that will infuse over a specific time.

> **RULE**
>
> To calculate IV volume:
> Total hours × mL/h = Total volume
> Or use ratio-proportion:
> Ratio for ordered mL/h = Ratio for X total volume per total hours
> $$\frac{mL}{h} = \frac{X\ Total\ mL}{Total\ h}$$

Example:

Your patient's IV is running on an infusion pump set at the rate of 100 mL/h. How much will be infused during the next 8 hours?

$$8\,h \times 100\ mL/h = 800\ mL$$

Or, use ratio-proportion:

$$\frac{100\ mL}{1\ h} \bowtie \frac{X\ mL}{8\ h}$$

$$X = 800\ mL$$

■ The formula to calculate IV infusion time, when mL is known:

$$\frac{\text{Total volume}}{\text{mL/h}} = \text{Total hours}$$

or use ratio-proportion: $\frac{\text{mL}}{\text{h}} = \frac{\text{Total mL}}{\text{X total h}}$

■ The formula to calculate IV infusion time, when flow rate in gtt/min, drop factor, and volume are known: $\frac{V}{T} \times C = R$; "T" is the unknown.

■ The formula to calculate total infusion volume, when mL/h are known:

Total hours $\times$ mL/h = Total volume

Or, use ratio-proportion: $\frac{\text{mL}}{\text{h}} = \frac{\text{X total mL}}{\text{Total h}}$

■ The formula to calculate IV volume, when flow rate (gtt/min), drop factor, and time are known: $\frac{V}{T} \times C = R$; "V" is the unknown.

REVIEW SET 42

Calculate the infusion time and rate (as requested) for the following IV orders:

1. Order: *500 mL D₅W at 30 gtt/min*

   Drop factor: 20 gtt/mL

   Time: _____ h and _____ min

2. Order: *1000 mL Lactated Ringer's at 25 gtt/min*

   Drop factor: 10 gtt/mL

   Time: _____ h and _____ min

3. Order: *800 mL D₅ Lactated Ringer's at 25 gtt/min*

   Drop factor: 15 gtt/mL

   Time: _____ h

4. Order: *120 mL Normal Saline to run at 20 mL/h*

   Drop factor: 60 microdrops/mL

   Time: _____ h

   Flow rate: _____ gtt/min

5. Order: *80 mL D₅W to run at 20 mL/h*

   Drop factor: 60 microdrops/mL

   Time: _____ h

   Flow rate: _____ gtt/min

Calculate the completion time for the following IVs.

6. At 1600 hours the nurse started an IV of 1200 mL D₅W at 27 gtt/min. The infusion set used is calibrated for a drop factor of 15 gtt/mL.

   Infusion time: _____ h

   Completion time: _____

7. At 1530 hours the nurse starts 2000 mL of D₅W to run at 125 mL/h. The infusion set used is calibrated for a drop factor of 10 gtt/mL.

   Infusion time: _____ h

   Completion time: _____

Calculate the total volume (mL) to be infused per 24 hours.

8. An IV of D_5 Lactated Ringer's is infusing on an electronic infusion pump @ 125 mL/h.

   Total volume: _____ mL/24 h

9. An IV is flowing at 12 gtt/min and the infusion set has a drop factor of 15 gtt/mL.

   Total volume: _____ mL/24 h

10. IV: D_5W

    Flow rate: 21 gtt/min

    Drop factor: 10 gtt/mL

    Total volume: _____ mL/24 h

Calculate IV volume for the following IVs.

11. *0.9% sodium chloride IV infusing at 65 mL/h for 4 h*

    Volume: _____ mL

12. *D_5W IV infusing at 150 mL/h for 2 h*

    Volume: _____ mL

13. *D_5LR IV at 75 mL/h for 8 h*

    Volume: _____ mL

14. *D_5 0.225 NaCl IV at 40 gtt/min for 8 h*

    Drop factor: 60 gtt/mL

    Infusion time: _____ min

    Volume: _____ mL

15. *0.45% NaCl IV at 45 gtt/min for 4 h*

    Drop factor: 20 gtt/mL

    Infusion time: _____ min

    Volume: _____ mL

After completing these problems, see pages 518-519 to check your answers.

CRITICAL THINKING SKILLS

It is important to know the equipment you are using. Let's look at an example in which the nurse was unfamiliar with the IV piggyback setup.

error

Failing to follow manufacturer's directions when using a new IV piggyback system.

possible scenario

Suppose the physician ordered Rocephin 1 g IV q.12h for an elderly patient with streptococcus pneumonia. The medication was sent to the unit by pharmacy utilizing the ADD-Vantage system. Rocephin 1 gram was supplied in a powder form and attached to a 50 mL IV bag of D_5W. The

(continues)

(continued)

directions for preparing the medication were attached to the label. The nurse, who was unfamiliar with the new ADD-Vantage system, hung the IV medication, calculated the drip rate, and infused the 50 mL of fluid. The nurse cared for the patient for three days. During walking rounds on the third day, the oncoming nurse noticed that the Rocephin powder remained in the vial and never was diluted in the IV bag. The nurse realized that the vial stopper inside of the IV bag was not open. Therefore, the medication powder was not mixed in the IV fluid during this shift for the past three days.

potential outcome

The omission by the nurse resulted in the patient missing three doses of the ordered IV antibiotic. The delay in the medication administration could have serious consequences for the patient, such as worsening of the pneumonia, septicemia, and even death, especially in the elderly. The patient received only one-half of the daily dose ordered by the physician for three days. The physician would be notified of the error and likely order additional diagnostic studies, such as chest X ray, blood cultures, and an additional one-time dose of Rocephin.

prevention

This error could easily have been avoided had the nurse read the directions for preparing the medication or consulted with another nurse who was familiar with the system.

PRACTICE PROBLEMS—CHAPTER 14

Compute the flow rate in drops per minute or milliliters per hour as requested. For these situations, hospital policy permits recalculating IVs when off schedule with a maximum variation in rate of 25 percent.

1. Order: *Ampicillin 500 mg dissolved in 200 mL D$_5$W IV to run for 2 h*

   Drop factor: 10 gtt/mL

   Flow rate: _____ gtt/min

2. Order: *1000 mL D$_5$W IV per 24h*

   Drop factor: 60 gtt/mL

   Flow rate: _____ gtt/min

3. Order: *1500 mL D$_5$LR IV to run for 12 h*

   Drop factor: 20 gtt/mL

   Flow rate: _____ gtt/min

4. Order: *200 mL D$_5$RL IV for 24 h*

   Drop factor: 60 gtt/mL

   Flow rate: _____ gtt/min

5. Order: *1 L D$_{10}$W IV to run from 1000 to 1800*

   Drop factor: On electronic infusion pump

   Flow rate: _____ mL/h

6. See question 5. At 1100 there are 800 mL remaining. Describe your nursing action now. _____

   _____

7. Order: *1000 mL NS followed by 2000 mL D$_5$W IV to run for 24 h*

   Drop factor: 15 gtt/mL

   Flow rate: _____ gtt/min

8. Order: *2.5 L NS IV to infuse at 125 mL/h*

   Drop factor: 20 gtt/mL

   Flow rate: _____ gtt/min

9. Order: *1000 mL D$_5$W IV for 6 h*

   Drop factor: 15 gtt/mL

   After 2 hours, 800 mL remain. Describe your nursing action now. _____

   _____

The IV tubing package in the accompanying figure is the IV system available in your hospital for manually regulated, straight gravity flow IV administration with macrodrop. The patient has an order for *500 mL D$_5$W IV q.4h* written at 1515 and you start the IV at 1530. Questions 10 through 20 refer to this situation.

10. How much IV fluid will the patient receive in 24 hours? _____ mL

11. Who is the manufacturer of the IV infusion set tubing? _____

12. What is the drop factor calibration for the IV infusion set tubing? _____

13. What is the drop factor constant for the IV infusion set tubing? _____

14. Using the shortcut (drop factor constant) method, calculate the flow rate of the IV as ordered. Show your work.

    Shortcut method calculation: _____

    Flow rate: _____ gtt/min

15. Using the formula method, calculate the flow rate of the IV as ordered. Show your work.

    Formula method calculation: _____

    Flow rate: _____ gtt/min

16. At what time should you anticipate the first IV bag of 500 mL D$_5$W will be completely infused?

    _____

17. How much IV fluid should be infused by 1730? _____ mL

18. At 1730 you notice that the IV has 210 mL remaining. After assessing your patient and confirming that his or her condition is stable, what should you do? _____

    _____

19. After consulting the physician, you decide to use an electronic controller to better regulate the flow rate. The physician orders that the controller be set to infuse 500 mL every 4 hours. You should set the controller for _____ mL/h

20. The next day the physician adds the order *Amoxicillin 250 mg in 50 mL D₅W IV PB to infuse in 30 min q.i.d.* The patient is still on the IV controller. To infuse the IV PB, set the controller for _____ mL/h

21. List the components and concentration strengths of the fluid $D_{2.5} \frac{1}{2}$ NS.

   _____

22. Calculate the amount of dextrose and sodium chloride in D_5NS 500 mL.

   dextrose _____ g

   NaCl _____ g

23. Define a central line. _____

   _____

24. Define a primary line. _____

   _____

25. Describe the purpose of a saline or heparin lock. _____

   _____

26. A safe IV push infusion rate of protamine sulfate is 5 mg/min. What is a safe infusion time to administer 50 mg? _____ min

   Protamine sulfate is available in a supply dosage of 10 mg/mL. To administer 50 mg IV push, prepare _____ mL and inject slowly IV at the rate of _____ mL/min or _____ mL/15 sec.

27. Describe the purpose of the PCA pump. _____

   _____

28. Identify two advantages of the syringe pump. _____

   _____

29. List two complications of IV sites. _____

   _____

30. How often should the IV site be monitored? _____

   _____

31. Describe the purpose of the Y-set IV system. _____

   _____

For each IV order in questions 32 through 47, use the drop factor to calculate the flow rate in gtt/min.

Order: *1 L hyperalimentation solution IV to infuse in 12 h*

32. Drop factor 10 gtt/mL   Flow rate: _____ gtt/min

33. Drop factor 15 gtt/mL   Flow rate: _____ gtt/min

34. Drop factor 20 gtt/mL   Flow rate: _____ gtt/min

35. Drop factor 60 gtt/mL   Flow rate: _____ gtt/min

Order: *2 L D₅NS IV to infuse in 20 h*

36. Drop factor 10 gtt/mL   Flow rate: _____ gtt/min

37. Drop factor 15 gtt/mL   Flow rate: _____ gtt/min

38. Drop factor 20 gtt/mL   Flow rate: _____ gtt/min

39. Drop factor 60 gtt/mL   Flow rate: _____ gtt/min

Order: *1000 mL of 0.45% NaCl IV @ 200 mL/h*

40. Drop factor 10 gtt/mL   Flow rate: _____ gtt/min

41. Drop factor 15 gtt/mL   Flow rate: _____ gtt/min

42. Drop factor 20 gtt/mL   Flow rate: _____ gtt/min

43. Drop factor 60 gtt/mL   Flow rate: _____ gtt/min

Order: *540 mL D₅ 0.33% NaCl IV @ 45 mL/h*

44. Drop factor 10 gtt/mL   Flow rate: _____ gtt/min

45. Drop factor 15 gtt/mL   Flow rate: _____ gtt/min

46. Drop factor 20 gtt/mL   Flow rate: _____ gtt/min

47. Drop factor 60 gtt/mL   Flow rate: _____ gtt/min

48. You make rounds before your lunch break and find that a patient has 150 mL of IV fluid remaining. The flow rate is 25 gtt/min. The drop factor is 10 gtt/mL. What volume will be infused during the hour that you are at lunch? _____ mL What should you alert your relief nurse to watch for while you are off the unit? _____

49. Your shift is 0700–1500. You make rounds at 0730 and find an IV of D_5 0.45% NaCl is regulated on an electronic infusion pump at the ordered rate of 75 mL/h with 400 mL remaining. The order specifies a continuous infusion. At what time should you anticipate hanging the next IV bag?

_____

50. Critical Thinking Skill: Describe the strategy you would implement to prevent this medication error.

possible scenario

Suppose the physician ordered *D₅LR at 125 mL/h* for an elderly patient just returning from the OR following abdominal surgery. The nurse gathered the IV solution and IV tubing, which had a drop factor of 20 gtt/mL. The nurse did not check the package for the drop factor and assumed it was 60 gtt/mL. The manual rate was calculated this way:

$$\frac{125 \text{ mL}}{60 \text{ min}} \times 60 \text{ gtt/mL} = 125 \text{ gtt/min}$$

The nurse infused the D_5LR at 125 gtt/min for 8 hours. While giving report to the oncoming nurse, the patient called for the nurse, complaining of shortness of breath. On further assessment the nurse heard crackles in the patient's lungs and noticed that the patient's third 1000 mL bottle of D_5LR this shift was nearly empty already. At this point the nurse realized the IV rate was in error. The nurse was accustomed to using the 60 gtt/mL IV set up and therefore calculated the drip rate using the 60 gtt/mL (microdrop) drop factor. However, the tubing used delivered 20 gtt/mL (macrodrop) drop factor. The nurse never looked at the drop factor on the IV set package and assumed it was a 60 gtt/mL set.

potential outcome

The patient developed signs of fluid overload and could have developed congestive heart failure due to the excessive IV rate. The physician would have been notified and likely ordered Lasix (a diuretic) to help eliminate the excess fluid. The patient likely would have been transferred to the ICU for closer monitoring.

prevention

_____

_____

Upon completion of these problems, see pages 519–521 to check your answers.

Body Surface Area and Advanced Pediatric Calculations

OBJECTIVES

Upon mastery of Chapter 15, you will be able to perform advanced calculations for children and apply these advanced concepts across the life span. To accomplish this you will also be able to:

● Determine the body surface area (BSA) using a calculation formula or a nomogram scale.
● Compute the safe amount of drug to be administered when ordered according to the BSA.
● Calculate intermittent intravenous (IV) medications administered with IV infusion control sets.
● Calculate the amount to mix proportionate IV additive medications into small volume IV solutions.
● Calculate the minimal and maximal dilution in which an IV medication can be safely prepared and delivered, such as via a syringe pump.
● Calculate pediatric IV maintenance fluids.

This chapter will focus on additional and more advanced calculations used frequently by pediatric nurses. It will help you understand the unique drug and fluid management required by a growing child. Further, these concepts, which are most commonly related to children, are also applied to adults in special situations. Let's start by looking at the BSA method of calculating a dosage and checking for accuracy and safety of a particular drug order.

BODY SURFACE AREA METHOD

The BSA is an important measure in calculating dosages for infants and children. BSA is also used for selected adult populations, such as those undergoing open-heart surgery or radiation therapy, severe burn victims, and those with renal disease. Regardless of age, antineoplastic agents (chemotherapy drugs) and an increasing number of other highly potent drug classifications are being prescribed based on BSA.

BSA is a mathematical estimate using the patient's *height* and *weight*. BSA is expressed in square meters (m^2). BSA can be determined by formula calculation or by using a chart, referred to as a *nomogram*, that estimates the BSA. Because drug dosages recommended by BSA measurement are very potent, and because the formula calculation is the most accurate, we will begin with the formulas. In most situations, the prescribing practitioner will compute the BSA for drugs ordered by this method. However, the nurse who administers the drug is responsible for verifying safe dosage, which may require calculating the BSA.

BSA Formula

One BSA formula is based on metric measurement of height in centimeters and weight in kilograms. The other is based on household measurement of height in inches and weight in pounds. Either is easy to compute using the square root function on a calculator.

> **RULE**
>
> To calculate BSA in m^2 based on *metric measurement* of height and weight:
>
> - BSA $(m^2) = \sqrt{\dfrac{\text{ht (cm)} \times \text{wt (kg)}}{3600}}$
>
> To calculate BSA in m^2 based on *household measurement* of height and weight:
>
> - BSA $(m^2) = \sqrt{\dfrac{\text{ht (in)} \times \text{wt (lb)}}{3131}}$

Let's apply both formulas, and see how the BSA measurements compare.

> **MATH TIP**
>
> Notice that in addition to metric versus household measurement, the other difference between the two BSA formulas is in the denominators of the fraction within the square root sign.

Example 1:

Use the metric formula to calculate the BSA of an infant whose length is 50 cm (20 in) and weight is 6.8 kg (15 lb).

$$\text{BSA } (m^2) = \sqrt{\frac{\text{ht (cm)} \times \text{wt (kg)}}{3600}} = \sqrt{\frac{50 \times 6.8}{3600}} = \sqrt{\frac{340}{3600}} = \sqrt{0.094} = 0.307 \; m^2 = 0.31 \; m^2$$

> **MATH TIP**
>
> To perform BSA calculations using the metric formula on most calculators, follow this sequence: multiply height in *cm* by weight in *kg*, divide by 3600, press =, then press $\sqrt{}$ to arrive at m^2. Round m^2 to hundredths (two decimal places). For Example 1, enter 50 × 6.8 ÷ 3600 = 0.094, and press $\sqrt{}$ to arrive at 0.307, rounded to 0.31 m^2.

Or use the BSA formula based on household measurement.

$$\text{BSA } (m^2) = \sqrt{\frac{\text{ht (in)} \times \text{wt (lb)}}{3131}} = \sqrt{\frac{20 \times 15}{131}} = \sqrt{\frac{300}{3131}} = \sqrt{0.095} = 0.309 \; m^2 = 0.31 \; m^2$$

> **MATH TIP**
>
> To use the calculator, follow this sequence: multiply height in *inches* by weight in *pounds*, divide by 3131, press =, then press $\sqrt{}$ to arrive at the m^2. Round m^2 to hundredths (two decimal places). For Example 1, enter 20 × 15 ÷ 3131 = 0.095, and press $\sqrt{}$ to arrive at 0.309, rounded to 0.31 m^2.

Example 2:

Calculate the BSA of a child whose height is 105 cm (42 inches) and weight is 31.8 kg (70 lb).

Metric:

$$\text{BSA } (m^2) = \sqrt{\frac{\text{ht (cm)} \times \text{wt (kg)}}{3600}} = \sqrt{\frac{105 \times 31.8}{3600}} = \sqrt{\frac{3339}{3600}} = \sqrt{0.927} = 0.963 \; m^2 = 0.96 \; m^2$$

Household:

$$\text{BSA } (m^2) = \sqrt{\frac{\text{ht (in)} \times \text{wt (lb)}}{3131}} = \sqrt{\frac{42 \times 70}{3131}} = \sqrt{\frac{2940}{3131}} = \sqrt{0.938} = 0.969 \; m^2 = 0.97 \; m^2$$

#%
MATH TIP

There is a slight variation in m^2 calculated by the metric and household methods because of the rounding used to convert centimeters and inches; more precisely, 1 in = 2.54 cm, which is rounded to 2.5 cm. The results of the two methods are approximate equivalents.

Example 3:

Calculate the BSA of an adult whose height is 173 cm (69 inches) and weight is 88.6 kg (195 lb).

Metric:

$$BSA\ (m^2) = \sqrt{\frac{ht\ (cm) \times wt\ (kg)}{3600}} = \sqrt{\frac{173 \times 88.6}{3600}} = \sqrt{\frac{15327.8}{3600}} = \sqrt{4.257} = 2.063\ m^2 = 2.06\ m^2$$

Household:

$$BSA\ (m^2) = \sqrt{\frac{ht\ (in) \times wt\ (lb)}{3131}} = \sqrt{\frac{68 \times 195}{3131}} = \sqrt{\frac{13260}{3131}} = \sqrt{4.235} = 2.057\ m^2 = 2.06\ m^2$$

These examples show that either metric or household measurements of height and weight result in essentially the same calculated BSA value.

BSA Nomogram

Some practitioners use a chart called a *nomogram* that *estimates* the BSA by plotting the height and weight and simply connecting the dots with a straight line. Figure 15-1 shows the most well-known BSA chart, the West Nomogram. It is used for both children and adults for heights up to 240 cm (95 inches) and weights up to 80 kg (180 lb).

CAUTION

Notice that the increments of measurement and the spaces on the BSA nomogram are not consistent. Be sure you correctly read the numbers and the calibration values between them.

For a child of normal height and weight, the BSA can be determined on the West Nomogram using the weight alone. Notice the enclosed column to the center left. Normal height and weight standards can be found on pediatric growth and development charts.

CAUTION

To use the normal column on the West Nomogram, you must be familiar with normal height and weight standards for children. If you are unsure, use both height and weight to estimate BSA. Do not guess.

QUICK REVIEW

- BSA is used to calculate select dosages across the life span, most often for children.
- BSA is calculated by height and weight and expressed in m^2.
- The following metric and household formulas are the preferred methods of calculating BSA:

  Metric: $BSA\ (m^2) = \sqrt{\frac{ht\ (cm) \times wt\ (kg)}{3600}}$

  Household: $BSA\ (m^2) = \sqrt{\frac{ht\ (in) \times wt\ (lb)}{3131}}$

- Nomograms can be used to estimate BSA, by correlating height and weight measures to m^2.

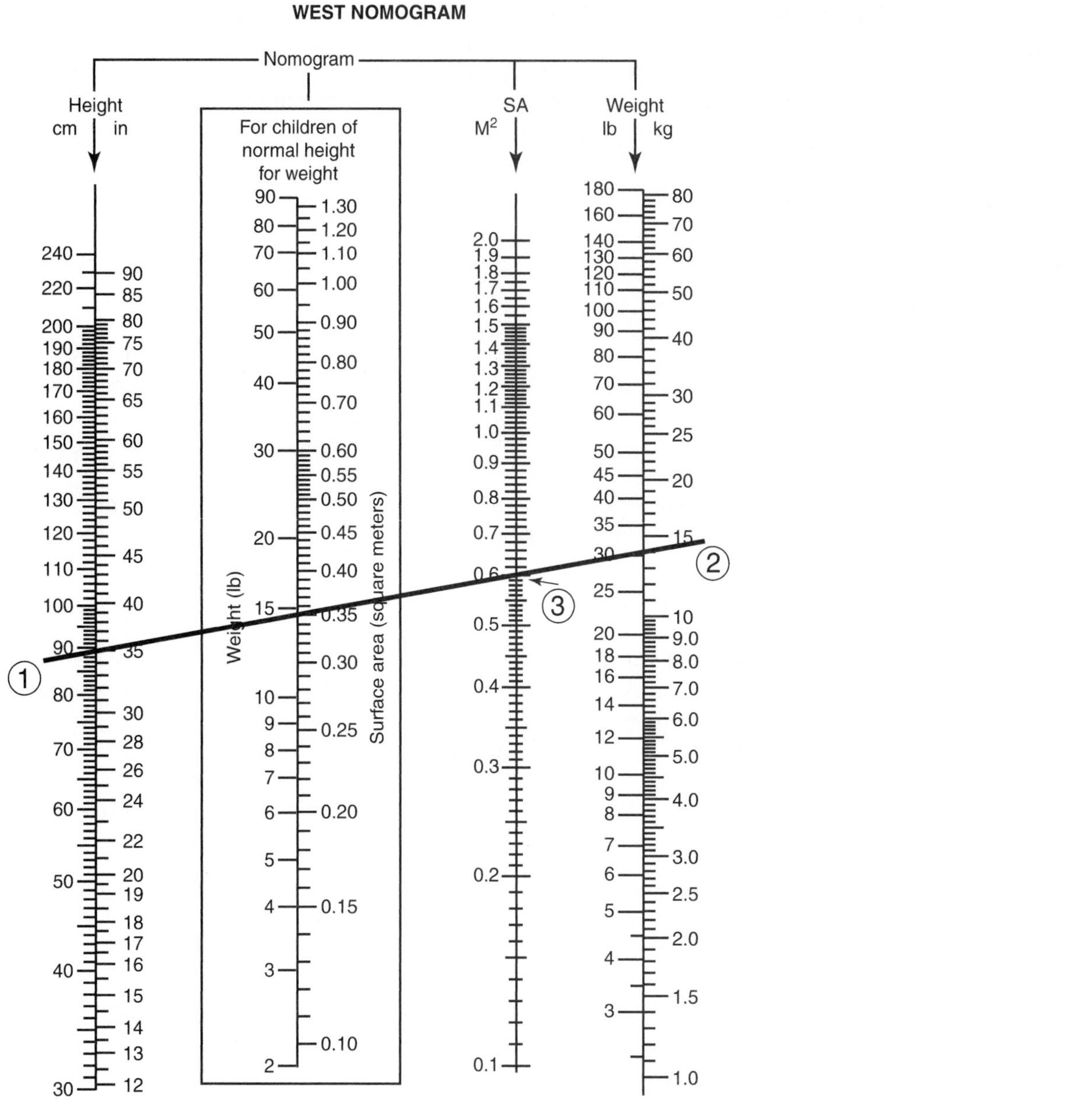

WEST NOMOGRAM

FIGURE 15-1 Body surface area (BSA) is determined by drawing a straight line from the patient's height (1) in the far left column to his or her weight (2) in the far right column. Intersection of the line with surface area (SA) column (3) is the estimated BSA (m^2). For infants and children of normal height and weight, BSA may be estimated from weight alone by referring to the enclosed area. (From *Nelson Textbook of Pediatrics* (16th ed) by R. E. Behrman, R. M. Kleigman, & H. B. Jenson, 2000, Philadelphia: Saunders. Reprinted with permission.)

REVIEW SET 43

Use the formula method to determine the BSA. Round to 2 decimal places.

1. A child measures 36 inches tall and weighs 40 lb. _____ m^2

2. An adult measures 190 cm tall and weighs 105 kg. _____ m^2

3. A child measures 94 cm tall and weighs 18 kg. _____ m^2

4. A teenager measures 153 cm tall and weighs 46 kg. _____ m^2

5. An adult measures 175 cm tall and weighs 85 kg. _____ m^2

6. A child measures 41 inches tall and weighs 76 lb. _____ m^2

7. An adult measures 62 inches tall and weighs 140 lb. _____ m^2

8. A child measures 28 inches tall and weighs 18 lb. _____ m^2

9. A teenager measures 160 cm tall and weighs 64 kg. _____ m^2

10. A child measures 65 cm tall and weighs 15 kg. _____ m^2

11. A child measures 55 inches tall and weighs 70 lb. _____ m^2

12. A child measures 92 cm tall and weighs 24 kg. _____ m^2

Find the BSA on the West Nomogram (Figure 15-1) for a child of normal height and weight.

13. 4 lb _____ m^2 14. 42 lb _____ m^2 15. 17 lb _____ m^2

Find the BSA on the West Nomogram (Figure 15-1) for children with the following height and weight.

16. 41 inches and 32 lb _____ m^2

17. 21 inches and 8 lb _____ m^2

18. 140 cm and 30 kg _____ m^2

19. 80 cm and 11 kg _____ m^2

20. 106 cm and 25 kg _____ m^2

After completing these problems, see page 521 to check your answers.

BSA Dosage Calculations

Once the BSA is obtained, the drug dosage can be verified by consulting a reputable drug resource for the recommended dosage. Package inserts, the *Hospital Formulary*, or other dosage handbooks contain pediatric and adults dosages. Remember to carefully read the reference to verify if the drug dosage is calculated in *m^2 per dose* or *m^2 per day*.

> ### RULE
>
> To verify safe pediatric dosage based on BSA:
> 1. Determine BSA in m^2.
> 2. Calculate the safe dosage based on **BSA: mg/m^2 × m^2 = X mg**
> 3. Compare the ordered dosage to the recommended dosage, and decide if the dosage is safe.
> 4. If the dosage is safe, calculate the amount to give and administer the dose. If the dosage seems unsafe, consult with the ordering practitioner before administering the drug.
> Note: Recommended dosage may specify mg/m^2, mcg/m^2, g/m^2, U/m^2, mU/m^2, or mEq/m^2.

Example 1:

A child is 126 cm tall and weighs 23 kg. The drug order reads: *Oncovin 1.8 mg IV at 10 AM.* Is this dosage safe for this child? The recommended dosage as noted on the package insert is 2 mg/m². Supply: See label, Figure 15-2.

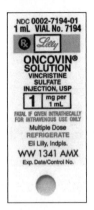

FIGURE 15-2 Oncovin Label

1. **Determine BSA.** The child's BSA is 0.9 m² (using the metric BSA formula).

$$\text{BSA (m}^2) = \sqrt{\frac{\text{ht (cm)} \times \text{wt (kg)}}{3600}} = \sqrt{\frac{126 \times 23}{3600}} = \sqrt{\frac{2898}{3600}} = \sqrt{0.805} = 0.897 \text{ m}^2 = 0.9 \text{ m}^2$$

2. **Calculate recommended dosage.** mg/m² × m² = 2 mg/m² × 0.9 m² = 1.8 mg

3. **Decide if the dosage is safe.** The dosage ordered is 1.8 mg and 1.8 mg is the amount recommended by BSA. The dosage is safe. How much should you give?

4. **Calculate one dose.**

Step 1   Convert   No conversion is necessary.

Step 2   Think   You want to give more than 1 mL and less than 2 mL.

Step 3   Calculate $\frac{\text{D}}{\text{H}} \times \text{Q} = \frac{1.8 \text{ mg}}{X \text{ mg}} \times X \text{mL} = 1.8 \text{ mL}$

Or, use ratio-proportion.

$$\frac{1 \text{ mg}}{1 \text{ mL}} \diagtimes \frac{1.8 \text{ mg}}{X \text{ mL}}$$

X = 1.8 mL

Example 2:

A 2-year-old child with herpes simplex is 35 inches tall and weighs 30 lb. The drug order reads *acyclovir 100 mg IV b.i.d.* Is this order safe? The drug reference recommends 250 mg/m² q.8h for children less than 12 years and more than 6 months. Acyclovir is supplied as Zovirax 500 mg injection with directions to reconstitute with 10 mL sterile water for injection for a concentration of 50 mg/mL.

1. **Determine BSA.** The child's BSA is 0.6 m^2 (using the West Nomogram, Figure 15-1).

2. **Calculate recommended dosage.** mg/m^2 $\times$ m^2 = 250 mg/m^2 $\times$ 0.6 m^2 = 150 mg

3. **Decide if the dosage is safe.** The dosage of 100 mg b.i.d. is not safe—the single dosage is too low. Further, the drug should be administered 3 times per day q.8h, not b.i.d. or 2 times per day.

4. **Confer with the prescriber.**

QUICK REVIEW

Safe dosage based on BSA: mg/m^2 $\times$ m^2, compared to recommended dosage.

REVIEW SET 44

1. What is the dosage of one dose of interferon alpha-2b required for a child with a BSA of 0.82 m^2 if the recommended dosage is 2 million U/m^2? _____ U

2. What is the total daily dosage range of mitomycin required for a child with a BSA of 0.59 m^2 if the recommended dosage range is 10 to 20 mg/m^2/day? _____ mg/day to _____ mg/day

3. What is the dosage of calcium EDTA required for an adult with a BSA of 1.47 m^2 if the recommended dosage is 500 mg/m^2? _____ mg

4. What is the total daily dosage of Thioplex required for a adult with a BSA of 2.64 m^2 if the recommended dosage is 6 mg/m^2/day? _____ mg. After 4 full days of therapy, this patient will have received a total of _____ mg of Thioplex.

5. What is the dosage of acyclovir required for a child with a BSA of 1 m^2, if the recommended dosage is 250 mg/m^2? _____ mg

6. Child is 30 inches tall and weighs 25 pounds.

    Order: *Zovirax 122.5 mg IV q.8h*

    Supply: Zovirax 500 mg with directions to reconstitute with 10 mL sterile water for injection for a final concentration of 50 mg/mL.

    Recommended dosage from drug insert: 250 mg/m^2

    BSA = _____ m^2

    Recommended dosage for this child: _____ mg

    Is the ordered dosage safe? _____

    If safe, give _____ mL

    If not safe, what should you do? _____

7. Child is 45 inches tall and weighs 55 pounds.

    Order: *methotrexate 2.9 mg IV q.d.*

    Supply: methotrexate 2.5 mg/mL

    Recommended dosage from drug insert: 3.3 mg/m^2

    BSA = _____ m^2

    Recommended dosage for this child: _____ mg

    Is the ordered dosage safe? _____

If safe, give _____ mL

If not safe, what should you do? _____

8. Order: *Benoject 22 mg IV q.8h.* Child has BSA of 0.44 m². Recommended safe dosage of Benoject is 150 mg/m²/day in divided dosages every 6 to 8 hours.

   Recommended daily dosage for this child: _____ mg/day

   Recommended single dosage for this child: _____ mg/dose

   Is the ordered dosage safe? _____

   If not safe, what should you do? _____

9. Order: *quinidine 198 mg p.o. q.d. for 5 days.* Child has BSA of 0.22 m². Recommended safe dosage of quinidine is 900 mg/m²/day given in 5 daily doses.

   Recommended dosage for this child: _____ mg/dose

   Is the dosage ordered safe? _____

   If not safe, what should you do? _____

   How much quinidine would this child receive over 5 days of therapy? _____ mg

10. Order: *deferoxamine mesylate IV per protocol.* Child has BSA of 1.02 m².

    Protocol: 600 mg/m² initially followed by 300 mg/m² at 4-hour intervals for 2 doses; then give 300 mg/m² q.12 h for 2 days. Calculate the total dosage received.

    Initial dosage: _____ mg

    Two q.4h dosages: _____ mg

    Two days of q.12h dosages: _____ mg

    Total dosage child would receive: _____ mg

11. Protocol: *Fludara 10 mg/m² bolus over 15 minutes followed by a continuous IV infusion of 30.5 mg/m²/day.* Child has BSA of 0.81 m². The bolus dosage is _____ mg, and the continuous 24-hour IV infusion will contain _____ mg of Fludara.

12. Order: *Accutane 83.75 mg IV q.12h* for a child with a BSA of 0.67 m². The recommended dosage range is 100 to 250 mg/m²/day in 2 divided doses.

    Recommended daily dosage range for this child: _____ mg/day to _____ mg/day

    Recommended single dosage range for this child: _____ mg/dose to _____ mg/dose

    Is the ordered dosage safe? _____

    If not, what should you do? _____

13. Order: *Cerubidine 9.6 mg IV on day 1 and day 8 of cycle.*

    Protocol: 25 to 45 mg/m² on days 1 and 8 of cycle. Child has BSA of 0.32 m².

    Recommended dosage range for this child: _____ mg/dose to _____ mg/dose

    Is the ordered dosage safe? _____

    If not safe, what should you do? _____

Answer questions 14 and 15 based on the following information.

The recommended dosage of Oncaspar is 2500 U/m^2/dose IV daily $\times$ 14 days for adults and children with a BSA > 0.6 m^2.

Supply: Oncaspar 750 U/mL with directions to dilute in 100 mL D$_5$W and give over 2 hours. You will administer the drug via infusion pump.

14. Order: *Give Oncaspar 2050 U IV today @ 1600.* Child is 100 cm tall and weighs 24 kg. The child's BSA is _____ m^2.

    The recommended dosage for this child is _____ U. Is the ordered dosage of Oncaspar safe? _____

    If yes, add _____ mL of Oncaspar for a total IV fluid volume of _____ mL. Set the IV infusion pump at _____ mL/h.

    If the order is not safe, what should you do? _____

15. Order: *Oncaspar 4050 U IV stat* for an adult patient who is 162 cm tall and weighs 58.2 kg. The patient's BSA is _____ m^2. The recommended dosage of Oncaspar for this adult is _____ U.

    Is the ordered dosage of Oncaspar safe? _____

    If safe, you would add _____ mL of Oncaspar for a total IV fluid volume of _____ mL. Set the infusion pump at _____ mL/h.

    If the order is not safe, what should you do? _____

After completing these problems, see pages 521–522 to check your answers.

PEDIATRIC VOLUME CONTROL SETS

Volume control sets, Figure 15-3, are most frequently used to administer hourly fluids and intermittent IV medications to children. The fluid chamber will hold 100 to 150 milliliters of fluid to be infused in a specified time period as ordered, usually 60 minutes or less. The medication is added to the IV fluid in the chamber for a prescribed dilution volume.

The volume of fluid in the chamber is filled by the nurse every 1 to 2 hours or as needed. Only small, ordered quantities of fluid are added, and the clamp above the chamber is fully closed. The IV bag acts only as a reservoir to hold future fluid infusions. The patient is protected from receiving more volume than intended. This is especially important for children, because they can tolerate only a narrow range of fluid volume. This differs from standard IV infusions that run directly from the IV bag through the drip chamber and IV tubing into the patient's vein.

Volume control sets may also be used to administer intermittent IV medications to adults with fluid restrictions, such as for heart or kidney disease. An electronic controller or pump may also be used to regulate the flow rate. When used, the electronic device will alarm when the chamber empties.

Intermittent IV Medication Infusion via Volume Control Set

Children receiving IV medications may have a saline or heparin lock in place of a continuous IV infusion. The nurse will inject the medication into the volume control set chamber, add an appropriate volume of IV fluid to dilute the drug, and attach the IV tubing to the child's IV lock to infuse over a specified period of time. After the chamber has emptied and the medication has infused, a flush of IV fluid is given to be sure all the medication has cleared the tubing. Realize that when the chamber empties, some medication still remains in the drip chamber, IV tubing, and the IV lock above the

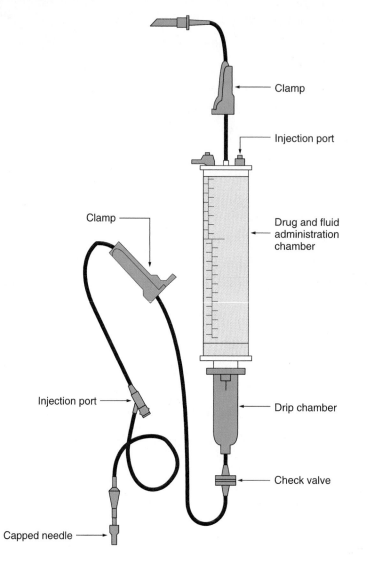

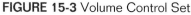

FIGURE 15-3 Volume Control Set

child's vein. There is no standard amount of fluid used to flush peripheral or central IV lines. Because tubing varies by manufacturer, the flush can vary from 15 mL to as much as 50 mL, according to the overall length of the tubing and extra extensions added. Verify your hospital policy on the correct volume to flush peripheral and central IV lines in children. For the purpose of sample calculations, this text uses a 15 mL volume to flush a peripheral IV line, unless specified otherwise.

To calculate the IV flow rate for the volume control set, you must consider the total fluid volume of the medication, the IV fluid used for dilution, and the volume of IV flush fluid. Volume control sets are microdrip sets with a drop factor of 60 gtt/mL.

Example:

Order: *Claforan 250 mg IV q.6h in 50 mL*
$D_5\frac{1}{4}NS$ *to infuse in 30 min followed by a*
15 mL flush. Child has a saline lock.

Supply: See label

Instructions from package insert for IV use:
Add 10 mL diluent for a total volume of
11 mL with a concentration of 180 mg/mL.

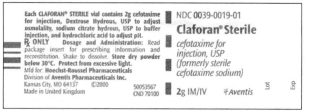

Each CLAFORAN® STERILE vial contains 2g cefotaxime for injection, Dextrose Hydrous, USP to adjust osmolality, sodium citrate hydrous, USP to buffer injection, and hydrochloric acid to adjust pH.
℞ ONLY   Dosage and Administration: Read package insert for prescribing information and reconstitution. Shake to dissolve. **Store dry powder below 30°C. Protect from excessive light.**
Mfd for: **Hoechst-Roussel Pharmaceuticals**
Division of **Aventis Pharmaceuticals Inc.**
Kansas City, MO 64137   ©2000
Made in United Kingdom   50053567
                             CND 70100

NDC 0039-0019-01
Claforan® Sterile
cefotaxime for injection, USP
(formerly sterile cefotaxime sodium)
2g IM/IV   ⚜*Aventis*   Lot   Exp

Step 1 Calculate the total volume of the intermittent IV medication and the IV flush.
50 mL + 15 mL = 65 mL

Step 2 Calculate the flow rate of the IV medication and the IV flush. Remember: The drop factor is 60 gtt/mL.

$$\frac{V}{T} \times C = \frac{65 \; \cancel{mL}}{\underset{1}{\cancel{30} \; min}} \times \overset{2}{\cancel{60}} \; gtt/\cancel{mL} = 130 \; gtt/min$$

Step 3 Calculate the volume of the medication to be administered.

$$\frac{D}{H} \times Q = \frac{250 \; \cancel{mg}}{180 \; \cancel{mg}} \times 1 \; mL = 1.38 \; mL = 1.4 \; mL$$

Step 4 Add 1.4 mL Claforan 2 g to the chamber and fill with IV fluid to a volume of 50 mL. This provides the prescribed total volume of 50 mL in the chamber.

Step 5 Set the flow rate of the 50 mL of intermittent IV medication for 130 gtt/min. Follow with the 15 mL flush also set at 130 gtt/min. When complete, detach IV tubing, and follow saline lock policy.

The patient may also have an intermittent medication ordered as part of a continuous infusion at a prescribed IV volume per hour. In such cases the patient is to receive the same fluid volume each hour, regardless of the addition of intermittent medications. This means that the total prescribed fluid volume must include the intermittent IV medication volume.

Example:

Order: *D_5NS IV at 30 mL/h for continuous infusion and gentamicin 30 mg IV q.8h over 30 min*

Supply: See label, Figure 15-4

An infusion controller is in use with the volume control set.

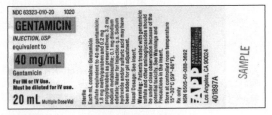

FIGURE 15-4 Gentamicin Label

Step 1 Calculate the dilution volume required to administer the gentamicin at the prescribed continuous flow rate of 30 mL/h.

    Think   If 30 mL infuses in 1 h, then $\frac{1}{2}$ of 30, or 15 mL, will infuse in $\frac{1}{2}$ h or 30 min.

    Calculate   Use ratio-proportion to verify your estimate.

$$\frac{30 \; mL}{60 \; min} \underset{\times}{\diagup} \frac{X \; mL}{30 \; min}$$

$$60X = 900$$

$$\frac{60X}{60} = \frac{900}{60}$$

$$X = 15 \; mL \; in \; 30 \; min$$

Therefore, the IV fluid dilution volume required to administer 30 mg of gentamicin in 30 minutes is 15 mL to maintain the prescribed, continuous infusion rate of 30 mL/h.

Step 2   Determine the volume of gentamicin and IV fluid to add to the volume control chamber.

$$\frac{D}{H} \times Q = \frac{\overset{3}{\cancel{30} \text{ mg}}}{\underset{4}{\cancel{40} \text{ mg}}} \times 1\text{ mL} = \frac{3}{4}\text{ mL} = 0.75\text{ mL}$$

Add 0.75 mL gentamicin and fill the chamber with D_5NS to the total volume of 15 mL.

Step 3   Set the controller to 30 mL/h in order to deliver 15 mL of intermittent IV gentamicin solution in 30 minutes. Resume the regular IV, which will also flush out the tubing. The continuous flow rate will remain at 30 mL/h.

QUICK REVIEW

- Volume control sets have a drop factor of 60 gtt/mL.
- The total volume of the medication, IV dilution fluid, and the IV flush fluid must be considered to calculate flow rates when using volume control sets.
- Use ratio-proportion to calculate flow rates for intermittent medications when a continuous IV rate in mL/h is prescribed.

REVIEW SET 45

Calculate the IV flow rate to administer the following IV medications by using a volume control set, and determine the amount of IV fluid and medication to be added to the chamber. The ordered time includes the flush volume.

1. Order: *Antibiotic X 60 mg IV q.8h in 50 mL $D_5\frac{1}{3}NS$ over 45 min. Flush with 15 mL.*

    Supply: Antibiotic X 60 mg/2 mL

    Flow rate: _____ gtt/min

    Add _____ mL medication and _____ mL IV fluid to the chamber.

2. Order: *Medication Y 75 mg IV q.6h in 60 mL $D_5\frac{1}{4}NS$ over 60 min. Flush with 15 mL.*

    Supply: Medication Y 75 mg/3 mL

    Flow rate: _____ gtt/min

    Add _____ mL medication and _____ mL IV fluid to the chamber.

3. Order: *Antibiotic Z 15 mg IV b.i.d. in 25 mL 0.9% NaCl over 20 min. Flush with 15 mL.*

    Supply: Antibiotic Z 15 mg 3 mL

    Flow rate: _____ gtt/min

    Add _____ mL medication and _____ mL IV fluid to the chamber.

4. Order: *Ancef 0.6 g IV q.12h in 50 mL D_5NS over 60 min on an infusion pump. Flush with 30 mL.*

    Supply: Ancef 1 g/10 mL

    Flow rate: _____ mL/h

    Add _____ mL medication and _____ mL IV fluid to the chamber.

5. Order: *Cleocin 150 mg IV q.8h in 32 mL D$_5$NS over 60 min on an infusion pump. Flush with 28 mL.*

   Supply: Cleocin 150 mg/mL

   Flow rate: _____ mL/h

   Add _____ mL medication and _____ mL IV fluid to the chamber.

   Total IV Volume after 3 doses are given is _____ mL.

Calculate the amount of IV fluid to be added to the volume control chamber.

6. Order: *0.9% NaCl at 50 mL/h for continuous infusion with Ancef 250 mg IV q.8h to be infused over 30 min by volume control set.*

   Supply: Ancef 125 mg/mL

   Add _____ mL medication and _____ mL IV fluid to the chamber.

7. Order: *D$_5$W at 30 mL/h for continuous infusion with Medication X 60 mg q.6h to be infused over 20 min by volume control set.*

   Supply: Medication X 60 mg/2 mL

   Add _____ mL medication and _____ mL IV fluid to the chamber.

8. Order: *D$_5$ 0.225% NaCl IV at 85 mL/h with erythromycin 600 mg IV q.6h to be infused over 40 min by volume control set.*

   Supply: erythromycin 50 mg/mL

   Add _____ mL medication and _____ mL IV fluid to the chamber.

9. Order: *D$_5$ 0.33% NaCl IV at 66 mL/h with Fortaz 720 mg IV q.8h to be infused over 40 min by volume control set.*

   Supply: Fortaz 1 g/10 mL

   Add _____ mL medication and _____ mL IV fluid to the chamber.

10. Order: *D$_5$ 0.45% NaCl IV at 48 mL/h with Vibramycin 75 mg IV q.12h to be infused over 2 h by volume control set.*

    Supply: Vibramycin 100 mg/10 mL

    Add _____ mL medication and _____ mL IV fluid to the chamber.

After completing these problems, see page 522 to check your answers.

PREPARING PEDIATRIC IVs

The physician may order a medication such as potassium chloride (KCl) to be added to each liter of IV fluid for continuous infusion. The volume of the IV solution bag selected for children is usually smaller than that for adults, since the total volume required per 24 hours is less. Therefore, the amount of medication to be added must be adjusted proportionately to the total volume of the IV bag. Use ratio-proportion to determine the appropriate amount of medication to add to the prescribed dilution.

Example:

Order: $D_5 \frac{1}{2}$ NS IV $\bar{c}$ KCl 20 mEq per L to infuse at 30 mL/h

The child's length is 64 cm and weight is 7.2 kg.

1. Should you choose a 1 liter (1000 mL) or 500 mL bag of IV fluid?

    30 mL/$\cancel{h}$ × 24 $\cancel{h}$ = 720 mL

    At the rate of 30 mL/h, the child would receive only 720 mL in 24 hours, so you should choose a 500 mL bag of $D_5 \frac{1}{2}$ NS rather than a 1 liter or 1000 mL bag. Otherwise, the same 1000 mL bag of IV fluid would be infusing for more than 24 hours, which is unsafe.

2. How many mEq of KCl should you add to the 500 mL bag?

    Step 1 Convert $1 \text{ L} = 1000 \text{ mL}$

    Step 2 Think 500 mL is $\frac{1}{2}$ of 1000 mL, so you would need $\frac{1}{2}$ of the 20 mEq of KCl or 10 mEq.

    Step 3 Calculate $\dfrac{20 \text{ mEq}}{1000 \text{ mL}} \quad\rlap{\diagup}{\diagdown}\quad \dfrac{\text{X mEq}}{500 \text{ mL}}$

    $$1000X = 10,000$$

    $$\frac{1000X}{1000} = \frac{10,000}{1000}$$

    $$X = 10 \text{ mEq}$$

3. Potassium chloride is available in 2 mEq per mL. How much KCl should you add to the *500 mL* IV bag? Remember that you will add 10 mEq to 500 mL IV solution.

    Step 1 Convert No conversions are needed.

    Step 2 Think You want to give more than 1 mL. In fact, you want to give 5 times 1 mL or 5 mL.

    Step 3 Calculate $\dfrac{D}{H} \times Q = \dfrac{\overset{5}{\cancel{10} \text{ mEq}}}{\underset{1}{\cancel{2} \text{ mEq}}} \times 1 \text{ mL} = 5 \text{ mL}$

4. How many mEq of potassium chloride would the child receive per hour?

    Total IV volume: 500 mL + 5 mL = 505 mL

    $\dfrac{10 \text{ mEq}}{505 \text{ mL}} \quad\rlap{\diagup}{\diagdown}\quad \dfrac{\text{X mEq}}{30 \text{ mL}}$

    $$505X = 300$$

    $$\frac{500 \text{ X}}{505} = \frac{300}{505}$$

    X = 0.59 mEq or 0.6 mEq of KCl per hour

5. The recommended dosage for children is *up to* 3 mEq/kg/day or 40 mEq/m^2/day. Based on the child's BSA, is the dosage ordered safe?

    First determine the amount of potassium chloride the child will receive per day.

    $$0.6 \text{ mEq/}\cancel{h} \times \frac{24 \cancel{h}}{24 \cancel{h}\backslash\text{day}} = 14.4 \text{ mEq/day}$$

Then determine the child's BSA and how many mEq the child should receive as recommended.

$$\text{BSA (m}^2\text{)} = \sqrt{\frac{\text{ht (cm)} \times \text{wt (kg)}}{3600}} = \sqrt{\frac{64 \times 7.2}{3600}} = \sqrt{\frac{460.8}{3600}} = \sqrt{0.128} = 0.357 \text{ m}^2 = 0.36 \text{ m}^2$$

40 mEq/m²/day × 0.36 m² = 14.4 mEq/day is recommended and 14.4 mEq/day will be infused.

Yes, the dosage ordered is safe. Add 5 mL of KCl 2 mEq/mL to each 500 mL of IV fluid to infuse 0.6 mEq/h or 14.4 mEq/day.

QUICK REVIEW

To determine the drug dosage required to prepare a prescribed dilution:
- use ratio-proportion

REVIEW SET 46

Use the following information to answer questions 1 through 7.

> Order: $D_5W\frac{1}{2}$ NS IV c̄ 20 mEq KCl per L to infuse at 15 mL/h
>
> Supply: 250 mL and 500 mL bags of $D_5W\frac{1}{2}$ NS and KCl 2 mEq/mL
>
> The infant is 18 in long and weighs 5 lb.

1. At the rate ordered, how many mL of IV fluid will this child receive per day? _____ mL/day

2. What volume IV solution bag (250 mL or 500 mL) should you select? _____ mL

   Explain. _____

3. How many mEq of KCl should be added to the 250 mL bag? _____ mEq

4. How many mL of KCl should be added to the 250 mL bag to fill the order? _____ mL

5. How many mEq of KCl would the infant receive per hour? _____ mEq/h

6. How many mEq of KCl would this infant receive per day? _____ mEq/day

7. The recommended dosage of KCl is up to 40 mEq/m²/day.

   Child's BSA: _____ m²

   Recommended maximum daily dosage for this infant: _____ mEq/day

   Is the ordered dosage safe? _____

   If not safe, what should you do? _____

Calculate the ordered medication for each of the following IV bags to achieve the ordered concentration. Supply: KCl 2 mEq/mL

8. Order: Add 10 mEq KCl per L of IV fluid

   Supply: 480 mL IV solution. Add: _____ mEq; _____ mL

9. Order: Add 30 mEq KCl per L of IV fluid

   Supply: 600 mL IV solution. Add: _____ mEq; _____ mL

10. Order: Add 15 mEq KCl per L of IV fluid

    Supply: 850 mL IV solution. Add: _____ mEq; _____ mL

After completing these problems, see page 523 to check your answers.

MINIMAL DILUTIONS FOR IV MEDICATIONS

Intravenous medications in infants and young children (or adults on limited fluids) are often ordered to be given in the smallest volume or *maximal safe concentration* to prevent fluid overload. Consult a pediatric reference, *Hospital Formulary*, or drug insert to assist you in problem solving. These types of medications are usually given via an electronic pump.

Many pediatric IV medications allow a dilution *range* or a minimum and maximum allowable concentration. A solution of *lower* concentration may be given if the patient can tolerate the added volume (called *minimal safe concentration*, *maximal dilution*, or *largest volume*). A solution of *higher* concentration (called *maximal safe concentration*, *minimal dilution*, or *smallest volume*) must not exceed the recommended dilution instructions. Recall that the greater the volume of diluent or solvent, the less concentrated the resulting solution. Likewise, less volume of diluent or solvent results in a more concentrated solution.

> **CAUTION**
>
> An excessively high concentration of an IV drug can cause vein irritation and potentially life-threatening toxic effects. Dilution calculations are critical skills.

Let's examine how to follow the drug reference recommendations for a minimal IV drug dilution, when a minimal and maximal range is given for an IV drug dilution.

> **RULE**
>
> Ratio for recommended drug dilution equals ratio for desired drug dilution.

Example 1:

The physician orders *Vancocin 40 mg IV q.12h* for an infant who weighs 4000 g. What is the minimal amount of IV fluid in which the Vancocin can be safely diluted? The package insert is provided for your reference, Figure 15-5. It states that a "concentration of no more than 10 mg/mL is recommended." This is the *maximal safe concentration*.

$$\frac{10 \text{ mg}}{1 \text{ mL}} \;\diagdown\!\!\!\!\diagup\; \frac{40 \text{ mg}}{X \text{ mL}}$$

$$10X = 40$$

$$\frac{10X}{10} = \frac{40}{10}$$

$X = 4$ mL (This is the minimal amount of IV fluid.)

```
                    8:12                  PA 8289 AMP
                    VIALS
              VANCOCIN® HCl
         STERILE VANCOMYCIN HYDROCHLORIDE, USP
                  INTRAVENOUS


                DOSAGE AND ADMINISTRATION
     A concentration of no more than 10 mg/mL is recommended. An infusion of 10 mg/min or
   less is associated with fewer infusion-related events (see Adverse Reactions).
     Patients With Normal Renal Function
     Adults—The usual daily intravenous dose is 2 g divided either as 500 mg every 6 hours or 1 g
   every 12 hours. Each dose should be administered over a period of at least 60 minutes. Other
   patient factors, such as age or obesity, may call for modification of the usual daily intravenous
   dose.
     Children—The total daily intravenous dosage of Vancocin HCl, calculated on the basis of
   40 mg/kg of body weight, can be divided and incorporated into the child's 24-hour fluid
   requirement. Each dose should be administered over a period of at least 60 minutes.
     Infants and Neonates—In neonates and young infants, the total daily intravenous dosage
   may be lower. In both neonates and infants, an initial dose of 15 mg/kg is suggested, followed
   by 10 mg/kg every 12 hours for neonates in the 1st week of life and every 8 hours thereafter
   up to the age of 1 month. Close monitoring of serum concentrations of vancomycin may be war-
   ranted in these patients.
```

FIGURE 15-5 Portion of Vancocin Package Insert

Example 2:

The physician orders *Claforan 1.2 g IV q.8h* for a child who weighs 36 kg. The recommended safe administration of Claforan for intermittent IV administration is a final concentration of 20 to 60 mg/mL to infuse over 15 to 30 minutes. What is the minimal amount of IV fluid to safely dilute this dosage? (*Remember this represents the **maximal safe concentration.***)

Step 1 Convert $1.2 \text{ g} = 1.2 \times 1000 = 1200 \text{ mg}$

Step 2 Think   1200 is more than 10 times 60, in fact it is 20 times 60. So you need at least 20 mL to dilute the drug.

Step 3 Calculate $\dfrac{60 \text{ mg}}{1 \text{ mL}} \Large\times \normalsize \dfrac{1200 \text{ mg}}{X \text{ mL}}$

$60X = 1200$

$\dfrac{60X}{60} = \dfrac{1200}{60}$

$X = 20 \text{ mL}$ (minimal dilution for maximal safe concentration)

What is the maximal amount of IV fluid recommended to safely dilute this drug to the minimal safe concentration?

Step 1 Convert $1.2 \text{ g} = 1.2 \times 1000 = 1200 \text{ mg}$

Step 2 Think   1200 is more than 50 times 20; in fact, it is 60 times 20. So you can use up to 60 mL to dilute the drug.

Step 3 Calculate $\dfrac{20 \text{ mg}}{1 \text{ mL}} \Large\times \normalsize \dfrac{1200 \text{ mg}}{X \text{ mL}}$

$20X = 1200$

$\dfrac{20X}{20} = \dfrac{1200}{20}$

$X = 60 \text{ mL}$ (maximal dilution for minimal safe concentration)

CALCULATION OF DAILY VOLUME FOR MAINTENANCE FLUIDS

Another common pediatric IV calculation is to calculate 24-hour maintenance IV fluids for children.

RULE

Use this formula to calculate the daily rate of pediatric maintenance IV fluids:
- 100 mL/kg/day for first 10 kg of body weight
- 50 mL/kg/day for next 10 kg of body weight
- 20 mL/kg/day for each kg above 20 kg of body weight

This formula uses the child's weight in kilograms to estimate the 24-hour total fluid need, including oral intake. It does not include replacement for losses, such as diarrhea, vomiting, or fever. This accounts only for fluid needed to maintain normal cellular metabolism and fluid turnover.

Pediatric IV solutions that run over 24 hours usually include a combination of glucose, saline, and potassium chloride and are *hypertonic* solutions (see Figure 14-1, page 325). Dextrose (glucose) for energy is usually concentrated between 5% and 12% for peripheral infusions. Sodium chloride is usually concentrated between 0.225% and 0.9% ($\frac{1}{4}$ NS up to NS). Further, 20 mEq per liter of potassium chloride (20 mEq KCl/L) are usually added to continuous pediatric infusions. Any dextrose and saline combination without potassium should be used only as an intermittent or short-term IV fluid in children. Be wary of isotonic solutions like 5% dextrose in water and 0.9% sodium chloride. They do not contribute enough electrolytes and can quickly lead to water intoxication.

CAUTION

A *red flag* should go up in your mind if either plain 5% dextrose in water or 0.9% sodium chloride (normal saline) are running continuously on an infant or child. Consult the ordering practitioner immediately!

Let's examine the daily rate of maintenance fluids and the hourly flow rate for the children in the following examples.

Example 1:

Child who weighs 6 kg

100 mL/kg/day $\times$ 6 kg = 600 mL/day or per 24h

$\frac{600\ mL}{24\ h}$ = 25 mL/h

Example 2:

Child who weighs 12 kg

100 mL/kg/day $\times$ 10 kg = 1000 mL/day (for first 10 kg)

50 mL/kg/day $\times$ 2 kg = 100 mL/day (for the remaining 2 kg)

Total: 1000 mL/day + 100 mL/day = 1100 mL/day or per 24 h

$\frac{1100\ mL}{24\ h}$ = 45.8 mL/h = 46 mL/h

Example 3:

Child who weighs 24 kg

100 mL/kg/day $\times$ 10 kg = 1000 mL/day (for first 10 kg)

50 mL/kg/day $\times$ 10 kg = 500 mL/day (for next 10 kg)

20 mL/kg/day $\times$ 4 kg = 80 mL/day (for the remaining 4 kg)

Total: 1000 mL/day + 500 mL/day + 80 mL/day = 1580 mL/day or per 24 h

$$\frac{1580 \text{ mL}}{24 \text{ h}} = 65.8 \text{ mL/h} = 66 \text{ mL/h}$$

QUICK REVIEW

- Minimal and maximal dilution volumes for some IV drugs are recommended to prevent fluid overload and to minimize vein irritation and toxic effects.
- The ratio for recommended dilution equals the ratio for desired drug dilution.
- When mixing IV drug solutions,
  - the *smaller* the added volume, the *stronger* or *higher* the resulting *concentration* (minimal dilution).
  - the *larger* the added volume, the *weaker (more dilute)* or *lower* the resulting *concentration* (maximal dilution).
- Daily volume of pediatric maintenance IV fluids based on body weight is:
  - 100 mL/kg/day for first 10 kg.
  - 50 mL/kg/day for next 10 kg.
  - 20 mL/kg/day for each kg above 20.

REVIEW SET 47

1. If a child is receiving chloramphenicol 400 mg IV q.6h and the maximum concentration is 100 mg/mL, what is the minimum volume of fluid in which the medication can be safely diluted? _____ mL

2. If a child is receiving gentamicin 25 mg IV q.8h and the minimal concentration is 1 mg/mL, what is the maximum volume of fluid in which the medication can be safely diluted? _____ mL

3. Calculate the total volume and hourly IV flow rate for a 25 kg child receiving maintenance IV fluids. Infuse _____ mL @ _____ mL/h

4. Calculate the total volume and hourly IV flow rate for a 13 kg child receiving maintenance IV fluids. Infuse _____ mL @ _____ mL/h

5. Calculate the total volume and hourly IV flow rate for a 77 lb child receiving maintenance fluids. Infuse _____ mL @ _____ mL/h

6. Calculate the total volume and hourly IV flow rate for a 3500 g infant receiving maintenance fluids. Infuse _____ mL @ _____ mL/h

7. A child is receiving 350 mg IV of a certain medication, and the minimal and maximal dilution range is 30 to 100 mg/mL. What is the minimum volume (maximal concentration) and the maximum volume (minimal concentration) for safe dilution? _____ mL (minimum volume); _____ mL (maximum volume).

8. A child is receiving 52 mg IV of a certain medication, and the minimal and maximal dilution range is 0.8 to 20 mg/mL. What is the minimum volume and the maximum volume of fluid for safe dilution? _____ mL (minimum volume); _____ mL (maximum volume).

9. A child is receiving 175 mg IV of a certain medication, and the minimal and maximal dilution range is 5 to 75 mg/mL. What is the minimum volume and the maximum volume of fluid for safe dilution? _____ mL (minimum volume); _____ mL (maximum volume).

10. You are making rounds on your pediatric patients and notice that a 2-year-old child who weighs 14 kg has 1000 mL of Normal Saline infusing at the rate of 50 mL/h. You decide to question this order. What is your rationale? _____

_____

After completing these problems, see pages 523–524 to check your answers.

_____

CRITICAL THINKING SKILLS

Let's look at an example in which the nurse *prevents* a medication error by calculating the safe dosage of a medication before administering the drug to a child.

error

Dosage that is too high for a child.

possible scenario

Suppose a physician ordered *KCl 25 mEq IV per 500 mL of* $D_5\frac{1}{2}$ *NS to infuse at the rate of 20 mL/h*. The infant weighs 10.5 lb and is 24 in long. KCl for IV injection is supplied as 2 mEq/mL. The nurse looked up potassium chloride in a drug reference and noted that the safe dosage of potassium chloride is up to 3 mg/kg or 40 mEq/m²/day. The nurse calculated the child's dosage as 14.4 mEq/day based on body weight and 11.2 mEq/day based on BSA.

$10.5 \text{ lb} = \frac{10.5}{2.2} = 4.8 \text{ kg}$

$3 \text{ mEq/kg/day} \times 4.8 \text{ kg} = 14.4 \text{ mEq/day}$

$\text{BSA (m}^2\text{)} = \sqrt{\frac{\text{ht (in)} \times \text{wt (lb)}}{3131}} = \sqrt{\frac{10.5 \times 24}{3131}} = \sqrt{\frac{252}{3131}} = \sqrt{0.08} = 0.283 \text{ m}^2 = 0.28 \text{ m}^2$

$40 \text{ mEq/m}^2\text{/day} \times 0.28 \text{ m}^2 = 11.2 \text{ mEq/day}$

The nurse further calculated that at the rate ordered, the child would receive 480 mL of IV fluid per day, which is a reasonable daily rate of pediatric maintenance IV fluids.

$20 \text{ mL/h} \times \frac{24 \text{ h}}{24 \text{ h day}} = 480 \text{ mL/day}$

Maintenance pediatric IV fluids:
100 mL/kg/day for first 10 kg: 100 mL/kg/day × 4.8 kg = 480 mL/day

But then the nurse calculated that to add 25 mEq KCl to the 500 mL IV bag would require 12.5 mL of KCl 2 mEq/mL.

$\frac{D}{H} \times Q = \frac{25 \text{ mEq}}{2 \text{ mEq}} \times 1 \text{ mL} = 12.5 \text{ mL}$

(continues)

(continued)

The total volume would be 512.5 mL (500 mL IV solution + 12.5 mL KCl) and the child would receive 0.98 or approximately 1 mEq KCl per hour.

$$\frac{25 \text{ mEq}}{512.5 \text{ mL}} \times \frac{X \text{ mEq}}{20 \text{ mL}}$$

$$\frac{512.5 \text{ X}}{512.5} = \frac{500}{512.5}$$

512.5 X = 500

X = 0.975 mEq = 0.98 mEq (approximately 1 mEq per hour)

Finally, the nurse calculated that at this rate the infant would receive 23.5 or 24 mEq/day, which is approximately twice the safe dosage. Therefore, the order is unsafe.

0.98 mEq/h̶r̶ × 24 h̶r̶/day = 23.5 mEq/day (approximately 24 mEq/day)

The nurse notified the physician and questioned the order. The physician responded, "Thank you, you are correct. I intended to order one-half that amount of KCl or 25 mEq per L, which should have been 12.5 mEq per 500 mL. This was my error and I am glad you caught it."

potential outcome

If the nurse had not questioned the order, the infant would have received twice the safe dosage. The baby likely would have developed signs of hyperkalemia that could lead to ventricular fibrillation, muscle weakness progressing to flaccid quadriplegia, respiratory failure, and death.

prevention

In this instance, the nurse prevented a medication error by checking the safe dosage and notifying the physician before administering the infusion. Let this be you!

PRACTICE PROBLEMS—CHAPTER 15

Calculate the volume for one dose of safe dosages. Refer to the BSA formulas or the West Nomogram on the next page as needed to answer questions 1 through 20.

1. Order: *vincristine 2 mg direct IV stat* for a child who weighs 85 pounds and is 50 inches tall.

   Recommended dosage of vincristine for children: 1.5–2 mg/m^2 1 time/week; inject slowly over a period of 1 minute.

   Supply: vincristine 1 mg/mL

   BSA (per formula) of this child: _____ m^2

   Recommended dosage range for this child: _____ mg to _____ mg

   Is the ordered dosage safe? _____

   If safe, give _____ mL/min or _____ mL/15 sec.

   If not, what should you do? _____

2. Use the BSA nomogram to calculate the safe oral dosage and amount to give of mercaptopurine for a child of normal proportions who weighs 25 pounds.

   Recommended dosage: 80 mg/m^2/day once daily p.o.

   Supply: mercaptopurine 50 mg/mL

   BSA: _____ m^2

   Safe dosage: _____ mg

3. Use the BSA nomogram to calculate the safe IV dosage of sargramostim for a 1-year-old child who is 25 inches tall and weighs 20 pounds.

   Recommended dosage: 250 mcg/m²/day once daily IV

   BSA: _____ m²

   Safe dosage: _____ mcg

4. Sargramostim is available in a solution strength of 500 mcg/10 mL. Calculate one dose for the child in question 3.

   Give: _____ mL

5. Use the BSA nomogram to determine the BSA for a child who is 35 inches tall and weighs 40 pounds.

   BSA: _____ m²

Metric:

$$BSA\ (m^2) = \sqrt{\frac{ht\ (cm) \times wt\ (kg)}{3600}}$$

Household:

$$BSA\ (m^2) = \sqrt{\frac{ht\ (in) \times wt\ (lb)}{3131}}$$

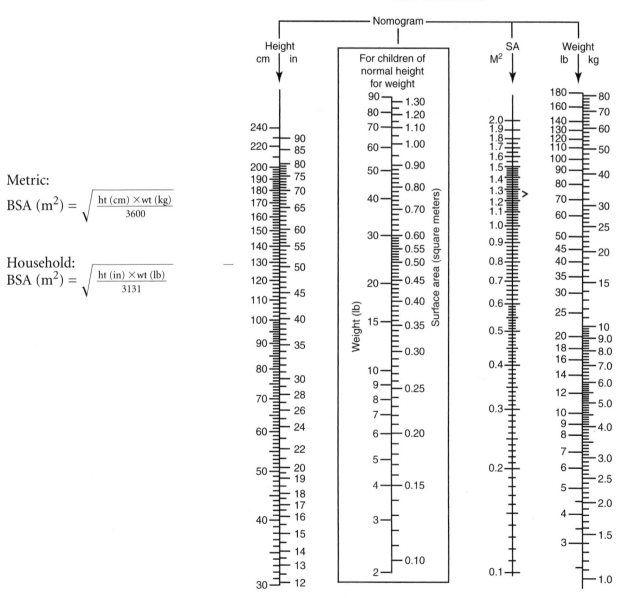

WEST NOMOGRAM

West Nomogram for Estimation of Body Surface Area. (From *Nelson Textbook of Pediatrics* (16th ed) by R. E. Behrman, R. M. Kleigman & H. B. Jenson, 2000, Philadelphia: Saunders. Reprinted with permission.)

6. The child in question 5 will receive levodopa. The recommended oral dosage of levodopa is 0.5 g/m^2. What is the safe dosage for this child?

   Safe dosage: _____ mg

7. Ledvodopa is supplied in 100 mg and 250 mg capsules. Calculate one dose for the child in question 6.

   Give: _____ of the _____ mg capsule(s)

8. Use the BSA nomogram to determine the safe IM dosage of Oncaspar for a child who is 42 inches tall and weighs 45 pounds. The recommended IM dosage is 2500 U/m^2/dose.

   BSA: _____ m^2

   Safe dosage: _____ U

9. Oncaspar is reconstituted to 750 U per 1 mL. Calculate one dose for the child in question 8.

   Give: _____ mL

10. Should the Oncaspar in question 9 be given in one injection? _____

11. A child is 140 cm tall and weighs 43.5 kg. The recommended IV dosage of Adriamycin is 20 mg/m^2. Use the BSA formula to calculate the safe IV dosage of Adriamycin for this child.

    BSA: _____ m^2

    Safe dosage: _____ mg

12. Calculate the dose amount of Adriamycin for the child in question 11.

    Supply: Adriamycin 2 mg/mL

    Give: _____ mL

For questions 13 through 20, use the BSA formulas to calculate the BSA value.

13. Height: 5 ft 6 in   Weight: 136 lb   BSA: _____ m^2

14. Height: 4 ft   Weight: 80 lb   BSA: _____ m^2

15. Height: 60 cm   Weight: 6 kg   BSA: _____ m^2

16. Height: 68 in   Weight: 170 lb   BSA: _____ m^2

17. Height: 164 cm   Weight: 58 kg   BSA: _____ m^2

18. Height: 100 cm   Weight: 17 kg   BSA: _____ m^2

19. Height: 64 in   Weight: 63 kg   BSA: _____ m^2

20. Height: 85 cm   Weight: 11.5 kg   BSA: _____ m^2

21. What is the safe dosage of one dose of interferon alpha-2b required for a child with a BSA of 0.28 m^2 if the recommended dosage is 2 million U/m^2? _____ U

22. What is the safe dosage of calcium EDTA required for an adult with a BSA of 2.17 m^2 if the recommended dosage is 500 mg/m^2? _____ mg or _____ g

23. What is the total daily dosage range of mitomycin required for a child with a BSA of 0.19 m^2 if the recommended dosage range is 10 to 20 mg/m^2/day? _____ to _____ mg/day

24. What is the total safe daily dosage of Thioplex required for a adult with a BSA of 1.34 m^2 if the recommended dosage is 6 mg/m^2/day? _____ mg/day

25. After 5 full days of therapy receiving the recommended dosage, the patient in question 24 will have received a total of _____ mg of Thioplex.

26. Order: *Ancef 0.42 g IV q.12 h in 30 mL D$_5$NS over 30 min by volume control set on an infusion controller. Flush with 15 mL.*

    Supply: Ancef 500 mg/5 mL

    Total IV fluid volume: _____ mL

    Flow rate: _____ mL/h

    Add _____ mL Ancef and _____ mL D$_5$NS to the chamber.

27. After 7 days of IV therapy, the patient referred to in question 26 will have received a total of _____ mL of Ancef.

28. Order: *clindaycin 285 mg IV q.8h in 45 mL D$_5$NS over 60 min by volume control set on an infusion controller. Flush with 15 mL.*

    Supply: clindamycin 75 mg/0.5 mL

    Total IV fluid volume: _____ mL

    Flow rate: _____ mL/h

    Add _____ mL clindamycin and _____ mL D$_5$NS to the chamber.

29. When the patient in item 28 has received 4 days therapy of clindamycin, he will have received a total IV medication volume of _____ mL.

30. Order: *D$_5$ 0.33% NaCl IV at 65 mL/h with erythromycin 500 mg IV q.6h to be infused over 40 min*

    You will use a volume control set and flush with 15 mL.

    Supply: erythromycin 50 mg/mL

    Add _____ mL of erythromycin and _____ mL D$_5$ 0.33% NaCl to the chamber.

31. Order: *D$_5$ 0.45% NaCl IV at 66 mL/h with Fortaz 620 mg IV q.8h to be infused over 40 min*

    You will use a volume control set and flush with 15 mL.

    Supply: Fortaz 0.5 g/5 mL

    Add _____ mL Fortaz and _____ mL D$_5$ 0.45% NaCl to the chamber.

For questions 32 through 34, calculate the ordered medication for each of the following IV bags to achieve the ordered concentration. Supply: KCl 2 mEq/mL

32. Order: *Add 30 mEq KCl per L of IV fluid*

    Supply: 360 mL IV solution   Add: _____ mEq; _____ mL

33. Order: *Add 20 mEq KCl per L of IV fluid*

    Supply: 700 mL IV solution   Add: _____ mEq; _____ mL

34. Order: *Add 15 mEq KCl per L of IV fluid*

    Supply: 250 mL IV solution   Add: _____ mEq; _____ mL

To calculate the daily volume of pediatric maintenance IV fluids, allow:

    100 mL/kg/day for first 10 kg of body weight

    50 mL/kg/day for next 10 kg of body weight

    20 mL/kg/day for each kg of body weight above 20 kg

35. Calculate the total volume and hourly IV flow rate for a 21 kg child receiving maintenance fluids.

    Infuse _____ mL @ _____ mL/h

36. Calculate the total volume and hourly IV flow rate for a 78 lb child receiving maintenance fluids.

    Infuse _____ mL @ _____ mL/h

37. Calculate the total volume and hourly IV flow rate for a 33 lb child receiving maintenance fluids.

    Infuse _____ mL @ _____ mL/h

38. Calculate the total volume and hourly IV flow rate for a 2400 g infant receiving maintenance fluids.

    Infuse _____ mL @ _____ mL/h

For questions 39 through 49, verify the safety of the following pediatric dosages ordered. If the dosage is safe, calculate one dose and the IV volume to infuse one dose.

Order for a child weighing 15 kg:

D_5 0.45% NaCl IV at 53 mL/h $\bar{c}$ ampicillin 275 mg IV q.4h infused over 40 min by volume control set

Recommended dosage: ampicillin 100–125 mg/kg/day in 6 divided doses

Supply: ampicillin 1 g/10 mL

39. Safe daily dosage range for this child: _____ mg/day to _____ mg/day

    Safe single dosage range for this child: _____ mg/dose to _____ mg/dose

    Is the ordered dosage safe? _____ If safe, give _____ mL/dose.

    If not safe, describe your action. _____

40. IV fluid volume to be infused in 40 min: _____ mL

    Add _____ mL ampicillin and _____ mL D_5 0.45% NaCl to the chamber.

Order for a child who weighs 27 lb:

D_5 0.33% NaCl IV at 46 mL/h $\bar{c}$ oxacillin 308 mg IV q.6h to be infused over 30 min by volume control set

Recommended dosage: oxacillan 100 mg/kg/day in 4 divided doses

Supply: oxacillan 500 mg/10 mL

41. Child's weight: _____ kg

    Safe daily dosage for this child: _____ mg/day

    Safe single dosage for this child: _____ mg/dose

    Is the ordered dosage safe? _____ If safe, give _____ mL/dose.

    If not safe, describe your action. _____

42. IV fluid volume to be infused in 30 min: _____ mL

    Add _____ mL oxacillan and _____ mL D_5 0.33% NaCl to the chamber.

Order for a child who weighs 22 kg:

D₅ 0.225% NaCl IV at 50 mL/h c̄ Amikin 165 mg IV q.8h to be infused over 30 min by volume control set

Recommended dosage: Amikin 15–22.5 mg/kg/day in 3 divided doses q.8h

Supply: Amikin 100 mg/2 mL

43. Safe daily dosage range for this child: _____ mg/day to _____ mg/day

    Safe single dosage range for this child: _____ mg/dose to _____ mg/dose

    Is the ordered dosage safe? _____ If safe, give _____ mL/dose.

    If not safe, describe your action. _____

44. IV fluid volume to be infused in 30 min: _____ mL

    Add _____ mL Amikin and _____ mL D₅ 0.225% NaCl to the chamber.

Order for a child who weighs 9 kg:

D₅ 0.33% NaCl IV at 38 mL/h c̄ Ticar 800 mg IV q.4h to be infused over 40 min by volume control set

Recommended dosage: Ticar 200–300 mg/kg/day in 6 divided doses every 4 hours

Supply: Ticar 200 mg/mL

45. Safe daily dosage range for this child: _____ mg/day to _____ mg/day

    Safe single dosage range for this child: _____ mg/dose to _____ mg/dose

    Is the ordered dosage safe? _____ If safe, give _____ mL/dose.

    If not safe, describe your action. _____

46. IV fluid volume to be infused in 40 min: _____ mL

    Add _____ mL Ticar and _____ mL D₅ 0.33% NaCl to the chamber.

Order for a child who weighs 55 lbs:

D₅NS IV at 60 mL/h c̄ penicillin G potassium 525,000 U q.4h to be infused over 20 min by volume control set

Recommended dosage: penicillin G potassium 100,000–250,000 U/kg/day in 6 divided doses q.4h

Supply: penicillin G potassium 200,000 U/mL

47. Child's weight: _____ kg

    Safe daily dosage for this child: _____ U/day to _____ U/day

    Safe single dosage for this child: _____ U/dose to _____ U/dose

48. Is the ordered dosage safe? _____ If safe, give _____ mL/dose.

    If not safe, describe your action. _____

49. IV fluid volume to be infused in 20 min: _____ mL

    Add _____ mL penicillin G potassium and _____ mL D₅NS to the chamber.

50. Critical Thinking Skill: Describe the strategy you would implement to prevent this medication error.

possible scenario

Suppose the physician came to the pediatric oncology unit to administer chemotherapy to a critically ill child whose cancer symptoms had recurred suddenly. The nurse assigned to care for the child was floated from the adult oncology unit and was experienced in administering chemotherapy to adults. The physician, recognizing the nurse, said, "Oh good, you know how to calculate and prepare chemo. Go draw up 2 mg/m^2 of Oncovin for this child so I can get his chemotherapy started quickly." The nurse consulted the child's chart and saw the following weights written on his assessment sheet: 20/.45. No height was recorded.

On the adult unit, that designation means ____X____ kg or ____Y____ lb. The nurse took the West Nomogram and estimated the child's BSA based on his weight of 45 lb to be 0.82 m^2. The nurse calculated 2 mg/m^2 × 0.82 m^2 = 1.64 mg. Oncovin is supplied as 1 mg/1 mL, so the nurse further calculated 1.6 mL was the dose and drew it up in a 3 mL syringe. As the nurse handed the syringe to the physician, the amount looked wrong. The physician asked the nurse how that amount was obtained. When the nurse told the physician the estimated BSA from the child's weight (45 pounds) is 0.82 m^2, and the dosage is 2 mg/m^2 × 0.82 m^2 = 1.64 mg or 1.6 mL, the physician said, "No! This child's *BSA is 0.45 m^2*. I wrote it myself next to his weight—20 pounds." The physician, despite the need to give the medication as soon as possible, took the necessary extra step and examined the amount of medication in the syringe. Though the physician knew and trusted the nurse, the amount of medication in the syringe did not seem right. Perhaps the physician had figured a "ball park" amount of about 1 mL, and the volume the nurse brought in made the physician question what was calculated. The correct dosage calculations are:

$$2 \text{ mg/m}^2 \times 0.45 \text{ m}^2 = 0.9 \text{ mg}$$

$$\frac{D}{H} \times Q = \frac{0.9 \text{ mg}}{1 \text{ mg}} \times 1 \text{ mL} = 0.9 \text{ mL}$$

potential outcome

The child, already critically ill, could have received almost double the amount of medication had the physician rushed to give the dose calculated and prepared by someone else. This excessive amount of medication probably could have caused a fatal overdose. What should have been done to prevent this error?

prevention

_____

_____

After completing these problems, see pages 524-526 to check your answers.

Advanced Adult Intravenous Calculations

OBJECTIVES

Upon mastery of Chapter 16, you will be able to perform advanced adult intravenous calculations and apply these skills to patients across the life span. To accomplish this you will also be able to:

- Calculate and assess safe hourly heparin dosage.
- Calculate heparin IV flow rate.
- Calculate the flow rate and assess safe dosages for critical care IV medications administered over a specified time period.
- Calculate the flow rate for primary IV and IVPB solutions for patients with restricted fluid intake requirements.

Nurses are becoming increasingly more responsible for the administration of intravenous (IV) medications in the critical care areas as well as on general nursing units. Patients in life-threatening situations require thorough and timely interventions that frequently involve specialized, potent drugs. This chapter focuses on advanced adult IV calculations with special requirements that can be applied to patients across the life span.

IV HEPARIN

Heparin is an anticoagulant for the prevention of clot formation. It is measured in USP units (Figure 16-1). Intravenous heparin is frequently ordered in *units per hour (U/h)* and as such should be administered by an electronic infusion device. Because of the potential for hemorrhage or clots with incorrect dosage, careful monitoring of patients receiving heparin is a critical nursing skill. The nurse is responsible for administering the correct dosage and for ensuring that the dosage is safe.

> **CAUTION**
>
> Heparin order, dosage, vial, and amount to give should be checked by another nurse before administering the dose.

Calculating Safe IV Heparin Flow Rate

When IV heparin is ordered in U/h, use $\frac{D}{H} \times Q = R$ or ratio-proportion to calculate the flow rate in mL/h.

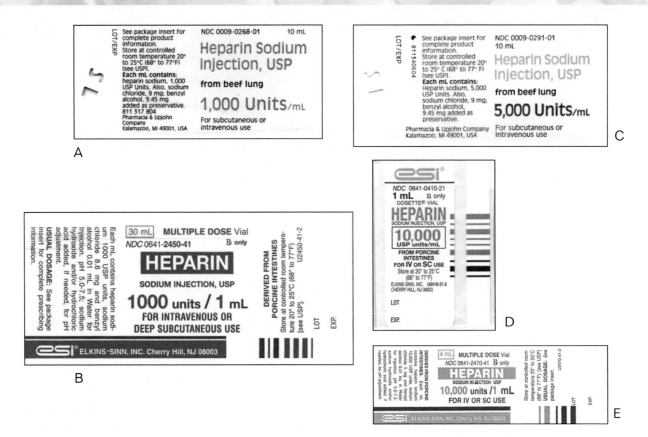

FIGURE 16-1 Various Heparin Dosage Strengths and Container Volumes

---

RULE

To calculate IV heparin flow rate in mL/h:

$$\frac{\text{D (U/h desired)}}{\text{H (U you have on hand)}} \times \text{Q (mL you have on hand)} = \text{R (mL/h)}$$

Or, ratio of supply dosage is equivalent to ratio of desired dosage rate

$$\frac{\text{Supply U}}{\text{Supply mL}} = \frac{\text{Desired U/h}}{\text{X mL/h}}$$

Note: This rule applies to drugs ordered in U/h, mU/h, mg/h, mcg/h, g/h, or mEq/h.

Let's apply the rule to some examples.

Example 1:

Order: D_5W 500 mL $\bar{c}$ heparin 25,000 U IV at 1000 U/h

What is the flow rate in mL/h?

$$\frac{D}{H} \times Q = \frac{1000 \text{ U/h}}{25,000 \text{ U}} \times 500 \text{ mL} = R \text{ (mL/h)}$$

MATH TIP

Units (U) cancel out to leave mL/h in the $\frac{D}{H} \times Q = R$ formula.

$$\frac{1000 \cancel{U}/h}{\underset{50}{\cancel{25,000\ \cancel{U}}}} \times \overset{1}{\cancel{500}} \text{ mL} = \frac{\overset{20}{\cancel{1000}}}{\underset{1}{\cancel{50}}} \text{ mL/h} = 20 \text{ mL/h}$$

Or, use ratio-proportion to calculate the flow rate in mL/h, which will administer 1000 U/h.

$$\frac{25,000 \text{ U}}{500 \text{ mL}} \Large\times\normalsize \frac{1000 \text{ U/h}}{X \text{ mL/h}}$$

$$25,000 \text{ X} = 500,000$$

$$\frac{25,000 \text{ X}}{25,000} = \frac{500,000}{25,000}$$

$$X = 20 \text{ mL/h}$$

Look at the labels in Figure 16-1, representing the various supply dosages of heparin you have available. Often, IV solutions with heparin additive come premixed. But, if you have to mix the solution, what label would you select to prepare the heparin infusion as ordered? The best answer is label E: 4 mL vial of heparin 10,000 U/mL. This is necessary because to add 25,000 U of heparin to 500 mL of IV solution, you would need 2.5 mL of heparin.

$$\frac{D}{H} \times Q = \frac{25,000 \cancel{U}}{10,000 \cancel{U}} \times 1 \text{ mL} = 2.5 \text{ mL}$$

However, notice that you could also select label B and prepare 25 mL of heparin 1000 U/mL, or label C and prepare 5 mL of heparin 5000 U/mL. Labels A and D do not have sufficient volume to fill the dosage required.

Example 2:

Order: D_5W 500 mL $\bar{c}$ heparin 25,000 U IV at 850 U/h

Calculate the flow rate in mL/h.

$$\frac{D}{H} \times Q = \frac{850 \cancel{U}/h}{\underset{50}{\cancel{25,000\ \cancel{U}}}} \times \overset{1}{\cancel{500}} \text{ mL} = \frac{\overset{17}{\cancel{850}}}{\underset{1}{\cancel{50}}} \text{ mL/h} = 17 \text{ mL/h}$$

Or, use ratio-proportion.

$$\frac{25,000 \text{ U}}{500 \text{ mL}} \Large\times\normalsize \frac{850 \text{ U/h}}{X \text{ mL/h}}$$

$$25,000 \text{ X} = 425,000$$

$$\frac{25,000 \text{ X}}{25,000} = \frac{425,000}{25,000}$$

$$X = 17 \text{ mL/h}$$

Example 3:

D_5W 500 mL with heparin 25,000 U IV is currently infusing at 850 U/h, or 17 mL/h. Based on laboratory results, it is determined that the patient's infusion must be increased by 120 U/h, so that it should now be infusing at 970 U/h.

Calculate the flow rate in mL/h.

$$\frac{D}{H} \times Q = \frac{970 \, \cancel{U}/h}{\underset{50}{\cancel{25,000} \, \cancel{U}}} \times \overset{1}{\cancel{500}} \text{ mL} = \frac{970}{50} \text{ mL/h} = 19.4 \text{ mL/h} = 19 \text{ mL/h}$$

Or, use ratio-proportion.

$$\frac{25,000 \text{ U}}{500 \text{ mL}} = \frac{970 \text{ U/h}}{X \text{ mL/h}}$$

$$25,000 \, X = 485,000$$

$$\frac{25,000 \, X}{25,000} = \frac{485,000}{25,000}$$

$$X = 19.4 = 19 \text{ mL/h}$$

You would need to increase the infusion from 17 mL/h (850 U/h) to 19 mL/h (970 U/h).

IV Heparin Protocol

Because patients vary significantly in weight, the intravenous heparin dosage is individualized based on patient weight. Many hospitals have standard protocols related to intravenous heparin administration. Figure 16-2 shows a sample protocol. Note that the bolus or loading dosage and the initial infusion dosage of heparin are based on the patient's weight. Line 10 indicates that for this protocol, the standard heparin bolus dosage is 80 U/kg and the infusion rate is 18 U/kg/h. When the patient's response to heparin therapy changes, as measured by the APTT blood clotting value (activated partial thromboplastin time measured in seconds), the heparin dosage is adjusted as indicated in lines 11–15. These orders in Figure 16-2 are based on patient weight rounded to the nearest 10 kg. Some facilities use the patient's exact weight in kilograms. It is very important to know the protocol for your clinical setting. Let's work through some examples of calculation of heparin dosage based on patient weight and a standardized heparin dosage protocol.

Example 1:

Protocol: *Bolus patient with heparin 80 U/kg body weight and start drip at 18 U/kg/h*

Patient's weight: 110 lb

How many units of heparin should the patient receive?

Step 1   Calculate patient's weight in kilograms. Conversion: 1 kg = 2.2 lb

$$110 \text{ lb} = \frac{110}{2.2} = 50 \text{ kg}$$

Step 2   Calculate the heparin bolus dosage.

$$80 \text{ U/}\cancel{kg} \times 50 \, \cancel{kg} = 4000 \text{ U}$$

This patient should receive 4000 U IV heparin as a bolus.

Standard Weight Based Heparin Protocol

For all patients on heparin drips:

1. Weight in KILOGRAMS. Required for order to be processed: _____ kg
2. Heparin 25,000 U in 250 mL of $\frac{1}{2}$NS. Boluses to be given as 1000 U/mL.
3. APTT q.6h or 6 hours after rate change; q.d. after two consecutive therapeutic APTTs.
4. CBC initially and repeat every _____ days(s).
5. Obtain APTT and PT/INR on day one prior to initiation of therapy.
6. Guaiac stool initially then every _____ day(s) until heparin discontinued. Notify if positive.
7. Neuro checks every _____ hours while on heparin. Notify physician of any changes.
8. D/C APTT and CBC once heparin drip is discontinued, unless otherwise ordered.
9. Notify physician of any bleeding problems.
10. Bolus with 80 U/kg. Start drip at 18 U/kg/h.
11. If APTT is < 35 secs: Rebolus with 80 U/kg and increase rate by 4 U/kg/h
12. If APTT is 36–44 secs: Rebolus with 40 U/kg and increase rate by 2 U/kg/h
13. If APTT is 45–75 secs: Continue current rate
14. If APTT is 76–90 secs: Decrease rate by 2 U/kg/h
15. If APTT is > 90 secs: Hold heparin for 1 hour and decrease rate by 3 U/kg/h

FIGURE 16-2 Sample Orders for Patient on Heparin Therapy

Step 3 Calculate the number of milliliters to administer for the bolus.

Supply: heparin 1000 U/mL, as recommended by the protocol (see line 2, Figure 16-2)

Think: You want to give 4000 U, which is 4 times 1000 U/mL, so you want to give 4 times 1 mL or 4 mL.

$$\frac{D}{H} \times Q = \frac{\overset{4}{\cancel{4000}\ \cancel{U}}}{\underset{1}{\cancel{1000}\ \cancel{U}}} \times 1\ mL = 4\ mL$$

Administer 4 mL of heparin for the bolus.

Step 4 Calculate the infusion rate for the heparin IV drip.

Protocol: *Start drip at 18 U/kg/h* (see line 10, Figure 16-2)

Supply: heparin 25,000 U/250 mL (see line 2, Figure 16-2) or 100 U/mL

18 U/$\cancel{kg}$/h × 50 $\cancel{kg}$ = 900 U/h

Think: You want to administer 9 times 1 mL or 9 mL for the IV heparin infusion.

$$\frac{D}{H} \times Q = \frac{\overset{9}{\cancel{900}\ \cancel{U}/h}}{\underset{1}{\cancel{100}\ \cancel{U}}} \times 1\ mL = 9\ mL/h$$

Example 2:

After 6 hours, the patient in Example 1 has an APTT of 43 secs. According to the protocol, you will *rebolus with 40 U/kg and increase the amount of IV heparin by 2 U/kg/h* (see line 12, Figure 16-2).

Step 1 You already know the patient's weight: 50 kg

Step 2 Calculate the heparin rebolus dosage.

40 U/kg × 50 kg = 2000 U

Step 3 Calculate the number of milliliters to prepare.

Supply: Heparin 1000 U/mL, as recommended by the protocol

Think: You want to give 2 times 1 mL or 2 mL.

$$\frac{D}{H} \times Q = \frac{\overset{2}{\cancel{2000}\ \cancel{U}}}{\underset{1}{\cancel{1000}\ \cancel{U}}} \times 1\ \text{mL} = 2\ \text{mL}$$

Administer 2 mL of heparin for the rebolus.

Step 4 Calculate the number of units the patient's IV heparin will be increased.

2 U/kg/h × 50 kg = 100 U/h

Step 5 Calculate the new infusion rate.

Supply: Heparin 25,000 U/250 mL (see line 2, Figure 16-2) or 100 U/mL

Think: You want to administer 100 U/h and you have 100 U/mL, so you want to increase the infusion by 1 mL/h.

$$\frac{D}{H} \times Q = \frac{\overset{1}{\cancel{100}\ \cancel{U}/h}}{\underset{1}{\cancel{100}\ \cancel{U}}} \times 1\ \text{mL} = 1\ \text{mL/h}$$

9 mL/h + 1 mL/h = 10 mL/h

Reset the infusion rate to 10 mL/h.

QUICK REVIEW

- Use $\frac{D}{H} \times Q = R$ of ratio-proportion to calculate mL/h when you know U/h and U/mL.
- Many hospitals use standard protocols to initiate and maintain heparin therapy.
- The protocols are based on patient weight in kilograms, and adjustments are made based on laboratory results (usually APTT).

REVIEW SET 48

Calculate the flow rate.

1. Order: *1000 mL 0.45% NS c̄ heparin 25,000 U to infuse at 1000 U/h.*

    Flow rate: _____ mL/h

2. Order: *500 mL D₅W IV c̄ heparin 40,000 U to infuse at 1100 U/h.*

    Flow rate: _____ mL/h

3. Order: *500 mL 0.45% NS IV c̄ heparin 25,000 U to infuse at 500 U/h.*

   Flow rate: _____ mL/h

4. Order: *500 mL D₅W IV c̄ heparin 40,000 U to infuse at 1500 U/h.*

   Flow rate: _____ mL/h

5. Order: *1 L D₅W IV c̄ heparin 25,000 U to infuse at 1200 U/h.* On rounds, you assess the patient and observe that the infusion pump is set at 120 mL/h.

   At what rate should the pump be set? _____ mL/h

   What should your action be? _____

6. Order: *500 mL D₅W with heparin 25,000 U to infuse at 800 U/h*

   Flow rate: _____ mL/h

Questions 7 through 10 refer to a patient who weighs 165 lb and has IV heparin ordered per the following Weight Based Heparin Protocol.

Weight Based Heparin Protocol:

Heparin IV infusion: heparin 25,000 U in 250 mL of $\frac{1}{2}$NS

IV Boluses: Use heparin 1000 U/mL

Calculate the patient's weight in kg. Weight: _____ kg

Bolus with heparin 80 U/kg. Then initiate heparin drip at 18 U/kg/h. Obtain APTT every 6 hours and adjust dosage and rate as follows:

If APTT is < 35 seconds: Rebolus with 80 U/kg and increase rate by 4 U/kg/h.

If APTT is 36–44 seconds: Rebolus with 40 U/kg and increase rate by 2 U/kg/h.

If APTT is 45–75 seconds: Continue current rate.

If APTT is 76–90 seconds: Decrease rate by 2 U/kg/h.

If APTT is > 90 seconds: Hold heparin for 1 hour and then decrease rate by 3 U/kg/h.

7. Convert the patient's weight to kg: _____ kg

   Calculate the initial heparin bolus dosage: _____ U

   Calculate the bolus dose: _____ mL

   Calculate the initial heparin infusion rate: _____ U/h or _____ mL/h

8. At 0900, the patient's APTT is 33 seconds. According to the protocol, what will your action be?

   Rebolus with _____ U or _____ mL

   Reset infusion rate to _____ U/h or _____ mL/h

9. At 1500, the patient's APTT is 40 seconds. According to the protocol, what will your action be?

   Rebolus with _____ U or _____ mL

   Reset infusion rate to _____ U/h or _____ mL/h

10. At 2100, the patient's APTT is 60 seconds. What will your action be according to the protocol? _____

The same method can be used to calculate flow rates for other medications ordered at a specified dosage unit per hour. Calculate flow rate for questions 11 through 15.

11. Order: *500 mL 0.9% NaCl IV c̄ Humulin R Regular U-100 insulin 500 U to infuse at 10 U/h.*

    Flow rate: _____ mL/h

12. Order: *1 L D₅W IV c̄ KCl 40 mEq to infuse at 2 mEq/h.*

    Flow rate: _____ mL/h

13. Order: *100 mL D₅W c̄ Cardizem 125 mg to infuse at 5 mg/h*

    Flow rate: _____ mL/h

14. Order: *250 mL NS c̄ Cardizem 125 mg to infuse at 10 mg/h*

    Flow rate: _____ mL/h

15. Order: *500 mL 0.9% NaCl c̄ Humulin R Regular U-100 insulin 300 U to infuse at 5 U/h*

    Flow rate: _____ mL/h

After completing these problems, see pages 526–527 to check your answers.

CRITICAL CARE IV CALCULATIONS: CALCULATING FLOW RATE OF AN IV MEDICATION TO BE GIVEN OVER A SPECIFIED TIME PERIOD

With increasing frequency, medications are ordered for patients in critical care situations as a prescribed amount to be administered in a specified time period, such as *X mg per minute.* Such medications are usually administered by electronic infusion devices, programmed in mL/h. Careful monitoring of patients receiving life-threatening therapies is a critical nursing skill.

IV Medication Ordered "Per Minute"

> **RULE**
>
> To determine the flow rate (mL/h) for IV medications ordered per minute (such as mg/min):
>
> **Step 1**   Calculate the dosage in mL/min:
> $$\frac{D}{H} \times Q = R \text{ (mL/min)}$$
>
> **Step 2**   Calculate the flow rate of the quantity to administer in mL/h:
> mL/min × 60 min/h = mL/h
>
> Note: The order may specify mg/min, mcg/min, g/min, U/min, mU/min, or mEq/min.

In the formula $\frac{D}{H} \times Q = R$ (mL/min):

     D = Dosage *desired:* mg/min

     H = Dosage you *have* available

     Q = *Quantity* of solution you have available

     R = Flow *rate:* mL/min

Example 1:

Order: *lidocaine 2 g IV in 500 mL D₅W at 2 mg/min via infusion pump.* You must prepare and hang 500 mL of D_5W IV solution that has 2 g of lidocaine added to it. Then, you must regulate the flow rate so the patient receives 2 mg of the lidocaine every minute. Determine the flow rate in mL/h.

Step 1 Calculate mL/min.

Apply the formula $\frac{D}{H} \times Q = R$ (mL/min).

D = dosage desired = 2 mg/min

H = dosage you have available = 2 g = 2 × 1000 = 2000 mg

Q = quantity of available solution = 500 mL

$$\frac{D}{H} \times Q = \frac{2 \text{ mg/min}}{2000 \text{ mg}} \times 500 \text{ mL} = R$$

MATH TIP

$\frac{\text{mg/min}}{\text{mg}} \times \text{mL} = \text{mL/min}$ because mg cancel out.

$$\frac{2 \text{ mg/min}}{\underset{4}{\cancel{2000} \text{ mg}}} \times \frac{\overset{1}{\cancel{500} \text{ mL}}}{1} = \frac{2}{4} \text{ mL/min} = 0.5 \text{ mL/min}$$

Step 2 Determine the flow rate (mL/h).

mL/min × 60 min/h = mL/h

0.5 mL/min × 60 min/h = X mL/h

MATH TIP

$\frac{\text{mL}}{\text{min}} \times \frac{\text{min}}{\text{h}} = \text{mL/h}$ because "min" cancel out.

$$\frac{0.5 \text{ mL}}{\text{min}} \times \frac{60 \text{ min}}{\text{h}} = 30 \text{ mL/h}$$

Or, you can use ratio-proportion.

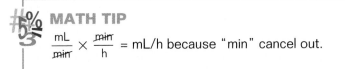

X = 30 mL (per 60 min or 30 mL/h)

MATH TIP

In the original ratio, $\frac{X \text{ mL}}{60 \text{ min}}$ means X mL/60 min or X mL/h.

Regulate the flow rate to 30 mL/h to deliver 2 mg/min of the drug.

Example 2:

Order: *nitroglycerin 125 mg IV in 500 mL D₅W to infuse at 42 mcg/min*

Calculate the flow rate in mL/h to program the infusion pump.

Step 1   Calculate mL/min.

Convert mg to mcg: 1 mg = 1000 mcg; 125 mg = 125 × 1000 = 125,000 mcg

$$\frac{D}{H} \times Q = \frac{42 \text{ mcg/min}}{\underset{250}{125,000 \text{ mcg}}} \times \overset{1}{500} \text{ mL} = \frac{42}{250} \text{ mL/min} = 0.168 \text{ mL/min} = 0.17 \text{ mL/min}$$

Step 2   Calculate mL/h. You know that 1 h = 60 min.

mL/min × 60 min/h = mL/h

0.17 mL/min × 60 min/h = 10.2 mL/h = 10 mL/h

Or, you can use ratio-proportion.

$$\frac{0.17 \text{ mL}}{1 \text{ min}} \diagdown\diagup \frac{X \text{ mL}}{60 \text{ min}}$$

X = 10.2 mL = 10 mL

Rate is 10 mL/60 min or 10 mL/h.

Regulate the flow rate to 10 mL/h to deliver 42 mcg/min of the drug.

IV Medication Ordered "Per Kilogram Per Minute"

The physician may also order the amount of medication in an IV solution that a patient should receive in a specified time period per kilogram of body weight. An electronic infusion device is usually used to administer these orders.

> **RULE**
>
> To calculate flow rate (***mL/h***) for IV medications ordered by weight per minute (such as ***mg/kg/min***):
> **Step 1**   Convert to like units, such as mg to mcg or lb to kg.
> **Step 2**   Calculate desired dosage per minute.
> **Step 3**   Calculate the desired dosage in mL/min: $\frac{D}{H} \times Q = R$ (mL/min).
> **Step 4**   Calculate the flow rate of the quantity to administer in mL/h.
> Note: The order may specify mg/kg/min, mcg/kg/min, g/kg/min, U/kg/min, mU/kg/min, or mEq/kg/min.

Example 1:

Order: *250 mL of IV solution with 225 mg of a medication to infuse at 3 mcg/kg/min via infusion pump* for a person who weighs 110 lb.

Determine the flow rate (mL/h).

Step 1   Convert mg to mcg: 1 mg = 1000 mcg; 225 mg = 225 × 1000 = 225,000 mcg

Convert lb to kg: 1 kg = 2.2 lb; 110 lb = $\frac{110}{2.2}$ = 50 kg

Step 2 Calculate desired mcg/min.

$$3 \text{ mcg/kg/min} \times 50 \text{ kg} = 150 \text{ mcg/min}$$

Step 3 Calculate mL/min.

$$\frac{D}{H} \times Q = \frac{150 \text{ mcg/min}}{\frac{225,000 \text{ mcg}}{900}} \times \overset{1}{250} \text{ mL} = \frac{150}{900} \text{ mL/min} = 0.166 \text{ mL/min} = 0.17 \text{ mL/min}$$

Step 4 Calculate mL/h. You know that 1 h = 60 min.

$$\text{mL/min} \times 60 \text{ min/h} = 0.17 \text{ mL/min} \times 60 \text{ min/h} = 10.2 \text{ mL/h} = 10 \text{ mL/h}$$

Or you can use ratio-proportion.

$$\frac{0.17 \text{ mL}}{1 \text{ min}} \bowtie \frac{X \text{ mL}}{60 \text{ min}}$$

$$X = 10.2 \text{ mL} = 10 \text{ mL}$$

Rate is 10 mL/60 min or 10 mL/h.

Regulate the flow rate to 10 mL/h to deliver 150 mcg/min of the drug.

Titrating IV Drugs

Sometimes IV medications may be ordered to be administered at an initial dosage over a specified time period and then continued at a different dosage and time period. These situations are common in obstetrics and critical care. Medications, such as magnesium sulfate, dopamine, Isuprel, and Pitocin, are ordered to be *titrated* or *regulated* to obtain measurable physiologic responses. Dosages will be adjusted until the desired effect is achieved. In some cases, a loading or bolus dose is infused and monitored closely. Most IV medications that require titration usually start at the lowest dosage and are increased or decreased as needed. An upper titration limit is usually set and is not exceeded unless the desired response is not obtained. A new drug order is then required.

Let's look at some of these situations.

> **RULE**
>
> To calculate flow rate (mL/h) for IV medications ordered over a specific time period (e.g., mg/min):
> **Step 1**   Calculate mg/mL.
> **Step 2**   Calculate mL/h.
> Note: The order may specify mg/min, mcg/min, g/min, U/min, mU/min, or mEq/min; or mg/h, mcg/h, g/h, U/h, mU/h, or mEq/h.

Example 1:

Order: *RL IV 1000 mL c̄ magnesium sulfate 20 g. Start with bolus of 4 g/30 min, then maintain a continuous infusion @ 2 g/h.*

1. What is the flow rate in mL/h for the bolus order?

Step 1 Calculate the bolus dosage in g/mL.

There are 20 g in 1000 mL. How many mL are necessary to infuse 4 g?

Desired = 4 g   Have = 20 g per 1000 mL (Q)

$$\frac{D}{H} \times Q = \frac{4 \text{ g}}{\underset{1}{20 \text{ g}}} \times \overset{50}{1000} \text{ mL} = 200 \text{ mL}$$

Or you can use ratio-proportion.

$$\frac{20\ g}{1000\ mL} \diagdown \frac{4\ g}{X\ mL}$$

$$20X = 4000$$

$$\frac{20\ X}{20} = \frac{4000}{20}$$

$$X = 200\ mL$$

Therefore, 200 mL contain 4 g, to be administered over 30 min.

Step 2   Calculate the bolus rate in mL/h.

What is the flow rate in mL/h to infuse 200 mL (which contain 4 g of magnesium sulfate)? Remember 1 h = 60 min.

$$\frac{Total\ mL}{Total\ min} \times 60\ min/h = \frac{200\ mL}{\overset{}{\underset{1}{30\ min}}} \times \frac{\overset{2}{60\ min}}{1\ h} = 400\ mL/h$$

Or you can use ratio-proportion.

$$\frac{200\ mL}{30\ min} \diagdown \frac{X\ mL}{60\ min}$$

$$30X = 12,000$$

$$\frac{30X}{30} = \frac{12,000}{30}$$

$$X = 400\ mL$$

Rate is 400 mL/60 min or 400 mL/h.

Set the infusion pump at 400 mL/h to deliver the bolus of 4 g/30 min as ordered.

Now calculate the continuous IV rate in mL/h.

2. What is the flow rate in mL/h for the continuous infusion of magnesium sulfate of 2 g/h? You know from the bolus dosage calculation that 200 mL contain 4 g.

Desired = 2 g/h   Have = 4 g per 200 mL (Q)

$$\frac{D}{H} \times Q = \frac{2\ g/h}{\underset{1}{4\ g}} \times \overset{50}{200}\ mL = 100\ mL/h$$

Or you can use ratio-proportion.

$$\frac{4\ g}{200\ mL} \diagdown \frac{2\ g/h}{X\ mL/h}$$

$$4X = 400$$

$$\frac{4X}{4} = \frac{400}{4}$$

$$X = 100\ mL/h$$

After the bolus has infused in the first 30 min, reset the infusion pump to 100 mL/h to deliver the continuous infusion of 2 g/h.

Let's look at an example using Pitocin (a drug used to induce or augment labor), measured in units and milliunits.

Example 2:

A drug order is written to induce labor: *LR 1000 mL IV c̄ Pitocin 20 U. Begin a continuous infusion IV @ 1 mU/min, increase by 1 mU/min q.15–30 min to a maximum of 20 mU/min.*

1. What is the flow rate in mL/h to deliver 1 mU/min?

In this example, the medication is measured in units (instead of g or mg).

Step 1 Calculate mU/mL.

Convert: $1U = 1000$ mU; 20 U $= 20 \times 1000 = 20,000$ mU

Desired $= 1$ mU   Have $= 20,000$ mU per 1000 mL (Q)

$$\frac{D}{H} \times Q = \frac{1\ \cancel{mU}}{\underset{20}{\cancel{20,000\ mU}}} \times \overset{1}{\cancel{1000}}\ mL = \frac{1}{20}\ mL = 0.05\ mL$$

Or you can use ratio-proportion.

$$\frac{20,000\ mU}{1000\ mL} \bowtie \frac{1\ mU}{X\ mL}$$

$20,000X = 1000$

$$\frac{20,000X}{20,000} = \frac{1000}{20,000}$$

$X = 0.05$ mL

Therefore, 0.05 mL contains 1 mU of Pitocin, or there is 1 mU/0.05 mL.

Step 2 Calculate mL/h.

What is the flow rate in mL/h to infuse 0.05 mL/min (which is 1 mU Pitocin/min)?

$$\frac{Total\ mL}{Total\ min} \times 60\ min/h = \frac{0.05\ mL}{1\ \cancel{min}} \times \frac{60\ \cancel{min}}{1\ h} = 3\ mL/h$$

Or you can use ratio-proportion.

$$\frac{0.05\ mL}{1\ min} \bowtie \frac{X\ mL}{60\ min}$$

$X = 3$ mL

Rate is 3 mL/60 min or 3 mL/h.

Set the infusion pump at 3 mL/h to infuse Pitocin 1 mU/min as ordered.

2. What is the maximum flow rate in mL/h that the Pitocin infusion can be set for the titration as ordered? Notice that the order allows a maximum of 20 mU/min. You know from the bolus dosage calculation that there is 1 mU per 0.05 mL.

Desired $= 20$ mU/min   Have $= 1$ mU per 0.05 mL (Q)

$$\frac{D}{H} \times Q = \frac{20\ \cancel{mU}/min}{1\ \cancel{mU}} \times 0.05\ mL = 1\ mL/min$$

Now convert mL/min to mL/h, so you can program the electronic infusion device.

mL/min $\times$ 60 min/h $= 1$ mL/$\cancel{min} \times 60\ \cancel{min}$/h $= 60$ mL/h

Or you can use ratio-proportion.

You know that 1 mU/min is infused at 3 mL/h.

$$\frac{3 \text{ mL/h}}{1 \text{ mU/min}} \bowtie \frac{X \text{ mL/h}}{20 \text{ mU/min}}$$

X = 60 mL/h

Rate of 60 mL/h will deliver 20 mU/min.

Verifying Safe IV Medication Dosage Recommended "Per Minute"

It is also a critical nursing skill to be sure that patients are receiving safe dosages of medications. Therefore, you must also be able to convert critical care IVs with additive medications to **mg/h** or **mg/min** to check safe or normal dosage ranges.

> **RULE**
>
> To check safe dosage of IV medications ordered in mL/h:
> **Step 1**   Calculate mg/h.
> **Step 2**   Calculate mg/min.
> **Step 3**   Compare recommended dosage and ordered dosage to decide if the dosage is safe.
> Note: The ordered and recommended dosages may specify mg/min, mcg/min, g/min, U/min, mU/min, or mEq/min.

Example:

The *Hospital Formulary* states that the recommended dosage of lidocaine is 1–4 mg/min. The patient has an order for *500 mL D$_5$W IV c̄ lidocaine 1 g to infuse at 30 mL/h*. Is the lidocaine dosage within the safe range?

Step 1 Calculate mg/h.

Convert: 1 g = 1000 mg

Desired = Unknown X mg/h   Have = 1000 mg per 500 mL (Q)

$$\frac{D}{H} \times Q = \frac{X \text{ mg/h}}{\underset{2}{\cancel{1000} \text{ mg}}} \times \overset{1}{\cancel{500}} \text{ mL} = 30 \text{ mL/h}$$

$$\frac{X}{2} = 30$$

$$\frac{X}{2} \bowtie \frac{30}{1}$$

X = 60 mg/h (You know the answer is in mg/h because "X" is measured in mg/h.)

Or you can use ratio-proportion.

$$\frac{1000 \text{ mg}}{500 \text{ mL}} \bowtie \frac{X \text{ mg/h}}{30 \text{ mL/h}}$$

500X = 30,000

$$\frac{500X}{500} = \frac{30,000}{500}$$

X = 60 mg/h   60 mg are administered in one hour when the flow rate is 30 mL/h.

Step 2 Calculate mg/min. THINK: It is obvious that 60 mg/h is the same as 60 mg/60 min or 1 mg/1 min.

$$1 \text{ h} = 60 \text{ min}$$

$$\frac{\text{mg/h}}{60 \text{ min/h}} = \text{mg/min}$$

$$\frac{\overset{1}{\cancel{60} \text{ mg/\cancel{h}}}}{\underset{1}{\cancel{60} \text{ min/\cancel{h}}}} = 1 \text{ mg/min}$$

Or you can use ratio-proportion.

$$\frac{60 \text{ mg}}{60 \text{ min}} \bowtie \frac{\text{X mg}}{1 \text{ min}}$$

$$60X = 60$$

$$\frac{60X}{60} = \frac{60}{60}$$

$$X = 1 \text{ mg}$$

Rate is 1 mg/min.

Step 3 Compare ordered and recommended dosages.

1 mg/min is within the safe range of 1 to 4 mg/min. The dosage is safe.

Likewise, IV medications ordered as mL/h and recommended in mg/kg/min require verification of their safety or normal dosage range.

RULE

To check safe dosage of IV medications recommended in mg/kg/min and ordered in mL/h:
Step 1 Convert to like units, such as mg to mcg or lb to kg.
Step 2 Calculate recommended mg/min.
Step 3 Calculate ordered mg/h.
Step 4 Calculate ordered mg/min.
Step 5 Compare ordered and recommended dosages. Decide if the dosage is safe.
Note: The ordered and recommended dosages may specify mg/kg/min, mcg/kg/min, g/kg/min, U/kg/min, mU/kg/min, or mEq/kg/min.

Example:

The recommended dosage range of Nitropress for adults is 0.3–10 mcg/kg/min. The patient has an order for *100 mL D$_5$W IV with Nitropress 420 mg to infuse at 1 mL/h*. The patient weighs 154 lb. Is the Nitropress dosage within the normal range?

Step 1 Convert lb to kg: $154 \text{ lb} = \frac{154}{2.2} = 70 \text{ kg}$

Convert mg to mcg: $420 \text{ mg} = 420 \times 1000 = 420,000 \text{ mcg}$

Step 2 Calculate recommended mcg/min range.

$$0.3 \text{ mcg/\cancel{kg}/min} \times 70 \text{ \cancel{kg}} = 21 \text{ mcg/min } \textit{minimum}$$

$$10 \text{ mcg/\cancel{kg}/min} \times 70 \text{ \cancel{kg}} = 700 \text{ mcg/min } \textit{maximum}$$

Step 3   Calculate ordered mcg/h.

Desired = Unknown X mcg/h   Have = 42,000 mcg per 100 mL (Q)

$$\frac{D}{H} \times Q = Rate$$

$$\frac{X \text{ mcg/h}}{\underset{420}{\cancel{42,000} \text{ mcg}}} \times \overset{1}{\cancel{100}} \text{ mL} = 1 \text{ mL/h}$$

$$\frac{X}{420} = 1$$

$$\frac{X}{420} \diagdown \frac{1}{1}$$

X = 420 mcg/h (You know the answer is in mcg/h because "X" is measured in mcg/h.)

Or you can use ratio-proportion.

$$\frac{420,000 \text{ mcg}}{100 \text{ mL}} \diagdown \frac{X \text{ mcg/h}}{1 \text{ mL/h}}$$

$$100 \text{ X} = 420,000$$

$$\frac{100 \text{ X}}{100} = \frac{420,000}{100}$$

X = 4200 mcg/h

Step 4   Calculate ordered mcg/min: 4200 mcg/h = 4200 mcg/60 min

$$\frac{4200 \text{ mcg}}{60 \text{ min}} = 70 \text{ mcg/min}$$

Step 5   Compare ordered and recommended dosages. Decide if the dosage is safe. 70 mcg/min is within the allowable range of 21 to 700 mcg/min. The ordered dosage is safe.

QUICK REVIEW

■ For IV medications ordered in mg/min:
  Step 1   Calculate mL/min, and then
  Step 2   Calculate mL/h.
■ To check safe dosages of IV medications recommended in mg/min and ordered in mL/h:
  Step 1   Calculate mg/h.
  Step 2   Calculate mg/min.
  Step 3   Compare recommended and ordered dosages. Decide if the dosage is safe.
■ To check safe dosage of IV medications recommended in mg/kg/min and ordered in mL/h:
  Step 1   Convert to like units, such as mg to mcg or lb to kg.
  Step 2   Calculate recommended mg/min.
  Step 3   Calculate ordered mg/h.
  Step 4   Calculate ordered mg/min.
  Step 5   Compare ordered and recommended dosages. Decide if the dosage is safe.

REVIEW SET 49

Compute the flow rate for each of these medications administered by infusion pump.

1. Order: *lidocaine 2 g IV per 1000 mL D$_5$W at 4 mg/min*

   Rate: _____ mL/min and _____ mL/h

2. Order: *Pronestyl 0.5 g IV per 250 mL D$_5$W at 2 mg/min*

   Rate: _____ mL/min and _____ mL/h

3. Order: *Isuprel 2 mg IV per 500 cc D$_5$W at 6 mcg/min*

   Rate: _____ mL/min and _____ mL/h

4. Order: *Medication "X" 450 mg IV per 500 mL NS at 4 mcg/kg/min*

   Weight: 198 lb

   Weight: _____ kg   Give: _____ mcg/min

   Rate: _____ mL/min and _____ mL/h

5. Order: *dopamine 800 mg in 500 mL NS IV at 15 mcg/kg/min*

   Weight: 70 kg

   Give: _____ mcg/min

   Rate: _____ mL/min and _____ mL/h

Refer to this order for questions 6 through 8.

Order: *500 mL D$_5$W IV c̄ Dobutrex 500 mg to infuse at 15 mL/h.* The patient weighs 125 lb.
Recommended range: 2.5–10 mcg/kg/min

6. What mcg/min range of Dobutrex should this patient receive?
   _____ to _____ mcg/min

7. What mg/min range of Dobutrex should this patient receive?
   _____ to _____ mg/min

8. Is the Dobutrex as ordered within the safe range? _____

Refer to this order for questions 9 and 10.

Order: *500 mL D$_5$W IV c̄ Pronestyl 2 g to infuse at 60 mL/h.* Normal range: 2–6 mg/min

9. How many mg/min of Pronestyl is the patient receiving? _____ mg/min

10. Is the dosage of Pronestyl within the normal range? _____

11. Order: *magnesium sulfate 20 g in LR 500 mL. Start with a bolus of 2 g to infuse over 30 min. Then maintain a continuous infusion at 1 g/h.*

    Rate: _____ mL/h for bolus

              _____ mL/h for continuous infusion

12. A drug order is written to induce labor as follows:

    Pitocin 15 U in LR 250 mL. Begin a continuous infusion at the rate of 1 mU/min.

    Rate: _____ mL/h

Refer to this order for questions 13 through 15.

Order: *1000 mL of D$_5$W IV with Brethine 10 mg to infuse at 150 mL/h.*

Normal dosage range: 10–80 mcg/min

13. How many mg/min of Brethine is the patient receiving? _____ mg/min

14. How many mcg/min of Brethine is the patient receiving? _____ mcg/min

15. Is the dosage of Brethine within the normal range? _____

After completing these problems, see pages 527–528 to check your answers.

LIMITING INFUSION VOLUMES

Calculating IV rates to include the IV PB volume may be necessary to limit the total volume of IV fluid a patient receives. To do this, you must calculate the flow rate for both the regular IV and the piggyback IV. In such instances of restricted fluids, the piggyback IVs are to be included as part of the total prescribed IV volume and time.

> ## RULE
>
> Follow these six steps to calculate the flow rate of an IV, which includes IV PB. Calculate:
>
> **Step 1**   *IV PB flow rate:* $\frac{V}{T} \times C = R$
>
> or use $\frac{mL/h}{\text{Drop factor constant}} = R$
>
> **Step 2**   *Total IV PB time:*   Time for one dose $\times$ # of doses in 24 h
> **Step 3**   *Total IV PB volume:*   Volume of one dose $\times$ # of doses in 24 h
> **Step 4**   *Total regular IV volume:*   Total volume – IV PB volume = Regular IV volume
> **Step 5**   *Total regular IV time:*   Total time – IV PB time = Regular IV time
> **Step 6**   *Regular IV flow rate:* $\frac{V}{T} \times C = R$
>
> or use $\frac{mL/h}{\text{Drop factor constant}} = R$

Example 1:

Order: *3000 mL D$_5$LR for 24 h with Kefzol 1 g IV PB/100 mL D$_5$W q.6h to run 1 hour. Limit total fluids to 3000 mL q.d.*

The drop factor is 10 gtt/mL.

NOTE: The order intends that the patient will receive a maximum of 3000 mL in 24 hours. Remember, when fluids are restricted, the piggybacks are to be *included* in the total 24-hour intake, not added to it.

Step 1   Calculate the flow rate of the IV PB.

$$\frac{V}{T} \times C = \frac{100 \text{ mL}}{\underset{6}{60 \text{ min}}} \times \overset{1}{10} \text{ gtt/mL} = \frac{100 \text{ gtt}}{6 \text{ min}} = 16.6 \text{ gtt/min} = 17 \text{ gtt/min}$$

or $\frac{mL/h}{\text{Drop factor constant}}$ = gtt/min (Drop factor constant is 6.)

$\frac{100 \text{ mL/h}}{6} = 16.6$ gtt/min = 17 gtt/min

Set the flow rate for the IV PB at 17 gtt/min to infuse 1 g Kefzol in 100 mL over one hour or 60 min.

Step 2   Calculate the total time the IV PB will be administered.

q.6h = 4 times/24 h; 4 $\times$ 1 h = 4 h

Step 3   Calculate the total volume of the IV PB.

100 mL $\times$ 4 = 400 mL IV PB per 24 hours.

Step 4   Calculate the volume of the regular IV fluids to be administered between IV PB. Total volume of regular IV minus total volume of IV PB: 3000 mL – 400 mL = 2600 mL.

Step 5   Calculate the total regular IV fluid time or the time between IV PB. Total IV time minus total IV PB time: 24 h – 4 h = 20 h

Step 6 Calculate the flow rate of the regular IV.

$$mL/h = \frac{2600 \text{ mL}}{20 \text{ h}} = 130 \text{ mL/h}$$

$$\frac{V}{T} \times C = \frac{130 \text{ mL}}{\frac{60 \text{ min}}{6}} \times \frac{1}{10} \text{ gtt/mL} = \frac{130 \text{ gtt}}{6 \text{ min}} = 21.6 \text{ gtt/min} = 22 \text{ gtt/min}$$

or $\frac{mL/h}{\text{Drop factor constant}} = \text{gtt/min}$ (Drop factor constant is 6.)

$$\frac{130 \text{ mL/h}}{6} = 21.6 \text{ gtt/min} = 22 \text{ gtt/min}$$

Set the regular IV of D_5LR at the flow rate of 22 gtt/min. Then after 5 hours, switch to the Kefzol IV PB at the flow rate of 17 gtt/min for one hour. Repeat this process 4 times in 24 hours.

Example 2:

Order: *2000 mL NS IV for 24 h with 80 mg gentamycin in 80 mL IV PB q.8h to run for 30 min. Limit fluid intake to 2000 mL q.d.*

Drop factor: 15 gtt/mL

Calculate the flow rate for the regular IV and for the IV PB.

Step 1 IV PB flow rate:

$$\frac{V}{T} \times C = \frac{80 \text{ mL}}{\frac{30 \text{ min}}{2}} \times \frac{1}{15} \text{ gtt/mL} = \frac{80 \text{ gtt}}{2 \text{ min}} = 40 \text{ gtt/min}$$

Step 2 Total IV PB time: q.8h = 3 times/24 h; $3 \times 30 \text{ min} = 90 \text{ min} = \frac{90}{60} = 1\frac{1}{2} \text{ h}$

Step 3 Total IV PB volume: $80 \text{ mL} \times 3 = 240 \text{ mL}$

Step 4 Total regular IV volume: $2000 \text{ mL} - 240 \text{ mL} = 1760 \text{ mL}$

Step 5 Total regular IV time: $24 \text{ h} - 1\frac{1}{2} \text{ h} = 22\frac{1}{2} \text{ h} = 22.5 \text{ h}$

Step 6 Regular IV flow rate:

$$mL/h = \frac{1760 \text{ mL}}{22.5 \text{ h}} = 78.2 = 78 \text{ mL/h}$$

$$\frac{V}{T} \times C = \frac{78 \text{ mL}}{\frac{60 \text{ min}}{4}} \times \frac{1}{15} \text{ gtt/mL} = \frac{78 \text{ gtt}}{4 \text{ min}} = 19.5 \text{ gtt/min} = 20 \text{ gtt/min}$$

or $\frac{mL/h}{\text{Drop factor constant}} = R$ (Drop factor constant is 4.)

$$\frac{78 \text{ mL/h}}{4} = 19.5 \text{ gtt/min} = 20 \text{ gtt/min}$$

Set the regular IV of NS at the flow rate of 20 gtt/min. After $7\frac{1}{2}$ hours, switch to the gentamycin IV PB at the flow rate of 40 gtt/min for 30 minutes. Repeat this process 3 times in 24 hours.

Patients receiving a primary IV at a specific rate via an infusion controller or pump may require that the infusion rate be altered when a secondary (piggyback) medication is being administered. To do this, calculate the flow rate of the secondary medication in mL/h as you would for the primary IV, and reset the infusion device.

Some infusion controllers or pumps allow you to set the flow rate for the secondary IV independent of the primary IV. Upon completion of the secondary infusion, the infusion device automatically returns to the original flow rate. If this is not the case, be sure to manually readjust the primary flow rate after the completion of the secondary set.

QUICK REVIEW

■ To calculate the flow rate of a regular IV with an IV PB and restricted fluids, calculate:
Step 1   IV PB flow rate
Step 2   Total IV PB time
Step 3   Total IV PB volume
Step 4   Total regular IV volume
Step 5   Total regular IV time
Step 6   Regular IV flow rate

REVIEW SET 50

Calculate the flow rates for the IV and IV PB orders. These patients are on limited fluid volume (restricted fluids).

1. Orders: *3000 mL NS IV for 24 h*

   Limit total IV fluids to 3000 mL q.d.

   penicillin G 1,000,000 U IV PB q.4h in 100 mL NS to run for 30 min

   Drop factor: 10 gtt/mL

   IV PB flow rate: _____ gtt/min

   IV flow rate: _____ gtt/min

2. Orders: *1000 mL D$_5$W IV for 24 h*

   Limit total IV fluids to 1000 mL q.d.

   Garamycin 40 mg q.i.d. in 40 mL IV PB to run 1 h

   Drop factor: 60 gtt/mL

   IV PB flow rate: _____ gtt/min

   IV flow rate: _____ gtt/min

3. Orders: *3000 mL D$_5$ LR IV for 24 h*

   Limit total IV fluids to 3000 mL q.d.

   ampicillin 0.5 g q.6h IV PB in 50 mL D$_5$W to run 30 min

   Drop factor: 15 gtt/mL

   IV PB flow rate: _____ gtt/min

   IV flow rate: _____ gtt/min

4. Orders: 2000 mL $\frac{1}{2}$ NS IV for 24 h

   Limit total IV fluids to 2000 mL q.d.

   Chloromycetin 500 mg/50 mL NS IV PB q.6h to run 1 h

   Drop factor: 60 gtt/mL

   IV PB flow rate: _____ gtt/min

   IV flow rate: _____ gtt/min

5. Orders: 1000 mL LR IV for 24 h

   Limit total IV fluids to 1000 mL q.d.

   Kefzol 250 mg IV PB/50 mL D_5W q.8h to run 1 h

   Drop factor: 60 gtt/mL

   IV PB flow rate: _____ gtt/min

   IV flow rate: _____ gtt/min

6. Orders: 2400 cc of D_5 LR for 24 h

   Limit total IV fluids to 2400 mL q.d.

   Ancef 1 g IV PB q.6h in 50 cc D_5W to run 30 min

   Drop factor: On infusion pump

   IV PB flow rate: _____ mL/h

   IV flow rate: _____ mL/h

7. Orders: 2000 cc NS for 24 h

   Limit total IV fluids to 2000 mL q.d.

   Garamycin 100 mg IV PB q.8h in 100 cc D_5W to run in over 30 min

   Drop factor: On infusion controller

   IV PB flow rate: _____ mL/h

   IV flow rate: _____ mL/h

8. Orders: 3000 cc D_5 0.45% NS to run 24 h

   Limit total IV fluids to 3000 mL q.d.

   Zantac 50 mg q.6h in 50 cc D_5W to infuse 15 min

   Drop factor: On infusion controller

   IV PB flow rate: _____ mL/h

   IV flow rate: _____ mL/h

9. Orders: 1500 cc D_5 NS to run 24 h

   Limit total IV fluids to 1500 mL q.d.

   Kefzol 500 mg IV PB/50 mL D_5W q.8 h to run 1 h

   Drop factor: 20 gtt/mL

   IV PB flow rate: _____ gtt/min

   IV flow rate: _____ gtt/min

10. Orders: *2700 cc NS IV for 24 h*

    Limit total IV fluids to 2700 mL q.d.

    gentamycin 60 mg in 60 mL D$_5$W IV PB q.8h to run for 30 min

Drop factor: On infusion pump

IV PB flow rate: _____ mL/h

IV flow rate: _____ mL/h

After completing these problems, see pages 528–530 to check your answers.

CRITICAL THINKING SKILLS

The importance of knowing the therapeutic dosage of a given medication is a critical nursing skill. Let's look at an example in which the order was unclear, and the nurse did not verify the order with the appropriate person.

error

Failing to clarify an order.

possible scenario

Suppose the physician ordered a heparin infusion for a patient with thrombophlebitis who weighs 100 kg. The facility uses the Standard Weight Based Heparin Protocol as seen in Figure 16-2, page 405. The order was written this way:

heparin 25,000 U in 250 mL $\frac{1}{2}$ NS at 18000/h.

The order was difficult to read and the nurse asked a co-worker to help her decipher it. They both agreed that it read 18,000 units per hour. The nurse calculated mL/h to be:

$$\frac{18,000 \text{ U}}{25,000 \text{ U}} \times 250 \text{ mL} = 180 \text{ mL/h}$$

She proceeded to start the heparin drip at 180 mL/h. The patient's APTT prior to initiation of the infusion was 37 seconds. Six hours into the infusion, an APTT was drawn according to protocol. The nurse was shocked when the results returned and were 95 seconds, which is abnormally high. She called the physician, who asked, "What is the rate of the heparin drip?" The nurse replied, "I have the infusion set at 180 mL/h so the patient receives the prescribed amount of 18,000 units per hour." The physician was astonished and replied, "I ordered the drip at 1800 units per hour, not 18,000 units per hour."

potential outcome

The physician would likely have discontinued the heparin; ordered protamine sulfate, the antidote for heparin overdosage; and obtained another APTT. The patient may have started to show signs of abnormal bleeding, such as blood in the urine, bloody nose, and increased tendency to bruise.

prevention

When the physician wrote the order for 1800 U/h, the U looked like an 0 and the nurse misinterpreted the order as 18,000. The nurse missed three opportunities to prevent this error. The order as written is unclear, unsafe, and incomplete. Contacting the physician and requesting a clarification of the order are appropriate actions for several reasons. First, the writing is unclear, which is an automatic caution to contact the prescribing practitioner for clarification. Guessing about the exact meaning of an order is dangerous, as this scenario demonstrates.

(continues)

(continued)

Second, the Standard Weight Based Heparin Protocol recommends a safe heparin infusion rate of 1800 U/h or 18 mL/h (with a supply dosage of 25,000 U/250 mL = 100 U/mL) for an individual weighing 100 kg. It is the responsibility of the individual administering a medication to be sure the Six Rights of medication administration are observed. The first three Rights state that the "*right* patient must receive the *right* drug in the *right* amount." The order of 18,000 U as understood by the nurse was unsafe. The patient was overdosed by 10 times the recommended amount of heparin.

Third, if the nurse clearly interpreted the order as 18,000, then no units were specified, which is a medication error that requires contact with the physician for correction. An incomplete order must not be filled.

PRACTICE PROBLEMS—CHAPTER 16

You are working on the day shift 0700–1500 hours. You observe that one of the patients assigned to you has an intravenous infusion with a volume control set. His orders include:

D₅W IV @ 50 mL/h for continuous infusion

Pipracil 1 g IV q.6h

The pharmacy supplies the Pipracil in a prefilled syringe labeled *1 g per 5 mL* with instructions to "add Pipracil to volume control set, and infuse over 30 minutes." Answer questions 1 through 5.

1. What is the drop factor of the volume control set? _____ gtt/mL

2. What amount of Pipracil will you add to the chamber? _____ mL

3. How much D₅W IV fluid will you add to the chamber with the Pipracil? _____ mL

4. To maintain the flow rate at 50 mL/h, you will time the IV Pipracil to infuse at _____ gtt/min.

5. The medication administration record indicates that the patient received his last dose of IV Pipracil at 0600. How many doses of Pipracil will you administer during your shift? _____

6. Order: *heparin 25,000 U in 250 mL 0.45% NS to infuse at 1200 U/h*

   Drop factor: On infusion controller

   Flow rate: _____ mL/h.

7. Order: *thiamine 100 mg per L D₅W IV to infuse at 5 mg/h*

   Drop factor: On infusion pump

   Flow rate: _____ mL/h

8. Order: *magnesium sulfate 4 g in 500 mL D₅W at 500 mg/h*

   Drop factor: On infusion pump

   Flow rate: _____ mL/h

9. A patient is to receive *D₅W 500 mL c̄ heparin 20,000 U at 1400 U/h.*

   Set the infusion pump at _____ mL/h.

10. At the rate of 4 mL/min, how long will it take to administer 1.5 L of IV fluid? _____ h and _____ min

11. Order: *lidocaine drip IV to run @ 4 mg/min*

    Supply: 500 mL D$_5$W with Lidocaine 2 g added

    Drop factor: On infusion pump

    Flow rate: _____ mL/h

12. Order: *Xylocaine 1 g IV in 250 mL D$_5$W at 3 mg/min*

    Drop factor: On infusion controller

    Flow rate: _____ mL/h

13. Order: *procainamide 1 g in 500 cc D$_5$W to infuse at 2 mg/min*

    Drop factor: On infusion pump

    Flow rate: _____ mL/h

14. Order: *dobutamine 250 mg in 250 cc D$_5$W to infuse at 5 mcg/kg/min*

    Weight: 80 kg

    Drop factor: On infusion controller

    Flow rate: _____ mL/h

15. Your patient has *1 L D$_5$W with 2 g lidocaine added infusing at 75 mL/h.* The recommended continuous IV dosage of Lidocaine is 1–4 mg/min. Is this dosage safe? _____

16. Order: *Restricted fluids: 3000 mL D$_5$ NS IV for 24 h*

    Chloromycetin 1 g IV PB in 100 mL NS q.6h to run 1 h

    Drop factor: 10 gtt/mL

    Flow rate: _____ gtt/min IV PB and _____ gtt/min primary IV

17. Order: *Restricted fluids: 3000 mL D$_5$W IV for 24 h*

    ampicillin 500 mg in 50 mL D$_5$W IV PB q.i.d. for 30 min

    Drop factor: On infusion pump

    Flow rate: _____ mL/h IV PB and _____ mL/h primary IV

18. Order: *50 mg Nitropress IV in 500 mL D$_5$W to infuse at 3 mcg/kg/min*

    Weight: 125 lb

    Drop factor: On infusion pump

    Flow rate: _____ mL/h

19. Order: *KCl 40 mEq to each liter IV fluid*

    Situation: IV discontinued with 800 mL remaining

    How much KCl infused? _____

20. A patient's infusion rate is 125 mL/h. The rate is equivalent to _____ mL/min

21. Order: *1500 mL $\frac{1}{2}$ NS to run at 100 mL/h.* Calculate the infusion time. _____ h

Use the infusion set that follows to calculate the information requested for questions 22 and 23.

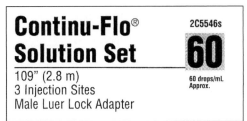

22. Order: *KCl 40 mEq/L D₅W IV to infuse at 2 mEq/h*

    Rate: _____ mL/h

    Rate: _____ gtt/min

23. Order: *heparin 50,000 U/L D₅W to infuse at 3750 U/h*

    Rate: _____ mL/h

    Rate: _____ gtt/min

24. If the minimal dilution for tobramycin is 5 mg/mL and you are giving 37 mg, what is the least amount of fluid in which you could safely dilute the dosage? _____ mL

25. Order: *oxytocin 10 U in 500 mL NS. Infuse 4 mU/min for 20 min, followed by 6 mU/min for 20 min. Use electronic infusion pump.*

    Rate: _____ mL/h for first 20 min

    Rate: _____ mL/h for next 20 min

26. Order: *magnesium sulfate 20 g IV in 500 mL of LR solution. Start with a bolus of 3 g to infuse over 30 min. Then maintain a continuous infusion at 2 g/h.*

    You will use an electronic infusion pump.

    Rate: _____ mL/h for bolus

    Rate: _____ mL/h for continuous infusion

27. Order: *Pitocin 15 U in 500 mL of LR solution. Infuse @ 1 mU/min*

    You will use an electronic infusion pump.

    Rate: _____ mL/h

28. Order: *heparin drip 40,000 U/L D₅W to infuse at 1400 U/h*

    Drop factor: On infusion pump

    Flow rate: _____ mL/h

Refer to this order for questions 29 and 30.

Order: *magnesium sulfate 4 g in 500 mL D₅W at 500 mg/h on an infusion pump*

29. What is the solution concentration? _____ mg/mL

30. What is the hourly flow rate? _____ mL/h

Calculate the drug concentration of the following IV solutions as requested.

31. A solution containing 80 U of oxytocin in 1000 mL of D₅W: _____ mU/mL

32. A solution containing 200 mg of nitroglycerin in 500 mL of D₅W: _____ mg/mL

33. A solution containing 4 mg of Isuprel in 1000 mL of D₅W: _____ mcg/mL

34. A solution containing 2 g of lidocaine in 500 mL of D₅W: _____ mg/mL

Refer to this order for questions 35 through 37.

Order: *Norcuron IV 1 mg/kg/min* to control respirations for a ventilated patient.

35. The patient weighs 220 pounds, which are equal to _____ kg.

36. The available Norcuron 20 mg is dissolved in 100 mL NS. This available solution concentration is _____ mg/mL, which is equivalent to _____ mcg/mL.

37. The IV is infusing at the rate of 1 mcg/kg/min on an infusion pump. The hourly rate is _____ mL/h.

Refer to this order for questions 38 through 43.

Order: *Restricted fluids: 3000 mL/24 h. Primary IV of D_5LR running via infusion pump.*
    ampicillin 3 g IV PB q.6h in 100 mL of D_5W over 30 min
    gentamycin 170 mg IV PB q.8h in 50 mL of D_5W to infuse in 1 h.

38. Calculate the IV PB flow rates. ampicillin: _____ mL/h; gentamycin: _____ mL/h

39. Calculate the total IV PB time. _____ h

40. Calculate the total IV PB volume. _____ mL

41. Calculate the total regular IV volume. _____ mL

42. Calculate the total regular IV time. _____ h

43. Calculate the regular IV flow rate. _____ mL/h

44. A 190 lb patient in renal failure receives *dopamine 800 mg in 500 mL of D_5W IV at 4 mcg/kg/min.* As the patient's blood pressure drops, the nurse titrates the drip to *12 mcg/kg/min* as ordered.

    What is the initial flow rate? _____ mL/h

    After titration, what is the flow rate? _____ mL/h

Questions 45 through 49 refer to your patient who has left leg deep vein thrombosis. He has orders for IV heparin therapy. He weighs 225 lb. On admission his APTT is 25 seconds. You initiate therapy at 1130 on 5/10/xx. Follow the "Standard Weight Based Heparin Protocol" on the next page. Record your answers on the "Standard Weight Based Heparin Protocol Worksheet" on page 428.

45. What is the patient's weight in kilograms? _____ kg (Round to the nearest 10 kg and record on the worksheet.) What does the protocol indicate for the standard bolus dosage of heparin? _____ U/kg

46. Calculate the dosage of heparin that should be administered for the bolus for this patient. _____ U (Record on the worksheet.)

    What does the protocol indicate as the required solution concentration (supply dosage) of heparin to use for the bolus? _____ U/mL

    Calculate the dose volume of heparin that should be administered for the bolus for this patient. _____ mL (Record on the worksheet.)

47. What does the protocol indicate for the initial infusion rate? _____ U/kg/h

    Calculate the dosage of heparin this patient should receive each hour. _____ U/h (Record on the worksheet.)

    What does the protocol indicate as the required solution concentration (supply dosage) of heparin to use for the initial infusion? _____ U/mL

    Calculate the heparin solution volume this patient should receive each hour to provide the correct infusion for his weight. _____ mL/h (Record on the worksheet.)

48. According to the protocol, how often should the patient's APTT be checked? q._____ h

    At 1730, the patient's APTT is 37 seconds. Rebolus with heparin _____ U (_____ mL) (Record on the worksheet.)

    How much should you change the infusion rate? _____ increase or _____ decrease heparin _____ U/h and _____ mL/h (Record on the worksheet.)

    The new infusion rate will be heparin _____ mL/h (Record on the worksheet.)

49. At 2330, the patient's APPT is 77 seconds. What should you do now? _____

    _____

    The infusion rate will be heparin _____ mL/h (Record on the worksheet.)

Standard Weight Based Heparin Protocol

For all patients on heparin drips:

1. Weight in KILOGRAMS. Required for order to be processed: _____ kg
2. Heparin 25,000 U in 250 mL of $\frac{1}{2}$NS. Boluses to be given as 1000 U/mL.
3. APTT q.6h or 6 hours after rate change; q.d. after two consecutive therapeutic APTTs.
4. CBC initially and repeat every _____ days(s).
5. Obtain APTT and PT/INR on day one prior to initiation of therapy.
6. Guaiac stool initially then every _____ day(s) until heparin discontinued. Notify if positive.
7. Neuro checks every _____ hours while on heparin. Notify physician of any changes.
8. D/C APTT and CBC once heparin drip is discontinued, unless otherwise ordered.
9. Notify physician of any bleeding problems.
10. Bolus with 80 U/kg. Start drip at 18 U/kg/h.
11. If APTT is < 35 secs: Rebolus with 80 U/kg and increase rate by 4 U/kg/h
12. If APTT is 36–44 secs: Rebolus with 40 U/kg and increase rate by 2 U/kg/h
13. If APTT is 45–75 secs: Continue current rate
14. If APTT is 76–90 secs: Decrease rate by 2 U/kg/h
15. If APTT is > 90 secs: Hold heparin for one hour and decrease rate by 3 U/kg/h

STANDARD WEIGHT BASED HEPARIN PROTOCOL WORKSHEET

Round Patient's Total Body Weight to Nearest 10 kg: _____ kg

DO NOT Change the Weight Based on Daily Measurements

FOUND ON THE ORDER FORM
Initial Bolus (80 U/kg) _____ U _____ mL
Initial Infusion Rate (18 U/kg/h) _____ U/h _____ mL/h

Make adjustments to the heparin drip rate as directed by the order form.

ALL DOSES ARE ROUNDED TO THE NEAREST 100 UNITS

Date	Time	APTT	Bolus	Rate Change U/h	mL/h	New Rate	RN 1	RN 2

If APTT is	Then
< 35 secs:	Rebolus with 80 U/kg and increase rate by 4 U/kg/h
36–44 secs:	Rebolus with 40 U/kg and increase rate by 2 U/kg/h
45–75 secs:	Continue current rate
76–90 secs:	Decrease rate by 2 U/kg/h
> 90 secs:	Hold heparin for one hour and decrease rate by 3 U/kg/h

Signatures _____ Initials _____

_____ _____

_____ _____

_____ _____

_____ _____

50. Critical Thinking Skill: Describe the strategy you would implement to prevent this medication error.

possible scenario

Suppose the physician writes an order to induce labor, as follows: *Pitocin 20 U added to 1 liter of LR beginning at 1 mU/min, then increase by 1 mU/min q 15–30 min to a maximum of 20 mU/min until adequate labor is reached.* The labor and delivery unit stocks Pitocin ampules 10 U per mL in boxes of 50 ampules. The nurse preparing the IV solution misread the order as "20 mL of Pitocin added to 1 liter of lactated Ringer's . . ." and pulled 20 ampules of Pitocin from the supply shelf. Another nurse, seeing this nurse drawing up medication from several ampules, asked what the nurse was preparing. When the nurse described the IV solution being prepared, he suddenly realized he had misinterpreted the order.

potential outcome

The amount of Pitocin that was being drawn up (20 mL) to be added to the IV solution would have been 10 U/mL $\times$ 20 mL = 200 U of Pitocin, 10 times the ordered amount of 20 U. Starting this Pitocin solution, even at the usual slow rate, would have delivered an excessively high amount of Pitocin that could have led to fatal consequences for both the fetus and laboring mother. What should the nurse have done to avoid this type of error?

prevention

After completing these problems, see pages 530–534 to check your answers.

SECTION 4 SELF-EVALUATION

Chapter 14: Intravenous Solutions, Equipment, and Calculations

1. Which of the following IV solutions is Normal Saline? _____ 0.45% NaCl

   _____ 0.9% NaCl   _____ D_5W

2. What is the solute and concentration of 0.9% NaCl? _____

3. What is the solute and concentration of 0.45% NaCl? _____

Use the following information to answer questions 4 and 5.

Order: *1000 mL of D_5 0.33% NaCl IV solution*

4. The IV solution contains _____ g dextrose.

5. The IV solution contains _____ g sodium chloride.

6. An order specifies *500 mL 0.45% NS IV.* The IV solution contains _____ g sodium chloride.

Refer to this order for questions 7 and 8.

Order: *750 mL D_{10} 0.9% NaCl IV*

7. The IV solution contains _____ g dextrose.

8. The IV solution contains _____ g sodium chloride.

9. Are most electronic infusion devices calibrated in gtt/min, mL/h, mL/min, or gtt/mL? _____

Use the following information to answer questions 10 and 11.

Mrs. Wilson has an order to receive *2000 mL of IV fluids over 24 h.* The IV tubing is calibrated for a drop factor of 15 gtt/mL.

10. Calculate the "watch count" flow rate for Mrs. Wilson's IV. _____ gtt/min

11. An infusion controller becomes available, and you decide to use it to regulate Mrs. Wilson's IV. Set the controller at _____ mL/h.

12. Mrs. Hawkins returns from the delivery room at 1530 with 400 mL D_5LR infusing at 24 gtt/min with your hospital's standard macrodrop infusion control set calibrated at 15 gtt/mL. You anticipate that Mrs. Hawkins's IV will be complete at _____ (hours).

13. You start your shift at 3:00 PM. On your nursing assessment rounds, you find that Mr. Johnson has an IV of $D_5 \frac{1}{2}$ NS infusing at 32 gtt/min. The tubing is calibrated for 10 gtt/mL. Mr. Johnson will receive _____ mL during your 8-hour shift.

Use the following information to answer questions 14 through 16.

As you continue on your rounds, you find Mr. Boyd with an infiltrated IV and decide to restart it and regulate it on an electronic infusion pump. The orders specify:
1000 mL NS IV c̄ 20 mEq KCl q.8h
Kefzol 250 mg IV PB/100 mL NS q.8h over 30 min
Limit IV total fluids to 3000 mL q.d.

14. Interpret Mr. Boyd's IV and medication order. _____

   _____

15. Regulate the electronic infusion pump for Mr. Boyd's standard IV at _____ mL/h.

16. Regulate the electronic infusion pump for Mr. Boyd's IV PB at _____ mL/h.

17. Order: *D₅LR 1200 mL IV @ 100 mL/h.* You start this IV at 1530 and regularly observe the IV and the patient. The IV has been infusing as scheduled, but during your nursing assessment at 2200, you find 650 mL remaining. The flow rate is 100 gtt/min using a microdrip infusion set. Describe your action now. _____

_____

Chapter 15: Body Surface Area and Advanced Pediatric Calculations

18. Order: *20 mEq KCl/L D₅NS IV continuous infusion at 20 mL/h*

Because this is a child, you choose a 250 mL IV bag of D_5W. The KCL is available in a solution strength of 2 mEq/mL. Add _____ mL KCL to the 250 mL bag of D_5W.

Calculate the hourly maintenance IV rate for the children described in questions 19 through 22. Use the following recommendations:

First, 10 kg of body weight: 100 mL/kg/day

Second, 10 kg of body weight: 50 mL/kg/day

Each additional kg over 20 kg of body weight: 20 mL/kg/day

19. A 40 lb child requires _____ mL/day for maintenance IV fluids.

20. The infusion rate for the same 40 lb child is _____ mL/h.

21. An 1185 g infant requires _____ mL/day for maintenance IV fluids.

22. The infusion rate for the same 1185 g infant is _____ mL/h.

Use the BSA formula method (next page) to answer questions 23 and 24.

23. Height: 30 in   Weight: 24 lb   BSA: _____ m²

24. Height: 155 cm   Weight: 39 kg   BSA: _____ m²

Questions 25 through 31 refer to the following situation.

A child who is 28 in tall and weighs 25 lb will receive one dosage of cisplatin IV. The recommended dosage is 37 to 75 mg/m² once every 2 to 3 weeks. The order reads *cisplatin 18.5 mg IV @ 1 mg/min today at 1500 hours.* You have available a 50 mg vial of cisplatin. Reconstitution directions state to add 50 mL of sterile water to yield 1 mg/mL. Minimal dilution instructions require 2 mL of IV solution for every 1 mg of cisplatin.

25. According to the nomogram (next page), the child's BSA is _____ m².

26. The safe dosage range for this child is _____ to _____ mg.

27. Is this dosage safe? _____.

28. If safe, you will prepare _____ mL. If not, describe your action. _____

_____

29. How many mL of IV fluid are required for safe dilution of the cisplatin? _____ mL

30. Given the ordered rate of 1 mg/min, set the infusion pump at _____ mL/h.

31. How long will this infusion take? _____ min

WEST NOMOGRAM

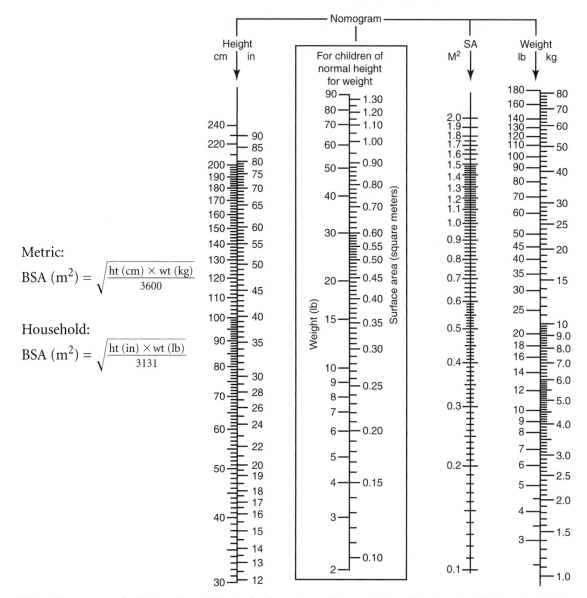

Metric:

$$BSA\ (m^2) = \sqrt{\frac{ht\ (cm) \times wt\ (kg)}{3600}}$$

Household:

$$BSA\ (m^2) = \sqrt{\frac{ht\ (in) \times wt\ (lb)}{3131}}$$

West Nomogram for Estimation of Body Surface Area. (From *Nelson Textbook of Pediatrics* (16th ed) by R. E. Behrman, R. M. Kleigman & H. B. Jenson, 2000, Philadelphia: Saunders. Reprinted with permission.)

Questions 32 through 35 refer to the following situation.

Order: *Oncovin 1.6 mg IV stat*. The child is 50 inches tall and weighs 40 lb. The following label represents the Oncovin solution you have available. The recommended dosage of Oncovin is 2 mg/m² q.d.

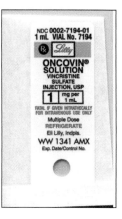

32. According to the nomogram, the child's BSA is _____ m².

33. The recommended safe dosage for this child is _____ mg.

34. Is the dosage ordered safe? _____

35. If safe, you will prepare _____ mL Oncovin to add to the IV. If not safe, describe your action. _____

36. Order: *NS IV for continuous infusion at 40 mL/h c̄ Ancef 250 mg IV q.8h over 30 min by volume control set*

    Available: Ancef 125 mg/mL

    Add _____ mL NS and _____ mL Ancef to the chamber to infuse at 40 mL/h.

37. Order: *ticarcillin 750 mg IV q.6h. Recommended minimal dilution (maximal concentration) is 100 mg/mL.* Calculate the number of mL to be used for minimal dilution of the ticarcillin as ordered. _____ mL

Chapter 16: Advanced Adult Intravenous Calculations

Use the following information to answer questions 38 through 41.

Mr. Smith is on restricted fluids. His IV order is: *1500 mL NS IV/24 h c̄ 300,000 U penicillin G potassium IV PB 100 mL NS q.4h over 30 min.* The infusion set is calibrated at 60 gtt/mL.

38. Set Mr. Smith's regular IV at _____ gtt/min.
39. Set Mr. Smith's IV PB at _____ gtt/min.
40. Later during your shift, an electronic infusion pump becomes available. You decide to use it to regulate Mr. Smith's IVs. Regulate Mr. Smith's regular IV at _____ mL/h.
41. Regulate Mr. Smith's IV PB at _____ mL/h.
42. Order: *KCl 40 mEq/L D_5W IV @ 2 mEq/h.*
    Regulate the infusion pump at _____ mL/h.
43. Order: *nitroglycerin 25 mg/L D_5W IV @ 5 mcg/min*
    Regulate the infusion pump at _____ mL/h.

Refer to this order for questions 44 through 47.

Order: *Induce labor c̄ Pitocin 15 U/L LR IV continuous infusion @ 2 mU/min; increase by 1 mU/min q.30 min to a maximum of 20 mU/min*

44. The initial concentration of Pitocin is _____ mU/mL.
45. The initial Pitocin order will infuse at the rate of _____ mL/min.
46. Regulate the electronic infusion pump at _____ mL/h to initiate the order.
47. The infusion pump will be regulated at a maximum of _____ mL/h to infuse the maximum of 20 mU/min.

Use the following information to answer questions 48 and 49.

Order for Ms. Hill, who weighs 150 lb: *dopamine 400 mg/0.5 L D_5W at 4 mcg/kg/min titrated to 12 mcg/kg/min to stabilize blood pressure*

48. Regulate the electronic infusion pump for Ms. Hill's IV at _____ mL/h to initiate the order.
49. Anticipate that the maximum flow rate for Ms. Hill's IV to achieve the maximum safe titration would be _____ mL/h.
50. Mr. Black has a new order for *heparin 10,000 U in 500 mL NS IV at 750 U/h.* Regulate the infusion pump at _____ mL/h.

After completing these problems, refer to pages 534–536 to check your answers. Give yourself two points for each correct answer.

Perfect score = 100   My score = _____

Minimum mastery score = 86 (43 correct)

Essential Skills Evaluation

This evaluation is designed to assess your mastery of essential dosage calculation skills. It is similar to the type of entry-level test given by hospitals and health care agencies during orientation for new graduates and new employees. It excludes the advanced calculation skills presented in Chapters 15 and 16.

You are assigned to give "Team Medications" on a busy Adult Medical Unit. The following labels represent the medications available in your medication cart to fill the orders given in questions 1 through 17. Calculate the amount you will administer for one dose. Assume that all tablets are scored. Draw an arrow on the appropriate syringe to indicate how much you will prepare for parenteral medications.

1. Order: *Phenergan 12.5 mg IM q.3–4h p.r.n., nausea*

   Give: _____ mL

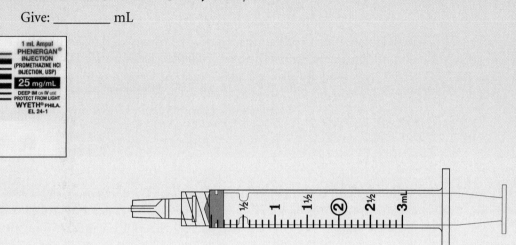

2. Order: *Thorazine 35 mg IM stat*

   Give: _____ mL

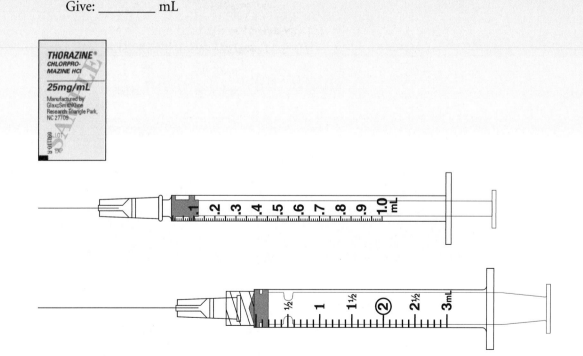

3. Order: *Dilantin 50 mg IV push q.8h*
   (administer at the rate recommended on the label)

   Give: _____ mL at _____ mL/min or
   _____ mL/15 sec

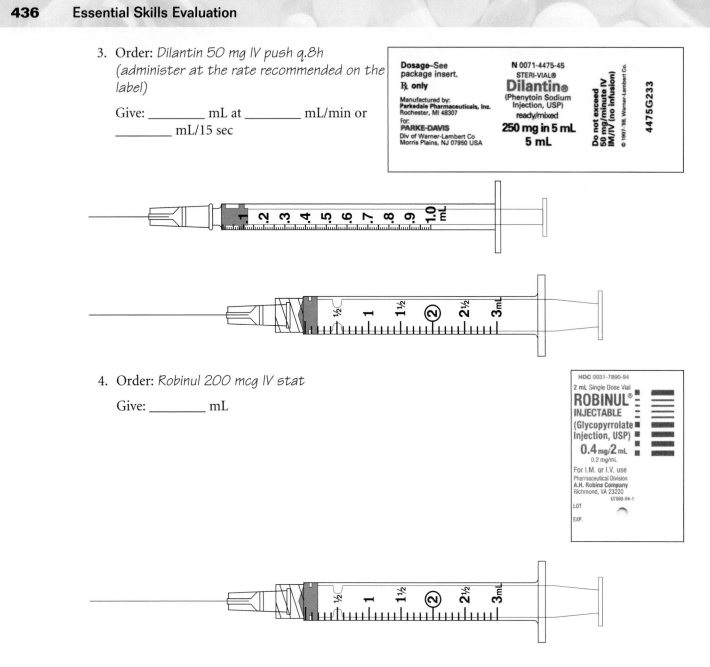

4. Order: *Robinul 200 mcg IV stat*

   Give: _____ mL

5. Order: *Lortab 7.5 mg p.o. q.3h p.r.n., pain*

   Dosage is based on hydrocodone.

   Give: _____ tablet(s)

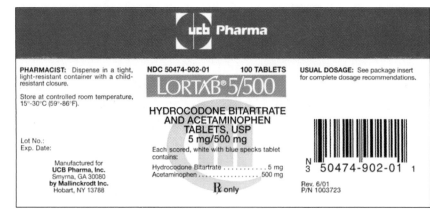

6. Order: *Lanoxin 0.125 mg IV q. AM*

   Give: _____ mL

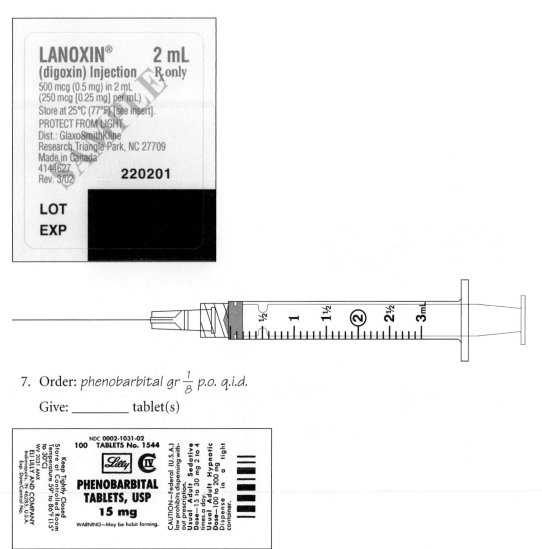

7. Order: *phenobarbital gr $\frac{1}{8}$ p.o. q.i.d.*

   Give: _____ tablet(s)

8. Order: *Kantrex 350 mg IM b.i.d.*

   Give: _____ mL

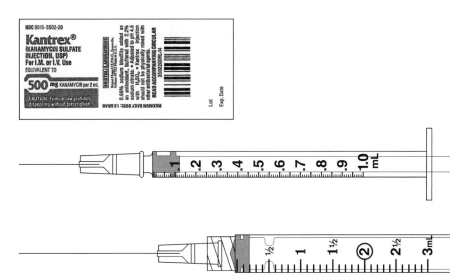

9. Order: *Novolin L Lente U-100 insulin 46 U c̄ Novolin R Regular U-100 insulin 22 U SC stat*

You will give _____ U total.

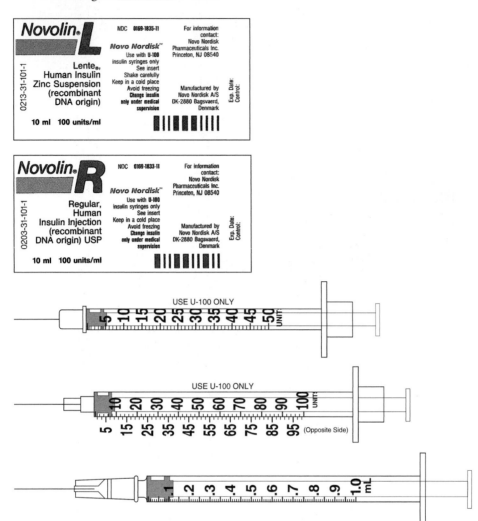

10. Order: *Synthroid 0.3 mg p.o. q. AM*

Give: _____ tablet(s)

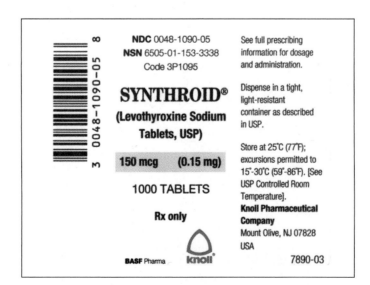

11. Order: *Calan 40 mg p.o. t.i.d.*

    Give: _____ tablet(s)

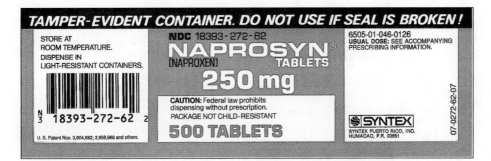

12. Order: *Naprosyn 375 mg p.o. b.i.d.*

    Give: _____ tablet(s)

13. Order: *Phenergan 40 mg IM stat*

    Give: _____ mL

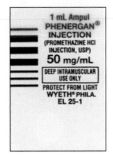

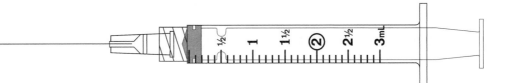

14. Order: *Stadol 3 mg IM stat*

Give: _____ mL

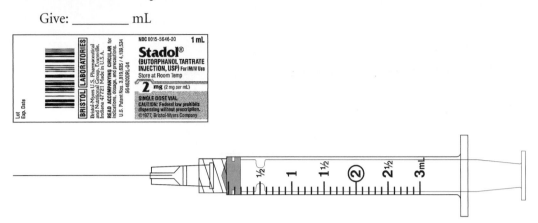

15. Order: *Augmentin 100 mg p.o. q.8h*

Give: _____ mL

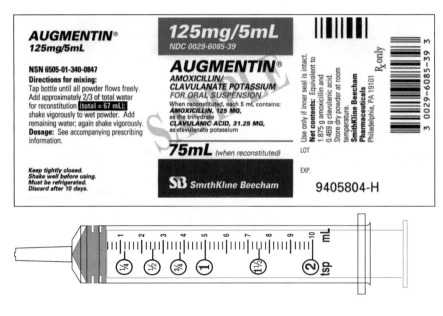

16. Order: *atropine gr $\frac{1}{100}$ IM stat*

Give: _____ mL

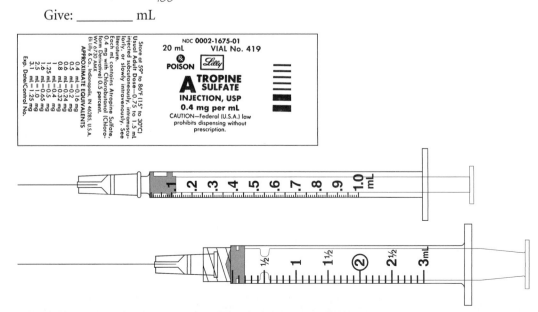

17. Order: *Zantac 35 mg in 100 mL D₅W IV PB over 20 min*

    Add _____ mL Zantac to the IV fluid, and set the flow rate to _____ gtt/min.

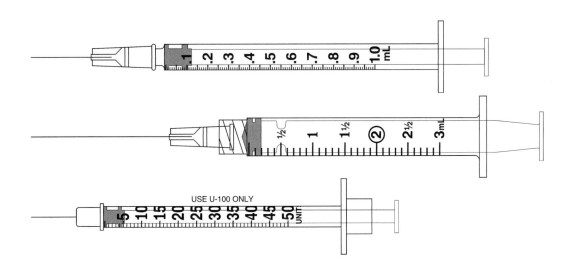

Refer to the MAR on the next page to answer questions 18 through 22.

Mrs. Betty Smedley in Room 217A is assigned to your team. She is hospitalized with osteoarthritis. The medications available from the pharmacy are noted on the MAR.

18. Mrs. Smedley had her last dose of Tylenol at 2110 hours. It is now 0215 hours, and her temperature is 39°C. Is Tylenol indicated? _____

    Explain: _____

    _____

19. How many tablets of Tylenol should she receive for each dose? _____ tablet(s)

20. Mrs. Smedley had 60 mg of Toradol at 1500 hours. At 2130 hours she is complaining of severe pain again. How much Toradol in the prefilled syringe will you give her now? Give _____ of the syringe amount.

21. Mrs. Smedley is complaining of itching. What p.r.n. medication would you select, and how much will you administer? Select _____, and give _____ mL. Draw an arrow on the appropriate syringe to indicate how much you will give.

09/15/xx
08:26
CHECKED BY: — — — — — — — — — — — — — — — —

2ND	241
217A	532729
	Smedley, Betty

MEDICATION ADMINISTRATION RECORD

PAGE: 1
REPT: PHR20B

DIAGNOSIS: 71590
ALLERGIES: NKA
NOTES:

DX: OSTEOARTHRITIS-UNSPEC

DIET: Regular
ADMIT: 09/15/xx
WT: 154 lb

ADMINISTRATION PERIOD:	07:30	09/15/xx	TO	07:29	09/16/xx

ORDER # DRUG NAME, STRENGTH, DOSAGE FORM DOSE RATE ROUTE SCHEDULE	START	STOP	TIME PERIOD 07:30 TO 15:29	TIME PERIOD 15:30 TO 23:29	TIME PERIOD 23:30 TO 07:29
NURSE:					
• • • PRN's FOLLOW • • •		• • • PRN's FOLLOW • • •			
264077 TYLENOL 325 MG TABLET PRN **650 MG** ORAL Q4H/PRN FOR TEMP > 101 F	09:30 09/15/xx		*0930* *GP*	*2110* *GP*	
264147 TORADOL 60 MG SYRINGE PRN **60 MG** IM PRN GIVE 60 MG FOR BREAKTHROUGH PAIN X1 DOSE THEN 30 MG Q6H/PRN	15:00 09/15/xx			*1500* *MS*	
264148 TORADOL 60 MG SYRINGE PRN **30 MG** IM Q6H/PRN GIVE 6 HOURS AFTER 60 MG DOSE FOR BREAK- THROUGH PAIN.	15:00 09/15/xx				
264151 INAPSINE 2.5 MG/ML AMPULE PRN **SEE NOTE** IV Q6H/PRN SAME AS DROPERIDOL; DOSE IS 0.625 MG TO 1.25 MG (0.5-1.0 ML) FOR NAUSEA	15:00 09/15/xx				
264152 BENADRYL 50 MG/ML AMPULE PRN **35 MG** IV Q4H/PRN FOR ITCHING	15:00 09/15/xx				
264153 NARCAN 0.4 MG/ML AMPULE PRN **0.4 MG** IV PRN FOR RR< 8 AND IF PT. IS UNAROUSABLE	15:00 09/15/xx				
NURSE:					
NURSE:					

INITIALS	SIGNATURE	INITIALS	SIGNATURE	NOTES
GP	G. Pickar, R.N.			
MS	M. Smith, R.N.			

| 217A | Betty Smedley | | AGE: 73 | SEX: F | PHYSICIAN: J. Physician, MD |

22. Mrs. Smedley's respiratory rate (R.R.) is 7, and she is difficult to arouse. What medication is indicated? _____ Give _____ mL. Draw an arrow on the syringe to indicate how much of this medication you will give.

Refer to the following MAR to answer questions 23 through 27.

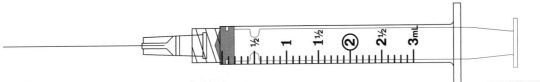

PAGE _____ of _____

MEDICATION ADMINISTRATION RECORD

ORIGINAL ORDER DATE	DATE STARTED/RENEWED	MEDICATION - DOSAGE	ROUTE	SCHEDULE 11-7	SCHEDULE 7-3	SCHEDULE 3-11	DATE 3-10-xx 11-7	DATE 3-10-xx 7-3	DATE 3-10-xx 3-11	DATE 3-11-xx 11-7	DATE 3-11-xx 7-3	DATE 3-11-xx 3-11	DATE 3-12-xx 11-7	DATE 3-12-xx ;7-3	DATE 3-12-xx 3-11	DATE 3-14-xx 11-7	DATE 3-14-xx 7-3	DATE 3-14-xx 3-11
3-10-xx	3-10	Theophylline 100 mg in 50 mL D₅W x 30 min q.6h	IV PB	12 6	12	6		GP 12	MS 6	JJ12 JJ6									
3-10-xx	3-10	Solu-Medrol 125 mg q.6h	IV	12 6	12	6		GP 12	MS 6	JJ12 JJ6									
3-10-xx	3-10	Carafate 1 g 15 min ac & hs	PO	7:45 11:45	5:45 10:00		GP7:45 GP11:45	MS5:45 MS10:00										
3-10-xx	3-10	Novulin R Regular U-100 insulin 30 min ac per sliding scale: Blood sugar Units	SC	7:30 11:30	5:30		GP7:30 GP11:30	MS5:30										
		0-150 0 U																
		151-250 8 U																
		251-350 13 U																
		351-400 18 U																
		>400 Call M.D.																

PRN

INJECTION SITES

B - RIGHT ARM
C - RIGHT ABDOMEN
D - RIGHT ANTERIOR THIGH
G - LEFT ARM
H - LEFT ABDOMEN
J - LEFT ANTERIOR THIGH
L - LEFT BUTTOCKS
M - RIGHT BUTTOCKS

DATE GIVEN	TIME	INT.	ONE - TIME MEDICATION - DOSAGE	RT.	11-7	7-3	3-11	11-7	7-3	3-11	11-7	7-3	3-11	11-7	7-3	3-11	11-7	7-3	3-11
					SCHEDULE			DATE			DATE			DATE			DATE		

SIGNATURE OF NURSE ADMINISTERING MEDICATIONS

11-7	JJ J.Jones LPN
7-3	GP G.Pickar,RN
3-11	MS M.Smith,RN

| DATE GIVEN | TIME | INT | MEDICATION-DOSAGE-CONT. | RT. |

LITHO IN U.S.A. K6508 (7-92) D395538

RECOPIED BY:

CHECKED BY:

Beck, John
ID #76834-21

ALLERGIES:

①

602-31 (7-xx) (MPC# 1355)

ORIGINAL COPY

John Beck, 19 years old, is diabetic. He is admitted to the medical unit with asthma. You are administering his medications. The MAR on page 443 is in the medication notebook on your medication cart. The labels represent the infusion set available and the medications in his medication cart drawer. Questions 23 through 27 refer to John.

23. Theophylline is available in a solution strength of 80 mg/15 mL. There will be _____ mL theophylline in the IV PB. Set the flow rate at _____ gtt/min.

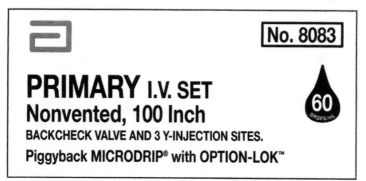

24. An infusion pump becomes available, and you decide to use it for John's IV. It is calibrated in mL/h. To administer the theophylline by infusion pump, set the pump at _____ mL/h.

25. Reconstitute the Solu-Medrol with _____ mL diluent, and give _____ mL.

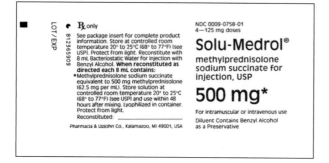

26. Mealtimes and bedtime are 8 AM, 12 NOON, 6 PM, and 10 PM. Using international time, give _____ tablet(s) of Carafate per dose each day at _____, _____, _____, and _____ hours.

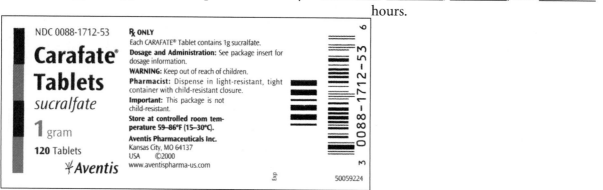

27. At 0730 John's blood sugar is 360. You will give him _____ U of insulin by the _____ route. Draw an arrow on the appropriate syringe to indicate the correct dosage.

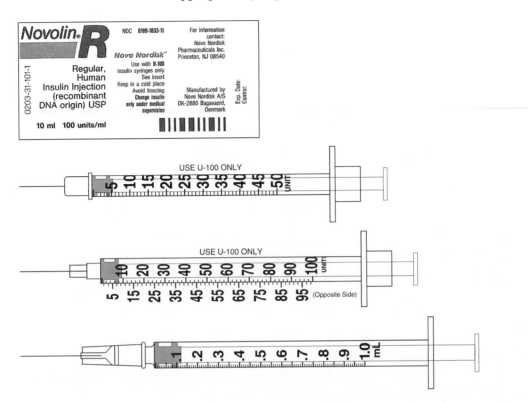

Jimmy Bryan is brought to the pediatric clinic by his mother. He is a 15 lb baby with an ear infection. Questions 28 through 31 refer to Jimmy.

28. The physician orders *amoxicillin 50 mg p.o. q.8h* for Jimmy. To reconstitute the amoxicillin, add _____ mL water.

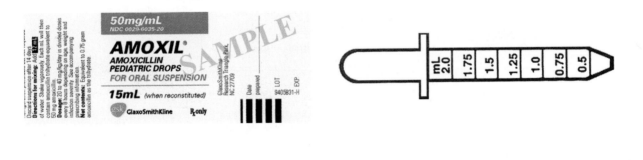

29. Is Jimmy's amoxicillin order safe and reasonable? _____ Explain: _____

_____

30. The physician asks you to give Jimmy one dose of the amoxicillin stat. You will give Jimmy _____ mL.

31. The physician also asks you to instruct Jimmy's mother about administering the medication at home. Tell Jimmy's mother to give the baby _____ dropperful to the _____ mL line for each dose. How often? _____

32. Jill Jones is a 16-year-old, 110 lb teenager with a duodenal ulcer and abdominal pain. Order: *cimetidine 250 mg q.6h in 50 mL D$_5$W IV PB to be infused in 20 min*

    The recommended cimetidine dosage is 20 to 40 mg/kg/day in 4 divided doses. Available is cimetidine for injection, 300 mg/2 mL. The label represents the infusion set available. What is the safe single dosage range for this child? _____ mg/dose to _____ mg/dose. Is this ordered dosage safe? _____

    If safe, add _____ mL cimetidine, and set the flow rate at _____ gtt/min.

33. The doctor writes a new order for strict intake and output assessment for a child. During your 8-hour shift, in addition to his IV fluids of 200 mL D$_5$NS, he consumed the following oral fluids:

    gelatin—ℨ iv

    water—ℨ iii × 2

    apple juice—pt i

    What is his total fluid intake during your shift? _____ mL

Use the following information to answer questions 34 through 36.

Order for a child with severe otitis media (inner ear infection) who weighs 40 lb: *Augmentin 240 mg p.o. q.8h.* The following Augmentin label represents the dosage you have available. Recommended Augmentin dosage is 40 mg/kg/day q.8h in divided doses.

34. Is the ordered dosage safe? _____

35. If it is safe, how much would you administer to the child? _____ mL per dose. If it is not safe, what would you do next? _____

36. The physician has ordered *washed, packed red blood cells 2 units (600 mL) IV to infuse in 4 h.* The IV tubing has a drop factor of 15 gtt/mL. You will regulate the IV flow rate at _____ gtt/min.

Use the following information to answer questions 37 and 38.

A child who weighs 61 lb 8 oz has an elevated temperature. For hyperthermia in children, the recommended dosage of acetaminophen is 10 to 15 mg/kg p.o. q.4–6h, not to exceed 5 doses per day.

37. What is the safe single dosage range of acetaminophen for this child? _____ mg/dose to _____ mg/dose

38. If the physician orders the maximum safe dosage and acetaminophen is available as a suspension of 80 mg/2.5 mL, how many mL will you give per dose? _____ mL

Use the following information to answer questions 39 and 40 for a child who weighs 52 lb.

Order: *Benadryl 25 mg IV q.6h*

Supply: Benadryl 10 mg/mL

Recommended dosage: 5 mg/kg/day in 4 divided doses

39. A safe single dosage for this child is _____ mg/dose. Is the order safe? _____

40. If safe, administer _____ mL. If not safe, what should you do? _____

_____

Use the following information to answer questions 41 through 44.

At 1430, a patient is started on *Demerol PCA IV pump at 10 mg q.10 min.* The Demerol syringe in the pump contains 300 mg/30 mL.

41. The patient can receive _____ mL every 10 minutes.

42. If the patient attempts 5 doses this hour, he would receive _____ mg and _____ mL of Demerol.

43. Based on the amount of Demerol in the syringe in the PCA pump, how many total doses can the patient receive? _____ dose(s)

44. If the patient receives 5 doses every hour, the Demerol will be empty at _____ hours. Convert this time to traditional AM/PM time. _____

45. Order: *Aldomet 250 mg stat in 100 mL D₅W IV PB, infuse over 30 min*

    Regulate the electronic infusion pump at _____ mL/h.

Use the following information to answer questions 46 through 49.

Order: *Fortaz 0.5 g IV q.8h*

The following label represents the drug you have available. You reconstitute the drug at 1400 on 1/30/xx.

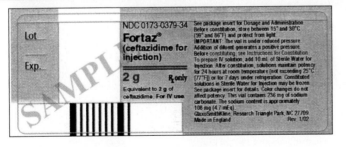

46. The total volume of Fortaz after reconstitution is _____ mL.

47. The resulting dosage strength of Fortaz is _____ mg per _____ mL.

48. Give _____ mL of Fortaz.

49. Prepare a reconstitution label for Fortaz.

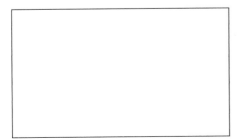

50. Critical Thinking Skill: Describe the strategy you would implement to prevent this medication error.

    possible scenario

    Order: *Decadron 4 mg IV q.6h*

    Day 1 Supply: Decadron 4 mg/mL

    Student nurse prepared and administered 1 mL.

    Day 2 Supply: Decadron 10 mg/mL

    Student nurse prepared 1 mL.

    potential outcome

    Day 2, the student's instructor asked the student to recheck the order, think about the action, check the calculation, and provide the rationale for the amount prepared. The student was alarmed at the possibility of administering 2.5 times the prescribed dosage. The student insisted that the pharmacy should consistently supply the same unit dosage. The instructor advised the student of the possibility that different pharmacy technicians could be involved, or possibly the original supply dosage was not available.

    prevention

    _____

    _____

After completing these problems, see pages 537–541 to check your answers. Give yourself two points for each correct answer.

Perfect score = 100   My score = _____

Minimum mastery score = 90 (45 correct)

Comprehensive Skills Evaluation

This evaluation is a comprehensive assessment of your mastery of the concepts presented in all 16 chapters of *Dosage Calculations*.

Donna Smith, a 46-year-old patient of Dr. J. Physician, has been admitted to the Progressive Care Unit (PCU) with complaints of an irregular heartbeat, shortness of breath, and chest pain relieved by nitroglycerin. Questions 1 through 14 refer to the admitting orders on the next page for Mrs. Smith. The labels shown represent available medications and infusion set.

1. How many capsules of nitroglycerin will you give Mrs. Smith?

    Give: _____ capsules

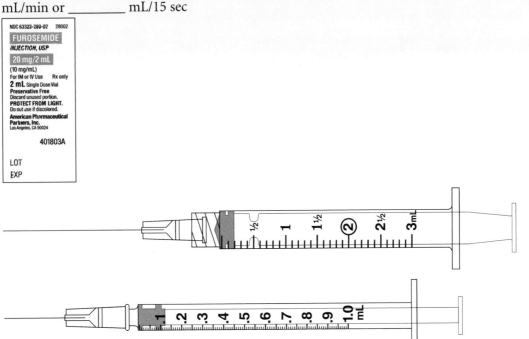

2. Sometimes nitroglycerin is ordered by the SL route. "SL" is the medical abbreviation for _____ Explain: _____

3. How much and at what rate will you administer Mrs. Smith's first dose of furosemide? Draw an arrow on the appropriate syringe to indicate how much you will prepare. The recommended direct IV administration rate for furosemide is 40 mg/2 min. Give: _____ mL at the rate of _____ mL/min or _____ mL/15 sec

ENTERED	FILLED	CHECKED	VERIFIED
			—

NOTE: A NON-PROPRIETARY DRUG OF EQUAL QUALITY MAY BE DISPENSED - IF THIS COLUMN IS NOT CHECKED!

DATE	TIME WRITTEN	PLEASE USE BALL POINT - PRESS FIRMLY	✓	TIME NOTED	NURSES SIGNATURE
9/3/xx	1600	Admit to PCU, monitored bed	✓		
		Bedrest c̄ bathroom privileges	✓		
		nitroglycerin 13 mg p.o. q.8h	✓		
		furosemide 20 mg IV Push stat, then 20 mg p.o. b.i.d.	✓		
		digoxin 0.25 mg IV Push stat, repeat in 4 hours,	✓	1610 GP	
		then 0.125 mg p.o. q.d.			
		KCl 10 mEq per L D$_5$ ½ NS IV @ 80 cc/h	✓		
		acetaminophen 1 g q.4h p.r.n, headache	✓		
		Labwork: Electrolytes and CBC in am	✓		
		Soft diet, advance as tolerated	✓		
		Dr. J. Physician			

AUTO STOP ORDERS: UNLESS REORDERED, FOLLOWING WILL BE D/C'D AT 0800 ON:

DATE	ORDER		
		☐ CONT	PHYSICIAN SIGNATURE
		☐ D/C	
		☐ CONT	PHYSICIAN SIGNATURE
		☐ D/C	
		☐ CONT	PHYSICIAN SIGNATURE
		☐ D/C	

CHECK WHEN ANTIBIOTICS ORDERED   ☐ Prophylactic   ☐ Empiric   ☐ Therapeutic

Allergies: None Known

Chest Pain

PATIENT DIAGNOSIS

Smith, Donna
ID #257-226-3

HEIGHT 5' 6"   WEIGHT 110 lb

FORM 959-708 (8xx)   **PHYSICIAN'S ORDER**   Reynolds + Reynolds LITHO IN U.S.A. K41814 (7/00) D330080

①

4. After the initial dose of furosemide, how much will you administer for each subsequent dose?

Give: _____ tablet(s)

NDC 0039-0067-50

Lasix® 20 mg
furosemide
500 Tablets ⦿Aventis

0039-0067-50

℞ ONLY
Each LASIX® Tablet contains 20mg furosemide. **Dosage and Administration:** See package insert for dosage information. **WARNING:** Keep out of reach of children. Do not use if bottle closure seal is broken. **Pharmacist:** Dispense in well-closed, light-resistant container with child-resistant closure. **Store at room temperature.**
Hoechst-Roussel Pharmaceuticals
Division of Aventis Pharmaceuticals Inc.
Kansas City, MO 64137 USA   ©2000
www.aventispharma-us.com

50058803 50058803 50058803

5. How much and at what rate will you administer the IV Lanoxin on admission? Draw an arrow on the syringe to indicate how much you will prepare. The recommended direct IV rate for digoxin (Lanoxin) is 0.25 mg in 4 mL NS administered IV at the rate of 0.25 mg/5 min.

   Give: _____ mL at the rate of _____ mL/min or _____ mL/15 sec

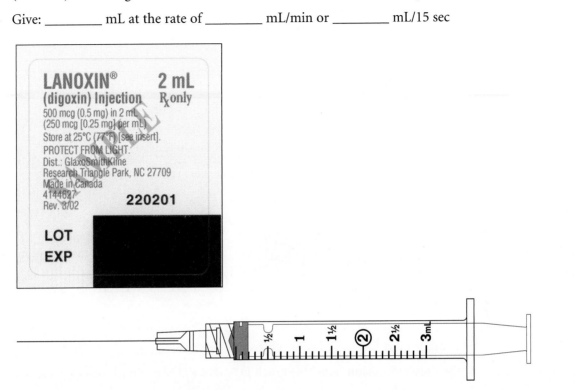

6. How many digoxin tablets will you need for a 24-hour supply of the p.o. order? _____ tablet(s)

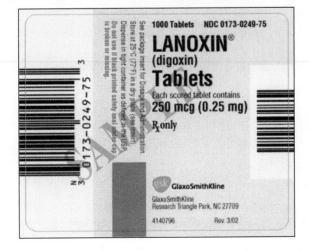

7. Calculate the "watch count" flow rate for the IV fluid ordered. _____ gtt/min

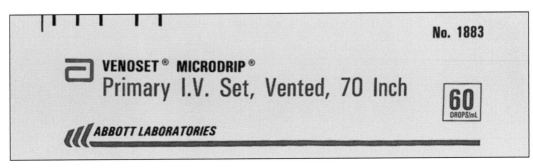

8. How much KCl will you add to the IV? Draw an arrow on the appropriate syringe to indicate the amount. Add: _____ mL

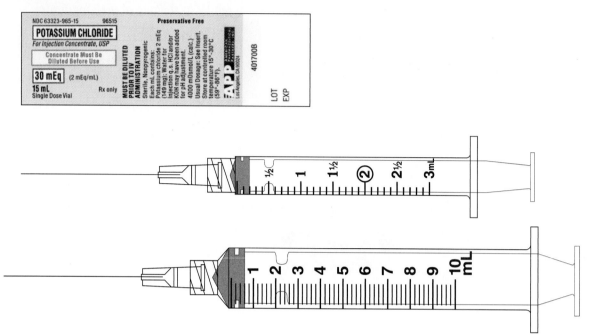

9. How many mEq KCl will Mrs. Smith receive per hour? _____ mEq/h

10. At the present infusion rate, how much $D_5 \frac{1}{2}$ NS will Mrs. Smith receive in a 24-hour period? _____ mL/day

11. The IV is started at 1630. Estimate the time and date that you should plan to hang the next liter of $D_5 \frac{1}{2}$ NS. _____ hours _____ date

12. Mrs. Smith has a headache. How much acetaminophen will you give her?

    Give: _____ tablet(s)

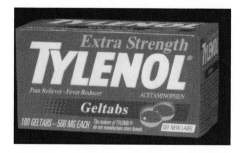

13. You have located an infusion controller for Mrs. Smith's IV. At what rate will you set the controller? _____ mL/h

14. Compare the drug order and the labels to determine which of Mrs. Smith's medications are ordered by their generic or chemical names. _____

    _____

Despite your excellent care, Mrs. Smith's condition worsens. She is transferred into the coronary care unit (CCU) with the following medical orders. Questions 15 through 20 refer to these orders. She weighs 110 lb.

			ENTERED	FILLED	CHECKED	VERIFIED

NOTE: A NON-PROPRIETARY DRUG OF EQUAL QUALITY MAY BE DISPENSED - IF THIS COLUMN IS NOT CHECKED!

DATE	TIME WRITTEN	PLEASE USE BALL POINT - PRESS FIRMLY	✓	TIME NOTED	NURSES SIGNATURE
9/4/xx	2230	Transfer to CCU	✓		
		NPO	✓		
		Discontinue Nitro-Bid	✓		
		lidocaine bolus 50 mg IV stat, then begin	✓		
		lidocaine drip 2 g in 500 cc D_5W			
		@ 2 mg/min by infusion pump			
		Increase lidocaine to 4 mg/min if PVCs	✓		
		(premature ventricular contractions)			
		persist		2235 MS	
		dopamine 400 mg IV PB in 250 cc D_5W	✓		
		@ 500 mcg/min by infusion pump			
		Increase KCl to 20 mEq per L D_5W	✓		
		1/2 NS IV @ 50 cc/h			
		Increase furosemide to 40 mg IV q.12h	✓		
		O_2 @ 30% p̄ ABGs (arterial blood gases)	✓		
		Labwork: Electrolytes stat and in am and	✓		
		ABGs stat & p.r.n.			
		Dr. J. Physician			

AUTO STOP ORDERS: UNLESS REORDERED, FOLLOWING WILL BE D/C'D AT 0800 ON:

DATE	ORDER		
		☐ CONT	PHYSICIAN SIGNATURE
		☐ D/C	
		☐ CONT	PHYSICIAN SIGNATURE
		☐ D/C	
		☐ CONT	PHYSICIAN SIGNATURE
		☐ D/C	

CHECK WHEN ANTIBIOTICS ORDERED　　☐ Prophylactic　　☐ Empiric　　☐ Therapeutic

Allergies:
None Known

Chest Pain
PATIENT DIAGNOSIS

Smith, Donna
ID #257-226-3

HEIGHT　5' 6"　　WEIGHT　110 lb

FORM 959-708 (8xx)　　**PHYSICIAN'S ORDER**　　Reynolds + Reynolds　LITHO IN U.S.A. K41814 (7-90)　D339366

①

15. You have lidocaine 10 mg/mL available. How much lidocaine will you give for the bolus? Draw an arrow on the appropriate syringe to indicate the amount you will give.

    Give: _____ mL

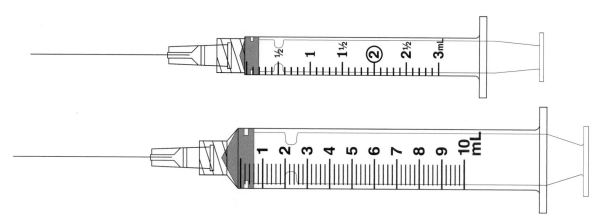

16. The infusion pump is calibrated to administer mL/h. At what rate will you initially set the infusion pump for the lidocaine drip? _____ mL/h

17. The recommended dosage of dopamine is 5–10 mcg/kg/min. Is the dosage ordered for Mrs. Smith safe? _____ If safe, how much dopamine will you add to mix the dopamine drip? You have dopamine 80 mg/mL available. Draw an arrow on the appropriate syringe to indicate the amount you will add. Add: _____ mL

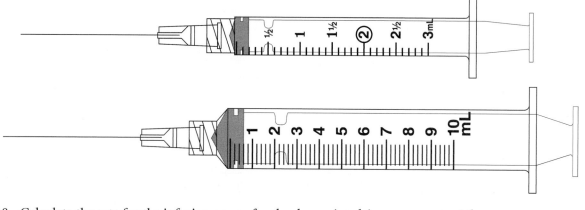

18. Calculate the rate for the infusion pump for the dopamine drip. _____ mL/h

19. How much dopamine will Mrs. Smith receive per hour? _____ mcg/h or _____ mg/h

20. Mrs. Smith is having increasing amounts of PVCs. To increase her lidocaine drip to 4 mg/min, you will now change the IV infusion pump setting to _____ mL/h.

21. Julie Thomas is a six-year-old pediatric patient who weighs 33 lb. She is in the hospital for fever of unknown origin. Julie complains of burning on urination and her urinalysis shows *E. coli* bacterial infection. The doctor prescribes Kantrex 75 mg IV q.8h to be administered by volume control set on an infusion pump in 25 mL D$_5$ $\frac{1}{2}$ NS followed by 15 mL flush over one hour. The maximum recommended dosage of Kantrex is 15 mg/kg/day IV in three doses.

    Is the order safe? _____ Explain: _____

If safe, add _____ mL Kantrex and _____ mL D$_5$W to the chamber, and set the flow rate for _____ mL/h.

22. Order: *Cardizem 125 mg in 100 mL D$_5$W IV @ 15 mg/h*

    Set the IV pump at _____ mL/h.

23. Jamie Smith is hospitalized with a staphylococcal bone infection. He weighs 66 lb.

    Orders: *D$_5\frac{1}{2}$ NS IV @ 50 mL/h for continuous infusion*

    Vancocin 300 mg IV q.6h

    Supply: Vancocin 500 mg/10 mL with instructions to "add to volume control set and infuse over 60 min."

    Recommended dosage: Vancomycin 40 mg/kg/day IV in 4 equally divided doses.

    Is this drug order safe? _____. Explain: _____

    If safe, how much Vancocin will you add to the chamber? _____ mL

    How much IV fluid will you add to the chamber with the Vancocin? _____ mL

    How much IV fluid will Jamie receive in 24 hours? _____ mL

24. You are preparing IV fluids for a young child according to the following order:

    D$_5\frac{1}{2}$ NS c̄ KCl 20 mEq/L IV at 30 cc/h

    You have chosen to use a 250 mL bag of D$_5\frac{1}{2}$ NS. How many mEq KCl will you add? _____ mEq

    Your supply of KCl is 2 mEq/mL. How much KCl will you add to the 250 mL bag? _____ mL

Use the related orders and labels to answer questions 25 through 29. Select and mark the dose volume on the appropriate syringe, as indicated.

25. Order: *Prostaphlin 500 mg IV q.6h in 50 mL D$_5$W IV by volume control set over 60 min. Follow with 15 mL IV flush.*

    Reconstitute with _____ mL diluent.

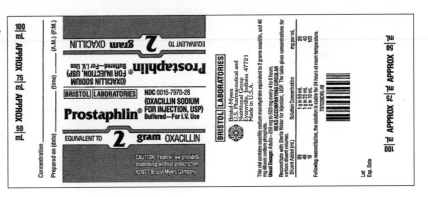

26. Prepare a reconstitution label for the Prostaphlin.

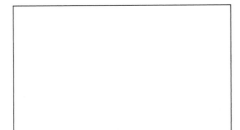

27. Add _____ mL Prostaphlin and _____ mL D$_5$W to the chamber.

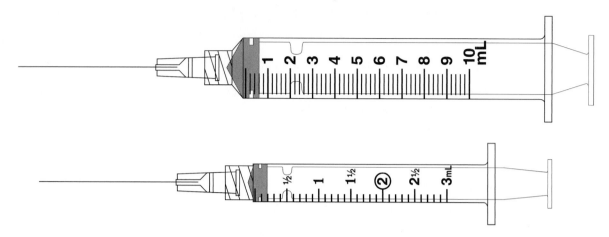

28. The IV Prostaphlin is regulated on an infusion pump. Set the volume control set flow rate at _____ mL/h.

29. Order: *heparin 10,000 U IV in 500 cc D$_5$W to infuse @ 1200 U/h.*

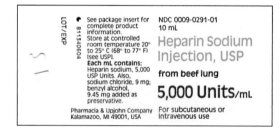

NDC 0009-0291-01
10 mL

LOT/EXP
811340604

● See package insert for complete product information.
Store at controlled room temperature 20° to 25° C (68° to 77° F) [see USP].
Each mL contains: Heparin sodium, 5,000 USP Units. Also, sodium chloride, 9 mg; benzyl alcohol, 9.45 mg added as preservative.
Pharmacia & Upjohn Company Kalamazoo, MI 49001, USA

Heparin Sodium Injection, USP

from beef lung

5,000 Units/mL

For subcutaneous or intravenous use

Add _____ mL heparin to the IV solution. Set the flow rate to _____ mL/h on an IV infusion pump.

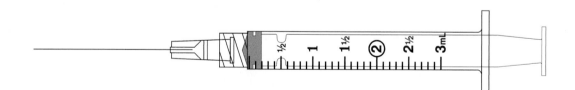

Questions 30 and 31 refer to a patient who weighs 125 lb and has IV heparin ordered per the following Weight Based Heparin Protocol.

Weight Based Heparin Protocol:

Heparin IV Infusion: *heparin 25,000 U in 250 mL of $\frac{1}{2}$ NS*

IV Boluses: Use heparin 1000 U/mL

Bolus with heparin 80 U/kg. Then initiate heparin drip at 18 U/kg/h. Obtain APTT every 6 hours and adjust dosage and rate as follows:

If APTT is < 35 seconds: Rebolus with 80 U/kg and increase rate by 4 U/kg/h.

If APTT is 36–44 seconds: Rebolus with 40 U/kg and increase rate by 2 U/kg/h.

If APTT is 45–75 seconds: Continue current rate.

If APTT is 76–90 seconds: Decrease rate by 2 U/kg/h.

If APTT is > 90 seconds: Hold heparin for one hour and then decrease rate by 3 U/kg/h.

30. Convert the patient's weight to kg: _____ kg

    Calculate the initial heparin bolus dosage: _____ U

    Calculate the bolus dose: _____ mL

    Calculate the initial heparin infusion rate: _____ U/h or _____ mL/h

31. At 0930, the patient's APTT is 77 seconds. According to the protocol, what will your action be?

    _____

    _____

    Reset infusion rate to _____ U/h or _____ mL/h.

32. Order: *Novolin R Regular U-100 insulin SC ac per sliding scale and blood sugar (BS) level. The patient's blood sugar at 1730 hours is 238.*

Sliding Scale	Insulin Dosage
BS: 0–150	0 U
BS: 151–250	8 U
BS: 251–350	13 U
BS: 351–400	18 U
BS: >400	Call M.D.

Give: _____ U, which equals _____ mL. (Mark dose on appropriate syringe.)

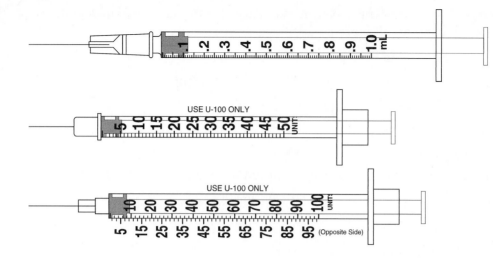

33. Order: *Humulin R Regular U-100 insulin 15 U c̄ Humulin N NPH U-100 insulin 45 U SC at 0730*

    You will give a total of _____ U insulin. (Mark dose on appropriate syringe, designating Regular and NPH insulin.)

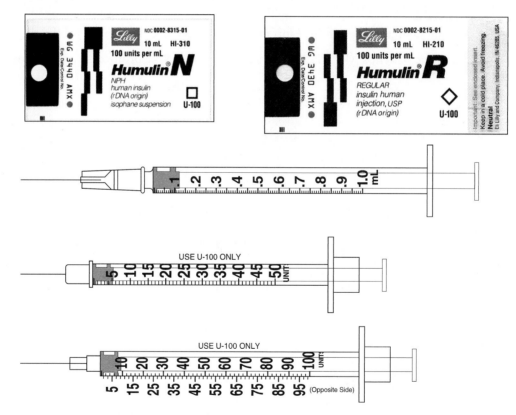

34. A patient with diabetes is receiving an insulin drip of *Humulin R Regular U-100 insulin 300 U in 150 mL NS infusing at 10 mL/h.* How many U/h of insulin is this patient receiving? _____ U/h

Questions 35 and 36 refer to an infant who weighs 16 lb and is admitted to the pediatric unit with vomiting and diarrhea for 3 days' duration.

Order: *¼ strength Isomil 80 cc q.3h for 4 feedings; if tolerated, increase Isomil to ½ strength 80 cc q.3h for 4 feedings*

Supply: Isomil Ready-to-Feed formula in 8 ounce cans

35. To reconstitute a full 8 ounce can of Isomil ready-to-feed to $\frac{1}{4}$ strength, you would add _____ mL water to mix a total of _____ mL $\frac{1}{4}$ strength reconstituted Isomil.

36. The child is not tolerating the oral feedings. Calculate this child's allowable daily and hourly IV maintenance fluids using the following recommendation. _____ mL/day or _____ mL/h.

    Daily rate of pediatric maintenance IV fluids:

    100 mL/kg for first 10 kg of body weight

    50 mL/kg for next 10 kg of body weight

    20 mL/kg for each kg above 20 kg of body weight

Use the following information and order to answer questions 37 and 38.

Metric: BSA $(\text{m}^2) = \sqrt{\dfrac{\text{ht (cm)} \times \text{wt (kg)}}{3600}}$ Household: BSA $(\text{m}^2) = \sqrt{\dfrac{\text{ht (in)} \times \text{wt (lb)}}{3131}}$

Order: *Mitomycin 28 mg IV Push stat*

Recommended dosage is 10–20 mg/m^2/single IV dose.

Patient is 5 ft 2 in tall and weighs 103 lb.

Mitomycin is available in a 40 mg vial with directions to reconstitute with 80 mL sterile water for injection and inject slowly over 10 minutes.

37. The patient's BSA is _____ m^2.

38. What is the recommended dosage of Mitomycin for this patient? _____ mg – _____ mg

    Is the ordered dosage safe? _____

    What is the concentration of Mitomycin after reconstitution? _____ mg/mL

    If the order is safe, administer _____ mL Mitomycin at the rate of _____ mL/min or _____ mL/15 sec.

39. A child's IV is *1 L D_5 0.33% NaCl.* Calculate the amount of solute in this IV solution. _____ g dextrose and _____ g NaCl.

40. An IV order says to *add 20 mEq KCl/L after first urination.* KCl is available as 40 mEq/20 mL. When it is time to add the KCl, there are 400 mL left in the IV bag. How many mEq of KCl will you add? _____ mEq   How much KCl will you add? _____ mL

Use the following order and label for the available drug to answer questions 41 and 42.

Order: *nafcillin 540 mg IV q.6h in IV fluid for total volume of 50 mL to infuse over 1 h via volume control set*

41. Add _____ mL nafcillin and _____ mL IV fluid to the chamber.

42. The minimal dilution (maximal concentration) of nafcillin is 40 mg/mL. Is the ordered amount of IV fluid sufficient to safely dilute the nafcillin? _____. Explain: _____

Use the following information to answer questions 43 and 44.

Order: *penicillin G potassium 400,000 U IV PB q.6h* for a child who weighs 10 kg.
Recommended dosage for children: Give penicillin G potassium 150,000–250,000 U/kg/day in divided doses q.6h; dilute with 100 mL NS and infuse over 60 minutes.

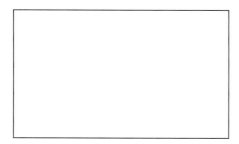

43. How many units per day of penicillin G potassium is this child ordered to receive? _____ U/day

Is the ordered dosage safe? _____ Explain: _____

If safe, reconstitute with _____ mL diluent for a concentration of _____ U/mL, and prepare a reconstitution label.

Prepare to give _____ mL.

If not safe, what should you do? _____

44. The child's IV is infusing on an electronic infusion pump. If the dosage is safe, set the IV flow rate at _____ mL/h.

Use the following patient situation to answer questions 45 through 48.

A patient has been admitted to the hospital with fever and chills, productive cough with yellow-green sputum, shortness of breath, malaise, and anorexia. Laboratory tests and X rays confirmed a diagnosis of pneumonia. The patient is complaining of nausea. The physician writes the following orders. The labels represent the drugs you have available.

NS 1000 mL IV @ 125 mL/h

Fortaz 1500 mg IV PB q.8h in 100 mL NS over 30 min

Phenergan 25 mg IV push q.4h p.r.n., nausea & vomiting

45. You can start the primary IV at 1:15 PM on an infusion pump. When do you estimate (using international time) the primary IV will be completely infused and have to be replaced? _____ hours

46. The recommendation for direct IV administration of Phenergan is at a rate not to exceed 25 mg/min. Give _____ mL Phenergan at the rate of _____ mL/min or _____ mL/15 sec.

47. You will give _____ mL Fortaz per dose.

48. Set the IV PB flow rate for each dose of Fortaz at _____ mL/h.

49. Critical Thinking Skill: Describe the strategy you would implement to prevent this medication error.

    possible scenario

    A student nurse was preparing for medication administration. One of the orders on the MAR was written as *Lanoxin 0.125 mg od.* The student nurse crushed the Lanoxin tablet. Prior to giving the medication, the nursing instructor checked the medications that the student had prepared. The instructor asked the student to explain the rationale for crushing the Lanoxin tablet. The student explained to the instructor that the Lanoxin order was for the right eye and the student planned to add a small amount of sterile water to the crushed tablet and put it in the patient's eye.

    potential outcome

    What is wrong with the Lanoxin order? _____

    _____

    What could be the result? _____

    prevention

    _____

    _____

50. Critical Thinking Skill: Describe the strategy you would implement to prevent this medication error.

    possible scenario

    Order: *Quinine 300 mg p.o. hs*

    Supply: Quinidine 300 mg tablets

    A student nurse administering medications noted the difference between the order and the supply drug, and queried the staff nurse about the order and what had been administered. The staff nurse at first dismissed it as only the brand name versus the generic name of the drug. Later the nurse realized that the student was exactly right to question the order and the drug supplied, and admitted to the student that the patient had been receiving the wrong drug all week.

    potential outcome

    The student referred to a drug reference book and compared the therapeutic and side effects of both drugs. The quinine was correctly ordered for leg cramps. Quinidine is an anti-arrhythmic heart medication. The student reviewed the patient's record and noted that the patient had been experiencing serious hypotension (a side effect of quinidine) for the past several days.

prevention

_____

_____

After completing these problems, see pages 541–547 to check your answers. Give yourself two points for each correct answer.

Perfect score = 100   My score = _____

Minimum mastery score = 90 (45 correct)

Mathematics Diagnostic Evaluation from pages 2–4

1) 1517.63 **2)** 20.74 **3)** 100.66 **4)** \$323.72 **5)** 46.11 **6)** 754.5 **7)** 16.91 **8)** 19,494.7 **9)** \$173.04 **10)** 403.26 **11)** 36 **12)** 2500

13) $\frac{2}{3}$ **14)** 6.25 **15)** $\frac{4}{5}$ **16)** 40% **17)** 0.4% **18)** 0.05 **19)** 1:3 **20)** 0.02 **21)** $1\frac{1}{4}$ **22)** $6\frac{13}{24}$ **23)** $1\frac{11}{18}$ **24)** $\frac{3}{5}$ **25)** $14\frac{7}{8}$ **26)** $\frac{1}{100}$

27) 0.009 **28)** 320 **29)** 3 **30)** 0.05 **31)** 4 **32)** 0.09 **33)** 0.22 **34)** 25 **35)** 4 **36)** 0.75 **37)** 3 **38)** 500 **39)** 18.24 **40)** 2.4 **41)** $\frac{1}{5}$

42) 1:50 **43)** 5 tablets **44)** 2 milligrams **45)** 30 kilograms **46)** 3.3 pounds **47)** $6\frac{2}{3}$ = 6.67 centimeters **48)** 7.5 centimeters

49) 90% **50)** 5:1

Solutions—Mathematics Diagnostic Evaluation

3)
```
    9.50
   17.06
   32.00
   41.11
    0.99
  ------
  100.66
```

6)
```
  1005.0
 - 250.5
 -------
   754.5
```

10)
```
    17.16
     23.5
   ------
     8580
    5148
   3432
 --------
 403.260 = 403.26
```

12)

$0.001\overline{)2.500.} = 2500$

19)

$\dfrac{33\frac{1}{3}}{100} = \dfrac{\frac{100}{3}}{100} = \dfrac{100}{3} \div \dfrac{100}{1} = \dfrac{100}{3} \times \dfrac{1}{100} = \dfrac{1}{3} = 1:3$

23)

$1\frac{5}{6} = 1\frac{15}{18}$
$-\frac{2}{9} = \frac{4}{18}$
$\overline{\qquad 1\frac{11}{18}}$

25) $4\frac{1}{4} \times 3\frac{1}{2} = \frac{17}{4} \times \frac{7}{2} = \frac{119}{8} = 14\frac{7}{8}$

29) $\dfrac{0.02 + 0.16}{0.4 - 0.34}$

```
  0.02      0.40
+ 0.16    - 0.34
------    ------
  0.18      0.06
```

$\dfrac{0.18}{0.16} = 0.06\overline{)0.18.} = 3$

32) $\frac{1}{2}\% = 0.5\% = 0.005$

```
      18
 × 0.005
 -------
   0.090 = 0.09
```

34) $\dfrac{\frac{1}{1000}}{\frac{1}{100}} \times 250 = \dfrac{1}{1000} \times \dfrac{100}{1} \times \dfrac{250}{1} = \dfrac{250}{10} = 25$

45) 66 pounds $= \dfrac{66}{2.2} = 30$ kilograms or

$\dfrac{2.2 \text{ pounds}}{1 \text{ kilogram}} \bowtie \dfrac{66 \text{ pounds}}{X \text{ kilograms}}$

$2.2X = 66$

$\dfrac{2.2X}{2.2} = \dfrac{66}{2.2}$

$X = 30$ kilograms

49)
```
   50
 -  5
 ----
   45
```
$\dfrac{45}{50} = \dfrac{9}{10} = 90\%$

Review Set 1 from pages 10–11

1) $\frac{6}{6}, \frac{7}{5}$ **2)** $\dfrac{\frac{1}{100}}{\frac{1}{150}}$ **3)** $\frac{1}{4}, \frac{1}{14}$ **4)** $1\frac{2}{9}, 1\frac{1}{4}, 5\frac{7}{8}$ **5)** $\frac{3}{4} = \frac{6}{8}, \frac{1}{5} = \frac{2}{10}, \frac{3}{9} = \frac{1}{3}$ **6)** $\frac{13}{2}$ **7)** $\frac{6}{5}$ **8)** $\frac{32}{3}$ **9)** $\frac{47}{6}$ **10)** $\frac{411}{4}$ **11)** 2 **12)** 1 **13)** $3\frac{1}{3}$ **14)** $1\frac{1}{3}$

15) $2\frac{3}{4}$ **16)** $\frac{6}{8}$ **17)** $\frac{4}{16}$ **18)** $\frac{8}{12}$ **19)** $\frac{4}{10}$ **20)** $\frac{6}{9}$ **21)** $\frac{1}{100}$ **22)** $\frac{1}{10,000}$ **23)** $\frac{5}{9}$ **24)** $\frac{3}{10}$ **25)** $\frac{2}{5}$ bottle **26)** $1\frac{1}{2}$ bottles **27)** $\frac{1}{20}$ of the class

are men **28)** $\frac{9}{10}$ of the questions were answered correctly **29)** $\frac{1}{2}$ dose **30)** $\frac{1}{2}$ teaspoon

Solutions—Review Set 1

8) $10\frac{2}{3} = \frac{(3\times 10)+2}{3} = \frac{32}{3}$

14) $\frac{100}{75} = 1\frac{25}{75} = 1\frac{1}{3}$

18) $\frac{2}{3} \times \frac{4}{4} = \frac{8}{12}$

25) 10 ounces – 6 ounces = 4 ounces remaining

$\frac{\overset{2}{\cancel{4}}}{\underset{5}{\cancel{10}}} = \frac{2}{5}$ bottle remaining

27)   57
      $\underline{+\ 3}$
      60   people in class

The men represent $\frac{3}{60}$ or $\frac{1}{20}$ of the class.

29) $\frac{80}{160} = \frac{1}{2}$ of a dose

30) $\frac{1}{2}$ of 1 teaspoon = $\frac{1}{2}$ teaspoon

Review Set 2 from page 14

1) $8\frac{7}{15}$ **2)** $1\frac{5}{12}$ **3)** $17\frac{5}{24}$ **4)** $1\frac{1}{24}$ **5)** $32\frac{5}{6}$ **6)** $5\frac{7}{12}$ **7)** $1\frac{1}{3}$ **8)** $5\frac{53}{72}$ **9)** 43 **10)** $5\frac{118}{119}$ **11)** $2\frac{8}{15}$ **12)** $\frac{53}{132}$ **13)** $\frac{1}{2}$ **14)** $4\frac{5}{6}$ **15)** $\frac{1}{24}$ **16)** $63\frac{2}{3}$
17) $299\frac{4}{5}$ **18)** $\frac{1}{6}$ **19)** $1\frac{2}{5}$ **20)** $7\frac{1}{16}$ **21)** $7\frac{2}{9}$ **22)** $1\frac{1}{4}$ **23)** $24\frac{6}{11}$ **24)** $\frac{7}{12}$ **25)** $\frac{1}{25}$ **26)** $\frac{7}{12}$ ounce **27)** $1\frac{1}{8}$ inches **28)** 8 inches
29) $21\frac{1}{2}$ pints **30)** $20\frac{1}{16}$ pounds

Solutions—Review Set 2

1) $7\frac{4}{5} + \frac{2}{3} = 7\frac{12}{15}$
       $+\ \frac{10}{15}$
       $\overline{7\frac{22}{15}} = 8\frac{7}{15}$

3) $4\frac{2}{3} + 5\frac{1}{24} + 7\frac{1}{2} = 4\frac{16}{24}$
         $5\frac{1}{24}$
       $+\ 7\frac{12}{24}$
       $\overline{16\frac{29}{24}} = 17\frac{5}{24}$

4) $\frac{3}{4} + \frac{1}{8} + \frac{1}{6} = \frac{18}{24} + \frac{3}{24} + \frac{4}{24} = \frac{18+3+4}{24} = \frac{25}{24} = 1\frac{1}{24}$

14) $8\frac{1}{12} - 3\frac{1}{4} = 8\frac{1}{12} - 3\frac{3}{12} = 7\frac{13}{12}$
        $-\ 3\frac{3}{12}$
        $\overline{4\frac{10}{12}} = 4\frac{5}{6}$

25) 50 pounds – 48 pounds = 2 pounds lost

$\frac{2}{50} = \frac{1}{25}$ of weight lost

26) $\frac{1}{4}$ ounce + $\frac{1}{3}$ ounce = $\frac{3}{12} + \frac{4}{12} = \frac{7}{12}$ ounce

29) $56 - 34\frac{1}{2} = 55\frac{2}{2}$
        $-\ 34\frac{1}{2}$
        $\overline{21\frac{1}{2}}$ pints

30) $30\frac{1}{8} - 10\frac{1}{16} = 30\frac{2}{16}$
        $-\ 10\frac{1}{16}$
        $\overline{20\frac{1}{16}}$ pounds

Review Set 3 from pages 18–19

1) $\frac{1}{40}$ **2)** $\frac{36}{125}$ **3)** $\frac{35}{48}$ **4)** $\frac{3}{100}$ **5)** 3 **6)** $1\frac{2}{3}$ **7)** $\frac{4}{5}$ **8)** $6\frac{8}{15}$ **9)** $\frac{1}{2}$ **10)** $23\frac{19}{36}$ **11)** $\frac{3}{32}$ **12)** $254\frac{1}{6}$ **13)** 3 **14)** $1\frac{34}{39}$ **15)** $\frac{3}{14}$ **16)** $\frac{1}{11}$ **17)** $\frac{1}{2}$
18) $\frac{1}{30}$ **19)** $3\frac{1}{3}$ **20)** $\frac{3}{20}$ **21)** $\frac{1}{3}$ **22)** $\frac{7}{12}$ **23)** $1\frac{1}{9}$ **24)** 60 calories **25)** 560 seconds **26)** 40 doses **27)** $31\frac{1}{2}$ tablets
28) 1275 milliliters **29)** $52\frac{1}{2}$ ounces **30)** 6 full days

Solutions—Review Set 3

3) $\frac{5}{8} \times 1\frac{1}{6} = \frac{5}{8} \times \frac{7}{6} = \frac{35}{48}$

5) $\frac{\frac{1}{6}}{\frac{1}{4}} \times \frac{\frac{3}{2}}{\frac{2}{3}} = \left(\frac{1}{6} \times \frac{4}{1}\right) \times \left(\frac{3}{1} \times \frac{3}{2}\right) = \frac{\overset{2}{\cancel{4}}}{\underset{3}{\cancel{6}}} \times \frac{9}{2} = \frac{\overset{3}{\cancel{18}}}{\underset{1}{\cancel{6}}} = 3$

16) $\frac{1}{33} \div \frac{1}{3} = \frac{1}{33} \times \frac{3}{1} = \frac{3}{33} = \frac{1}{11}$

19) $2\frac{1}{2} \div \frac{3}{4} = \frac{5}{2} \div \frac{3}{4} = \frac{5}{\underset{1}{\cancel{2}}} \times \frac{\overset{2}{\cancel{4}}}{3} = \frac{10}{3} = 3\frac{1}{3}$

27) $3 \times 7 = 21$ doses

$21 \times 1\frac{1}{2} = 21 \times \frac{3}{2} = \frac{63}{2} = 31\frac{1}{2}$ tablets

28) $850 \div \frac{2}{3} = \frac{\overset{425}{\cancel{850}}}{1} \times \frac{3}{\underset{1}{\cancel{2}}} = 1275$ milliliters

30)

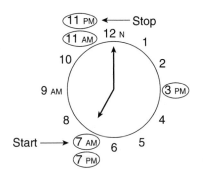

Daily doses would be taken at: 7 AM, 11 AM, 3 PM,

7 PM, and 11 PM for 5 doses/day.

5 doses/day $\times \frac{1}{2}$ ounce/dose $= \frac{5}{2} = 2\frac{1}{2}$ ounces/day

16 ounces $\div 2\frac{1}{2}$ ounces/day $= \frac{16}{1} \div \frac{5}{2} = \frac{16}{1} \times \frac{2}{5} = \frac{32}{5} =$

$6\frac{2}{5}$ days or 6 full days

Review Set 4 from pages 25–26

1) 0.2, two tenths **2)** $\frac{17}{20}$, 0.85 **3)** $1\frac{1}{20}$, one and five hundredths **4)** $\frac{3}{500}$, six thousandths **5)** 10.015, ten and fifteen thousandths **6)** $1\frac{9}{10}$, one and nine tenths **7)** $5\frac{1}{10}$, 5.1 **8)** 0.8, eight tenths **9)** $250\frac{1}{2}$, two hundred fifty and five tenths **10)** 33.03, thirty-three and three hundredths **11)** $\frac{19}{20}$, ninety-five hundredths **12)** 2.75, two and seventy-five hundredths **13)** $7\frac{1}{200}$, 7.005 **14)** 0.084, eighty-four thousandths **15)** $12\frac{1}{8}$, twelve and one hundred twenty-five thousandths **16)** $20\frac{9}{100}$, twenty and nine hundredths **17)** $22\frac{11}{500}$, 22.022 **18)** $\frac{3}{20}$, fifteen hundredths **19)** 1000.005, one thousand and five thousandths **20)** $4085\frac{3}{40}$, 4085.075 **21)** 0.0170 **22)** 0.25 **23)** 0.75 **24)** $\frac{9}{200}$ **25)** 0.120 **26)** 0.063 **27)** False **28)** False **29)** True **30)** 0.8 gram and 1.25 grams

Solutions—Review Set 4

4) $0.006 = \frac{6}{1000} = \frac{3}{500}$

8) $\frac{4}{5} = 5\overline{)4.0}$ 0.8

14) $\frac{21}{250} = 250\overline{)21.000}$
$$0.084$$
$$\underline{20\ 00}$$
$$1\ 000$$
$$\underline{1\ 000}$$

15) $12.125 = 12\frac{125}{1000} = 12\frac{1}{8}$

18) $0.15 = \frac{15}{100} = \frac{3}{20}$

30) 0.5 gram ≤ safe dose ≤ 2 grams

Safe doses: 0.8 grams and 1.25 grams

Note: "≤" means "less than or equal to"

Review Set 5 from pages 28–29

1) 22.585 **2)** 44.177 **3)** 12.309 **4)** 11.3 **5)** 175.199 **6)** 25.007 **7)** 0.518 **8)** $9.48 **9)** $18.91 **10)** $22.71 **11)** 6.403 **12)** 0.27 **13)** 4.15 **14)** 1.51 **15)** 10.25 **16)** 2.517 **17)** 374.35 **18)** 604.42 **19)** 27.449 **20)** 23.619 **21)** 0.697 gram **22)** 18.55 ounces **23)** $2,058.06 **24)** 12.3 grams **25)** 8.1 hours

Solutions—Review Set 5

2)
$$7.517$$
$$3.200$$
$$0.160$$
$$\underline{33.300}$$
$$44.177$$

9)
$$8\ 9\ 10$$
$$\$1\cancel{9}.\cancel{0}\cancel{0}$$
$$\underline{-\ 0.09}$$
$$\$18.91$$

25)
3 h 20 min
40 min
3 h 30 min
24 min
$\underline{12\ \text{min}}$
6 h 126 min = 8 h 6 min (60 minutes/hour)
$= 8\frac{6}{60} = 8\frac{1}{10} = 8.1$ hours

ANSWERS

Review Set 6 from page 34

1) 5.83 **2)** 2.20 **3)** 42.75 **4)** 0.15 **5)** 403.14 **6)** 75,100.75 **7)** 32.86 **8)** 2.78 **9)** 348.58 **10)** 0.02 **11)** 400 **12)** 3.74 **13)** 5

14) 2.98 **15)** 4120 **16)** 5.45 **17)** 272.67 **18)** 1.5 **19)** 50,020 **20)** 300 **21)** 562.50. = 56,250 **22)** 16.0. = 160 **23)** .025. = 0.025

24) .032.005 = 0.032005 **25)** .00.125 = 0.00125 **26)** 23.2.5 = 232.5 **27)** 71.7.717 = 71.7717 **28)** 83.1.6 = 831.6

29) 0.33. = 33 **30)** 14.106. = 14,106

Solutions—Review Set 6

10) $1.14 \times 0.014 = 0.01596 = 0.02$ **14)** $45.5 \div 15.25 = 2.983 = 2.98$

Practice Problems—Chapter 1 from pages 34–36

1) $\frac{7}{20}$ **2)** 0.375 **3)** LCD = 21 **4)** LCD = 55 **5)** LCD = 18 **6)** LCD = 15 **7)** $3\frac{7}{15}$ **8)** $7\frac{29}{60}$ **9)** $\frac{1}{2}$ **10)** $2\frac{7}{24}$ **11)** $\frac{7}{27}$ **12)** $10\frac{1}{8}$ **13)** $4\frac{4}{17}$

14) $\frac{39}{80}$ **15)** $5\frac{1}{55}$ **16)** $5\frac{5}{18}$ **17)** $2\frac{86}{87}$ **18)** $\frac{3}{20}$ **19)** $\frac{1}{3125}$ **20)** $\frac{1}{4}$ **21)** $1\frac{5}{7}$ **22)** $16\frac{1}{32}$ **23)** 60.27 **24)** 66.74 **25)** 42.98 **26)** 4833.92

27) 190.8 **28)** 19.17 **29)** 9.48 **30)** 7.7 **31)** 42.75 **32)** 300 **33)** 12,930.43 **34)** 3200.63 **35)** 2 **36)** 150.96 **37)** 9716 **38)** 0.5025

39) 25 **40)** 5750 **41)** 0.025 **42)** 115.25 **43)** 147 ounces **44)** 138 nurses; 46 maintenance/cleaners; 92 technicians; 92 others;

45) False **46)** $915.08 **47)** $1.46 **48)** 0.31 gram **49)** 800 mL **50)** 2.95 kilograms

Solutions—Practice Problems—Chapter 1

43) $3\frac{1}{2}$ ounces/feeding $\times$ 6 feedings/day =

21 ounces/day, and 21 ounces/day $\times$ 7 days/week =

147 ounces in one week

44) $\frac{3}{8} \times 368 = 138$ nurses

$\frac{1}{8} \times 368 = 46$ maintenance/cleaners

$\frac{1}{4} \times 368 = 92$ technicians and 92 others

45) $1\frac{2}{32} = 1.0625$; False, it's greater than normal.

46) 40 hours $\times$ $17.43/hour = $697.20

6.25 hours overtime $\times$ $34.86 =   + 217.88

(Overtime rate = $17.43 $\times$ 2 = $34.86) $915.08

47) A case of 12 boxes with 12 catheters/box =

144 catheters

By case: $975 \div 144 = $6.77/catheter

By box: $98.76 \div 12 = $8.23/catheter

$8.23
$- 6.77$
$1.46 savings/catheter

48) 0.065 gram/ounce $\times$ 4.75 ounces = 0.31 gram

49) 1200 milliliters $\times \frac{2}{3} = \frac{\overset{400}{\cancel{1200}}}{1} \times \frac{2}{\underset{1}{\cancel{3}}} = 800$ milliliters

50) 6.65 kilograms
$- 3.70$ kilograms
2.95 kilograms gained

Review Set 7 from page 41

1) $\frac{1}{50}$ **2)** $\frac{3}{5}$ **3)** $\frac{1}{3}$ **4)** $\frac{4}{7}$ **5)** $\frac{3}{4}$ **6)** 0.5 **7)** 0.15 **8)** 0.14 **9)** 0.07 **10)** 0.24 **11)** 25% **12)** 40% **13)** 12.5% **14)** 70% **15)** 50% **16)** $\frac{9}{20}$

17) $\frac{3}{5}$ **18)** $\frac{1}{200}$ **19)** $\frac{1}{100}$ **20)** $\frac{2}{3}$ **21)** 0.03 **22)** 0.05 **23)** 0.06 **24)** 0.33 **25)** 0.01 **26)** 4:25 **27)** 1:4 **28)** 1:2 **29)** 9:20 **30)** 3:50

31) 0.9 **32)** $\frac{1}{5}$ **33)** 0.25% **34)** 0.5 **35)** $\frac{1}{100}$

Solutions—Review Set 7

1) $\dfrac{\frac{3}{150}}{\frac{150}{50}} = \dfrac{\frac{1}{3}}{\underset{50}{\cancel{150}}} = \dfrac{1}{50}$ **3)** $\dfrac{0.05}{0.15} = \dfrac{\frac{1}{0.05}}{\underset{3}{0.15}} = \dfrac{1}{3}$

7) $\dfrac{\frac{1}{1000}}{\frac{1}{150}} = \dfrac{1}{1000} \times \dfrac{\overset{15}{\cancel{150}}}{1} = \dfrac{15}{100} = 0.15. = 0.15$

12) $2:5 = \dfrac{2}{5} = 0.4;\ 0.4 = \dfrac{4}{10} = \dfrac{40}{100} = 40\%$

13) $0.08 : 0.64 = \dfrac{0.08}{0.64} = \dfrac{1}{8} = 0.125;$

   $0.125 = \dfrac{125}{1000} = \dfrac{12.5}{100} = 12.5\%$

17) $60\% = \dfrac{60}{100} = \dfrac{3}{5}$

18) $0.5\% = \dfrac{0.5}{100} = 0.5 \div 100 = 0.00.5 = 0.005 = \dfrac{5}{1000} = \dfrac{1}{200}$

21) $2.94\% = \dfrac{2.94}{100} = 2.94 \div 100 = 0.02.94 = 0.029 = 0.03$

30) $6\% = \dfrac{6}{100} = \dfrac{3}{50} = 3{:}50$

31) Convert to decimals and compare:

   $0.9\% \quad = 0.009$

   $0.9 \quad\ \ = 0.900$ (largest)

   $1:9 \quad\ = 0.111$

   $1:90 \quad = 0.011$

Review Set 8 from page 45

1) 3 **2)** 3.3 **3)** 1.25 **4)** 5.33 **5)** 0.56 **6)** 1.8 **7)** 0.64 **8)** 12.6 **9)** 40 **10)** 0.48 **11)** 1 **12)** 0.96 **13)** 4.5 **14)** 0.94 **15)** 10 **16)** 0.4 **17)** 1.5 **18)** 10 **19)** 20 **20)** 1.8

Solutions—Review Set 8

2) $\dfrac{\frac{3}{4}}{\frac{1}{2}} \times 2.2 = X$

   $\dfrac{3}{4} \div \dfrac{1}{2} \times \dfrac{2.2}{1} = X$

   $\dfrac{3}{\underset{2}{\cancel{4}}} \times \dfrac{\overset{1}{\cancel{2}}}{1} \times \dfrac{2.2}{1} = X$

   $\dfrac{6.6}{2} = X$

   $X = 3.3$

4) $\dfrac{40\%}{60\%} \times 8 = X$

   $\dfrac{\underset{3}{\cancel{0.6}}}{\overset{2}{\cancel{0.4}}} \times 8 = X$

   $\dfrac{2}{3} \times \dfrac{8}{1} = X$

   $\dfrac{16}{3} = X$

   $X = 5.333$

   $X = 5.33$

6) $\dfrac{0.15}{0.1} \times 1.2 = X$

   $\dfrac{\overset{3}{\cancel{0.15}}}{\underset{2}{\cancel{0.10}}} \times \dfrac{1.2}{1} = X$

   $\dfrac{3}{2} \times \dfrac{1.2}{1} = X$

   $\dfrac{3.6}{2} = X$

   $X = 1.8$

8) $\dfrac{\overset{3}{\cancel{1,200,000}}}{\underset{1}{\cancel{400,000}}} \times 4.2 = X$

   $\dfrac{3}{1} \times \dfrac{4.2}{1} = X$

   $\dfrac{12.6}{1} = X$

   $X = 12.6$

10) $\dfrac{\overset{3}{\cancel{30}}}{\underset{5}{\cancel{50}}} \times 0.8 = X$

   $\dfrac{3}{5} \times \dfrac{0.8}{1} = X$

   $\dfrac{2.4}{5} = X$

   $X = 0.48$

14) $\dfrac{\overset{1}{\cancel{250,000}}}{\underset{8}{\cancel{2,000,000}}} \times 7.5 = X$

   $\dfrac{1}{8} \times \dfrac{7.5}{1} = X$

   $\dfrac{7.5}{8} = X$

   $X = 0.937$

   $X = 0.94$

20) $\dfrac{\frac{1}{100}}{\frac{1}{150}} \times 1.2 = X$

   $\dfrac{1}{100} \div \dfrac{1}{150} \times \dfrac{1.2}{1} = X$

   $\dfrac{1}{\underset{2}{\cancel{100}}} \times \dfrac{\overset{3}{\cancel{150}}}{1} \times \dfrac{1.2}{1} = X$

   $\dfrac{1}{2} \times \dfrac{3}{1} \times \dfrac{1.2}{1} = X$

   $\dfrac{3.6}{2} = X$

   $X = 1.8$

Review Set 9 from pages 49–50

1) 0.25 **2)** 1 **3)** 0.56 **4)** 1000 **5)** 0.7 **6)** 514.29 **7)** 2142.86 **8)** 500 **9)** 200 **10)** 10.5 **11)** 3 **12)** 0.63 **13)** 10 **14)** 0.67 **15)** 1.25
16) 31.25 **17)** 16.67 **18)** 240 **19)** 0.75 **20)** 2.27 **21)** 1 **22)** 6 **23)** 108 nurses **24)** 72 calories **25)** 81.82 milligrams/hour

Solutions—Review Set 9

4) $\dfrac{0.5}{2} \times \dfrac{250}{X}$

$0.5X = 500$

$\dfrac{0.5X}{0.5} = \dfrac{500}{0.5}$

$X = 1000$

6) $\dfrac{1200}{X} \times 12 = 28$

$\dfrac{1200}{X} \times \dfrac{12}{1} = 28$

$\dfrac{14{,}400}{X} \times \dfrac{28}{1}$

$28X = 14{,}400$

$\dfrac{28X}{28} = \dfrac{14{,}400}{28}$

$X = 514.285$

$X = 514.29$

9) $\dfrac{15}{500} \times X = 6$

$\dfrac{15X}{500} \times \dfrac{6}{1}$

$15X = 3000$

$\dfrac{15X}{15} = \dfrac{3000}{15}$

$X = 200$

10) $\dfrac{5}{X} \times \dfrac{10}{21}$

$10X = 105$

$\dfrac{10X}{10} = \dfrac{105}{10}$

$X = 10.5$

11) $\dfrac{250}{1} \times \dfrac{750}{X}$

$250X = 750$

$\dfrac{250X}{250} = \dfrac{750}{250}$

$X = 3$

14) $\dfrac{\frac{1}{100}}{1} \times \dfrac{\frac{1}{150}}{X}$

$\dfrac{1}{100}X = \dfrac{1}{150}$

$\dfrac{\frac{1}{100}X}{\frac{1}{100}} = \dfrac{\frac{1}{150}}{\frac{1}{100}}$

$X = \dfrac{1}{150} \div \dfrac{1}{100}$

$X = \dfrac{1}{\underset{3}{\cancel{150}}} \times \dfrac{\overset{2}{\cancel{100}}}{1}$

$X = \dfrac{2}{3} = 0.666 = 0.67$

22) $\dfrac{25\%}{30\%} = \dfrac{5}{X}$

$\dfrac{0.25}{0.3} \times \dfrac{5}{X}$

$0.25X = 1.5$

$\dfrac{0.25X}{0.25} = \dfrac{1.5}{0.25}$

$X = 6$

23) $\dfrac{45}{100} \times \dfrac{X}{240}$

$100X = 10{,}800$

$\dfrac{100X}{100} = \dfrac{10{,}800}{100}$

$X = 108$

Review Set 10 from page 51

1) 1.3 **2)** 4.75 **3)** 56 **4)** 0.43 **5)** 26.67 **6)** 15 **7)** 0.8 **8)** 2.38 **9)** 37.5 **10)** 112.5 **11)** 8 pills **12)** 720 milliliters **13)** $3,530.21
14) 7.2 ounces **15)** 700 calories

Solutions—Review Set 10

1) $0.0025 \times 520 = 1.3$

8) $0.07 \times 34 = 2.38$

11) 0.4×20 pills $= 8$ pills

13)   80% of \$17,651.07 $= 0.8 \times$ \$17,651.07 $=$ \$14,120.86

$$\begin{array}{r} \$17,651.07 \text{ total bill} \\ -\ 14,120.86 \text{ paid by insurance co.} \\ \hline \$3,530.21 \text{ paid by patient} \end{array}$$

14) 0.4×18 ounces $= 7.2$ ounces

15) 0.2×3500 calories $= 700$ calories

Practice Problems—Chapter 2 from pages 51–53

1) 0.4, 40%, 2:5 **2)** $\frac{1}{20}$, 5%, 1:20 **3)** 0.17, $\frac{17}{100}$, 17:100 **4)** 0.25, $\frac{1}{4}$, 25% **5)** 0.06, $\frac{3}{50}$, 3:50 **6)** 0.17, 17%, 1:6 **7)** 0.5, $\frac{1}{2}$, 1:2

8) 0.01, $\frac{1}{100}$, 1% **9)** $\frac{9}{100}$, 9%, 9:100 **10)** 0.38, 38%, 3:8 **11)** 0.67, $\frac{2}{3}$, 67% **12)** 0.33, 33%, 1:3 **13)** $\frac{13}{25}$, 52%, 13:25

14) 0.45, $\frac{9}{20}$, 45% **15)** 0.86, 86%, 6:7 **16)** 0.3, $\frac{3}{10}$, 30% **17)** 0.02, 2%, 1:50 **18)** $\frac{3}{5}$, 60%, 3:5 **19)** $\frac{1}{25}$, 4%, 1:25

20) 0.1, $\frac{1}{10}$, 1:10 **21)** 0.04 **22)** 1:40 **23)** 7.5% **24)** $\frac{1}{2}$ **25)** 3:4 **26)** 262.5 **27)** 3.64 **28)** 1.97 **29)** 1:4 **30)** 1:10 **31)** 84 **32)** 90,000

33) 1 **34)** 1.1 **35)** 100 **36)** 39 **37)** 0.75 **38)** 21 **39)** 120 **40)** 90 **41)** 25 grams protein; 6.25 grams fat **42)** 231 points

43) 60 minutes **44)** 50 milliliters **45)** 27 milligrams **46)** 5.4 grams **47)** 283.5 milligrams **48)** 6.5 pounds **49)** \$10.42

50) 6 total doses

Solutions—Practice Problems—Chapter 2

36) $\dfrac{3}{9} \diagdown\diagup \dfrac{X}{117}$

$9X = 351$

$\dfrac{9X}{9} = \dfrac{351}{9}$

$X = 39$

41) $125 \times 0.2 = 25$ grams protein

$125 \times 0.05 = 6.25$ grams fat

$$\begin{array}{r} 125 \\ \times\ 0.2 \\ \hline 25.0\ = 25 \end{array}$$

$$\begin{array}{r} 125 \\ \times\ 0.05 \\ \hline 6.25\ = 6.25 \end{array}$$

43) $\dfrac{90}{27} \diagdown\diagup \dfrac{200}{X}$

$90X = 5400$

$\dfrac{90X}{90} = \dfrac{5400}{90}$

$X = 60$

45) $60 \times 0.45 = 27$ milligrams

$$\begin{array}{r} 60 \\ \times\ 0.45 \\ \hline 300 \\ 240 \\ \hline 27.00 = 27 \end{array}$$

46) $\dfrac{2.7}{0.75} \diagdown\diagup \dfrac{X}{1.5}$

$0.75X = 4.05$

$\dfrac{0.75X}{0.75} = \dfrac{4.05}{0.75}$

$X = 5.4$

47) $\dfrac{6.75}{1} \diagdown\diagup \dfrac{X}{42}$

$X = 283.5$

48) $130 \times 0.05 = 6.5$ pounds

$$\begin{array}{r} 130 \\ \times\ 0.05 \\ \hline 6.50 = 6.5 \end{array}$$

49) $0.17 \times \$12.56 = \$2.14$

$$\begin{array}{r} \$12.56 \\ -\ 2.14 \\ \hline \$10.42 \end{array}$$

50) $10\% \text{ of } 150 = 0.10 \times 150 = 15;$

$$\begin{array}{r} 150 \text{ mg} \quad \text{first dose} \\ -\ 15 \\ \hline \end{array}$$
$$\begin{array}{r} 135 \text{ mg} \quad \text{second dose} \\ -\ 15 \\ \hline \end{array}$$
$$\begin{array}{r} 120 \text{ mg} \quad \text{third dose} \\ -\ 15 \\ \hline \end{array}$$
$$\begin{array}{r} 105 \text{ mg} \quad \text{fourth dose} \\ -\ 15 \\ \hline \end{array}$$
$$\begin{array}{r} 90 \text{ mg} \quad \text{fifth dose} \\ -\ 15 \\ \hline \end{array}$$
$$75 \text{ mg} \quad \text{sixth dose}$$

6 total doses

Section 1—Self-Evaluation from pages 54–55

1) 3.05 **2)** 4002.5 **3)** 0.63 **4)** 723.27 **5)** LCD = 12 **6)** LCD = 110 **7)** $\frac{11}{12}$ **8)** $\frac{47}{63}$ **9)** 1 **10)** $\frac{1}{2}$ **11)** 45.78 **12)** 0.02 **13)** 59.24
14) 0.09 **15)** 12 **16)** $\frac{2}{3}$ **17)** $\frac{1}{2}$ **18)** 0.64 **19)** $\frac{1}{10}, \frac{1}{6}, \frac{1}{5}, \frac{1}{3}, \frac{1}{2}$ **20)** $\frac{2}{3}, \frac{3}{4}, \frac{5}{6}, \frac{7}{8}, \frac{9}{10}$ **21)** 0.009, 0.125, 0.1909, 0.25, 0.3
22) $\frac{1}{2}$%, 0.9%, 50%, 100%, 500% **23)** 1:3 **24)** 1:600 **25)** 0.01 **26)** 0.04 **27)** 0.9% **28)** $\frac{1}{3}$ **29)** 5:9 **30)** $\frac{1}{20}$ **31)** 1:200
32) $\frac{2}{3}$ **33)** 75% **34)** 40% **35)** 0.17 **36)** 1.21 **37)** 1.3 **38)** 2.5 **39)** 0.67 **40)** 100 **41)** 4 **42)** 20,000 **43)** 3.3 **44)** 300 **45)** 8.33
46) 24 participants **47)** 2 holidays **48)** $2.42 **49)** 12 cans of water **50)** 8 centimeters

Solutions—Section 1—Self-Evaluation

16) $\dfrac{1}{150} \div \dfrac{1}{100} = \dfrac{1}{150} \times \dfrac{100}{1} = \dfrac{\overset{2}{\cancel{100}}}{\underset{3}{\cancel{150}}} = \dfrac{2}{3}$

18) $\dfrac{16\%}{\frac{1}{4}} = 16\% \times \dfrac{4}{1} = 0.16 \times 4 = 0.64$

33) $3:4 = \dfrac{3}{4} = 4\overline{)3.0}^{\,0.75} = 75\%$

37) $\dfrac{0.3}{2.6} \diagup\!\!\!\!\diagdown \dfrac{0.15}{X}$

$0.3X = 2.6 \times 0.15$

$0.3X = 0.39$

$\dfrac{0.3X}{0.3} = \dfrac{0.39}{0.3}$

$X = 1.3$

42) $\dfrac{10\%}{\frac{1}{2}\%} \times 1000 = X$

$\dfrac{0.1}{0.005} \times \dfrac{1000}{1} = X$

$\dfrac{100}{0.005} = X$

$X = 20,000$

46) $600 \times 0.04 = 24 \text{ participants}$

$$\begin{array}{r} 600 \\ \times\ 0.04 \\ \hline 24.00 \ = 24 \end{array}$$

Review Set 11 from pages 62–63

1) metric **2)** volume **3)** weight **4)** length **5)** $\frac{1}{1000}$ or 0.001 **6)** 1000 **7)** 10 **8)** kilogram **9)** milligram **10)** 1000 **11)** 1
12) 1000 **13)** 10 **14)** 0.3 g **15)** 1.33 mL **16)** 5 kg **17)** 1.5 mm **18)** 10 mg **19)** microgram **20)** milliliter **21)** cubic centimeter
22) gram **23)** millimeter **24)** kilogram **25)** centimeter

Review Set 12 from page 65

1) dram **2)** ounce **3)** minim **4)** one-half **5)** grain **6)** ℥ ss **7)** gr $\frac{1}{6}$ **8)** ℥ iv **9)** pt ii **10)** qt i $\frac{1}{4}$ **11)** gr x **12)** ℥ viiiss **13)** gr ii
14) pt 16 **15)** gr iii **16)** ℥ 32 **17)** gr viiss **18)** 32 **19)** i **20)** ii

Review Set 13 from page 68

1) twenty drops **2)** one thousand units **3)** ten milliequivalents **4)** four teaspoons **5)** ten tablespoons **6)** 4 gtt

7) 30 mEq **8)** 5 T **9)** 1500 U **10)** 10 t **11)** False **12)** False **13)** False **14)** units, U **15)** 3 **16)** 2 **17)** 1 **18)** 1 **19)** 1

20) international unit, IU

Practice Problems—Chapter 3 from pages 70–71

1) milli **2)** micro **3)** centi **4)** kilo **5)** 1 milligram **6)** 1 kilogram **7)** 1 microgram **8)** 1 centimeter **9)** meter **10)** gram

11) liter **12)** drop **13)** ounce **14)** ounce **15)** grain **16)** milligram **17)** microgram **18)** unit **19)** milliequivalent

20) teaspoon **21)** milliunit **22)** milliliter **23)** cubic centimeter **24)** pint **25)** tablespoon **26)** millimeter **27)** gram

28) centimeter **29)** liter **30)** meter **31)** kilogram **32)** international unit **33)** gr ss **34)** 2 t **35)** ʒ $\frac{1}{3}$ **36)** 500 mg **37)** 0.5 L

38) ʒ $\frac{1}{4}$ **39)** gr $\frac{1}{200}$ **40)** 0.05 mg **41)** eight and one-quarter ounces **42)** three hundred seventy-five international units

43) one one-hundred twenty-fifths of a grain **44)** two and six tenths milliliters **45)** twenty milliequivalents **46)** four tenths

of a liter **47)** four and one-half grains **48)** seventeen hundredths of a milligram

49)　Critical Thinking Skill: Prevention. This type of error can be prevented by avoiding the use of a decimal point or

　　　　extra zero when not necessary. In this instance the decimal point and zero serve no purpose and can easily be

　　　　misinterpreted, especially if the decimal point is difficult to see. Question any order that is unclear or unreasonable.

50)　Critical Thinking Skill: Prevention. This is both an error in notation and transcription. One grain should have been

　　　　written *gr i*. Health care facilities would be wise to require the use of metric notation, especially for narcotics. The

　　　　nurse's knowledge of correct notation as well as common dosages for pain medication should signal a problem.

　　　　Question any order that is unclear or unreasonable.

Review Set 14 from pages 76–77

1) divide **2)** multiply **3)** 3 **4)** 3 **5)** $3\frac{1}{2}$ **6)** 16 **7)** 72 **8)** $1\frac{1}{2}$ **9)** $\frac{2}{3}$ **10)** 52 **11)** $\frac{1}{4}$ **12)** 30 **13)** $3\frac{1}{3}$ **14)** 14 **15)** $\frac{3}{4}$ **16)** $\frac{1}{12}$ **17)** $\frac{2}{3}$

18) $\frac{1}{4}$ **19)** 40 **20)** $3\frac{1}{2}$ **21)** 20 servings **22)** 8 quarts **23)** 64¢ **24)** 20¢ **25)** 24¢

Solutions—Review Set 14

6)　　$32 \div 2 = 16$

8)　　$\frac{1}{2} \times 3 = \frac{3}{2} = 1\frac{1}{2}$

19)　　$2\frac{1}{2} \times 16 = \frac{5}{\underset{1}{2}} \times \frac{\overset{8}{16}}{1} = 40$

20)　　$\frac{126}{36} = 3\frac{18}{36} = 3\frac{1}{2}$

21)　　2 quarts = 8 cups

　　　　$\frac{1}{2}$ gallon = 8 cups

　　　　　　　　+ 4 cups

　　　　_____

　　　　　　20 cups or 20 1-cup servings

23)　　Store A: = $1.56 × 2 =　　$3.12/gallon

　　　　Store B: = $0.94 × 4 =　　$3.76/gallon

　　　　　　　　　　　　　　− $3.12

　　　　　　　　　　_____

　　　　　　　　　　$0.64 savings at Store A

24)　　$1.56 ÷ 8 = $0.195 or 19.5¢/cup or 20¢/cup

25)　　$0.94 ÷ 4 = $0.235 or 23.5¢/cup or 24¢/cup

Review Set 15 from page 80

1) 0.5 **2)** 15 **3)** 0.008 **4)** 0.01 **5)** 0.06 **6)** 0.3 **7)** 0.0002 **8)** 1200 **9)** 2.5 **10)** 65 **11)** 5 **12)** 1500 **13)** 2 **14)** 0.25 **15)** 2000

16) 56.08 **17)** 5 **18)** 1000 **19)** 1000 **20)** 0.001 **21)** 0.023 **22)** 0.00105 **23)** 0.018 **24)** 400 **25)** 0.025 **26)** 0.5 **27)** 10,000

28) 0.45 **29)** 0.005 **30)** 30,000

ANSWERS

Solutions—Review Set 15

2) $\underset{\smile}{0.015}$. g = 15 mg; g is larger than mg. To convert from larger to smaller unit, multiply. It takes more of mg (smaller) unit to make equivalent amount of g (larger) unit. Equivalent: 1 g = 1000 mg. Therefore, multiply by 1000 or move decimal point three places to right.

3) $\underset{\smile}{.008}$. mg = 0.008 g; mg is smaller unit than g. To convert from smaller to larger unit, divide. It takes fewer of g (larger) unit to make equivalent amount of mg (smaller) unit. Therefore, divide by 1000 or move decimal point three places to left.

7) $\underset{\smile}{.000.2}$ mg = 0.0002 g **9)** $\underset{\smile}{0.002.5}$ kg = 2.5 g **20)** $\underset{\smile}{.001}$. mL = 0.001 L **23)** $\underset{\smile}{.018}$. mcg = 0.018 mg

Review Set 16 from pages 84–86

1) 30, gr i = 60 mg **2)** 45, gr i = 60 mg **3)** 0.003, 1 kg = 1000 g **4)** 0.4, gr i = 60 mg **5)** 0.5, 1 g = gr xv **6)** $\frac{1}{4}$, gr i = 60 mg **7)** 65, 1 t = 5 mL **8)** ss, ℥ i = 30 cc **9)** 75, ℥ i = 30 mL **10)** iss, pt i = 500 mL **11)** 4, 1 t = 5 mL **12)** 60, 1 T = 15 mL **13)** 19.8, 1 kg = 2.2 lb **14)** viii, qt i = pt ii **15)** 96, 1 L = ℥ 32 **16)** 121, 1 kg = 2.2 lb **17)** 30, 1 in = 2.5 cm **18)** 2, qt i = 1 L **19)** 15, 1 t = 5 mL **20)** 45, 1 kg = 2.2 lb **21)** 300, gr i = 60 mg; or 325, gr i = 65 mg (in select cases) **22)** $\frac{1}{100}$, gr i = 60 mg **23)** 500, pt i = 500 mL **24)** 600, gr i = 60 mg; or 650, gr i = 65 mg (in select cases) **25)** v, gr i = 60 mg **26)** 12, 1 in = 2.5 cm **27)** iss, gr i = 60 mg **28)** ii, ℥ i = 30 mL **29)** 10, gr i = 60 mg **30)** i, gr i = 65 mg (only in select cases) **31)** 80, 1 in = 2.5 cm **32)** 14, 1 in = 2.5 cm, 1 cm = 10 mm **33)** 3, 1 in = 2.5 cm, 1 cm = 10 mm **34)** 50, 1 in = 2.5 cm, 1 cm = 10 mm **35)** 88, 1 kg = 2.2 lb **36)** 7160, 1 kg = 1000 g **37)** 50, 1 kg = 2.2 lb **38)** 7.7, 1 kg = 2.2 lb **39)** 28.64, 1 kg = 2.2 lb **40)** 53.75 **41)** 4, $\frac{1}{2}$ **42)** 15.75 **43)** 2430 **44)** 1.25 **45)** 10 **46)** Dissolve 2 teaspoons of Betadine concentrate in 1 pint or 2 cups of warm water. **47)** 2 **48)** 3 **49)** 16 **50)** 93.64

Solutions—Review Set 16

2) gr → mg; larger → smaller: (X)

$$gr\,\frac{3}{4} = \frac{3}{\overset{}{\underset{1}{4}}} \times \frac{\overset{15}{60}}{1} = 45\ mg$$

4) gr → mg; larger → smaller: (X)

$$gr\,\frac{1}{150} = \frac{1}{\underset{5}{150}} \times \frac{\overset{2}{60}}{1} = \frac{2}{5}\ mg = 0.4\ mg$$

5) gr → g; smaller → larger unit: (÷)

gr viiss = gr $7\frac{1}{2}$; gr 7.5 = 7.5 ÷ 15 = 0.5 g

6) mg → gr; smaller → larger: (÷)

15 mg = 15 ÷ 60 = gr $\frac{1}{4}$

9) ℥ → mL; larger → smaller: (X)

℥ iiss = ℥ $2\frac{1}{2}$; ℥ 2.5 = 2.5 × 30 = 75 mL

11) mL → t; smaller → larger: (÷)

20 mL = 20 ÷ 5 = 4 t

16) kg → lb; larger → smaller: (X)

55 kg = 55 × 2.2 = 121 lb

20) lb → kg; smaller → larger: (÷)

99 lb = 99 ÷ 2.2 = 45 kg

24) gr → mg; larger → smaller: (×)

gr x = gr 10; gr 10 = 10 × 60 = 600 mg

28) mL → ℥; smaller → larger: (÷)

60 mL = 60 ÷ 30 = ℥ 2 = ℥ ii

34) in → mm; larger → smaller: (×)

2 in = 2 × 2.5 = 5 cm

cm → mm; larger → smaller: (×)

5 cm = 5 × 10 = 50 mm

41) mL → oz; smaller → larger: (÷)

120 mL = 120 ÷ 30 = 4 = ℥ iv

℥ → cups; smaller to larger: (÷)

℥ iv = ℥ 4; ℥ 4 = 4 ÷ 8 = $\frac{1}{2}$ cup

42) m → km; smaller to larger: (÷)

500 m = 500 ÷ 1000 = 0.5 km

0.75	Day 1
+ .50	
1.25	Day 2
+ .50	
1.75	Day 3
+ .50	
2.25	Day 4
+ .50	
2.75	Day 5
+ .50	
3.25	Day 6
+ .50	
3.75	Day 7

Total kilometers walked in 7 days =

0.75 + 1.25 + 1.75 + 2.25 + 2.75 + 3.25 + 3.75 =

15.75 km

43) Add up the ounces: 81 ounces

ʒ → mL; larger → smaller: (×)

ʒ 81 = 81 × 30 = 2430 mL

44) lb → kg; smaller → larger: (÷)

55 kg = 55 ÷ 2.2 = 25 kg

0.05 mg/kg × 25 kg = 1.25 mg

45) Find the total number of mL per day and the total number of mL per bottle.

Per day: 12 mL × 4 = 48 mL

Per bottle: 16 ounces × 30 mL/ounce = 480 mL

480 mL ÷ 48 mL/day =

$\overset{10}{480 \text{ mL}} \times \frac{1 \text{ day}}{\underset{1}{48 \text{ mL}}} = 10 \text{ days}$

46) mL → t; smaller → larger (÷)

10 mL = 10 ÷ 5 = 2 t

500 mL = pt i or 2 cups water

Use 2 t Betadine concentrate in 1 pint or 2 cups of water.

48) qt i = ʒ 32 per container
4 oz/feeding × 8 feedings/day = ʒ 32 per day
She needs 3 containers for 3 days.

Review Set 17 from page 87

1) 30, 1 g = 1000 mg

2) 20, 1 in = 2.5 cm

3) 220, 1 kg = 2.2 lb

4) $\frac{3}{4}$, gr i = 60 mg

5) 0.175, 1 mg = 1000 mcg

6) 4.5, 1 kg = 2.2 lb

7) 15, 1 t = 5 mL

8) 2, qt i = 1 L

9) 3.5, 1 kg = 1000 g

10) 12, 1 in = 2.5 cm

11) 0.6, gr i = 60 mg

12) 0.00015, 1 g = 1000 mg; 1 mg = 1000 mcg

13) $\frac{1}{6}$, gr i = 60 mg

14) 2, 1 t = 5 mL

15) 2273, 1 kg = 2.2 lb; 1 kg = 1000 g

16) 375, 1 mg = 1000 mcg

17) 2.5, 1 t = 5 mL

18) 15, ʒ i = 30 mL

19) iiss, ʒ i = 30 mL

Solutions—Review Set 17

1) 0.03 g = 30 mg   1 g = 1000 mg

$\frac{0.03 \text{ g}}{1 \text{ g}} \times 1000 \text{ mg} = 30 \text{ mg}$

4) 45 mg = gr $\frac{3}{4}$ gr i = 60 mg

$\frac{45 \text{ mg}}{\underset{4}{60 \text{ mg}}} \times \text{gr i} = \text{gr} \frac{\overset{3}{}}{4}$

5) 175 mcg = 175 ÷ 1000 = 0.175 mg 1 mg = 1000 mcg

$\frac{175 \text{ mcg}}{1000 \text{ mcg}} \times 1 \text{ mg} = 0.175 \text{ mg}$

11) gr $\frac{1}{100}$ = 0.6 mg   gr i = 60 mg

$\frac{\text{gr} \frac{1}{100}}{\text{gr } 1} \times 60 \text{ mg} = \frac{60}{100} \text{ mg} = \frac{6}{10} \text{ mg} = 0.6 \text{ mg}$

12) 1 g = 1000 mg; 1 mg = 1000 mcg

150 mcg = 0.00015 g

$\frac{150 \text{ mcg}}{1000 \text{ mcg}} \times 1 \text{ mg} = 0.15 \text{ mg}$

$\frac{0.15 \text{ mg}}{1000 \text{ mg}} \times 1 \text{ g} = 0.00015 \text{ g}$

15) 1 kg = 2.2 lb;   1 kg = 1000 g   5 lb = 2273 g

$\frac{5 \text{ lb}}{2.2 \text{ lb}} \times 1 \text{ kg} = 2.2727 = 2.273 \text{ kg}$

$\frac{2.273 \text{ kg}}{1 \text{ kg}} \times 1000 \text{ g} = 2273 \text{ g}$

ANSWERS

Review Set 18 from page 90

1) 0.05, 1 L = 1000 mL **2)** 45, 1 g = gr 15 **3)** 38.18, 1 kg = 2.2 lb **4)** 1.33, 1 g = gr 15 **5)** 7.5, gr i = 60 mg;

6) iiss, ʒ i = 30 mL **7)** iss, pt i = 500 mL **8)** 45, ʒ i = 30 mL **9)** $\frac{1}{4}$, gr i = 60 mg **10)** 0.625, 1 mg = 1000 mcg

11) $\frac{1}{2}$, 1 t = 5 mL **12)** 30, gr i = 60 mg **13)** $\frac{1}{6}$, gr i = 60 mg **14)** $\frac{1}{100}$, gr i = 60 mg **15)** 3, 1 in = 2.5 cm

16) 16,000, 1 g = 1000 mg **17)** ss, ʒ i = 30 mL **18)** ss, qt i = ʒ 32 **19)** 2, qt i = 1 L **20)** ss, qt i = pt ii **21)** v, ʒ i =

30 mL **22)** 1, 1 t = 5 mL **23)** 8, 1 L = 1000 mL, 1 L = qt i, qt i = ʒ 32 **24)** 3; 1 t = 5 mL **25)** 15, gr i = 60 mg

Solutions—Review Set 18

3) $\frac{1 \text{ kg}}{2.2 \text{ lb}} \diagup\!\!\!\!\diagdown \frac{X \text{ kg}}{84 \text{ kg}}$

$$2.2X = 84$$

$$\frac{2.2X}{2.2} = \frac{84}{2.2}$$

$$X = 38.18 \text{ kg}$$

5) $\frac{\text{gr i}}{60 \text{ mg}} \diagup\!\!\!\!\diagdown \frac{\text{gr}\frac{1}{8}}{X \text{ mg}}$

$$X = 60 \times \frac{1}{8}$$

$$X = \frac{60}{8} \text{ mg} = 7.5 \text{ mg}$$

7) $\frac{500 \text{ mL}}{\text{pt i}} \diagup\!\!\!\!\diagdown \frac{750 \text{ mL}}{\text{pt X}}$

$$500X = 750$$

$$\frac{500X}{500} = \frac{750}{500}$$

$$X = \text{pt } 1\frac{1}{2}$$

$$X = \text{pt iss}$$

14) $\frac{\text{gr i}}{60 \text{ mg}} \diagup\!\!\!\!\diagdown \frac{X \text{ gr}}{0.6 \text{ mg}}$

$$60X = 0.6$$

$$\frac{60X}{60} = \frac{0.6}{60}$$

$$X = \text{gr } 0.01 = \text{gr } \frac{1}{100}$$

23) 2000 mL = 2 L

$$2 \text{ L} = \text{qt ii} = 64 \text{ oz}$$

$\frac{8 \text{ oz}}{1 \text{ cup}} \diagup\!\!\!\!\diagdown \frac{64 \text{ oz}}{X \text{ cup}}$

$$8X = 64$$

$$\frac{8X}{8} = \frac{64}{8}$$

$$X = 8 \text{ cups or 8 8-oz glasses}$$

Practice Problems—Chapter 4 from pages 91–92

1) 500 **2)** 10 **3)** 7.5 **4)** 3 **5)** 0.004 **6)** 0.5 **7)** ss **8)** 0.3 **9)** 70 **10)** 149.6 **11)** 180 **12)** 105 **13)** 0.3 **14)** 15 **15)** 6 **16)** 90

17) 32.05 **18)** 7.99 **19)** 0.008 **20)** 2 **21)** 95 **22)** *v*iiss **23)** $\frac{1}{100}$ **24)** 0.67 **25)** 68.18 **26)** i **27)** 1 **28)** 500 **29)** 2 **30)** iii **31)** 30

32) 30 **33)** 1 **34)** 1 **35)** 1 **36)** 1500 **37)** 45 **38)** iss **39)** $\frac{1}{6}$ **40)** 0.025 **41)** 4300 **42)** 0.06 **43)** 15 **44)** 45 **45)** 0.8 **46)** 9 **47)** 8

48) 840 **49)** 100%; all of it

50) Critical Thinking Skill: Prevention. The nurse didn't use the conversion rules correctly. The nurse divided instead of multiplying. Further, the conversion factor is 1000, not 2. This type of medication error is avoided by double checking your dosage calculations and asking yourself, "Is this dosage reasonable?" Certainly you know if there are 1000 mg in 1 g, and you want to give 2 g, then you need *more* than 1000 milligrams, not less. Remember: To convert from a larger unit (g) to a smaller unit (mg), *multiply* by the conversion factor. Larger → Smaller: (×).

Solutions—Practice Problems—Chapter 4

46) Per bottle: ʒ i*v* = 4 × 30 = 120 mL (ʒ i = 30 mL)

Each dose: $2\frac{1}{2}$ t = $2\frac{1}{2}$ × 5 = 12.5 mL (1 t = 5 mL)

Bottle holds 120 mL; each dose is 12.5 mL.

120 m̶L̶ ÷ 12.5 m̶L̶/dose = 9.6 doses or 9 *full* doses

47) 120 m̶L̶ ÷ 15 m̶L̶/dose = 8 doses (1 T = 15 mL)

48) $4 + 8 + 6 + 10 = 28$ oz ; $28 \text{ oz} \times 30 \text{ mL/oz} = 840 \text{ mL}$ ($\overline{3}$ i = 30 mL)

49) gr $\frac{1}{6} = \frac{1}{6} \times \frac{60}{1} = \frac{60}{6}$ mg = 10 mg ordered (gr i = 60 mg)

The ampule contains 10 mg, and the doctor orders gr $\frac{1}{6}$ or 10 mg; therefore, the patient should receive all of the solution in the ampule.

Review Set 19 from page 96

1) 12:32 AM 2) 7:30 AM 3) 4:40 PM 4) 9:21 PM 5) 11:59 PM 6) 12:15 PM 7) 2:20 AM 8) 10:10 AM 9) 1:15 PM 10) 6:25 PM

11) 1330 12) 0004 13) 2145 14) 1200 15) 2315 16) 0345 17) 2400 18) 1530 19) 0620 20) 1745

21) "zero-six-twenty-three" 22) "zero-zero-forty-one" 23) "nineteen-zero-three" 24) "twenty-three-eleven"

25) "zero-three hundred"

Review Set 20 from pages 98–99

1) –17.8 2) 185 3) 212 4) 89.6 5) 22.2 6) 37.2 7) 39.8 8) 104 9) 176 10) 97.5 11) 37.8 12) 66.2 13) 39.2 14) 34.6

15) 39.3 16) 35.3 17) 44.6 18) 31.1 19) 98.6 20) 39.7

Solutions—Review Set 20

1)
$$°C = \frac{°F - 32}{1.8}$$
$$°C = \frac{0 - 32}{1.8}$$
$$°C = \frac{-32}{1.8}$$
$$°C = -17.8°$$

2)
$$°F = 1.8°C + 32$$
$$°F = (1.8 \times 85) + 32$$
$$°F = 153 + 32$$
$$°F = 185°$$

Practice Problems—Chapter 5 from pages 99–100

1) 2:57 AM 2) 0310 3) 1622 4) 8:01 PM 5) 11:02 AM 6) 0033 7) 0216 8) 4:42 PM 9) 11:56 PM 10) 0420 11) 1931

12) 2400 or 0000 13) 0645 14) 9:15 AM 15) 9:07 PM 16) 6:23 PM 17) 5:40 AM 18) 1155 19) 2212 20) 2106 21) 4 h 22) 7 h

23) 8 h 30 min 24) 12 h 15 min 25) 14 h 50 min 26) 4 h 12 min 27) 4 h 48 min 28) 3 h 41 min 29) 6 h 30 min

30) 16 h 38 min 31) False 32) a. AM; b. PM; c. AM; d. PM 33) 37.6 34) 97.7 35) 102.6 36) 37.9 37) 36.7 38) 99.3

39) 32 40) 40 41) 36.6 42) 95.7 43) 39.7 44) 77 45) 212 46) 5.6 47) –7.8 48) 37.2, 99 (98.96° rounds to 99.0°F) 49) True

50) Critical Thinking Skill: Prevention. Such situations can be easily prevented by accurately applying the complete formula for temperature conversion. Guessing is not acceptable in medical and health care calculations. Temperature conversion charts are readily available in most health care settings, but, when they are not, the conversion formulas should be used.

Solutions—Practice Problems—Chapter 5

24)
$$\begin{array}{r} 2150 \\ -\ 0935 \\ \hline 1215 = 12 \text{ h } 15 \text{ min} \end{array}$$

26) 2316 = 11:16 PM, 0328 = 3:28 AM
11:16 PM $\rightarrow$ 3:16 AM = 4 h
$$\begin{array}{r} 3:16 \text{ AM} \rightarrow 3:28 \text{ AM} = 12 \text{ min} \\ \hline 4 \text{ h } 12 \text{ min} \end{array}$$

28)
4:35 PM $\rightarrow$ 7:35 PM = 3 h
$$\begin{array}{r} 7:35 \text{ PM} \rightarrow 8:16 \text{ PM} = 41 \text{ min} \\ \hline 3 \text{ h } 41 \text{ min} \end{array}$$

48)
$$\frac{37.6 + 35.5 + 38.1 + 37.6}{4} = \frac{148.8}{4} = 37.2°C \text{ (average)}$$
$$°F = 1.8(37.2) + 32 = 99°$$

Review Set 21 from pages 110–112

1) 1 mL(tuberculin) 2) a. yes; b. Round 1.25 to 1.3 and measure on the mL scale as 1.3 mL. 3) No 4) 0.5 cc 5) a. False; b. The size of the drop varies according to the diameter of the tip of the dropper. 6) No 7) Measure the oral liquid in a 3 mL syringe, which is not intended for injections. 8) 5 9) Discard the excess prior to injecting the patient. 10) To prevent needlestick injury.

11)

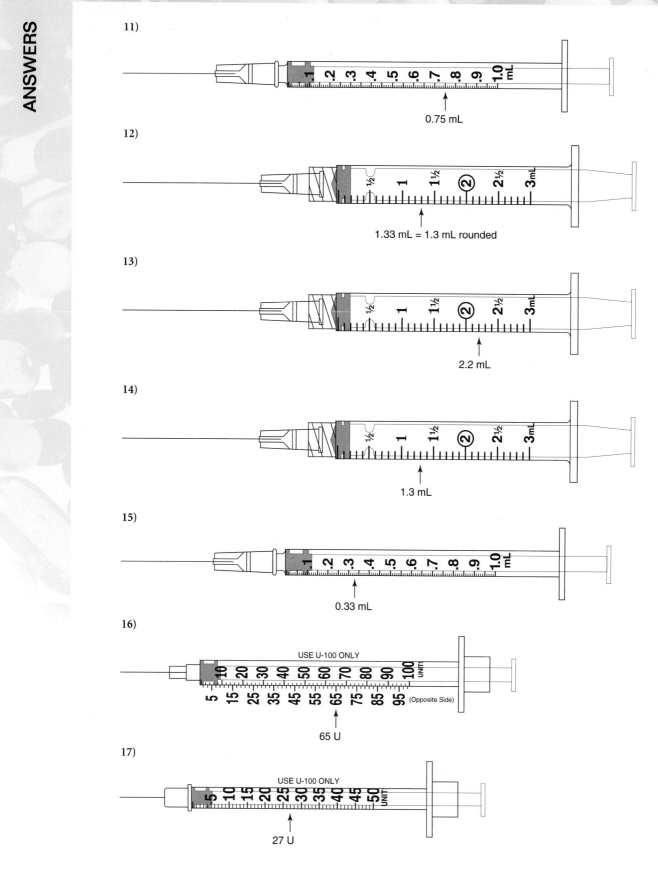

0.75 mL

12)

1.33 mL = 1.3 mL rounded

13)

2.2 mL

14)

1.3 mL

15)

0.33 mL

16)

USE U-100 ONLY

(Opposite Side)

65 U

17)

USE U-100 ONLY

27 U

18)

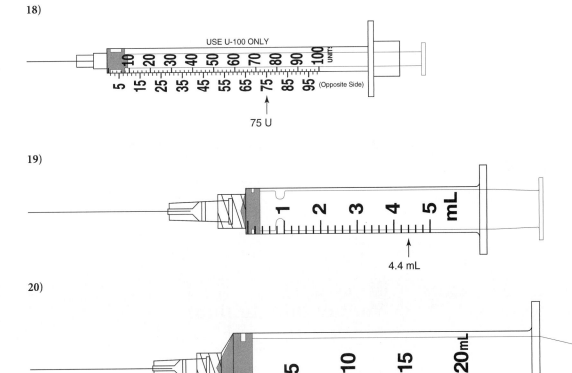

75 U

19)

4.4 mL

20)

16 mL

21) 0.2 mL 22) 1 mL 23) 0.2 mL

Practice Problems—Chapter 6 from pages 113–116

1) 1 2) hundredths or 0.01 3) No. The tuberculin syringe has a maximum capacity of 1 mL. 4) Round to 1.3 mL and measure at 1.3 mL. 5) 30 mL or 1 oz 6) 1 mL 7) 0.75 8) False 9) False 10) True 11) To prevent accidental needle sticks during intravenous administration 12) top ring 13) 10 14) True 15) standard 3 mL, 1 mL, and insulin

16)

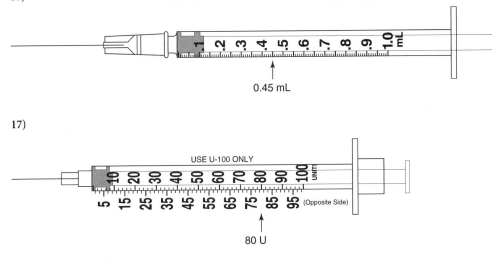

0.45 mL

17)

USE U-100 ONLY

80 U

18)

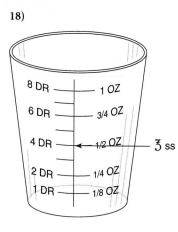

19)

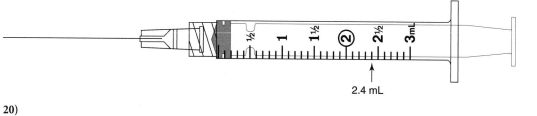

2.4 mL

20)

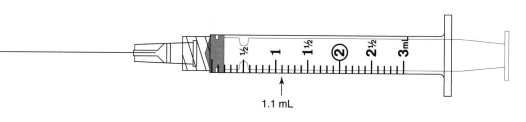

1.1 mL

21)

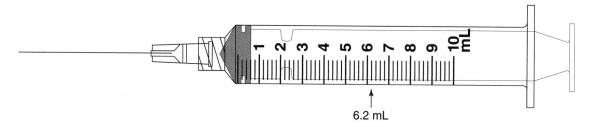

6.2 mL

22)

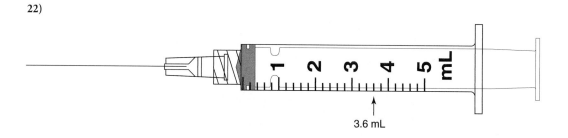

3.6 mL

23)

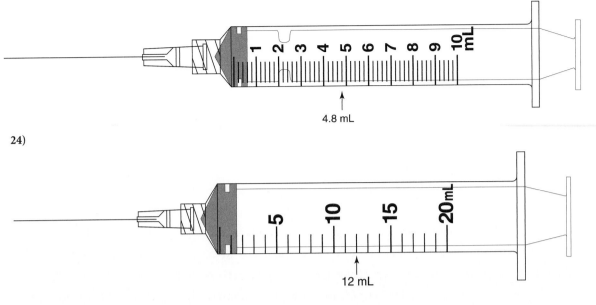

4.8 mL

24)

12 mL

25) Critical Thinking Skill: Prevention. This error could have been avoided by following the principle of not putting oral drugs in syringes intended for injection. Instead, place the medication in an oral syringe to which a needle cannot be attached. In addition, the medication should have been labeled for oral use only. The medication was ordered orally, not by injection. The alert nurse would have noticed the discrepancy. Finally, but just as important, a medication should be administered only by the nurse who prepared it.

26) Critical Thinking Skill: Prevention. The nurse needs to recognize the difference between an oral and a parenteral syringe. Look at the syringe markings that are typically for oral measurement and the absence of the luerlock hub, found on parenteral injection syringes. The nurse must remove the cap on the oral syringe prior to administering the medication, so that the child cannot choke on the cap. Also, a needle should not be applied to the syringe.

Review Set 22 from pages 120–121

1) Give 250 milligrams of naproxen orally 2 times a day. 2) Give 30 units of Humulin N NPH U-100 insulin subcutaneously every day 30 minutes before breakfast. 3) Give 500 milligrams of Ceclor orally immediately, and then give 250 milligrams every 8 hours. 4) Give 25 micrograms of Synthroid orally once a day. 5) Give 10 milligrams of Ativan intramuscularly every 4 hours as necessary for agitation. 6) Give 20 milligrams of furosemide intravenously (slowly) immediately. 7) Give 10 milliliters of Gelusil orally at bedtime. 8) Give 2 drops of 1% atropine sulfate ophthalmic in the right eye every 15 minutes for 4 applications. 9) Give $\frac{1}{4}$ grain of morphine sulfate intramuscularly every 3 to 4 hours as needed for pain. 10) Give 0.25 milligram of Lanoxin orally once a day. 11) Give 250 milligrams of tetracycline orally 4 times a day. 12) Give $\frac{1}{400}$ grain of nitroglycerin sublingually immediately. 13) Give 2 drops of Cortisporin otic suspension in both ears 3 times a day and at bedtime. 14) The abbreviation t.i.d. means three times a day with no specific interval between times. An attempt is made to give the three doses during waking hours. The abbreviation q.8h means every 8 hours. These doses would be given around the clock at 8-hour intervals. For example, administration times for t.i.d. might be 0800, 1200, 1700; administration times for q.8h could be 0800, 1600, 2400. 15) Contact the physician for clarification. 16) No, q.i.d. orders are given 4 times in 24 hours with no specific interval between times indicated in order, typically during waking hours; whereas q.4h orders are given 6 times in 24 hours at 4-hour intervals. 17) Determined by hospital or institutional policy. 18) Patient, drug, dosage, route, frequency, date and time written, signature of physician/writer. 19) Parts 1–5 20) The right patient must receive the right drug in the right amount by the right route at the right time, followed by the right documentation.

Review Set 23 from pages 126–127

1) 6 AM, 12 noon, 6 PM, 12 midnight 2) 9 AM 3) 7:30 AM, 11:30 AM, 4:30 PM, 9 PM 4) 9 AM, 5 PM 5) every

4 hours, as needed for severe pain 6) 9/7/xx at 0900 or 9 AM 7) sublingual, under the tongue 8) once a day 9) 125 mcg

10) nitroglycerin, Darvocet-N 100, meperidine (Demerol), promethazine (Phenergan) 11) subcutaneous injection

12) once 13) Keflex 14) before breakfast (at 7:30 AM) 15) milliequivalent 16) Keflex and Slow-K 17) Tylenol 18) twice

19) 0900 and 2100 20) 2400, 0600, 1200, and 1800 21) In the "One-Time Medication Dosage" section, lower left corner.

Practice Problems—Chapter 7 from pages 127–131

1) ounce 2) per rectum 3) before meals 4) after 5) three times a day 6) every four hours 7) when necessary 8) by mouth,

orally 9) once a day, every day 10) right eye 11) immediately 12) freely, as desired 13) hour of sleep, bedtime

14) intramuscular 15) without 16) ss 17) gtt 18) mL 19) gr 20) g 21) q.i.d. 22) O.U. 23) SC 24) t 25) b.i.d. 26) q.3h

27) p.c. 28) $\bar{a}$ 29) kg 30) Give 60 milligrams of Toradol intramuscularly immediately and every 6 hours. 31) Give

300,000 units of procaine penicillin G intramuscularly 4 times a day. 32) Give 5 milliliters of Mylanta orally 1 hour before

and 1 hour after meals, at bedtime, and every 2 hours as needed at night. 33) Give 25 milligrams of Librium orally every

6 hours when necessary for agitation. 34) Give 5,000 units of heparin subcutaneously immediately. 35) Give 50 milligrams

of Demerol intramuscularly every 3–4 hours when necessary for pain. 36) Give 0.25 milligram of digoxin orally every day.

37) Give 2 drops of 10% Neosynephrine ophthalmic to the left eye every 30 minutes for 2 applications. 38) Give

40 milligrams of Lasix intramuscularly immediately. 39) Give 4 milligrams of Decadron intravenously twice a day.

40) 12:00 midnight, 8:00 AM, 4:00 PM 41) 20 units 42) SC, subcutaneous 43) Give 500 milligrams of Cipro orally every

12 hours. 44) 8:00 AM, 12:00 noon, 6:00 PM 45) digoxin (Lanoxin) 0.125 mg p.o. q.d. 46) with, $\bar{c}$ 47) Give 150 milligrams

of ranitidine tablets orally twice daily with breakfast and supper. 48) Vancomycin 49) 12 hours

50) Critical Thinking Skill: Prevention. This error could have been avoided by paying careful attention to the ordered frequency and by writing the frequency on the MAR.

Review Set 24 from pages 142–145

1) B 2) D 3) C 4) A 5) E 6) F 7) G 8) 5 mL 9) IM or IV 10) A, B, C, D, E, F, G—all of the labels 11) Filmtab means

film sealed tablet. 12) 1 mg per mL 13) 2 tablets 14) penicillin G potassium 15) Pfizerpen 16) 5,000,000 units per vial;

reconstituted to 250,000 U/mL, 500,000 U/mL, or 1,000,000 U/mL 17) IM or IV 18) 0049-0520-83 19) Pfizer-Roerig

20) 1% 21) 1 g per 100 mL 22) 10 mg per mL

Practice Problems—Chapter 8 from pages 146–149

1) 50 mEq/50 mL or 1 mEq/mL 2) 63323-006-50 3) 84 mg/mL 4) cefpodoxime proxetil 5) "Shake bottle to loosen

granules. Add approximately $\frac{1}{2}$ the total amount of distilled water required for constitution (total water = 29 mL). Shake

vigorously to wet the granules. Add remaining water and shake vigorously." 6) Pharmacia and Upjohn 7) 10 mL

8) 25 mg/mL 9) 1 mL 10) Nebcin 11) tobramycin 12) 0002-7090-01 13) injection solution 14) 10 mL

15) intramuscular 16) Ayerst Laboratories, Inc. 17) tablet 18) Store at room temperature; approximately 25°C

19) 12/2007 20) 2 mEq per mL 21) I 22) H 23) H 24) oral 25) 0666060 26) 2% 27) 2 g per 100 mL, or 20 mg per mL

28) Critical Thinking Skill: Prevention. This error could have been prevented by carefully comparing the drug label and dosage to the MAR drug and dosage three times while preparing the medication. In this instance both the incorrect drug and the incorrect dosage strength sent by the pharmacy should have been noted by the nurse. Further, the nurse should have asked for clarification of the order.

29) Critical Thinking Skill: Prevention. The nurse should have recognized that the patient was still complaining of signs and symptoms that the medication was ordered to treat.

30) If the order was difficult to read, the physician should have been called to clarify the order. Was the dosage of 100 mg a usual dosage for Celexa? The nurse should have consulted a drug guide to ensure that the dosage was appropriate. Also, if the patient wasn't complaining of depression, the nurse should have questioned why Celexa was ordered.

Section 2—Self-Evaluation from pages 150–153

1) gr $\frac{2}{3}$ 2) 4 t 3) gr $\frac{1}{300}$ 4) 0.5 mL 5) ℥ ss 6) four drops 7) four hundred fifty milligrams 8) one one-hundredth of a grain 9) seven and one-half grains 10) twenty-five hundredths of a liter 11) (7.13 kg) = 7130 g = 7,130,000 mg = 7,130,000,000 mcg 12) 0.000000925 kg = 0.000925 g = 0.925 mg = (925 mcg) 13) 0.000125 kg = 0.125 g = (125 mg) = 125,000 mcg 14) 0.0164 kg = (16.4 g) = 16,400 mg = 16,400,000 mcg 15) 10 mg = 0.01 g 16) 0.02 g = gr $\frac{1}{3}$ 17) 12 t = 60 mL 18) 9 L = 9000 mL 19) 37.5 cm = 375 mm 20) 5.62 cm = 2.25 in = $2\frac{1}{4}$ in 21) 90 kg = 90,000 g 22) 11,590 g = 25.5 lb = $25\frac{1}{2}$ lb 23) iii 24) 360 25) 0.2 26) 6, vi 27) 455 28) 2335 29) 6:44 PM 30) 0417 31) 8:03 AM 32) 100.4 33) 38.6 34) 99

35)

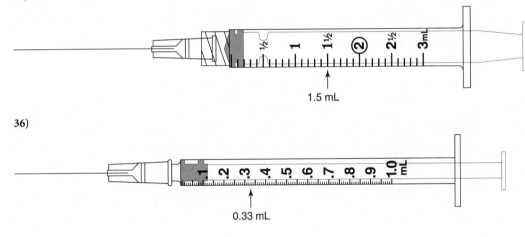

1.5 mL

36)

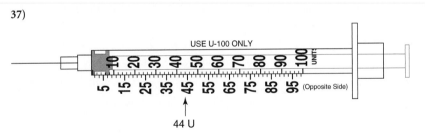

0.33 mL

37)

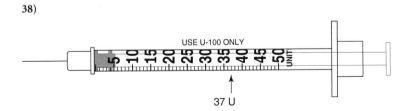

USE U-100 ONLY

(Opposite Side)

44 U

38)

USE U-100 ONLY

37 U

39)

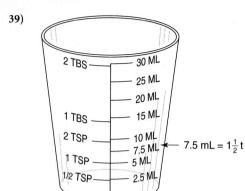

7.5 mL = $1\frac{1}{2}$ t

40) neomycin and polymixin B sulfates and hydrocortisone 41) Use in ears only. 42) 10 mL 43) Give 2 drops of Cortisporin otic solution in both ears every 15 minutes for 3 doses. 44) 5000 units per mL 45) 63323-262-01

46) Give 3750 units of heparin subcutaneously every 8 hours. 47) Ceclor 48) 250 mg per 5 mL

49) a. 2.5 mL; b. $\frac{1}{2}$ t

c.

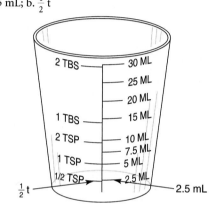

$\frac{1}{2}$ t   2.5 mL

50) Give 250 mg of Amoxil by mouth 3 times per day.

Solutions—Section 2—Self-Evaluation

15) gr → mg or larger → smaller: (×);

gr $\frac{1}{6} = \frac{1}{6} \times 60 = 10$ mg

mg → g or smaller → larger: (÷)

10 mg = 10 ÷ 1000 = 0.01 g

21) lb → kg or smaller → larger: (÷)

198 lb = 198 ÷ 2.2 = 90 kg

kg → mg or larger → smaller: (×)

90 kg = 90 × 1000 = 90,000 g

24) gr → mg or larger → smaller: (X)

gr $\frac{3}{4} = \frac{3}{4} \times 60 = \frac{180}{4} = 45$ mg; q.3h = 8 doses/24 h;

45 mg/dose × 8 doses = 360 mg

27) 15 oz = 15 × 30   = 450 mL

1 t   = 5 mL

total   = 455 mL

Review Set 25 from pages 167–169

1) 1 2) 1 3) $1\frac{1}{2}$ 4) $\frac{1}{2}$ 5) $\frac{1}{2}$ 6) 2 7) 2 8) 2 9) $1\frac{1}{2}$ 10) 2 11) 1 12) $\frac{1}{2}$ 13) 2 14) 2 15) 2 16) $1\frac{1}{2}$ 17) 10, 1 18) 10 and 5; 1 of each, 4 19) 15, 1 20) 60, 1 21) B, 1 caplet 22) I, 2 tablets 23) F, 1 tablet 24) H, 2 tablets 25) C, 1 tablet
26) E, 2 capsules 27) D, 2 tablets 28) G, 2 tablets 29) A, 1 tablet 30) C, 1 tablet

Solutions—Review Set 25

1) Order: 0.1 g = 0.1 × 1000 = 100 mg
Supply: 100 mg/tab

$$\frac{D}{H} \times Q = \frac{\overset{1}{\cancel{100\,mg}}}{\underset{1}{\cancel{100\,mg}}} \times 1\ tab = 1\ tab$$

5) Order: 0.125 mg
Supply: 0.25 mg/tab = 0.250 mg/tab

$$\frac{D}{H} \times Q = \frac{\overset{1}{\cancel{0.125\,mg}}}{\underset{2}{\cancel{0.250\,mg}}} \times 1\ tab = \frac{1}{2}\ tab$$

10) Order: 5 mg = 5.0 mg
Supply: 2.5 mg/tab

$$\frac{D}{H} \times Q = \frac{\overset{2}{\cancel{5.0\,mg}}}{\underset{1}{\cancel{2.5\,mg}}} \times 1\ tab = 2\ tab$$

14) Order: 0.1 mg = 0.1 × 1000 = 100 mcg
Supply: 50 mcg/tab

$$\frac{D}{H} \times Q = \frac{\overset{2}{\cancel{100\,mcg}}}{\underset{1}{\cancel{50\,mcg}}} \times 1\ tab = 2\ tab$$

17) Order: gr $\frac{1}{6} = \frac{1}{\cancel{6}} \times \overset{10}{\cancel{60}} = 10\,mg$ (gr i = 60 mg)

Supply: 10 mg and 2.5 mg/tab
Select: 10 mg and give 1 tab

$$\frac{D}{H} \times Q = \frac{\overset{1}{\cancel{10\,mg}}}{\underset{1}{\cancel{10\,mg}}} \times 1\ tab = 1\ tab$$

28) Order: 0.5 mg = 0.5 × 1000 = 500 mcg
Supply: 250 mcg/tab

$$\frac{D}{H} \times Q = \frac{\overset{2}{\cancel{500\,mcg}}}{\underset{1}{\cancel{250\,mcg}}} \times 1\ tab = 2\ tab$$

Review Set 26 from pages 173–177

1) 7.5 **2)** 5 **3)** 20 **4)** 4 **5)** 1 **6)** 20 **7)** 2 **8)** 7.5 **9)** 3 **10)** 2.5 **11)** 22.5 **12)** 7.5 **13)** 2 **14)** 2.5 **15)** 5 **16)** ss **17)** $1\frac{1}{2}$ **18)** i **19)** 15
20) 1 **21)** 2 **22)** B; 2.5 mL ($\frac{1}{2}$ t) **23)** C; 2 mL **24)** A; 2 mL **25)** 5 **26)** 0.75 **27)** 10; 48 **28)** 3 **29)** 4 **30)** 0900, 1300, 1900

Solutions—Review Set 26

2) Order: gr $\frac{1}{6} = \frac{1}{\cancel{6}} \times \frac{\overset{10}{\cancel{60}}}{1} = 10\,mg$ (gr i = 60 mg)

Supply: 10 mg/5mL

$$\frac{D}{H} \times Q = \frac{\overset{1}{\cancel{10\,mg}}}{\underset{1}{\cancel{10\,mg}}} \times 5\ mL = 5\ mL$$

4) Order: 100 mg
Supply: 125 mg/5mL

$$\frac{D}{H} \times Q = \frac{\overset{4}{\cancel{100\,mg}}}{\underset{5}{\cancel{125\,mg}}} \times 5\ mL = \frac{\overset{4}{\cancel{20}}}{\underset{1}{\cancel{5}}}\ mL = 4\ mL$$

6) Order: 25 mg
Supply: 6.25 mg/t = 6.25 mg/5 mL (1 t = 5 mL)

$$\frac{D}{H} \times Q = \frac{25\,\cancel{mg}}{6.25\,\cancel{mg}} \times 5\ mL = \frac{125}{6.25}\ mL = 20\ mL$$

7) Order: 125 mg
Supply: 62.5 mg/5 mL

$$\frac{D}{H} \times Q = \frac{\overset{2}{\cancel{25\,mg}}}{\underset{1}{\cancel{62.5\,mg}}} \times 5\ mL = 10\ mL$$

$$10\ mL = \frac{10}{5} = 2\ t\ (1\ t = 5\ mL)$$

11) Order: 0.24 g = 0.24 × 1000 = 240 mg
Supply: 80 mg/7.5 mL

$$\frac{D}{H} \times Q = \frac{\overset{3}{\cancel{240\,mg}}}{\underset{1}{\cancel{80\,mg}}} \times 7.5\ mL = 22.5\ mL$$

15) Order: 0.25 mg = 0.25 × 1000 = 250 mcg
Supply: 50 mcg/mL

$$\frac{D}{H} \times Q = \frac{\overset{5}{\cancel{250\,mcg}}}{\underset{1}{\cancel{50\,mcg}}} \times 1\ mL = 5\ mL$$

17) Order: 375 mg
Supply: 250 mg/5 mL

$$\frac{D}{H} \times Q = \frac{375\,\cancel{mg}}{\underset{50}{\cancel{250\,mg}}} \times \overset{1}{\cancel{5}}\ mL = \frac{375}{50}\ mL = 7.5\ mL$$

$$7.5\ mL = \frac{7.5}{5} = 1\frac{1}{2}\ t\ (1\ t = 5\ mL)$$

19) Order: 1.2 g = 1.2 × 1000 = 1200 mg
Supply: 400 mg/5 mL

$$\frac{D}{H} \times Q = \frac{\overset{3}{\cancel{1200\,mg}}}{\underset{1}{\cancel{400\,mg}}} \times 5\ mL = 15\ mL$$

20) Order: 0.25 g = 0.25 × 1000 = 250 mg

Supply: 125 mg/2.5 mL

$$\frac{D}{H} \times Q = \frac{\overset{2}{\cancel{250 \text{ mg}}}}{\underset{1}{\cancel{125 \text{ mg}}}} \times 2.5 \text{ mL} = 5 \text{ mL} = 1 \text{ t}$$

21) Order: 100 mg

Supply: 250 mg/5 mL

$$\frac{D}{H} \times Q = \frac{100 \text{ mg}}{\underset{50}{\cancel{250 \text{ mg}}}} \times \overset{1}{\cancel{5}} \text{ mL} = \frac{\overset{2}{\cancel{100}}}{\underset{1}{\cancel{50}}} \text{ mL} = 2 \text{ mL}$$

Practice Problems—Chapter 9 from pages 178–186

1) $\frac{1}{2}$ 2) 2 3) $\frac{1}{2}$ 4) 2.5 5) 10 6) 2 7) 8 8) $1\frac{1}{2}$ 9) 1 10) $\frac{1}{2}$ 11) $1\frac{1}{2}$ 12) 1 13) $1\frac{1}{2}$ 14) 1 15) 1 16) 5; $1\frac{1}{2}$ 17) 7.5 18) $1\frac{1}{2}$
19) 2 20) 3 21) 0.75; 1 22) $\frac{1}{2}$ 23) 2 24) 2 25) 2 26) 2 27) 15 and 30; one of each 28) 2.4 29) 5 30) 3 31) D; 2 tablets
32) A; 1 capsule 33) C; 1 tablet 34) B; 2 tablets 35) I; 2 tablets 36) G; 2 tablets 37) F; 2 tablets 38) H; 1 tablet
39) M; 2 tablets 40) L; 2 tablets 41) E; 30 mL 42) K; 1 tablet 43) J; 2 tablets 44) N; 2 tablets 45) O; 1 tablet
46) Q; 2 tablets 47) P; 4 tablets 48) R; 1 tablet 49) S; 1 tablet

50) Critical Thinking Skill: Prevention. This medication error could have been prevented if the nurse had more carefully read the physician's order as well as the medication label. The doctor's order misled the nurse by noting the volume first and then the drug dosage. If confused by the order, the nurse should have clarified the intent with the physician. By focusing on the volume, the nurse failed to follow the steps in dosage calculation. Had the nurse noted 250 mg as the desired dosage and the supply (or on-hand) dosage as 125 mg per 5 mL, the correct amount to be administered would have been clear. Slow down and take time to compare the order with the labels. Calculate each dose carefully before preparing and administering both solid and liquid form medications.

Solutions—Practice Problems—Chapter 9

2) Order: gr ss = $\dfrac{1}{\underset{1}{\cancel{2}}} \times \dfrac{\overset{30}{\cancel{60}}}{1} = 30 \text{ mg}$

Supply: 15 mg/tab

$$\frac{D}{H} \times Q = \frac{\overset{2}{\cancel{30 \text{ mg}}}}{\underset{1}{\cancel{15 \text{ mg}}}} \times 1 \text{ tab} = 2 \text{ tab}$$

3) Order: 0.075 mg = 0.075 × 1000 = 75 mcg

Supply: 150 mcg/tab

$$\frac{D}{H} \times Q = \frac{\overset{1}{\cancel{75 \text{ mcg}}}}{\underset{2}{\cancel{150 \text{ mcg}}}} \times 1 \text{ tab} = \frac{1}{2} \text{ tab}$$

8) Order: 150 mg

Supply: 0.1 g/tab = 0.1 × 1000 = 100 mg/tab

$$\frac{D}{H} \times Q = \frac{\overset{3}{\cancel{150 \text{ mg}}}}{\underset{2}{\cancel{100 \text{ mg}}}} \times 1 \text{ tab} = 1\frac{1}{2} \text{ tab}$$

9) Order: gr v = 5 × 60 = 300 mg

Supply: 325 mg/tab

$$\frac{D}{H} \times Q = \frac{300 \text{ mg}}{325 \text{ mg}} \times 1 \text{ tab} = 0.92 \text{ tab}$$

0.92 tablet is not a reasonable dosage. Remember, in some instances gr i = 65 mg is more appropriate for conversions from grains to milligrams.

Order: gr v = 5 × 65 = 325 mg

Supply: 325 mg/tab

$$\frac{D}{H} \times Q = \frac{\overset{1}{\cancel{325 \text{ mg}}}}{\underset{1}{\cancel{325 \text{ mg}}}} \times 1 \text{ tab} = 1 \text{ tab}$$

14) Order: gr $\dfrac{1}{8} = \dfrac{1}{\underset{2}{\cancel{8}}} \times \dfrac{\overset{15}{\cancel{60}}}{1} = \dfrac{15}{2} = 7.5 \text{ mg}$

Supply: 7.5 mg/tab

$$\frac{D}{H} \times Q = \frac{\cancel{7.5 \text{ mg}}}{\cancel{7.5 \text{ mg}}} \times 1 \text{ tab} = 1 \text{ tab}$$

19) Order: 0.25 mg = 0.250 mg

Supply: 0.125 mg/tab

$$\frac{D}{H} \times Q = \frac{\overset{2}{\cancel{0.250 \text{ mg}}}}{\underset{1}{\cancel{0.125 \text{ mg}}}} \times 1 \text{ tab} = 2 \text{ tab}$$

27) gr $\dfrac{3}{4} = \dfrac{3}{\underset{1}{\cancel{4}}} \times \dfrac{\overset{15}{\cancel{60}}}{1} = 45 \text{ mg}$

Supply: 15 mg, 30 mg, and 60 mg tablets

Select: 1 15-mg tablet and 1 30-mg tablet for 45 mg

Remember: If you have a choice, give whole tablets and as few as possible.

Review Set 27 from pages 193–199

1) 2.5

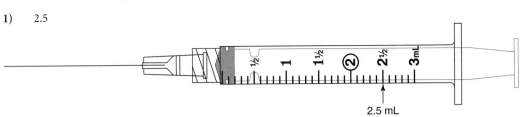

2.5 mL

2) 4 (4 mL divided into 2 syringes)

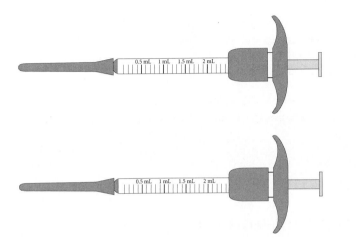

3) 2.4

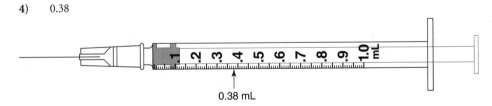

2.4 mL

4) 0.38

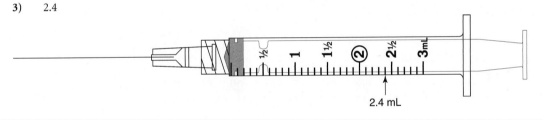

0.38 mL

The route is IM; the needle may need to be changed to an appropriate gauge and length.

5) 2

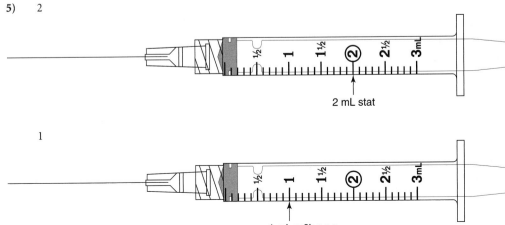

2 mL stat

1

1 mL q.6h p.r.n.

ANSWERS

6)   0.8

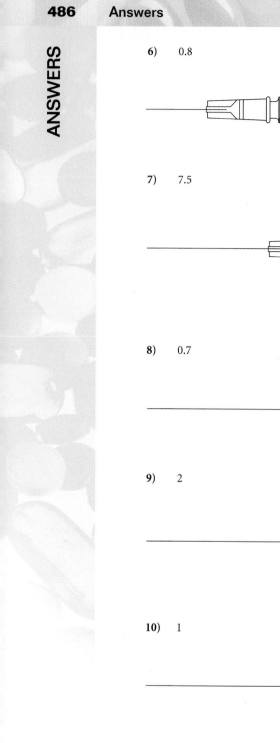

0.8 mL

7)   7.5

7.5 mL
(7.6 would be closest calibration on this syringe)

8)   0.7

0.7 mL

9)   2

2 mL

10)   1

1 mL

11)   1.2

1.2 mL

12)   0.9

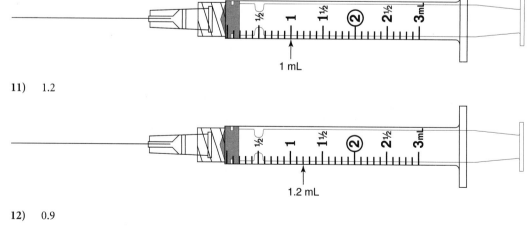

0.9 mL

13) 0.5

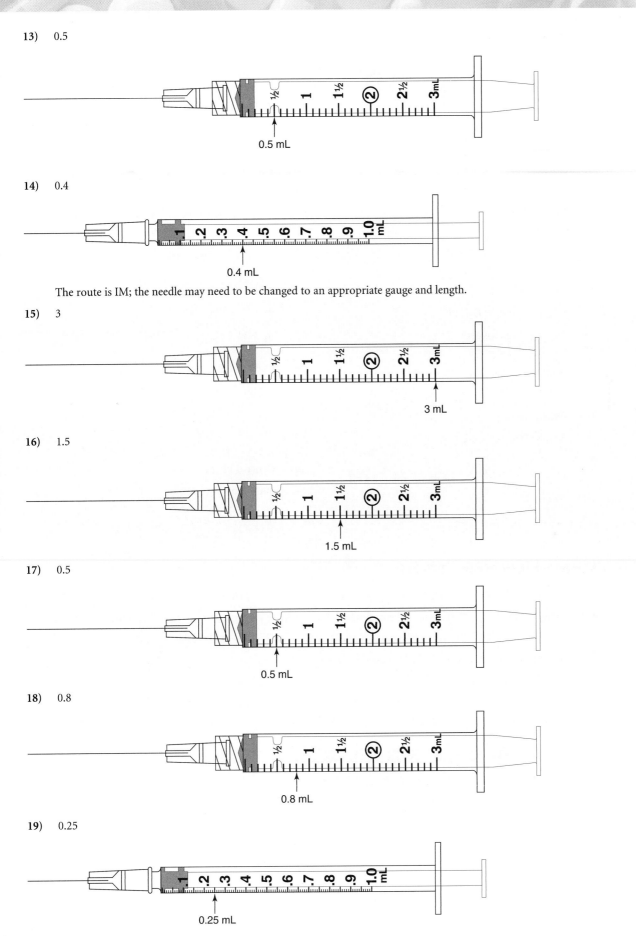

0.5 mL

14) 0.4

0.4 mL

The route is IM; the needle may need to be changed to an appropriate gauge and length.

15) 3

3 mL

16) 1.5

1.5 mL

17) 0.5

0.5 mL

18) 0.8

0.8 mL

19) 0.25

0.25 mL

The route is IM; the needle may need to be changed to an appropriate gauge and length.

20) 1.5

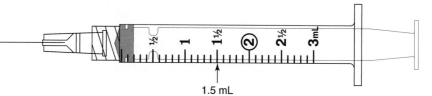

1.5 mL

Solutions—Review Set 27

1) Order: 1 g = 1000 mg

Supply: 400 mg/mL

$$\frac{D}{H} \times Q = \frac{\overset{5}{\cancel{1000 \text{ mg}}}}{\underset{2}{\cancel{400 \text{ mg}}}} \times 1 \text{ mL} = \frac{5}{2} \text{ mL} = 2.5 \text{ mL}$$

2) Order: 2,400,000 U

Supply: 1,200,000 U/2 mL

$$\frac{D}{H} \times Q = \frac{\overset{2}{\cancel{2,400,000 \text{ U}}}}{\underset{1}{\cancel{1,200,000 \text{ U}}}} \times 2 \text{ mL} = 4 \text{ mL}$$

4 mL divided into
2 doses of 2 mL each

3) Order: 600 mcg

Supply: 500 mcg/2 mL

$$\frac{D}{H} \times Q = \frac{\overset{6}{\cancel{600 \text{ mcg}}}}{\underset{5}{\cancel{500 \text{ mcg}}}} \times 2 \text{ mL} = \frac{12}{5} \text{ mL} = 2.4 \text{ mL}$$

6) Order: 4000 U

Supply: 5000 U/mL

$$\frac{D}{H} \times Q = \frac{\overset{4}{\cancel{4000 \text{ U}}}}{\underset{5}{\cancel{5000 \text{ U}}}} \times 1 \text{ mL} = \frac{4}{5} \text{ mL} = 0.8 \text{ mL}$$

10) Order: gr $\frac{1}{4} = \frac{1}{4} \times 60 = 15$ mg

Supply: 15 mg/mL

$$\frac{D}{H} \times Q = \frac{\cancel{15 \text{ mg}}}{\cancel{15 \text{ mg}}} \times 1 \text{ mL} = 1 \text{ mL}$$

11) Order: 30 mg

Supply: 25 mg/mL

$$\frac{D}{H} \times Q = \frac{\overset{6}{\cancel{30 \text{ mg}}}}{\underset{5}{\cancel{25 \text{ mg}}}} \times 1 \text{ mL} = \frac{6}{5} \text{ mL} = 1.2 \text{ mL}$$

19) Order: 12.5 mg

Supply: 50 mg/mL

$$\frac{D}{H} \times Q = \frac{\overset{1}{\cancel{12.5 \text{ mg}}}}{\underset{4}{\cancel{50 \text{ mg}}}} \times 1 \text{ mL} = 0.25 \text{ mL}$$

Review Set 28 from pages 207–211

1) Humulin R Regular, Rapid-acting **2)** Novolin N, Intermediate-acting   **3)** Humulin U Ultralente, Long-acting

4) Humalog, Rapid-acting **5)** Humulin L Lente, Intermediate-acting **6)** Standard, dual-scale 100 unit/mL U-100 syringe;

Lo-dose, 50 unit/0.5 mL U-100 syringe; Lo-dose, 30 unit/0.3 mL U-100 syringe **7)** Lo-dose, 30 unit U-100 syringe

8) Lo-dose, 50 unit U-100 syringe **9)** 0.6 **10)** 0.25 **11)** Standard dual-scale 100 unit U-100 syringe **12)** False **13)** 68

14) 15 **15)** 23 **16)** 57

17)

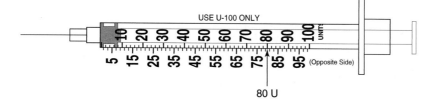

80 U

18)

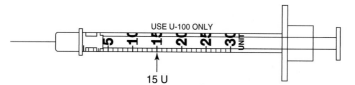

15 U

19)

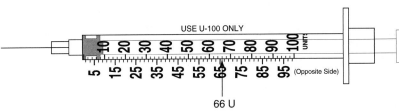

66 U

20)

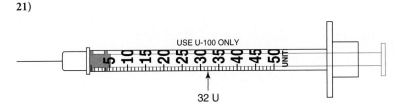

16 U

21)

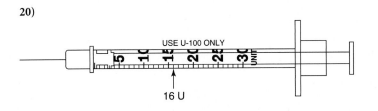

32 U

22)

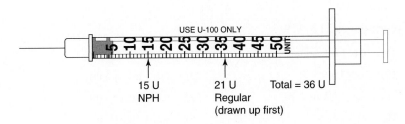

15 U   21 U   Total = 36 U
NPH   Regular
             (drawn up first)

23)

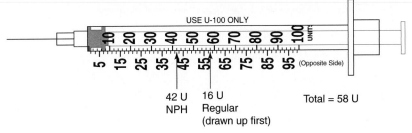

42 U   16 U   Total = 58 U
NPH   Regular
         (drawn up first)

24)

40 U   32 U   Total = 72 U
NPH   Regular
             (drawn up first)

25)

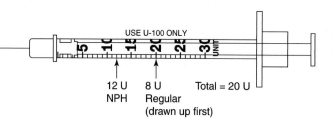

USE U-100 ONLY

12 U   8 U   Total = 20 U
NPH   Regular
       (drawn up first)

26) Before meals and before insulin administration.

27) Blood glucose levels of 160–400.

28) Administer 4 units of Humulin R Regular U-100 insulin.

29) None, do not administer insulin.

30) Contact the physician for further instructions.

Solutions—Review Set 28

9) Recall U-100 = 100 units per mL

$$\frac{\overset{6}{\cancel{60\,U}}}{\underset{10}{\cancel{100\,U}}} \times 1\ mL = 0.6\ mL$$

Practice Problems—Chapter 10 from pages 212–219

1) 0.4; 1 mL tuberculin

The route is IM; the needle may need to be changed to an appropriate gauge and length.

2) 1.5; 3 mL

3) 2.4; 3 mL

4) 0.6; 1 mL or 3 mL

5) 2; 3 mL

6) 15; 20 mL

7) 0.8; 1 mL or 3 mL

8) 1; 3 mL

9) 1; 3 mL

10) 0.5; 1 mL or 3 mL

11) 1.5; 3 mL

12) 0.6; 1 mL or 3 mL

13) 0.6; 1 mL or 3 mL

14) 1.9; 3 mL

15) 0.6; 1 mL or 3 mL

16) 1; 3 mL

17) 0.67; 1 mL

The route is IM; the needle may need to be changed to an appropriate gauge and length.

18) 1; 3 mL

19) 1.2; 3 mL

20) 0.7; 1 mL or 3 mL

21) 0.75; 1 mL

The route is IM; the needle may need to be changed to an appropriate gauge and length.

22) 1.5; 3 mL

23) 0.7; 1 mL or 3 mL

24) 0.8; 1 mL or 3 mL

25) 1.3; 3 mL

26) 1.6; 3 mL

27) 6; 10 mL

28) 0.8; 1 mL or 3 mL

29) 1.5; 3 mL

30) 2.5; 3 mL

31) 1; 3 mL

32) 0.7; 1 mL or 3 mL

33) 1; 3 mL

34) 30; 20 mL (2 syringes)

35) 16; 30 U Lo-Dose U-100 insulin

36) 25; 50 U Lo-Dose U-100 insulin

37) 0.3

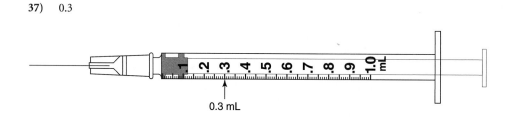

0.3 mL

The route is IM; the needle may need to be changed to an appropriate gauge and length.

38) 1.6

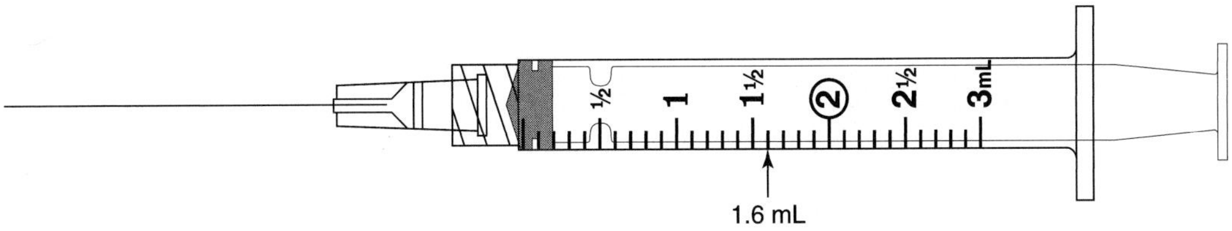

1.6 mL

39) 0.4

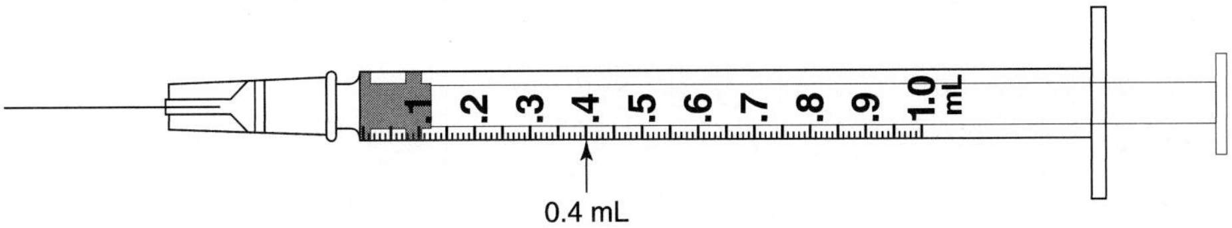

0.4 mL

40) 2.5

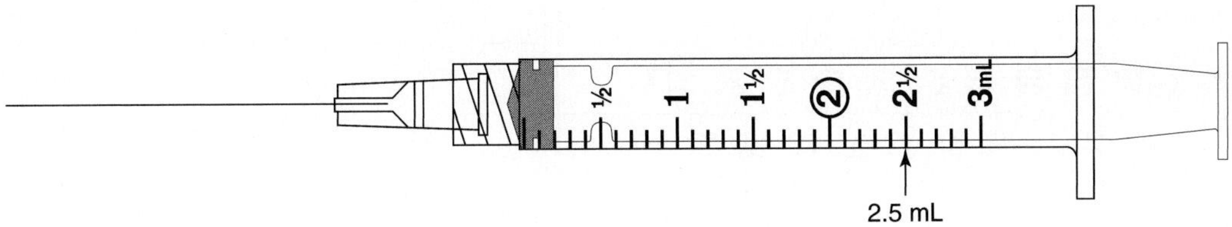

2.5 mL

41) 1.2

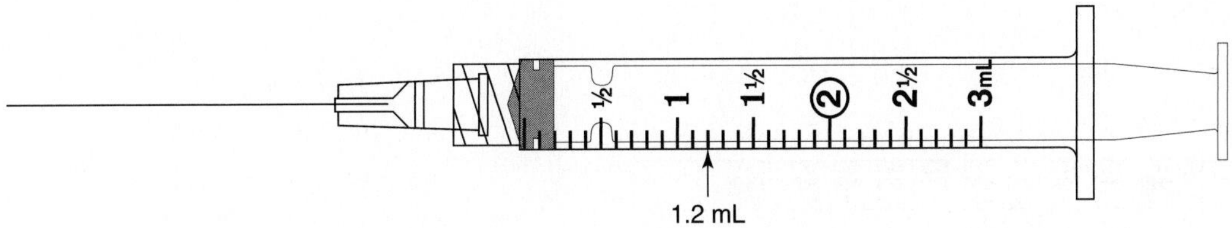

1.2 mL

42) 22

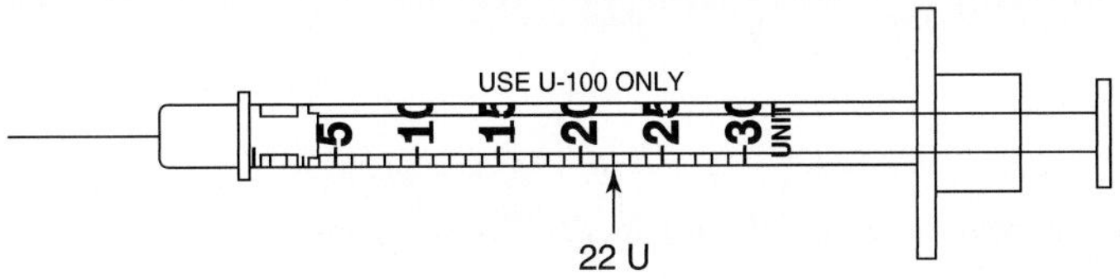

USE U-100 ONLY

22 U

43) 0.8

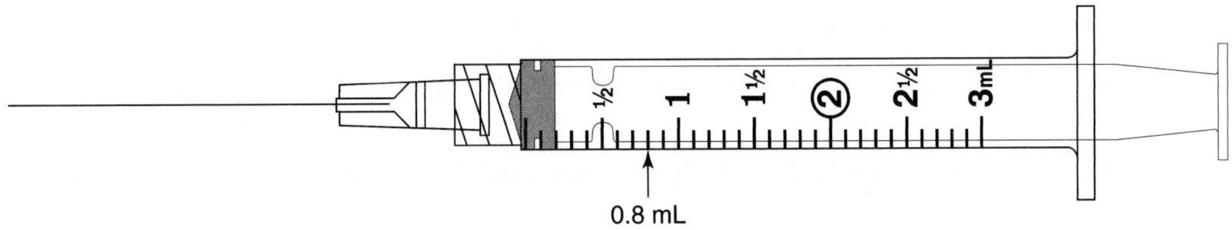

0.8 mL

44) 0.6

0.6 mL

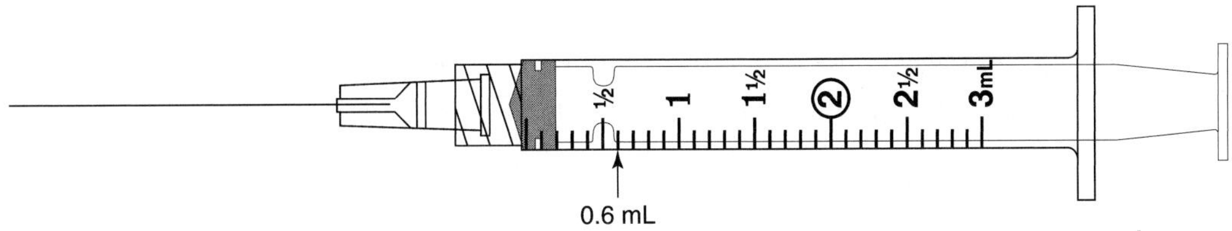

45) 1.4

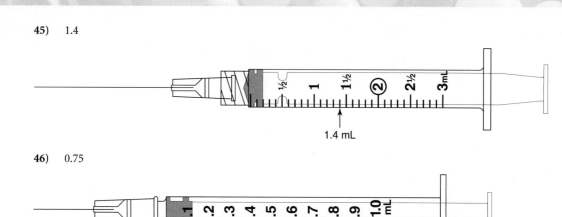

1.4 mL

46) 0.75

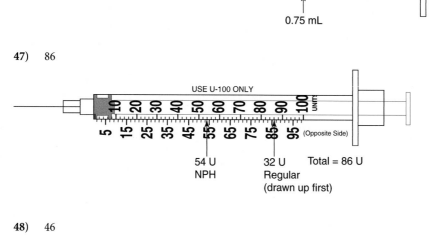

0.75 mL

47) 86

USE U-100 ONLY

54 U
NPH

32 U
Regular
(drawn up first)

Total = 86 U

48) 46

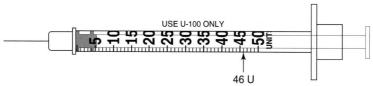

USE U-100 ONLY

46 U

49) Critical Thinking: Prevention.

This error could have been avoided had the nurse been more careful checking the label of the insulin vial and comparing the label to the order. The nurse should have checked the label three times as taught in nursing school. In addition, the nurse should have asked another nurse to double-check her as she was drawing up the insulin, as required. Such hospital policies and procedures are written to protect the patient and the nurse.

50) Critical Thinking: Prevention.

This insulin error should never occur. It is obvious that the nurse did not use Step 2 of the three-step method. The nurse did not stop to think of the reasonable dosage. If so, the nurse would have realized that the supply dosage of U-100 insulin is 100 U/mL, not 10 U/mL.

If you are unsure of what you are doing, you need to ask before you act. Insulin should only be given in an insulin syringe. The likelihood of the nurse needing to give insulin in a tuberculin syringe because an insulin syringe was unavailable is almost nonexistent today. The nurse chose the incorrect syringe. Whenever you are in doubt, you should ask for help. Further, if the nurse had asked another nurse to double-check the dosage, as required, the error could have been found before the patient received the wrong dosage of insulin. After giving the insulin, it is too late to rectify the error.

Solutions—Practice Problems—Chapter 10

3) Order: 0.6 mg = 0.6 × 1000 = 600 mcg

Supply: 500 mcg/2 mL

$$\frac{D}{H} \times Q = \frac{\overset{6}{\cancel{600 \text{ mcg}}}}{\underset{5}{\cancel{500 \text{ mcg}}}} \times 2 \text{ mL} = \frac{12}{5} \text{ mL} = 2.4 \text{ mL}$$

6) Order: 30 mEq

Supply: 2 mEq/mL

$$\frac{D}{H} \times Q = \frac{\overset{15}{\cancel{30 \text{ mEq}}}}{\underset{1}{\cancel{2 \text{ mEq}}}} \times 1 \text{ mL} = 15 \text{ mL}$$

Note: Route is IV, so this large dose is accepable.

11) Order: gr $\frac{1}{100} = \frac{1}{\underset{10}{\cancel{100}}} \times \frac{\overset{6}{\cancel{60}}}{1} = 0.6$ mg

Supply: 0.4 mg/mL

$$\frac{D}{H} \times Q = \frac{\overset{3}{\cancel{0.6 \text{ mg}}}}{\underset{2}{\cancel{0.4 \text{ mg}}}} \times 1 \text{ mL} = \frac{3}{2} \text{ mL} = 1.5 \text{ mL}$$

14) Order: 75 mg

Supply: 80 mg/2 mL

$$\frac{D}{H} \times Q = \frac{75 \text{ mg}}{\underset{40}{\cancel{80 \text{ mg}}}} \times \overset{1}{\cancel{2}} \text{ mL} = \frac{75}{40} \text{ mL} = 1.87 \text{ mL} = 1.9 \text{ mL}$$

15) Order: gr $\frac{1}{10} = \frac{1}{\underset{1}{\cancel{10}}} \times \frac{\overset{6}{\cancel{60}}}{1} = 6$ mg

Supply: 10 mg/mL

$$\frac{D}{H} \times Q = \frac{6 \text{ mg}}{10 \text{ mg}} \times 1 \text{ mL} = 0.6 \text{ mL}$$

19) Order: 60 mg

Supply: 75 mg/1.5 mL

$$\frac{D}{H} \times Q = \frac{\overset{4}{\cancel{60 \text{ mg}}}}{\underset{5}{\cancel{75 \text{ mg}}}} \times 1.5 \text{ mL} = \frac{6}{5} \text{ mL} = 1.2 \text{ mL}$$

26) Order: 0.4 mg = 0.4 × 1000 = 400 mcg

Supply: 500 mcg/2 mL

$$\frac{D}{H} \times Q = \frac{\overset{4}{\cancel{400 \text{ mcg}}}}{\underset{5}{\cancel{500 \text{ mcg}}}} \times 2 \text{ mL} = \frac{8}{5} \text{ mL} = 1.6 \text{ mL}$$

30) Order: 50 mg

Supply: 2% = 2 g/100 mL = 2000 mg/100 mL =

$$2 \times 1000 = \frac{2000 \text{ mg}}{100 \text{ mL}} = 20 \text{ mg/mL}$$

$$\frac{D}{H} \times Q = \frac{\overset{5}{\cancel{50 \text{ mg}}}}{\underset{2}{\cancel{20 \text{ mg}}}} \times 1 \text{ mL} = \frac{5}{2} \text{ mL} = 2.5 \text{ mL}$$

33) Order: 0.5 mg

Supply: 1:2000 = 1 g/2000 mL =

1000 mg/2000 mL = 0.5 mg/mL

$$\frac{D}{H} \times Q = \frac{0.5 \text{ mg}}{0.5 \text{ mg}} \times 1 \text{ mL} = 1 \text{ mL}$$

41) Order: 12,000 U

Supply: 10,000 U/mL

$$\frac{D}{H} \times Q = \frac{12,000 \text{ U}}{10,000 \text{ U}} \times 1 \text{ mL} = \frac{12}{10} \text{ mL} = 1.2 \text{ mL}$$

Review Set 29 from pages 237–248

1) 1.5; 280; 0.71; 2

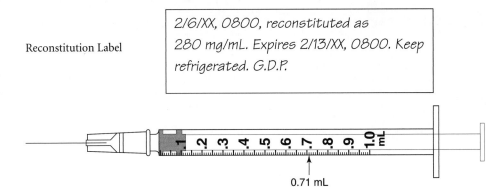

Reconstitution Label

2/6/XX, 0800, reconstituted as 280 mg/mL. Expires 2/13/XX, 0800. Keep refrigerated. G.D.P.

0.71 mL

The route is IM; the needle may need to be changed to an appropriate gauge and length.

2)   9.8; 5000; 0.5; 20

Reconstitution Label

> 2/6/XX, 0800, reconstituted as
> 5000 U/mL. Expires 2/13/XX, 0800. Keep
> refrigerated. G.D.P.

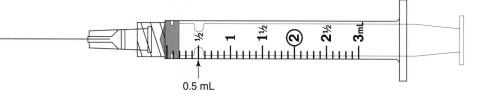

0.5 mL

3)   2; 100/2; 0.5

Four doses are available; however, the unused solution is to be discarded. No reconstitution label would be needed.

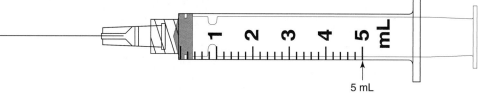

0.5 mL

4)   4.8; 100; 5

No reconstitution label is required; all of the medication will be used for 1 dose.

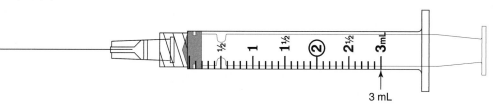

5 mL

5)   3.6; 250; 3; 1

3 mL

6)   18.2; 250,000; 4

8.2; 500,000; 2

3.2; 1,000,000; 1

Select 500,000 U/mL and give 2 mL. Either 1 mL or 2 mL is an appropriate amount to give IM depending on reconstitution, but 500,000 U/mL is less concentrated than 1,000,000 U/mL and is therefore less irritating to the muscle.

5 doses available in vial

Reconstitution Label

> 2/6/XX, 0800, reconstituted as
> 500,000 U/mL. Expires 2/13/XX, 0800.
> Keep refrigerated. G.D.P.

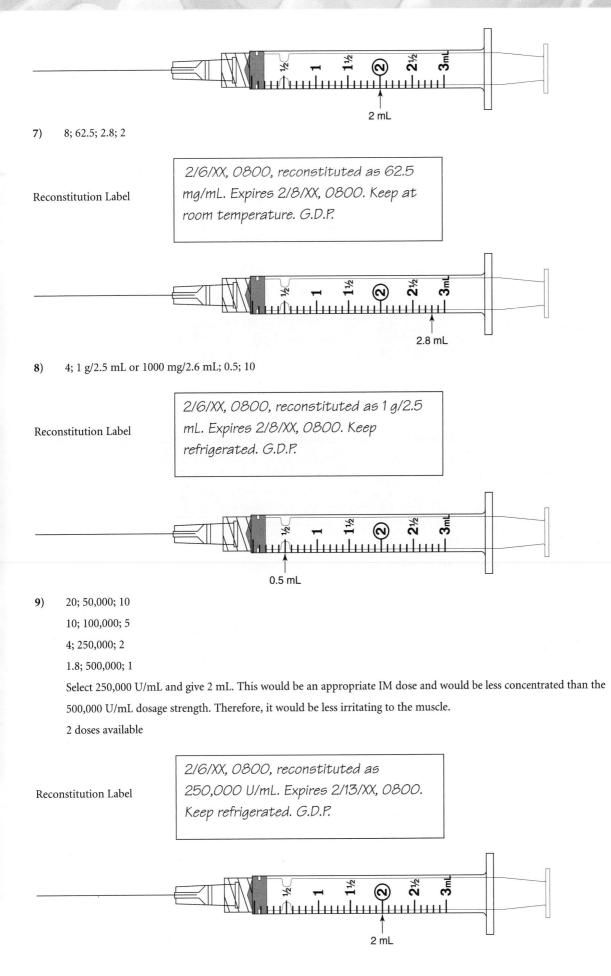

2 mL

7)   8; 62.5; 2.8; 2

Reconstitution Label

2/6/XX, 0800, reconstituted as 62.5 mg/mL. Expires 2/8/XX, 0800. Keep at room temperature. G.D.P.

2.8 mL

8)   4; 1 g/2.5 mL or 1000 mg/2.6 mL; 0.5; 10

Reconstitution Label

2/6/XX, 0800, reconstituted as 1 g/2.5 mL. Expires 2/8/XX, 0800. Keep refrigerated. G.D.P.

0.5 mL

9)   20; 50,000; 10
      10; 100,000; 5
      4; 250,000; 2
      1.8; 500,000; 1

Select 250,000 U/mL and give 2 mL. This would be an appropriate IM dose and would be less concentrated than the 500,000 U/mL dosage strength. Therefore, it would be less irritating to the muscle.

2 doses available

Reconstitution Label

2/6/XX, 0800, reconstituted as 250,000 U/mL. Expires 2/13/XX, 0800. Keep refrigerated. G.D.P.

2 mL

10) 3.2; 1.5/4; 375; 4; 1

(4 mL divided into 2 syringes)

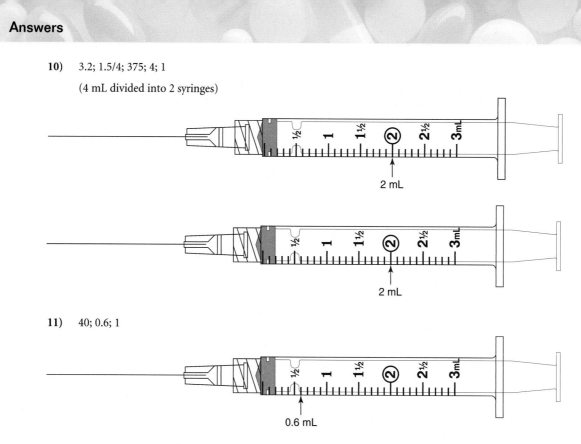

11) 40; 0.6; 1

12) 10; 2/10; 200; 1.3

Seven full doses of 1.3 mL are available. Because of the need to round 1.25 mL to 1.3 mL, there will be only 7 doses. Yes; the drug is ordered for administration twice a day; the 7 full doses would be given over $3\frac{1}{2}$ days and the solution is good for 7 days under refrigeration.

Reconstitution Label

> 2/6/XX, 0800, reconstituted as 200 mg/mL. Expires 2/13/XX, 0800. Keep refrigerated. G.D.P.

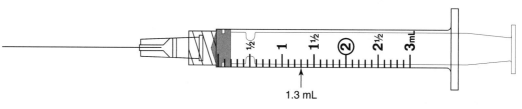

13) 19.2; 100; 15; 1

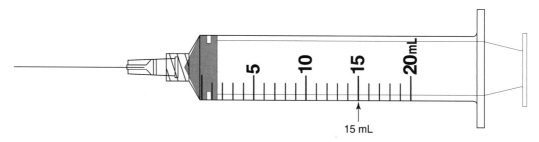

14)   30; 40; 5; 6

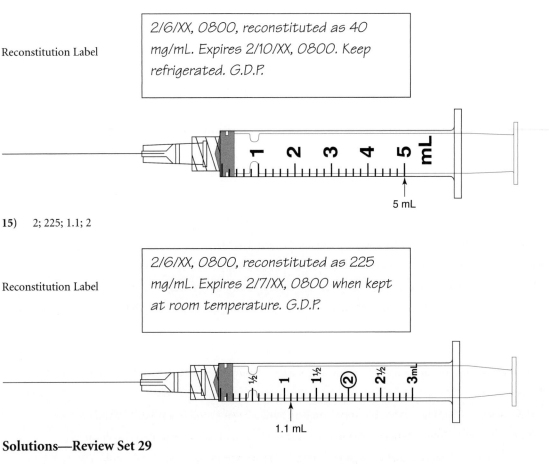

Reconstitution Label

> *2/6/XX, 0800, reconstituted as 40 mg/mL. Expires 2/10/XX, 0800. Keep refrigerated. G.D.P.*

5 mL

15)   2; 225; 1.1; 2

Reconstitution Label

> *2/6/XX, 0800, reconstituted as 225 mg/mL. Expires 2/7/XX, 0800 when kept at room temperature. G.D.P.*

1.1 mL

Solutions—Review Set 29

1)   Order: 200 mg

Supply: 280 mg/mL

$$\frac{D}{H} \times Q = \frac{200 \text{ mg}}{280 \text{ mg}} \times 1 \text{ mL} = 0.714 \text{ mL} = 0.71 \text{ mL}$$

500 mg/vial ÷ 200 mg/dose = 2.5 doses/vial = 2 full doses per vial available

2)   Order: 2500 U

Supply: 5000 U/mL

$$\frac{D}{H} \times Q = \frac{\overset{1}{2500} \text{ U}}{\underset{2}{5000} \text{ U}} \times 1 \text{ mL} = 0.5 \text{ mL}$$

50,000 U/vial ÷ 2500 U/dose = 20 doses/vial

6)   Order: 1,000,000 U

Supply: 250,000 U/mL

$$\frac{D}{H} \times Q = \frac{\overset{4}{1,000,000} \text{ U}}{\underset{1}{250,000} \text{ U}} \times 1 \text{ mL} = 4 \text{ mL}$$

Order: 1,000,000 U

Supply: 500,000 U/mL

$$\frac{D}{H} \times Q = \frac{\overset{2}{1,000,000} \text{ U}}{\underset{1}{500,000} \text{ U}} \times 1 \text{ mL} = 2 \text{ mL}$$

Order: 1,000,000 U

Supply: 1,000,000 U/mL

$$\frac{D}{H} \times Q = \frac{\overset{1}{1,000,000} \text{ U}}{\underset{1}{1,000,000} \text{ U}} \times 1 \text{ mL} = 1 \text{ mL}$$

5,000,000 U/vial ÷ 1,000,000 U/dose = 5 doses (available per vial)

8)   Order: 200 mg

Supply: 1000 mg/2.5 mL

$$\frac{D}{H} \times Q = \frac{\overset{1}{200} \text{ mg}}{\underset{5}{1000} \text{ mg}} \times 2.5 \text{ mL} = \frac{2.5}{5} \text{ mL} = 0.5 \text{ mL}$$

2 g/vial = 2 × 1000 = 2000 mg/vial

2000 mg/vial ÷ 200 mg/dose = 10 doses (available per vial)

12) Order: 250 mg

Supply: 200 mg/mL

$$\frac{\text{D}}{\text{H}} \times \text{Q} = \frac{\overset{5}{\cancel{250 \text{ mg}}}}{\underset{4}{\cancel{200 \text{ mg}}}} \times 1 \text{ mL} = \frac{5}{4} \text{ mL} = 1.25 \text{ mL} = 1.3 \text{ mL}$$

If looking at weight, there would be 8 doses available—2000 mg/vial ÷ 250 mg/dose = 8 doses/vial. However, because of the need to round the volume given, there will only be 7 doses available—10 mL/vial ÷ 1.3 mL/dose = 7.7 doses/vial = 7 full doses per vial

Review Set 30 from page 254

1) 160 mL hydrogen peroxide (solute) + 320 mL saline (solvent) = 480 mL $\frac{1}{3}$ strength solution.

2) 1 ounce hydrogen peroxide + 3 ounces saline = 4 ounces $\frac{1}{4}$ strength solution.

3) 180 mL hydrogen peroxide + 60 mL saline = 240 mL $\frac{3}{4}$ strength solution.

4) 8 ounces hydrogen peroxide + 8 ounces saline = 16 ounces $\frac{1}{2}$ strength solution.

5) 300 mL Ensure + 600 mL water = 900 mL $\frac{1}{3}$ strength Ensure; one 12-oz can. Discard 2 oz (60 mL).

6) 6 ounces (180 mL) Isomil + 18 ounces (540 mL) water = 24 ounces (720 mL) $\frac{1}{4}$ strength Isomil; one 6-oz can. No discard.

7) 800 mL Sustacal + 400 mL water = 1200 mL $\frac{2}{3}$ strength Sustacal; three 10-oz cans. Discard 100 mL.

8) 13 ounces Ensure + 13 ounces water = 26 ounces $\frac{1}{2}$ strength Ensure; one 12-oz can + one 4-oz can. Discard 3 oz (180 mL).

9) 500 mL Sustacal + 500 mL water = 1000 mL $\frac{1}{2}$ strength Sustacal; two 10-oz cans. Discard 100 mL.

10) 36 ounces Isomil + 12 ounces water = 48 ounces $\frac{3}{4}$ strength Isomil; use three 12-oz cans. No discard.

11) 4 ounces Ensure + 2 ounces water = 6 ounces $\frac{2}{3}$ strength Ensure; use one 4-oz can. No discard.

12) 4 ounces Ensure + 12 ounces water = 16 ounces (pt i) $\frac{1}{4}$ strength Ensure; use one 4-oz can. No discard.

Solutions—Review Set 30

1) $\text{D} \times \text{Q} = \frac{1}{\cancel{3}} \times \overset{160}{\cancel{480}} \text{ mL} = 160 \text{ mL solute}$

480 mL (quantity desired solution) – 160 mL (solute) = 320 mL (solvent)

5) $\text{D} \times \text{Q} = \frac{1}{\cancel{3}} \times \overset{300}{\cancel{900}} \text{ mL} = 300 \text{ mL Ensure}$

900 mL (total solution) – 300 mL (Ensure) = 600 mL (water)

one 12-oz can = 30 mL/oz × 12 oz/can = 360 mL/can

360 mL (full can) – 300 mL (Ensure needed) = 60 mL (discarded)

6) 4 oz q.4h = 4 oz/feeding × 6 feedings = 24 oz total;

$\text{D} \times \text{Q} = \frac{1}{\cancel{4}} \times \overset{6}{\cancel{24}} \text{ oz} = 6 \text{ oz (Isomil)}$

24 oz (solution) – 6 oz (Isomil) = 18 oz (water); use one 6-oz can.

12) $\text{D} \times \text{Q} = \frac{1}{4} \times 16 \text{ oz} = 4 \text{ oz Ensure}$

16 oz (solution) – 4 oz (Ensure) = 12 oz (water); use one 4-oz can Ensure. No discard.

Practice Problems—Chapter 11 from pages 255–262

1) 3.375/5; 3.7; 5 mL **2)** 2; 3 mL **3)** 1.5; 3 mL **4)** 19.2; 100; 7.5; 2; 10 mL

5) 1.8; 3 mL; 2

> *2/6/XX, 0800, reconstituted as 280 mg/mL.*
> *Expires 2/13/XX, 0800. Keep refrigerated. G.D.P.*

6) 3.8; 5 mL; 1 **7)** 2; 225; 1.3; 3 mL; 1; No **8)** 8; 125; 1.6; 3 mL; The vial states single-dose vial. If the vial was saved for additional doses, then a reconstitution label would be required. **9)** 1.5; 280; 1.3; 3 mL; 1; No **10)** 9.8; 5000; 1.5; 3 mL; 6; Yes **11)** 10; 2/10; 6.3; 10 mL; 1; No **12)** 30; 40; 3.8; 5 mL; 8; Yes **13)** 3.2; 1,000,000; 2; 3 mL; 2; Yes **14)** 1.8; 500,000; 2; 3 mL; 1; No **15)** 2; 225; 1.8; 3 mL; 1; No

16)   2 ounces hydrogen peroxide + 14 ounces normal saline = 16 ounces $\frac{1}{8}$ strength solution.

17)   120 mL hydrogen peroxide + 200 mL normal saline = 320 mL $\frac{3}{8}$ strength solution.

18)   50 mL hydrogen peroxide + 30 mL normal saline = 80 $\frac{5}{8}$ strength solution.

19)   12 ounces hydrogen peroxide + 6 ounces normal saline = 18 ounces $\frac{2}{3}$ strength solution.

20)   14 ounces hydrogen peroxide + 2 ounces normal saline = 16 ounces (1 pt) $\frac{7}{8}$ strength solution.

21)   250 mL hydrogen peroxide + 750 mL normal saline = 1000 mL (1 L) $\frac{1}{4}$ strength solution.

22)   30 mL Enfamil + 90 mL water = 120 mL $\frac{1}{4}$ strength Enfamil; one 3-oz bottle. Discard 2 oz (60 mL).

23)   270 mL Sustacal + 90 mL water = 360 mL $\frac{3}{4}$ strength Sustacal; one 10-oz can. Discard 1 oz (30 mL).

24)   300 mL Ensure + 150 mL water = 450 mL $\frac{2}{3}$ strength Ensure; two 8-oz cans. Discard 6 oz (180 mL).

25)   36 ounces Enfamil + 60 ounces water = 96 ounces $\frac{3}{8}$ strength Enfamil; six 6-oz bottles. No discard.

26)   20 mL Ensure + 140 mL water = 160 mL $\frac{1}{8}$ strength Ensure; one 4-oz can. Discard 100 mL.

27)   225 mL Ensure + 225 mL water = 550 mL $\frac{1}{2}$ strength Ensure; one 12-oz can. Discard 135 mL.

28)   2 cans are needed; $1\frac{1}{2}$ cans are used (12 oz Enfamil)

29)   36

30)   Critical Thinking: Prevention.

     This type of error could have been prevented had the nurse read the label carefully for the correct amount of diluent for the dosage of medication to be prepared. Had the nurse read the label carefully before the medication was prepared, medication, valuable time, health care resources, and patient expense charges would have been saved. Additionally, if the nurse had used Step 2 (Think) of the three-step method, the nurse would have realized earlier (before preparing it) that 4 mL would be an unreasonable volume for an IM injection.

Solutions—Practice Problems—Chapter 11

1)   Concentration is 3.375 g/5 mL

     Order: 2.5 g

     Supply: 3.375 g/5 mL

$$\frac{D}{H} \times Q = \frac{2.5\,g}{3.375\,g} \times 5\text{ mL} = 3.70\text{ mL} = 3.7\text{ mL}$$

4)   Order: 750 mg

     Supply: 100 mg/mL

$$\frac{D}{H} \times Q = \frac{750\,mg}{100\,mg} \times 1\text{ mL} = 7.5\text{ mL}$$

     Vial has 2 g Rocephin. Order is for 750 mg/dose.

     2 g/vial = 2 × 1000 = 2000 mg/vial; 2000 mg/vial ÷ 750 mg/dose = 2.6 doses/vial = 2 full doses/vial

6)   Order: 375 mg

     Supply: 100 mg/mL

$$\frac{D}{H} \times Q = \frac{375\,mg}{100\,mg} \times 1\text{ mL} = 3.75\text{ mL} = 3.8\text{ mL}$$

     500 mg/vial ÷ 375 mg/dose = 1.3 doses/vial = 1 full dose/vial available.

9)   Order: 350 mg

     Supply: 280 mg/mL

$$\frac{D}{H} \times Q = \frac{350\,mg}{280\,mg} \times 1\text{ mL} = 1.25\text{ mL} = 1.3\text{ mL}$$

     500 mg/vial ÷ 350 mg/dose = 1.4 doses/vial = 1 full dose/vial available.

14)   Order: 1,000,000 U

     Supply: 50,000 U/mL

$$\frac{D}{H} \times Q = \frac{\overset{20}{1,000,000\,U}}{\underset{1}{500,000\,U}} \times 1\text{ mL} = 20\text{ mL (too much for IM dose)}$$

     Order: 1,000,000 U

     Supply: 100,000 U/mL

$$\frac{D}{H} \times Q = \frac{\overset{10}{1,000,000\,U}}{\underset{1}{100,000\,U}} \times 1\text{ mL} = 10\text{ mL (too much for IM dose)}$$

Order: 1,000,000 U

Supply: 250,000 U/mL

$$\frac{D}{H} \times Q = \frac{\overset{4}{\cancel{1,000,000}\,U}}{\underset{1}{\cancel{250,000}\,U}} \times 1\ mL = 4\ mL \text{ (too much for IM dose--}$$
$$\text{3 mL or less is preferable)}$$

Order: 1,000,000 U

Supply: 500,000 U/mL

$$\frac{D}{H} \times Q = \frac{\overset{2}{\cancel{1,000,000}\,U}}{\underset{1}{\cancel{500,000}\,U}} \times 1\ mL = 2\ mL \text{ (acceptable}$$
$$\text{IM dose)}$$

22) 12 mL every hour for 10 hours = 12 × 10 = 120 mL total;

$$D \times Q = \frac{1}{\underset{1}{\cancel{4}}} \times \overset{30}{\cancel{120}}\ mL = 30\ mL\ Enfamil$$

120 mL (solution) – 30 mL (Enfamil) = 90 mL (water); one 3-oz bottle = 90 mL

90 mL (full bottle) – 30 mL (Enfamil needed) = 60 mL (2 oz discarded)

28) $D \times Q = \dfrac{1}{\underset{1}{\cancel{4}}} \times \overset{12}{\cancel{48}}\ oz = 12\ oz\ Enfamil;$

Need $1\frac{1}{2}$ cans (8 oz each can) of Enfamil for each infant.

29) 48 oz (solution) – 12 oz (Enfamil) = 36 oz (water)

Review Set 31 from page 268

1) 2 **2)** 2.5 **3)** 0.8 **4)** 0.7 **5)** 7.5 **6)** 0.6 **7)** $1\frac{1}{2}$ **8)** 3 **9)** 30 **10)** 1.6 **11)** 3 **12)** 0.5 **13)** 2 **14)** 250 mg; $\frac{1}{2}$ of 250 mg tab
15) 2.4 **16)** 2 **17)** 8 **18)** 1.3 **19)** 16 **20)** 7

Solutions—Review Set 31

2)
$$\frac{300\ mg}{5\ mL} \diagdown\!\!\!\!\diagup \frac{150\ mg}{X\ mL}$$

$$300X = 750$$

$$\frac{300X}{300} = \frac{750}{300}$$

$$X = 2.5\ mL$$

5)
$$\frac{8\ mEq}{5\ mL} \diagdown\!\!\!\!\diagup \frac{12\ mEq}{X\ mL}$$

$$8X = 60$$

$$\frac{8X}{8} = \frac{60}{8}$$

$$X = 7.5\ mL$$

6)
$$\frac{4\ mg}{1\ mL} \diagdown\!\!\!\!\diagup \frac{2.4\ mg}{X\ mL}$$

$$4X = 2.4$$

$$\frac{4X}{4} = \frac{2.4}{4}$$

$$X = 0.6\ mL$$

9)
$$\frac{80\ mg}{15\ mL} \diagdown\!\!\!\!\diagup \frac{160\ mg}{X\ mL}$$

$$80X = 2400$$

$$\frac{80X}{80} = \frac{2400}{80}$$

$$X = 30\ mL$$

13) A. Convert gr to mg; gr ss = gr $\frac{1}{2}$

$$\frac{gr\ i}{60\ mg} \diagdown\!\!\!\!\diagup \frac{gr\ ss}{X\ mg}$$

$$X = 60 \times \frac{1}{2}$$

$$X = 30\ mg$$

B.
$$\frac{15\ mg}{1\ tab} \diagdown\!\!\!\!\diagup \frac{30\ mg}{X\ tab}$$

$$15X = 30$$

$$\frac{15X}{15} = \frac{30}{15}$$

$$X = 2\ tab$$

16) A. Convert mcg to mg:

$$\frac{1\ mg}{1000\ mcg} \diagdown\!\!\!\!\diagup \frac{0.15\ mg}{X\ mcg}$$

$$X = 150\ mcg$$

B.
$$\frac{75\ mcg}{1\ tab} \diagdown\!\!\!\!\diagup \frac{150\ mcg}{X}$$

$$75X = 150$$

$$\frac{75X}{75} = \frac{150}{75}$$

$$X = 2\ tab$$

18) $\dfrac{80 \text{ mg}}{1 \text{ mL}} \diagdown \diagup \dfrac{100 \text{ mg}}{X \text{ mL}}$

$$80X = 100$$

$$\dfrac{80X}{80} = \dfrac{100}{80}$$

$$X = 1.25 \text{ mL} = 1.3 \text{ mL (measured in a 3 mL syringe)}$$

19) $\dfrac{2.5 \text{ mg}}{5 \text{ mL}} \diagdown \diagup \dfrac{8 \text{ mg}}{X \text{ mL}}$

$$2.5X = 40$$

$$\dfrac{2.5X}{2.5} = \dfrac{40}{2.5}$$

$$X = 16 \text{ mL}$$

Practice Problems—Chapter 12 from pages 270–272

1) 45 **2)** 2 **3)** 2 **4)** $\frac{1}{2}$ **5)** 2.5 **6)** 16 **7)** 1.4 **8)** 0.7 **9)** 2.3 **10)** 0.13 (measured in a 1 mL syringe) **11)** 1.6 **12)** 1.5 **13)** 1.3 **14)** 2.5 **15)** 1.6 **16)** 7.5 **17)** 1.6 **18)** 2 **19)** 8 **20)** 4.5 **21)** 30 **22)** 1.4 **23)** 15 **24)** 20 **25)** 12

26)   Critical Thinking: Prevention.

This type of calculation error occurred because the nurse set up the proportion incorrectly. In this instance the nurse mixed up the units with mg *and* mL in the numerators, and mg *and* mL in the denominators. The **mg** unit should be in both numerators of the proportion, and the **mL** unit in both denominators.

$\dfrac{125 \text{ mg}}{5 \text{ mL}} \diagdown \diagup \dfrac{50 \text{ mg}}{X \text{ mL}}$

$$125X = 250$$

$$\dfrac{125X}{125} = \dfrac{250}{125}$$

$$X = 2 \text{ mL}$$

In addition, **think first**. Then use ratio and proportion to calculate the dosage.

Solutions—Practice Problems—Chapter 12

1) $\dfrac{3.33 \text{ g}}{5 \text{ mL}} \diagdown \diagup \dfrac{30 \text{ g}}{X \text{ mL}}$

$$3.33X = 150$$

$$\dfrac{3.33X}{3.33} = \dfrac{150}{3.33}$$

$$X = 45 \text{ mL}$$

2) $\dfrac{5,000,000 \text{ U}}{20 \text{ mL}} \diagdown \diagup \dfrac{500,000 \text{ U}}{X \text{ mL}}$

$$5,000,000X = 10,000,000$$

$$\dfrac{5,000,000X}{5,000,000} = \dfrac{10,000,000}{5,000,000}$$

$$X = 2 \text{ mL}$$

6) $\dfrac{12.5 \text{ mg}}{5 \text{ mL}} \diagdown \diagup \dfrac{40 \text{ mg}}{X \text{ mL}}$

$$12.5X = 200$$

$$\dfrac{12.5X}{12.5} = \dfrac{200}{12.5}$$

$$X = 16 \text{ mL}$$

7) $\dfrac{500,000 \text{ U}}{2 \text{ mL}} \diagdown \diagup \dfrac{350,000 \text{ U}}{X \text{ mL}}$

$$500,000X = 700,000$$

$$\dfrac{500,000X}{500,000} = \dfrac{700,000}{500,000}$$

$$X = 1.4 \text{ mL}$$

8) $\dfrac{10 \text{ mg}}{2 \text{ mL}} \diagdown \diagup \dfrac{3.5 \text{ mg}}{X \text{ mL}}$

$$10X = 200$$

$$\dfrac{10X}{10} = \dfrac{7}{10}$$

$$X = 0.7 \text{ mL}$$

9) $\dfrac{80 \text{ mg}}{2 \text{ mL}} \diagdown \diagup \dfrac{90 \text{ mg}}{X \text{ mL}}$

$$80X = 180$$

$$\dfrac{80X}{80} = \dfrac{180}{80}$$

$$X = 2.25 \text{ mL} = 2.3 \text{ mL}$$

13)   A. Convert g to mg: 1 g = 1000 mg

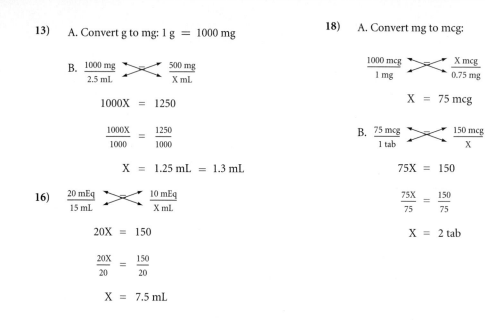

B. $\dfrac{1000 \text{ mg}}{2.5 \text{ mL}} \bowtie \dfrac{500 \text{ mg}}{X \text{ mL}}$

$$1000X = 1250$$

$$\dfrac{1000X}{1000} = \dfrac{1250}{1000}$$

$$X = 1.25 \text{ mL} = 1.3 \text{ mL}$$

16) $\dfrac{20 \text{ mEq}}{15 \text{ mL}} \bowtie \dfrac{10 \text{ mEq}}{X \text{ mL}}$

$$20X = 150$$

$$\dfrac{20X}{20} = \dfrac{150}{20}$$

$$X = 7.5 \text{ mL}$$

18)   A. Convert mg to mcg:

$\dfrac{1000 \text{ mcg}}{1 \text{ mg}} \bowtie \dfrac{X \text{ mcg}}{0.75 \text{ mg}}$

$$X = 75 \text{ mcg}$$

B. $\dfrac{75 \text{ mcg}}{1 \text{ tab}} \bowtie \dfrac{150 \text{ mcg}}{X}$

$$75X = 150$$

$$\dfrac{75X}{75} = \dfrac{150}{75}$$

$$X = 2 \text{ tab}$$

Review Set 32 from pages 288–293

1) 25; 312.5; 78.1; 625; 156.3; Yes **2)** 10 **3)** 2.2; 110; 55; Yes **4)** 0.55 **5)** 15; 120; Yes **6)** 6; 8 **7)** 32; 320; 480; Yes **8)** 15

9) 20; 500; 125; 1000; 250; Yes **10)** 5 **11)** 5; 7.5; 9.5; Yes

12)   0.8

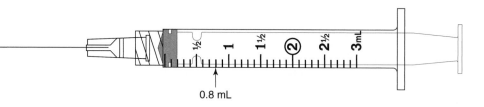

0.8 mL

13)   3.4; 51; 17; No

14)   The dosage of Kantrex 34 mg IV q.8h is higher than the recommended dosage. Therefore, the ordered dosage is not safe. The prescribing practitioner should be called and the order questioned.

15)   120; 60; 7.5; Yes

16)   7.5; $1\frac{1}{2}$

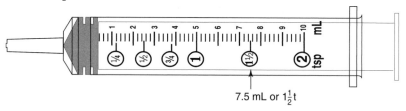

7.5 mL or $1\frac{1}{2}$ t

17)   1.8; 4.5; No

18)   The ordered dosage is too high and ordered to be given too frequently. The recommended dosage is 4.5 mg q.8h. The ordered dosage is 40 mg q.8h. The prescribing practitioner should be notified and the order questioned.

19)   31.8; 0.22; 0.11; 0.32; 0.16; Yes

20) 3

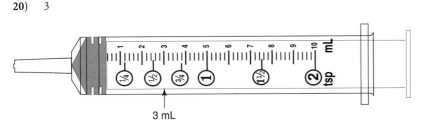

3 mL

21) 17.7; 354; 118; 708; 236; No

22) The dosage ordered of 100 mg q.8h does not fall within the recommended dosage range of 118–236 mg/dose. It is an underdosage and would not produce a therapeutic effect. The physician should be called for clarification.

23) 25; 375; 125; 625; 208.3; No

24) The ordered dosage of 100 mg q.8h does not fall within the recommended dosage range of 125–208.3 mg q.8h. It is an underdosage and the physician should be called for clarification.

25) No, the ordered dosage is not safe. The label states a maximum of 250 mg per single daily injection for children over 8 years of age. This child is only 7 and the order exceeds the maximum recommended dosage. The physician should be called to clarify the order.

26) 200–300 mg/kg/day by IV infusion in divided doses every 4 or 6 hours.

27) 150–200 mg/kg/day by IV infusion in divided doses every 4 or 6 hours.

28) 8.9; 11.8

29) 1.5; 2

30) 2.2; 3

Solutions—Review Set 32

1) 1 kg = 2.2 lb; smaller → larger: (÷)
   55 lb = 55 ÷ 2.2 = 25 kg

   Minimum daily dosage:

   125 mg/kg/day × 25 kg = 312 mg/day

   312.5 mg ÷ 4 doses = 78.12 mg/dose = 78.1 mg/dose

   Maximum daily dosage:

   25 mg/kg/day × 25 kg = 625 mg/day

   625 mg ÷ 4 doses = 156.25 mg/dose = 156.3 mg/dose

   Yes, dosage is safe.

2) $\dfrac{D}{H} \times Q = \dfrac{\overset{2}{\cancel{125 \text{ mg}}}}{\underset{1}{\cancel{62.5 \text{ mg}}}} \times 5 \text{ mL} = 10 \text{ mL}$

3) Convert g to kg: 2200 g = 2200 ÷ 1000 = 2.2 kg

   50 mg/kg/day × 2.2 kg = 110 mg/day

   110 mg ÷ 2 doses = 55 mg/dose; yes, dosage is safe

4) $\dfrac{D}{H} \times Q = \dfrac{55 \text{ mg}}{\underset{100}{\cancel{1000 \text{ mg}}}} \times \overset{1}{\cancel{10}} \text{ mL} = 0.55 \text{ mL}$

6) $\dfrac{D}{H} \times Q = \dfrac{\overset{6}{\cancel{120 \text{ mg}}}}{\underset{5}{\cancel{100 \text{ mg}}}} \times 5 \text{ mL} = \dfrac{\overset{6}{\cancel{30}}}{\underset{1}{\cancel{8}}} \text{ mL} = 6 \text{ mL}$

   50 mL ÷ 6 mL/dose = 8.3 doses or 8 full doses

7) Minimum dosage: 10 mg/kg/dose × 32 kg = 320 mg/dose

   Maximum dosage: 15 mg/kg/dose × 32 kg = 480 mg/dose

   Dosage is the *maximum* dosage (480 mg), and it is a safe dosage.

8) $\dfrac{D}{H} \times Q = \dfrac{\overset{3}{\cancel{480 \text{ mg}}}}{\underset{1}{\cancel{160 \text{ mg}}}} \times 5 \text{ mL} = 15 \text{ mL}$

13) 1 lb = 16 oz; 8 oz = 8 ÷ 16 = $\frac{1}{2}$ lb

    7 lb 8 oz = $7\frac{1}{2}$ lb = 7.5 ÷ 2.2 = 3.4 kg

    15 mg/kg/day × 3.4 kg = 51 mg/day

    51 mg ÷ 3 doses = 17 mg/dose, if administered q.8h

    Ordered dosage of 34 mg q.8h exceeds recommended dosage and is not safe.

19) 70 lb = 70 ÷ 2.2 = 31.8 kg

Minimum daily dosage:

7 mcg/kg/day × 31.8 kg = 222.6 mcg/day

Convert mcg to mg; 222.6 mcg/day =
222.6 ÷ 1000 = 0.2226 mg/day = 0.22 mg/day

Minimum single dosage:
0.22 mg ÷ 2 doses = 0.11 mg/dose

Maximum daily dosage:
10 mcg/kg/day × 31.8 kg = 318 mcg/day

Convert mcg to mg; 318 mcg/day =
318 ÷ 1000 = 0.318 mg/day = 0.32 mg/day

Maximum single dosage:
0.32 mg ÷ 2 doses = 0.16 mg/dose

Yes, dosage ordered is safe.

21) 39 lb = 39 ÷ 2.2 = 17.72 kg = 17.7 kg

Minimum daily dosage:
20 mg/kg/day × 17.7 kg = 354 mg/day

Minimum single dosage:
354 mg ÷ 3 doses = 118 mg/dose

Maximum daily dosage:
40 mg/kg/day × 17.7 kg = 708 mg/day

Maximum single dosage:
708 mg ÷ 3 doses = 236 mg/dose

The dosage of 100 mg q.8h is not safe. It is
an underdosage and would not produce a
therapeutic effect, as the recommended dosage range
is 118–236 mg/dose.

28) 130 lb = 130 ÷ 2.2 = 59.1 kg

150 mg/kg/day × 59.1 kg = 8865 mg/day

Convert mg to g: 8865 mg/day =
8865 ÷ 1000 = 8.865 g/day = 8.9 g/day

200 mg/kg/day × 59.1 kg = 11,820 mg/day

Convert mg to g: 11,820 mg/day =
11,820 ÷ 1000 = 11.82 g/day = 11.8 g/day

29) 8.9 g ÷ 6 doses = 1.5 g/dose

11.8 g ÷ 6 doses = 2 g/dose

30) 8.9 g ÷ 4 doses = 2.2 g/dose

11.8 g ÷ 4 doses = 3 g/dose

Practice Problems—Chapter 13 from pages 294–307

1) 5.5 **2)** 3.8 **3)** 1.6 **4)** 2.3 **5)** 15.5 **6)** 3 **7)** 23.6 **8)** 0.9 **9)** 240 **10)** 80 **11)** 19.5; 39; 48.8; Yes

12) 1

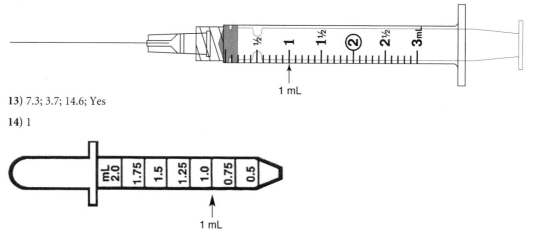

1 mL

13) 7.3; 3.7; 14.6; Yes

14) 1

1 mL

15) 18.2; 182; 91; 364; 182; Yes

16) 7.5

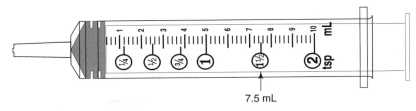

7.5 mL

17) 29.1; 291; 145.5; 436.5; 218.3; Yes

18) 3

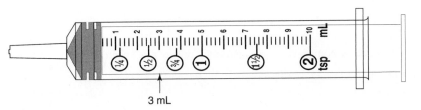

3 mL

19)   2.5; 2250; 750; Yes

20)   9.8; 10; 5000; 0.15

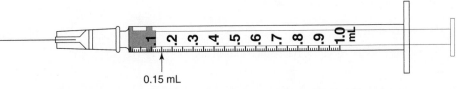

0.15 mL

Route is IM; needle may need to be changed to appropriate gauge and length.

21)   18.6; 372; 124; 744; 248; Yes

22)   6

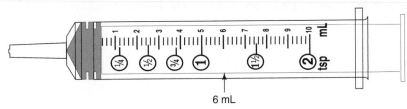

6 mL

23)   9.3; 372; 186; Yes, the ordered dosage is reasonably safe.

24)   5

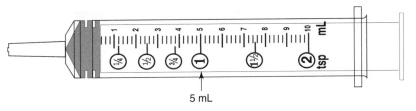

5 mL

25)   10; 0.1; Yes

26)   0.25

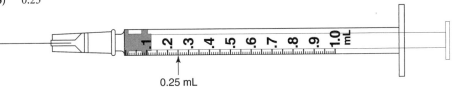

0.25 mL

27) 28; 35; Yes

28) 3.5

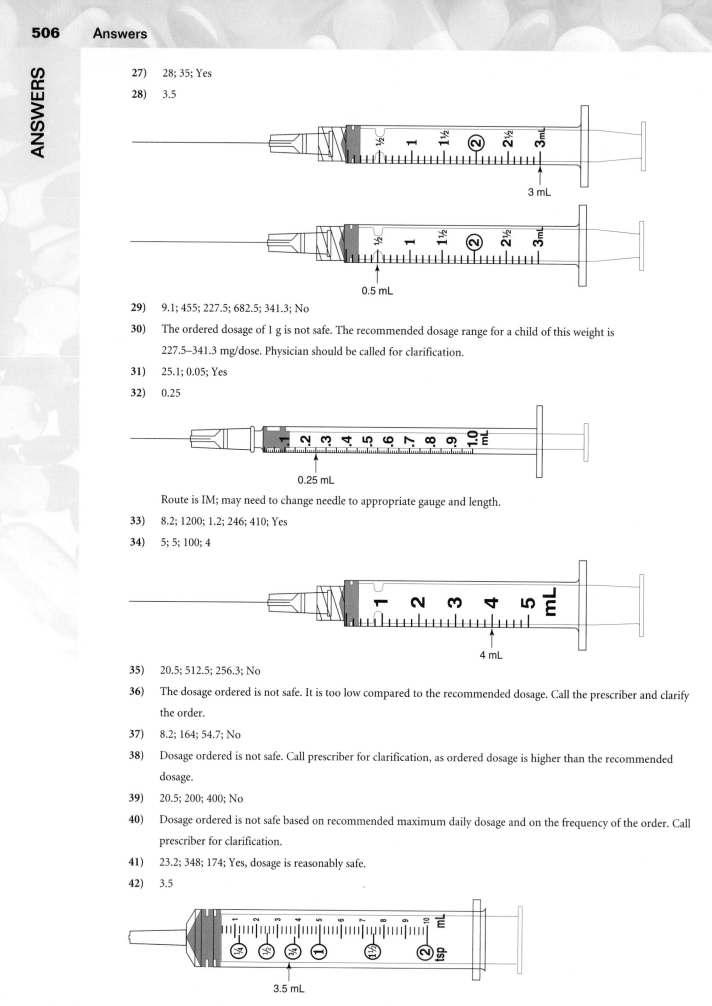

3 mL

0.5 mL

29) 9.1; 455; 227.5; 682.5; 341.3; No

30) The ordered dosage of 1 g is not safe. The recommended dosage range for a child of this weight is 227.5–341.3 mg/dose. Physician should be called for clarification.

31) 25.1; 0.05; Yes

32) 0.25

0.25 mL

Route is IM; may need to change needle to appropriate gauge and length.

33) 8.2; 1200; 1.2; 246; 410; Yes

34) 5; 5; 100; 4

4 mL

35) 20.5; 512.5; 256.3; No

36) The dosage ordered is not safe. It is too low compared to the recommended dosage. Call the prescriber and clarify the order.

37) 8.2; 164; 54.7; No

38) Dosage ordered is not safe. Call prescriber for clarification, as ordered dosage is higher than the recommended dosage.

39) 20.5; 200; 400; No

40) Dosage ordered is not safe based on recommended maximum daily dosage and on the frequency of the order. Call prescriber for clarification.

41) 23.2; 348; 174; Yes, dosage is reasonably safe.

42) 3.5

3.5 mL

43) 0.25

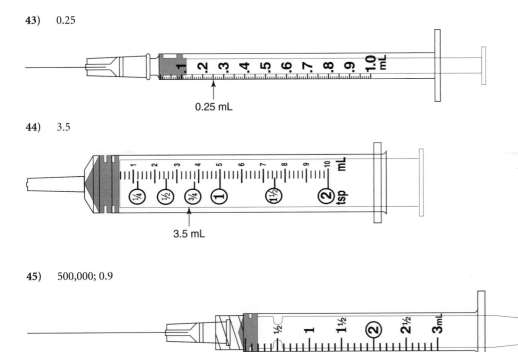

0.25 mL

44) 3.5

3.5 mL

45) 500,000; 0.9

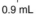

0.9 mL

Needle may need to be changed to appropriate gauge and length for this small child.

46) Dosage is not safe; this child is ordered a total of 2 mg/day, which is too high. Prescriber should be called to clarify.

47) The ordered dosage of 20 mg q.3–4h p.r.n. is too high when compared to the recommended dosage range for a child of this weight. The order should be clarified with the prescriber.

48) 0.76

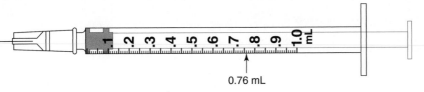

0.76 mL

Route is IM; needle may need to be changed to appropriate gauge and length.

49) #45 (penicillin G potassium) and #48 (Kefzol). (Note: #43 Solu-Medrol is a single-dose vial. Check package insert to determine if storage after mixing is safe.)

50) Critical Thinking: Prevention.

The child should have received 75 mg a day and no more than 25 mg per dose. The child received more than four times the safe dosage of tobramycin. Had the nurse calculated the safe dosage, the error would have been caught sooner, the resident consulted, and the dosage could have been adjusted before the child ever received the first dose. The pharmacist also should have caught the error but did not. In this scenario the resident, pharmacist, and nurse all committed medication errors. If the resident had not noticed the error, one can only wonder how many doses the child would have received. The nurse is the last safety net for the child when it comes to a dosage error, because the nurse administers the drug.

In addition, the nurse has to reconcile the fact that she actually gave the overdose. The nurse is responsible for whatever dosage is administered and must verify the safety of the order and the patient's 6 rights. We are all accountable for our actions. Taking shortcuts in administering medications to children can be disastrous. The time the nurse saved by not calculating the safe dosage was more than lost in the extra monitoring, not to mention the cost of follow-up to the medication error, *and most importantly*, the risk to the child.

Solutions—Practice Problems—Chapter 13

1)   1 kg = 2.2 lb; smaller → larger: (÷)

   12 lb = 12 ÷ 2.2 = 5.45 kg = 5.5 kg

2)   8 lb 4 oz = $8\frac{4}{16}$ lb = $8\frac{1}{4}$ lb = 8.25 lb

   8.25 lb = 8.25 ÷ 2.2 = 3.75 kg = 3.8 kg

3)   1570 g = 1570 ÷ 1000 = 1.57 kg = 1.6 kg

6)   1 lb = 16 oz; 10 oz = 10 ÷ 16 = $\frac{5}{8}$ lb

   6 lb 10 oz = $6\frac{5}{8}$ lb = 6.625 lb

   6.625 lb = 6.625 ÷ 2.2 = 3.01 kg = 3 kg

17)   64 lb = 64 ÷ 2.2 = 29.09 kg = 29.1 kg

   Minimum daily dosage:

   10 mg/kg/day × 29.1 kg = 291 mg/day

   Minimum single dosage: (based on b.i.d.)

   291 mg/2 doses = 145.5 mg/dose

   Maximum daily dosage:

   15 mg/kg/day × 29.1 kg = 436.5 mg/day

   Maximum single dosage: (based on b.i.d.)

   436.5 mg ÷ 2 doses = 218.25 = 218.3 mg/dose

   Dosage ordered is safe. Child will receive 300 mg in a 24-hour period in divided doses of 150 mg b.i.d. This falls within the recommended dosage range of 145.5 mg/dose to 218.3 mg/dose and does not exceed the maximum recommended single-dosage allowance of 250 mg/dose.

18) $\frac{D}{H} \times Q = \dfrac{\overset{3}{\cancel{150\,\text{mg}}}}{\underset{5}{\cancel{250\,\text{mg}}}} \times 5\,\text{mL} = \dfrac{3}{\cancel{5}} \times \cancel{5}\,\text{mL} = 3\,\text{mL}$

19)   2500 g = 2500 ÷ 1000 = 2.5 kg

   Recommended daily dosage:

   900 U/kg/day × 2.5 kg = 2250 U/day

   Recommended single dosage:

   2250 U ÷ 3 doses = 750 U/dose

   Ordered dosage is safe.

23)   20.5 lb = 20.5 ÷ 2.2 = 9.31 kg = 9.3 kg

   Recommended daily dosage:

   40 mg/kg/day × 9.3 kg = 372 mg/day

   Recommended single dosage:

   372 mg ÷ 2 doses = 186 mg/dose

   The ordered dosage of 187 mg p.o. is reasonably safe for this child.

24) $\frac{D}{H} \times Q = \dfrac{\overset{1}{\cancel{187\,\text{mg}}}}{\underset{1}{\cancel{187\,\text{mg}}}} \times 5\,\text{mL} = 5\,\text{mL}$

   If we used the recommended single dosage of 186 mg/dose, the calculation would be:

   $\frac{D}{H} \times Q = \dfrac{186\,\cancel{\text{mg}}}{187\,\cancel{\text{mg}}} \times 5\,\text{mL} = 4.9\,\text{mL}$;

   which we round to 5 mL to measure in the pediatric oral syringe; therefore, as stated above, the ordered dosage is reasonably safe.

25)   22 lb = 22 ÷ 2.2 = 10 kg

   0.01 mg/kg/dose × 10 kg = 0.1 mg/dose

   0.1 mg = 0.1 × 1000 = 100 mcg

   Ordered dosage is safe.

29)   20 lb = 20 ÷ 2.2 = 9.1 kg

   Recommended minimum daily dosage:

   50 mg/kg/day × 9.1 kg = 455 mg/day

   Recommended minimum single dosage:

   455 mg ÷ 2 doses = 227.5 mg/dose

   Recommended maximum daily dosage:

   75 mg/kg/day × 9.1 kg = 682.5 mg/day

   Recommended maximum single dosage:

   682.5 mg ÷ 2 doses = 341.3 mg/dose

   The dosage ordered (1 g q.12h) is not safe. The recommended dosage range for a child of this weight is 227.5–341.3 mg/dose. Physician should be called for clarification.

41) 51 lb = 51 ÷ 2.2 = 23.2 kg

Recommended daily dosage:

15 mg/kg/day × 23.2 kg = 348 mg/day

Recommended single dosage:

348 mg ÷ 2 doses = 174 mg/dose

Ordered dosage of 175 mg is reasonably safe as an oral medication and should be given.

43) 95 lb = 95 ÷ 2.2 = 43.2 kg

0.5 mg/kg/day × 43.2 kg = 21.6 mg/day

Since the recommended dosage is not less than 21.6 mg/day and the order is for 10 mg q.6h for a total of 40 mg/day, the order is safe.

$$\frac{D}{H} \times Q = \frac{\overset{1}{\cancel{10 \text{ mg}}}}{\underset{4}{\cancel{40 \text{ mg}}}} \times 1 \text{ mL} = 0.25 \text{ mL}$$

Section 3—Self-Evaluation from pages 308–319

1) C; 2 **2)** F; 1 **3)** J; 1 **4)** B; 7.5 **5)** H; 12 **6)** I; 2 **7)** E; 2 **8)** K; $\frac{1}{2}$ **9)** M; 1.25 **10)** L; 7.5 **11)** E; 0.2 **12)** C; 3.5 **13)** G; 0.2
14) A; 0.8 **15)** D; 1.5 **16)** F; 0.75 **17)** B; 0.6 **18)** H; 0.75

19)

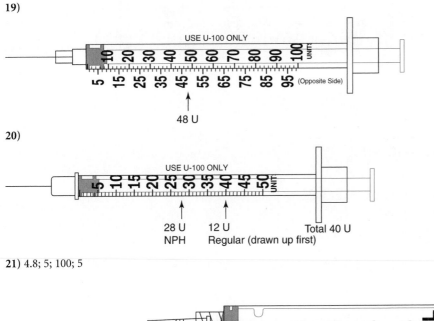

48 U

20)

28 U   12 U   Total 40 U
NPH   Regular (drawn up first)

21) 4.8; 5; 100; 5

5 mL

22) 20; 20; 1/20

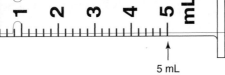

2/6/xx, 0800, reconstituted as 1 g/20 mL. Expires 2/20/xx, 0880. Keep refrigerated. G.D.P.

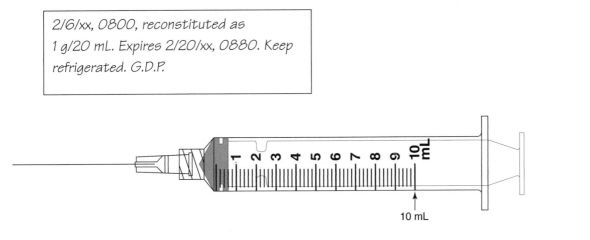

10 mL

23) 1.5; 1.8; 280; 0.71 (May need to change needles as this is an IM dose.)

> 2/6/xx, 0800, reconstituted as
> 280 mg/mL. Expires 2/13/xx, 0800. Keep
> refrigerated. G.D.P.

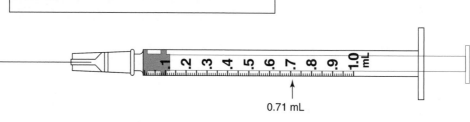

0.71 mL

24) 2.5; 3; 330; 2.3

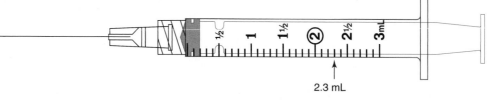

2.3 mL

25) 8; 8; 62.5; 4

> 2/6/xx, 0800, reconstituted as
> 62.5 mg/mL. Expires 2/8/xx, 0800. Keep
> at controlled room temperature 20–25°C
> (66-77°F). G.D.P.

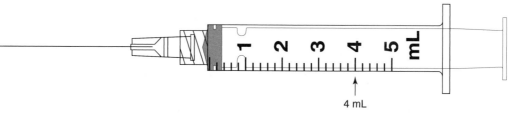

4 mL

26) 30; 30; 40; 2.5

> 2/6/xx, 0800, reconstituted as
> 40 mg/mL. Expires 2/10/xx, 0800. Keep
> refrigerated. G.D.P.

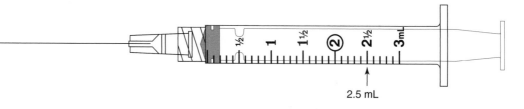

2.5 mL

27) 12 doses are available.

28) The medication supplied will be used up before it expires. It is good for 4 days (96 hours) under refrigeration. The medication is to be given every 8 hours; therefore in 4 days, 12 doses will be used before the expiration, providing the last dose is given on time.

29) 120; 240 **30)** 180; 60 **31)** 120 **32)** $1\frac{1}{2}$ 33) 3 **34)** 540 **35)** 0.8 **36)** 7 **37)** 0.3 **38)** 1.5 **39)** 0.6 **40)** 7 **41)** 2 **42)** 1 **43)** 3

44) 3.8

45) 0.75

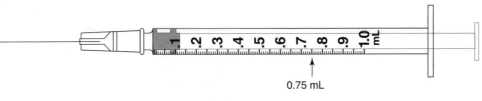

0.75 mL

46) 12; 15; 50; 1.5

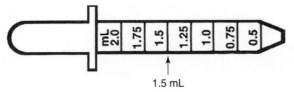

1.5 mL

47) Order of 100 mg t.i.d. is too high and the maximum recommended dosage is 100 mg/day for this child. The order is not safe. Physician should be called for clarification.

48) Order is too high and the maximum recommended dosage for this child is 292 mg/day. This order would deliver 748 mg/day. Recommended dosage is also twice daily and this order is for 4 times/day. This order is not safe. Physician should be called for clarification.

49) Order is too high and is not safe. Recommended dosage is 36.5 mg/dose, or 109.5 mg/day. Physician should be called for clarification.

50) 500

Solutions—Section 3—Self-Evaluation

5) Order: 16 mEq

Supply: 20 mEq/15 mL

$$\frac{D}{H} \times Q = \frac{\overset{4}{\cancel{16}}\,mEq}{\underset{5}{\cancel{20}}\,mEq} \times 15\ mL = \frac{4}{\cancel{5}} \times \frac{3}{\cancel{15}}\,mL = 12\ mL$$

7) Order: 0.05 mg = 0.05 × 1000 = 50 mcg

Supply: 25 mcg/tab

$$\frac{D}{H} \times Q = \frac{\overset{2}{\cancel{50}}\,mcg}{\underset{1}{\cancel{25}}\,mcg} \times 1\ tab = 2\ tab$$

Label N-Synthroid 100 mcg not selected because it is best to give whole tablets when possible rather than trying to split the tablet in half.

8) Convert: gr i = 60 mg

gr $\frac{1}{4} = \frac{1}{4} \times 60 = 15$ mg

Order: gr $\frac{1}{4}$ = 15 mg

Supply: 30 mg/tab

$$\frac{D}{H} \times Q = \frac{\overset{1}{\cancel{15}}\,mg}{\underset{2}{\cancel{30}}\,mg} \times 1\ tab = \frac{1}{2}\ tab$$

9) Order: 12.5 mg

Supply: 10 mg/mL

$$\frac{D}{H} \times Q = \frac{12.5\ \cancel{mg}}{10\ \cancel{mg}} \times 1\ mL = 1.25\ mL$$

Answer should be left at 1.25 mL as the dropper supplied with the medication will measure 1.25 mL. Notice the picture of the dropper on the label.

13) Order: 200 mcg

Supply: 1 mg/mL = 1000 mcg/mL

$$\frac{D}{H} \times Q = \frac{\overset{2}{\cancel{200\ mcg}}}{\underset{10}{\cancel{1000\ mcg}}} \times 1\ mL = \frac{2}{10}\ mL = 0.2\ mL$$

17) Order: gr $\frac{1}{10} = \frac{1}{10} \times 60 = 6$ mg

Supply: 10 mg/mL

$$\frac{D}{H} \times Q = \frac{6\ \cancel{mg}}{10\ \cancel{mg}} \times 1\ mL = \frac{6}{10}\ mL = 0.6\ mL$$

22) Order: 500 mg

Supply: 1 g/20 mL = 1000 mg/20 mL

$$\frac{D}{H} \times Q = \frac{500\ \cancel{mg}}{\underset{50}{\cancel{1000\ mg}}} \times \overset{1}{\cancel{20}}\ mL = \frac{\overset{10}{\cancel{500}}}{\underset{1}{\cancel{50}}}\ mL = 10\ mL$$

1 gram vial: $\dfrac{\overset{2}{\cancel{1000\ mg}}}{\underset{1}{\cancel{500\ mg}}} = 2$ (doses available)

25) Order: 250 mg

Supply: 62.5 mg/mL

$$\frac{D}{H} \times Q = \frac{250\ \cancel{mg}}{62.5\ \cancel{mg}} \times 1\ mL = 4\ mL$$

500 mg vial: $\dfrac{\overset{2}{\cancel{500\ mg}}}{\underset{1}{\cancel{250\ mg}}} = 2$ (doses available)

29) $D \times Q = \frac{1}{3} \times 360\ mL = 120\ mL$ hydrogen peroxide;

360 mL (total) – 120 mL (solute) = 240 mL (solvent)

31) 8 oz = 8 × 30 = 240 mL

$D \times Q = X$ (solve for Q)

$$\frac{2}{3} \times Q = 240$$

$$\frac{2}{3}\,Q = 240$$

$$\frac{\frac{2}{3}\,Q}{\frac{2}{3}} = \frac{240}{\frac{2}{3}}$$

$$Q = 240 \div \frac{2}{3} =$$

$$\frac{\overset{120}{\cancel{240}}}{1} \times \frac{3}{\underset{1}{\cancel{2}}} = 360\ mL\ \text{(total quantity)}$$

360 mL (total) – 240 mL (Ensure) = 120 mL (water)

33) 9 infants require 4 oz each = 4 oz × 9 = 36 oz total

$D \times Q = X$

$\frac{1}{2} \times 36$ oz = 18 oz (Isomil)

$\dfrac{18\ \cancel{oz}}{8\ \cancel{oz}/can} = 2\frac{1}{4}$ cans (you would need to open 3 cans)

34) 36 oz total solution – 18 oz solute (Isomil) = 18 oz

solvent (water)

18 $\cancel{oz}$ × 30 mL/$\cancel{oz}$ = 540 mL (water)

36) Order: 175 mg

Supply: 25 mg/mL

$$\frac{25\ mg}{1\ mL} \overset{=}{\underset{}{\bowtie}} \frac{175\ mg}{X\ mL}$$

$$25X = 175$$

$$\frac{25X}{25} = \frac{175}{25}$$

$$X = 7\ mL$$

40) Order: 350 mg

Supply: 500 mg/10 mL

$$\frac{50\ mg}{10\ mL} \overset{=}{\underset{}{\bowtie}} \frac{350\ mg}{X\ mL}$$

$$500X = 3500$$

$$\frac{500X}{500} = \frac{3500}{500}$$

$$X = 7\ mL$$

41) Order: gr $\frac{1}{100} = \frac{1}{100} \times 60 = 0.6$ mg

Supply: 0.3 mg/tab

$$\frac{0.3\ mg}{1\ tab} \overset{=}{\underset{}{\bowtie}} \frac{0.6\ mg}{X\ tab}$$

$$0.3X = 0.6$$

$$\frac{0.3X}{0.3} = \frac{0.6}{0.3}$$

$$X = 2\ tab$$

45) 67 lb = 67 ÷ 2.2 = 30.45 = 30.5 kg

Recommended dosage:

100 mcg/$\cancel{kg}$/dose × 30.5 $\cancel{kg}$ = 3050 mcg (minimum)

200 mcg/$\cancel{kg}$/dose × 30.5 $\cancel{kg}$ = 6100 mcg (maximum)

Order: gr $\frac{1}{10} = \frac{1}{10} \times 60 = 6$ mg = 6 × 1000 = 6000 mcg

This dosage is safe.

$$\frac{D}{H} \times Q = \frac{6\ \cancel{mg}}{8\ \cancel{mg}} \times 1\ mL = \frac{6}{8}\ mL = 0.75\ mL$$

46) 15 lb = 15 ÷ 2.2 = 6.81 kg = 6.8 kg

Minimum daily dosage:

20 mg/$\cancel{kg}$/day × 6.8 $\cancel{kg}$ = 136 mg/day

Minimum single dosage:

136 mg ÷ 3 doses = 45.3 mg/dose

Maximum daily dosage:

40 mg/$\cancel{kg}$/day × 6.8 $\cancel{kg}$ = 272 mg/day

Maximum single dosage:

272 mg ÷ 3 doses = 90.7 mg/dose

Dosage ordered is safe.

$$\frac{D}{H} \times Q = \frac{75 \text{ mg}}{50 \text{ mg}} \times 1 \text{ mL} = 1.5 \text{ mL}$$

47) Recommended dosage:

5 mg/kg/day × 20 kg = 100 mg/day

100 mg ÷ 3 doses = 33.3 mg/dose

Order of 100 mg t.i.d. is not safe. It is higher than the recommended dosage of 33.3 mg/dose.

48) 16 lb = 16 ÷ 2.2 = 7.27 kg = 7.3 kg

Recommended dosage:

40 mg/kg/day × 7.3 kg = 292 mg/day

Ordered dosage is not safe. The child would receive 187 mg × 4 doses or a total of 748 mg/day, which is over the recommended dosage of 292 mg/day.

49) 16 lb = 16 ÷ 2.2 = 7.27 kg = 7.3 kg

Recommended dosage:

15 mg/kg/day × 7.3 kg = 109.5 mg/day

109.5 mg ÷ 3 doses = 36.5 mg/dose

Dosage ordered is 60 mg q.8h, which is over the recommended dosage of 36.5 mg/dose. Although the total daily dosage is within limits, the q.8h dosage is too high and is not safe.

50) 275 lb = 275 ÷ 2.2 = 125 kg

15 mg/kg/day × 125 kg = 1875 mg/day

Because 1875 mg/day or 1.9 g/day exceeds the recommended maximum dose of 1.5 g/day, you would expect the order for this adult to be the maximum recommended dosage of 1.5 g/day or 1500 mg/day. This could be divided into 3 doses of 0.5 g q.8h or 500 mg q.8h.

Review Set 33 from page 327

1) C; sodium chloride 0.9%, 0.9 g/100 mL; 308 mOsm/L; isotonic

2) E; dextrose 5%, 5 g/100 mL; 252 mOsm/L; isotonic

3) G; dextrose 5%, 5 g/100 mL; sodium chloride 0.9%, 0.9 g/100 mL; 560 mOsm/L; hypertonic

4) D; dextrose 5%, 5 g/100 mL, sodium chloride 0.45%, 0.45 g/100 mL; 406 mOsm/L; hypertonic

5) A; dextrose 5%, 5 g/100 mL, sodium chloride 0.225%, 0.225 g/100 mL; 329 mOsm/L; isotonic

6) H; dextrose 5%, 5 g/100 mL; sodium lactate 0.31 g/100 mL, NaCl 0.6 g/100 mL; KCl 0.03 g/100 mL; CaCl 0.02 g/100 mL; 525 mOsm/L; hypertonic

7) B; dextrose 5%, 5 g/100 mL; sodium chloride 0.45%; 0.45 g/100 mL; potassium chloride 20 mEq per liter (0.149 g/100 mL); 447 mOsm/L; hypertonic

8) F; sodium chloride 0.45%, 0.45 g/100 mL; 154 mOsm/L; hypotonic

Review Set 34 from page 331

1) 50; 9 2) 25; 2.25 3) 25 4) 6.75 5) 25; 1.65 6) 150; 27 7) 50; 1.125 8) 36; 2.7 9) 100; 4.5 10) 3.375

Solutions—Review Set 34

1) D_5 NS = 5 g dextrose per 100 mL and 0.9 g NaCl per 100mL

Dextrose:

$$\frac{5 \text{ g}}{100 \text{ mL}} \times = \times \frac{X \text{ g}}{1000 \text{ mL}}$$

100X = 5000

$$\frac{100X}{100} = \frac{5000}{100}$$

X = 50 g

NaCl:

$$\frac{0.9 \text{ g}}{100 \text{ mL}} \times = \times \frac{X \text{ g}}{1000 \text{ mL}}$$

100X = 900

$$\frac{100X}{100} = \frac{900}{100}$$

X = 9 g

7) $D_{10}\frac{1}{4}$ NS = 10 g dextrose per 100 mL and 0.225 g NaCl per 100 mL

Dextrose:

$$\frac{10\text{ g}}{100\text{ mL}} \times = \times \frac{X\text{ g}}{500\text{ mL}}$$

$$100X = 5000$$

$$\frac{100X}{100} = \frac{5000}{100}$$

$$X = 50\text{ g}$$

NaCl:

$$\frac{0.225\text{ g}}{100\text{ mL}} \times = \times \frac{X\text{ g}}{500\text{ mL}}$$

$$100X = 112.5$$

$$\frac{100X}{100} = \frac{112.5}{100}$$

$$X = 1.125\text{ g}$$

Review Set 35 from page 340

1) 100 **2)** 120 **3)** 83 **4)** 200 **5)** 120 **6)** 125 **7)** 125 **8)** 200 **9)** 75 **10)** 125 **11)** 63 **12)** 24 **13)** 150 **14)** 125 **15)** 42

Solutions—Review Set 35

1) 1 L = 1000 mL

$$\frac{\text{Total mL}}{\text{Total h}} = \frac{1000\text{ mL}}{10\text{ h}} = 100\text{ mL/h}$$

3) $\dfrac{\text{Total mL}}{\text{Total h}} = \dfrac{2000\text{ mL}}{24\text{ h}} = 83.3\text{ mL/h} = 83\text{ mL/h}$

4) $\dfrac{100\text{ mL}}{\underset{1}{\cancel{30\text{ min}}}} \times \dfrac{\overset{2}{\cancel{60\text{ min}}}}{\text{h}} = 200\text{ mL/h}$

5) $\dfrac{30\text{ mL}}{\underset{1}{\cancel{15\text{ min}}}} \times \dfrac{\overset{4}{\cancel{60\text{ min}}}}{\text{h}} = 120\text{ mL/h}$

6) 2.5 L = 2.5 × 1000 = 2500 mL

$$\frac{\text{Total mL}}{\text{Total h}} = \frac{2500\text{ ml}}{20\text{ h}} = 125\text{ mL/h}$$

Review Set 36 from pages 342–343

1) 15 **2)** 10 **3)** 60 **4)** 60 **5)** 10

Review Set 37 from page 346

1) $\frac{V}{T} \times C = R$ **2)** 21 **3)** 50 **4)** 33 **5)** 25 **6)** 83 **7)** 26 **8)** 50 **9)** 50 **10)** 80 **11)** 20 **12)** 30 **13)** 17 **14)** 55 **15)** 40

Solutions—Review Set 37

1) $\dfrac{V}{T} \times C = R$ or $\dfrac{\text{Volume}}{\text{Time in min}} \times$ Drop Factor = Rate

Volume in mL divided by *time* in minutes, multiplied by the *drop factor calibration* in drops per milliliter, equals the flow *rate* in drops per minute.

2) $\dfrac{V}{T} \times C = \dfrac{125\text{ mL}}{\underset{6}{\cancel{60\text{ min}}}} \times \overset{1}{\cancel{10}}\text{ gtt/mL} = \dfrac{125\text{ gtt}}{6\text{ min}} = 20.8\text{ gtt/min}$

$= 21\text{ gtt/min}$

3) $\dfrac{V}{T} \times C = \dfrac{50\text{ mL}}{\underset{1}{\cancel{60\text{ min}}}} \times \cancel{60}\text{ gtt/mL} = 50\text{ gtt/min}$

Recall that when drop factor is 60 mL/h, then mL/h = gtt/min.

4) $\dfrac{V}{T} \times C = \dfrac{100\text{ mL}}{\underset{3}{\cancel{60\text{ min}}}} \times \overset{1}{\cancel{20}}\text{ gtt/mL} = \dfrac{100\text{ gtt}}{3\text{ min}} = 33.3\text{ gtt/min}$

$= 33\text{ gtt/min}$

6) Two 500 mL units of blood = 1000 mL total volume

$$\text{mL/h} = \frac{1000\text{ mL}}{4\text{h}} = 250\text{ mL/h}$$

$\dfrac{V}{T} \times C = \dfrac{250\text{ mL}}{\underset{3}{\cancel{60\text{ min}}}} \times \overset{1}{\cancel{20}}\text{ gtt/mL} = \dfrac{250\text{ gtt}}{3\text{ min}} = 83.3\text{ gtt/min}$

$= 83\text{ gtt/min}$

7) $\dfrac{\text{Total mL}}{\text{Total h}} = \dfrac{1240\text{ mL}}{12\text{ h}} = 103.3\text{ mL/h} = 103\text{ mL/h}$

$\dfrac{V}{T} \times C = \dfrac{103\text{ mL}}{\underset{4}{\cancel{60\text{ min}}}} \times \overset{1}{\cancel{15}}\text{ gtt/mL} = \dfrac{103\text{ gtt}}{4\text{ min}} = 25.7\text{ gtt/min}$

$= 26\text{ gtt/min}$

9) $\dfrac{150\text{ mL}}{\underset{3}{\cancel{45\text{ min}}}} \times \overset{1}{\cancel{15}}\text{ gtt/mL} = \dfrac{\overset{50}{\cancel{150}}\text{ gtt}}{\underset{1}{\cancel{3}}\text{ min}} = 50\text{ gtt/min}$

Review Set 38 from page 349

1) 60 **2)** 1 **3)** 3 **4)** 4 **5)** 6 **6)** $\dfrac{\text{mL/h}}{\text{drop factor constant}}$ = gtt/min **7)** 50 **8)** 42 **9)** 28 **10)** 60 **11)** 8 **12)** 31 **13)** 28

14) 25 **15)** 11

Solutions—Review Set 38

4) $\dfrac{60}{15} = 4$

7) $\dfrac{\text{mL/h}}{\text{drop factor constant}}$ = gtt/min: $\dfrac{200 \text{ mL/h}}{4} = 50$ gtt/min

8) $\dfrac{\text{mL/h}}{\text{drop factor constant}}$ = gtt/min: $\dfrac{125 \text{ mL/h}}{3} = 41.7$ gtt/min
= 42 gtt/min

9) $\dfrac{\text{mL/h}}{\text{drop factor constant}}$ = gtt/min: $\dfrac{165 \text{ mL/h}}{6} = 27.5$ gtt/min
= 28 gtt/min

10) $\dfrac{\text{mL/h}}{\text{drop factor constant}}$ = gtt/min: $\dfrac{60 \text{ mL/h}}{1} = 60$ gtt/min
(Set the flow rate at the same number of gtt/min as the number of mL/h when the drop factor is 60 gtt/mL because the drop factor constant is 1.)

14) 0.5 L = 500 mL; $\dfrac{500 \text{ mL}}{20 \text{ h}} = 25$ mL/h; since drop factor is 60 gtt/mL, then mL/h = gtt/min; so rate is 25 gtt/min.

15) 650 mL in 10 h = $\dfrac{650 \text{ mL}}{10 \text{ h}} = 65$ mL/h

$\dfrac{\text{mL/h}}{\text{drop factor constant}}$ = gtt/min: $\dfrac{65 \text{ mL/h}}{6} = 10.8$ gtt/min
= 11 gtt/min

Review Set 39 from pages 350–351

1) 125; 31 **2)** 100 **3)** 100; 33 **4)** 50 **5)** 125; 31 **6)** 125; 125 **7)** 35 **8)** 17 **9)** 25 **10)** 125 **11)** 83 **12)** 125 **13)** 200 **14)** 150

15) 200 **16)** 13.5 **17)** 20; 1.8 **18)** 22.5 **19)** 32.5; 2.145 **20)** 50; 2.25

Solutions—Review Set 39

1) $\dfrac{\text{Total mL}}{\text{Total h}} = \dfrac{3000 \text{ mL}}{24 \text{ h}} = 125$ mL/h

$\dfrac{V}{T} \times C = \dfrac{125 \text{ mL}}{\overset{\overset{1}{}}{\underset{4}{60 \text{ min}}}} \times 15 \text{ gtt/mL} = \dfrac{125 \text{ gtt}}{4 \text{ min}} = 31.3$ gtt/min
= 31 gtt/min

7) $\dfrac{\text{mL/h}}{\text{drop factor constant}}$ = gtt/min: $\dfrac{105 \text{ mL/h}}{3} = 35$ gtt/min

8) $\dfrac{\text{mL/h}}{\text{drop factor constant}}$ = gtt/min: $\dfrac{100 \text{ mL/h}}{6} = 16.6$ gtt/min
= 17 gtt/min

10) $\dfrac{\text{Total mL}}{\text{Total h}} = \dfrac{1000 \text{ mL}}{8 \text{ h}} = 125$ mL/h

13) $\dfrac{100 \text{ mL}}{\underset{1}{30 \text{ min}}} \times \dfrac{\overset{2}{60 \text{ min}}}{h} = 200$ mL/h

15) $\dfrac{150 \text{ mL}}{\underset{3}{45 \text{ min}}} \times \dfrac{\overset{4}{60 \text{ min}}}{h} = 200$ mL/h

16) $\frac{1}{2}$ NS = 0.45% NaCl = 0.45 g NaCl per 100 mL

$\dfrac{0.45 \text{ g}}{100 \text{ mL}} \underset{\times}{=} \dfrac{X \text{ g}}{3000 \text{ mL}}$

$100X = 1350$

$\dfrac{100X}{100} = \dfrac{1350}{100}$

$X = 13.5 \text{ g (NaCl)}$

17) $D_{10}NS$ = 10% dextrose = 10 g dextrose per 100 mL and 0.9% NaCl = 0.9 g NaCl per 100 mL

Dextrose:

$$\frac{10\ g}{100\ mL} \diagdown = \diagup \frac{X\ g}{200\ mL}$$

$$100X = 2000$$

$$\frac{100X}{100} = \frac{2000}{100}$$

$$X = 20\ g\ (dextrose)$$

$$NS = 0.9\%\ NaCl = 0.9\ g\ NaCl\ per\ 100\ mL$$

NaCl:

$$\frac{0.9\ g}{100\ mL} \diagdown = \diagup \frac{X\ g}{200\ mL}$$

$$100X = 180$$

$$\frac{100X}{100} = \frac{180}{100}$$

$$X = 1.8\ g\ (NaCl)$$

Review Set 40 from pages 354–356

1) 42; 6; 142; 47; 12%; reset to 47 gtt/min (12% increase is acceptable).

2) 42; 2; 180; 45; 7%; reset to 45 gtt/min (7% increase is acceptable).

3) 42; 4; 200; 67; 60%; recalculated rate 67 gtt/min (60% increase is unacceptable). Consult physician.

4) 28; 4; 188; 31; 11%; reset to 31 gtt/min (11% increase is acceptable).

5) 21; 4; 188; 31; 48%; (48% increase is unacceptable). Consult physician.

6) 31; 1350; 10; 135; 34; 10%; reset to 34 gtt/min (10% increase is acceptable).

7) 50; 3; 233; 78; 56%; (56% increase is unacceptable). Consult physician.

8) 33; 3; 83; 28; –15%; (–15% slower is acceptable). IV is ahead of schedule. Slow rate to 28 gtt/min, and observe patient's condition.

9) 13; 10; 60; 15; 15%; reset to 15 gtt/min (15% increase is acceptable).

10) 100; 5; 100; 100; 0%; IV is on time, so no adjustment is needed.

Solutions—Review Set 40

1) $\dfrac{V}{T} \times C = \dfrac{125\ \cancel{mL}}{\underset{3}{\cancel{60}\ min}} \times \overset{1}{\cancel{20}}\ gtt/\cancel{mL} = \dfrac{125\ gtt}{3\ min} = 41.6\ gtt/min = 42\ gtt/min\ (ordered\ rate)$

$12\ h - 6\ h = 6\ h$

$\dfrac{Remaining\ volume}{Remaining\ hours}$ = Recalculated mL/h; $\dfrac{850\ mL}{6\ h}$ = 141.6 mL/h = 142 mL/h

$\dfrac{V}{T} \times C = \dfrac{142\ \cancel{mL}}{\underset{3}{\cancel{60}\ min}} \times \overset{1}{\cancel{20}}\ gtt/\cancel{mL} = \dfrac{142\ gtt}{3\ min} = 47.3\ gtt/min = 47\ gtt/min\ (adjusted\ rate)$

$\dfrac{Adjusted\ gtt/min - Ordered\ gtt/min}{Ordered\ gtt/min}$ = % of variation; $\dfrac{47-42}{42} = \dfrac{5}{42} = 0.12 = 12\%$ (within the acceptable % of variation); reset rate to 47 gtt/min

3) $\dfrac{V}{T} \times C = \dfrac{125\ \cancel{mL}}{\underset{3}{\cancel{60}\ min}} \times \overset{1}{\cancel{20}}\ gtt/\cancel{mL} = \dfrac{125\ gtt}{3\ min} = 41.6\ gtt/min = 42\ gtt/min\ (ordered\ rate)$

$8\ h - 4\ h = 4\ h$

$\dfrac{800\ mL}{4\ h} = 200\ mL/h;\ \dfrac{V}{T} \times C = \dfrac{200\ \cancel{mL}}{\underset{3}{\cancel{60}\ min}} \times \overset{1}{\cancel{20}}\ gtt/\cancel{mL} = \dfrac{200\ gtt}{3\ min} = 66.6 = 67\ gtt/min\ (adjusted\ rate)$

$\dfrac{Adjusted\ gtt/min - Ordered\ gtt/min}{Ordered\ gtt/min}$ = % of variation; $\dfrac{67-42}{42} = \dfrac{25}{42} = 0.59 = 0.6 = 60\%$ faster; unacceptable % of variation—call physician for a revised order

6) $\dfrac{V}{T}\times C=\dfrac{125\ \text{mL}}{\underset{4}{60\ \text{min}}}\times\overset{1}{15}\ \text{gtt/mL}=\dfrac{125\ \text{gtt}}{4\ \text{min}}=31.3\ \text{gtt/min}=31\ \text{gtt/min (ordered rate)}$

2000 mL – 650 mL = 1350 mL remaining; 16 h – 6 h = 10 h

$\dfrac{1350\ \text{mL}}{10\ \text{h}}=135\ \text{mL/h};\ \dfrac{V}{T}\times C=\dfrac{135\ \text{mL}}{\underset{4}{60\ \text{min}}}\times\overset{1}{15}\ \text{gtt/mL}=\dfrac{135\ \text{gtt}}{4\ \text{min}}=33.7\ \text{gtt/min}=34\ \text{gtt/min}$

$\dfrac{\text{Adjusted gtt/min – Ordered gtt/min}}{\text{Ordered gtt/min}}=\%\text{ of variation};\ \dfrac{34-31}{31}=\dfrac{3}{31}=0.096=0.10=10\%$

(within acceptable % of variation); reset rate to 34 gtt/min

8) $\dfrac{V}{T}\times C=\dfrac{100\ \text{mL}}{\underset{3}{60\ \text{min}}}\times\overset{1}{20}\ \text{gtt/mL}=\dfrac{100\ \text{gtt}}{3\ \text{min}}=33.3\ \text{gtt/min}=33\ \text{gtt/min (ordered rate)}$

5 h – 2 h = 3 h

$\dfrac{250\ \text{mL}}{3\ \text{h}}=83.3\ \text{mL/h}=83\ \text{mL/h};\ \dfrac{V}{T}\times C=\dfrac{83\ \text{mL}}{\underset{3}{60\ \text{min}}}\times\overset{1}{20}\ \text{gtt/mL}=\dfrac{83\ \text{gtt}}{3\ \text{min}}=27.6\ \text{gtt/min}=28\ \text{gtt/min (adjusted rate)}$

$\dfrac{\text{Adjusted gtt/min – Ordered gtt/min}}{\text{Ordered gtt/min}}=\%\text{ of variation};\ \dfrac{28-33}{33}=\dfrac{-5}{33}=-0.15=-15\%$

(Remember the [–] sign indicates the IV is ahead of schedule and rate must be decreased.) Within the acceptable % of variation. Slow IV to 28 gtt/min, and closely monitor patient.

Review Set 41 from pages 360–363

1) 133 2) 133 3) 50 4) 200 5) 100 6) 25 7) 50 8) 200 9) 150 10) 167 11) 133 12) 25 13) 120 14) 56 15) 200 16) 12; 3; 1 17) 3; 3; 0.25 18) 0.6; 2; 24; 0.06 19) 2; 18; 19; 2.5 20) 1.5; 0.75; 0.19

Solutions—Review Set 41

1) $\dfrac{V}{T}\times C=\dfrac{100\ \text{mL}}{\underset{3}{45\ \text{min}}}\times\overset{4}{60}\ \text{gtt/mL}=\dfrac{400\ \text{gtt}}{3\ \text{min}}=133.3\ \text{gtt/min}$

$=133\ \text{gtt/min}$

2) $\dfrac{100\ \text{mL}}{45\ \text{min}}\ \underset{\times}{=}\ \dfrac{X\ \text{mL}}{60\ \text{min}}$

$45X=6000$

$\dfrac{45X}{45}=\dfrac{6000}{45}$

$X=133.3\ \text{mL}=133\ \text{mL}$

133 mL/60 min = 133 mL/h

3) $\dfrac{V}{T}\times C=\dfrac{50\ \text{mL}}{\underset{1}{15\ \text{min}}}\times\overset{1}{15}\ \text{gtt/mL}=50\ \text{gtt/min}$

4) $\dfrac{50\ \text{mL}}{15\ \text{min}}\ \underset{\times}{=}\ \dfrac{X\ \text{mL}}{60\ \text{min}}$

$15X=3000$

$\dfrac{15X}{15}=\dfrac{3000}{15}$

$X=200\ \text{mL}$

200 mL/60 min = 200 mL/h

11) $\dfrac{V}{T}\times C=\dfrac{100\ \text{mL}}{\underset{3}{15\ \text{min}}}\times\overset{4}{20}\ \text{gtt/mL}=\dfrac{400\ \text{gtt}}{3\ \text{min}}=133.3\ \text{gtt/min}$

$=133\ \text{gtt/min}$

16) $\dfrac{D}{H}\times Q=\dfrac{120\ \text{mg}}{10\ \text{mg}}\times 1\ \text{mL}=12\ \text{mL}$

$\dfrac{D}{H}\times Q=\dfrac{\overset{3}{120\ \text{mg}}}{\underset{1}{40\ \text{mg}}}\times 1\ \text{min}=3\ \text{min}$

Administer 12 mL over at least 3 min.

1 min = 60 sec

3 min = 3 × 60 = 180 sec

$\dfrac{12\ \text{mL}}{180\ \text{sec}}\ \underset{\times}{=}\ \dfrac{X\ \text{mL}}{15\ \text{sec}}$

$180X=180$

$\dfrac{180X}{180}=\dfrac{180}{180}$

$X=1\ \text{mL per 15 sec}$

17) $\dfrac{D}{H} \times Q = \dfrac{\overset{3}{\cancel{150}} \text{ mg}}{\underset{50}{\cancel{250}} \text{ mg}} \times \overset{1}{\cancel{5}} \text{ mL} = \dfrac{\overset{3}{\cancel{150}}}{\underset{1}{\cancel{50}}} \text{ mL} = 3 \text{ mL}$

$\dfrac{D}{H} \times Q = \dfrac{\overset{3}{\cancel{150}} \text{ mg}}{\underset{1}{\cancel{50}} \text{ mg}} \times 1 \text{ min} = 3 \text{ min}$

Administer 3 mL over 3 min.

1 min = 60 sec

3 min = 3 × 60 = 180 sec

$\dfrac{3 \text{ mL}}{180 \text{ sec}} \diagup\!\!\!\diagdown \dfrac{X \text{ mL}}{15 \text{ sec}}$

$180X = 45$

$\dfrac{180X}{180} = \dfrac{45}{180}$

$X = 0.25 \text{ mL (per 15 sec)}$

18) $\dfrac{D}{H} \times Q = \dfrac{6 \text{ mg}}{10 \text{ mg}} \times 1 \text{ mL} = \dfrac{6}{10} \text{ mL} = 0.6 \text{ mL}$

$\dfrac{D}{H} \times Q = \dfrac{6 \text{ mg}}{2.5 \text{ mg}} \times 1 \text{ min} = 2.4 \text{ min}$

1 min = 60 sec

2 min = 2 × 60 = 120 sec; 0.4 min = 0.4 × 60 = 24 sec

120 sec + 24 sec = 144 sec

$\dfrac{0.6 \text{ mL}}{144 \text{ sec}} \diagup\!\!\!\diagdown \dfrac{X \text{ mL}}{15 \text{ sec}}$

$144X = 9$

$\dfrac{144X}{144} = \dfrac{9}{144}$

$X = 0.06 \text{ mL (per 15 sec)}$

Review Set 42 from pages 366–367

1) 5 h and 33 min 2) 6 h and 40 min 3) 8 4) 6; 20 5) 4; 20 6) Approximately 11; 0300 the next morning

7) 16; 0730 the next morning 8) 3000 9) 1152 10) 3024 11) 260 12) 300 13) 600 14) 320 15) 540

Solutions—Review Set 42

1) $\dfrac{V}{T} \times C = R$; notice T is the missing quantity

$\dfrac{500 \text{ mL}}{T \text{ min}} \times 20 \text{ gtt/mL} = 30 \text{ gtt/min}$

$\dfrac{10{,}000}{T} \diagup\!\!\!\diagdown \dfrac{30}{1}$

$30T = 10{,}000$

$\dfrac{30T}{30} = \dfrac{10{,}000}{30}$

T = 333 min

$333 \text{ min} = \dfrac{333}{60} = 5 \text{ h and } 33 \text{ min}$

2) $\dfrac{V}{T} \times C = R$; notice T is the missing quantity

$\dfrac{1000 \text{ mL}}{T \text{ min}} \times 10 \text{ gtt/mL} = 25 \text{ gtt/min}$

$\dfrac{10{,}000}{T} \diagup\!\!\!\diagdown \dfrac{25}{1}$

$25T = 10{,}000$

$\dfrac{25T}{25} = \dfrac{10{,}000}{25}$

T = 400 min

$400 \text{ min} = \dfrac{400}{60} = 6 \text{ h and } 40 \text{ min}$

4) $\text{Time:} \dfrac{\text{Total vol}}{\text{mL/h}} = \text{Total h}$

$\dfrac{120 \text{ mL}}{20 \text{ mL/h}} = 6 \text{ h}$

$\dfrac{V}{T} \times C = \dfrac{20 \text{ mL}}{\underset{1}{\cancel{60}} \text{ min}} \times \overset{1}{\cancel{60}} \text{ gtt/mL} = 20 \text{ gtt/min}$

6) $\dfrac{V}{T} \times C = R$; notice T is the missing quantity

$\dfrac{1200 \text{ mL}}{T \text{ min}} \times 15 \text{ gtt/mL} = 27 \text{ gtt/min}$

$\dfrac{18{,}000}{T} \diagup\!\!\!\diagdown \dfrac{27}{1}$

$27T = 18{,}000$

$\dfrac{27T}{27} = \dfrac{18{,}000}{27}$

$T = 667 \text{ min}; 667 \text{ min} = \dfrac{667}{60} = 11 \text{ h and } 7 \text{ min}$
$\text{or } 11 \text{ h (rounded)}$

1600 + 1100 (11h) = 2700 − 2400 = 0300

7) $\text{Time:} \dfrac{\text{Total vol}}{\text{mL/h}} = \text{Total h}$

$\dfrac{2000 \text{ mL}}{125 \text{ mL/h}} = 16 \text{ h}$

1530 + 1600 = 3130 − 2400 = 0730

8) Total hours × mL/h = Total volume

$24 \text{ h} \times 125 \text{ mL/h} = 3000 \text{ mL}$

9) $\dfrac{V}{T} \times C = R$; notice V is the missing quantity

$\dfrac{V \text{ mL}}{1440 \text{ min}} \times 15 \text{ gtt/mL} = 12 \text{ gtt/min}$

$\dfrac{15V}{1440} \diagup\!\!\!\diagdown \dfrac{12}{1}$

$15V = 17{,}280$

$\dfrac{15V}{15} = \dfrac{17{,}280}{15}$

$V = 1152 \text{ mL}$

11) $65 \text{ mL/}\cancel{h} \times 4\cancel{h} = 260 \text{ mL}$

14) $8 \text{ h} = 8 \times 60 = 480 \text{ min}$

$\dfrac{V}{T} \times C = R$; notice V is the missing quantity

$\dfrac{V \text{ mL}}{480 \text{ min}} \times 60 \text{ gtt/mL} = 40 \text{ gtt/min}$

$\dfrac{60V}{480} \diagup\!\!\!\!\!= \diagup\!\!\!\!\! \dfrac{40}{1}$

$60V = 19{,}200$

$\dfrac{60V}{60} = \dfrac{19{,}200}{60}$

$V = 320 \text{ mL}$

15) $4 \text{ h} = 4 \times 60 = 240 \text{ min}$

$\dfrac{V}{T} \times C = R$; notice V is the missing quantity

$\dfrac{V \text{ ml}}{240 \text{ min}} \times 20 \text{ gtt/mL} = 45 \text{ gtt/min}$

$\dfrac{20V}{240} \diagup\!\!\!\!\!= \diagup\!\!\!\!\! \dfrac{45}{1}$

$20V = 10{,}800$

$\dfrac{20V}{20} = \dfrac{10{,}800}{20}$

$V = 540 \text{ mL}$

Practice Problems—Chapter 14 from pages 368–372

1) 17   **2)** 42   **3)** 42   **4)** 8   **5)** 125   **6)** Assess patient. If stable, recalculate and reset to 114 mL/h; observe patient closely.

7) 31   **8)** 42   **9)** Assess patient. If stable, recalculate and reset to 50 gtt/min; observe patient closely.   **10)** 3000   **11)** Abbott Laboratories   **12)** 15 gtt/mL   **13)** 4

14) $\text{mL/h} = \dfrac{500 \text{ mL}}{4 \text{ h}} = 125 \text{ mL/h}$

$\dfrac{\text{mL/h}}{\text{drop factor constant}} = \text{gtt/min}: \dfrac{125 \text{ mL/h}}{4} = 31.2 \text{ gtt/min} = 31 \text{ gtt/min}$

15) $\dfrac{V}{T} \times C = \dfrac{125 \,\cancel{\text{mL}}}{\underset{4}{\cancel{60} \text{ min}}} \times \overset{1}{\cancel{15}} \text{ gtt/}\cancel{\text{mL}} = \dfrac{125 \text{ gtt}}{4 \text{ min}} = 31.3 \text{ gtt/min} = 31 \text{ gtt/min}$

16) 1930 (or 7:30 PM)   **17)** 250   **18)** Recalculate 210 mL to infuse over remaining 2 hours. Reset IV to 26 gtt/min and observe patient closely.   **19)** 125   **20)** 100   **21)** Dextrose 2.5% (2.5 g/100 mL) and NaCl 0.45% (0.45 g/100 mL)   **22)** 25; 4.5   **23)** A central line is a special catheter inserted to access a large vein in the chest.   **24)** A primary line is the IV tubing used to set up a primary IV infusion.   **25)** The purpose of a saline/heparin lock is to administer IV medications when the patient does not require continuous IV fluids.   **26)** 10; 5; 0.5; 0.13   **27)** The purpose of the PCA pump is to allow the patient to safely self-administer IV pain medication without having to call the nurse for a p.r.n. medication.

28) Advantages of the syringe pump are that a small amount of medication can be delivered directly from the syringe, and a specified time can be programmed in the pump.   **29)** Phlebitis and infiltration   **30)** $q \frac{1}{2} - 1$ h, according to hospital policy   **31)** This IV tubing has 2 spikes—one for blood, the other for saline—that join at a common drip chamber or Y connection.   **32)** 14   **33)** 21   **34)** 28   **35)** 83   **36)** 17   **37)** 25   **38)** 33   **39)** 100   **40)** 33   **41)** 50   **42)** 67   **43)** 200   **44)** 8   **45)** 11

46) 15   **47)** 45   **48)** 150. The IV will finish in 1 hour. Leave a new IV bag in case you are delayed so the relief nurse can spike the new bag and continue the infusion.   **49)** 1250 (or 12:50 PM)

50)   Critical Thinking Skill: Prevention.

This error could have been prevented had the nurse carefully inspected the IV tubing package to determine the drop factor. Every IV tubing set has the drop factor printed on the package, so it is not necessary to memorize or guess the drop factor. The IV calculation should have looked like this:

$\dfrac{125 \,\cancel{\text{mL}}}{\underset{3}{\cancel{60} \text{ min}}} \times \overset{1}{\cancel{20}} \text{ gtt/}\cancel{\text{mL}} = \dfrac{125 \text{ gtt}}{3 \text{ min}} = 41.6 \text{ gtt/min} = 42 \text{ gtt/min}$

With the infusion set of 20 gtt/mL, a flow rate of 42 gtt/min would infuse 125 mL/h. At the 125 gtt/min rate the nurse calculated, the patient received three times the IV fluid ordered hourly. Thus, the patient actually received 375 mL/h of IV fluids.

Solutions—Practice Problems—Chapter 14

1) $\dfrac{\text{Total mL}}{\text{Total h}} = \dfrac{200 \text{ mL}}{2 \text{ h}} = 100 \text{ mL/h}$

$\dfrac{V}{T} \times C = \dfrac{100 \cancel{\text{ mL}}}{\underset{6}{\cancel{60} \text{ min}}} \times \cancel{10}^{1} \text{ gtt/}\cancel{\text{mL}} = \dfrac{100 \text{ gtt}}{6 \text{ min}} = 16.6 \text{ gtt/min}$

$= 17 \text{ gtt/min}$

2) $\dfrac{\text{Total mL}}{\text{Total h}} = \dfrac{1000 \text{ mL}}{24 \text{ h}} = 41.6 \text{ mL/h} = 42 \text{ mL/h}$

drop factor is 60 gtt/mL: 42 mL/h = 42 gtt/min

5) $\dfrac{\text{Total mL}}{\text{Total h}} = \dfrac{1000 \text{ mL}}{8 \text{ h}} = 125 \text{ mL/h}$

6) $\dfrac{\text{Total mL}}{\text{Total h}} = \dfrac{800 \text{ mL}}{7 \text{ h}} = 114.2 \text{ mL/h} = 114 \text{ mL/h}$

$\dfrac{\text{Adjusted gtt/min} - \text{Ordered gtt/min}}{\text{Ordered gtt/min}} = \% \text{ variation:}$

$\dfrac{144 - 25}{125} = \dfrac{-11}{125} = -0.088 = -9\% \text{ (decrease); within safe}$

limits of 25% variance.

Reset infusion rate to 114 mL/h.

7) 1000 mL + 2000 mL = 3000 mL;

$\dfrac{\text{Total mL}}{\text{Total h}} = \dfrac{3000 \text{ mL}}{24 \text{ h}} = 125 \text{ mL/h}$

$\dfrac{V}{T} \times C = \dfrac{125 \cancel{\text{ mL}}}{\underset{4}{\cancel{60} \text{ min}}} \times \cancel{15}^{1} \text{ gtt/}\cancel{\text{mL}} = \dfrac{125 \text{ gtt}}{4 \text{ min}} = 31.3 \text{ gtt/min}$

$= 31 \text{ gtt/min}$

8) $\dfrac{V}{T} \times C = \dfrac{125 \cancel{\text{ mL}}}{\underset{3}{\cancel{60} \text{ min}}} \times \cancel{20}^{1} \text{ gtt/}\cancel{\text{mL}} = \dfrac{125 \text{ gtt}}{3 \text{ min}} = 41.6 \text{ gtt/min}$

$= 42 \text{ gtt/min}$

9) $\dfrac{\text{Total mL}}{\text{Total h}} = \dfrac{1000 \text{ mL}}{6 \text{ h}} = 166.6 \text{ mL/h} = 167 \text{ mL/h}$

$\dfrac{V}{T} \times C = \dfrac{167 \cancel{\text{ mL}}}{\underset{4}{\cancel{60} \text{ min}}} \times \cancel{15}^{1} \text{ gtt/}\cancel{\text{mL}} = \dfrac{167 \text{ gtt}}{4 \text{ min}} = 41.7 \text{ gtt/min}$

$= 42 \text{ gtt/min}$

6 h − 2 h = 4 h remaining; $\dfrac{\text{Total mL}}{\text{Total h}} = \dfrac{\overset{200}{\cancel{800} \text{ mL}}}{\underset{1}{\cancel{4} \text{ h}}} = 200 \text{ mL/h}$

$\dfrac{V}{T} \times C = \dfrac{200 \cancel{\text{ mL}}}{\underset{4}{\cancel{60} \text{ min}}} \times \cancel{15}^{1} \text{ gtt/}\cancel{\text{mL}} = \dfrac{\overset{50}{\cancel{200} \text{ gtt}}}{\underset{1}{\cancel{4} \text{ min}}} = 50 \text{ gtt/min}$

$\dfrac{\text{Adjusted gtt/min} - \text{Ordered gtt/min}}{\text{Ordered gtt/min}} = \% \text{ variation:}$

$\dfrac{50 - 42}{42} = \dfrac{8}{42} = 0.19 = 19\% \text{ increase;}$

within safe limits of 25% variance

Reset infusion rate to 50 gtt/min.

10) q.4h = 6 times/24 h; 6 × 500 mL = 3000 mL

13) $\dfrac{60}{15} = 4$

16) 1530 + 4 h = 1530 + 0400 = 1930; 1930 − 1200 =

7:30 PM

17) $\dfrac{\text{Total mL}}{\text{Total h}} = \dfrac{500 \text{ mL}}{4 \text{ h}} = 125 \text{ mL/h}$

125 mL/$\cancel{\text{h}}$ × 2 $\cancel{\text{h}}$ = 250 mL

18) $\dfrac{\text{Total mL}}{\text{Total h}} = \dfrac{210 \text{ mL}}{2 \text{ h}} = 105 \text{ mL/h}$

$\dfrac{V}{T} \times C = \dfrac{105 \cancel{\text{ mL}}}{\underset{4}{\cancel{60} \text{ min}}} \times \cancel{15}^{1} \text{ gtt/}\cancel{\text{mL}} = \dfrac{105 \text{ gtt}}{4 \text{ min}} = 26.2 \text{ gtt/min}$

$= 26 \text{ gtt/min}$

$\dfrac{\text{Adjusted gtt/min} - \text{Ordered gtt/min}}{\text{Ordered gtt/min}} = \% \text{ variation:}$

$\dfrac{26 - 31}{31} = \dfrac{-5}{31} = -0.16 = -16\% \text{ decrease; within safe}$

limits

Reset infusion rate to 26 gtt/min.

19) $\dfrac{\text{Total mL}}{\text{Total h}} = \dfrac{500 \text{ mL}}{4 \text{ h}} = 125 \text{ mL/h}$

20) $\dfrac{50 \text{ mL}}{30 \text{ min}} \bowtie \dfrac{X \text{ mL}}{60 \text{ min}}$

30X = 3000

$\dfrac{30X}{30} = \dfrac{3000}{30}$

X = 100 mL/h

22) Dextrose 5% = 5 g/100 mL   NaCl 0.9% = 0.9 g/100 mL

Dextrose: NaCl:

$\dfrac{5 \text{ g}}{100 \text{ mL}} \bowtie \dfrac{X \text{ g}}{500 \text{ mL}}$ $\dfrac{0.9 \text{ g}}{100 \text{ mL}} \bowtie \dfrac{X \text{ g}}{500 \text{ mL}}$

100X = 2500   100X = 450

$\dfrac{100X}{100} = \dfrac{2500}{100}$ $\dfrac{100X}{100} = \dfrac{450}{100}$

X = 25 g   X = 4.5 g

26) $\dfrac{5 \text{ mg}}{1 \text{ min}} \bowtie \dfrac{50 \text{ mg}}{X \text{ min}}$

5X = 50

$\dfrac{5X}{5} = \dfrac{50}{5}$

X = 10 min

$\dfrac{D}{H} \times Q = \dfrac{\overset{5}{\cancel{50} \text{ mg}}}{\underset{1}{\cancel{10} \text{ mg}}} \times 1 \text{ mL} = 5 \text{ mL}$

Give 50 mg/10 min or 5 mL/10 min; 0.5 mL/min

1 min = 60 sec

10 min = 10 × 60 = 600 sec

$\dfrac{5 \text{ mL}}{600 \text{ sec}} \bowtie \dfrac{X \text{ mL}}{15 \text{ sec}}$

600X = 75

$\dfrac{600X}{600} = \dfrac{75}{600}$

X = 0.13 mL/15 sec

32) $\dfrac{\text{Total mL}}{\text{Total h}} = \dfrac{1000 \text{ mL}}{12 \text{ h}} = 83.3 \text{ mL/h} = 83 \text{ mL/h}; \dfrac{V}{T} \times C =$

$\dfrac{83 \cancel{\text{ mL}}}{\underset{6}{\cancel{60} \text{ min}}} \times \cancel{10}^{1} \text{ gtt/}\cancel{\text{mL}} = \dfrac{83 \text{ gtt}}{6 \text{ min}} = 13.8 \text{ gtt/min} = 14 \text{ gtt/min}$

33) $\dfrac{V}{T} \times C = \dfrac{\cancel{83}\,\cancel{mL}}{\underset{4}{\cancel{60}\,min}} \times \overset{1}{\cancel{15}}\,gtt/\cancel{mL} = \dfrac{83\,gtt}{4\,min} = 20.7\,gtt/min$

$= 21\,gtt/min$

34) $\dfrac{V}{T} \times C = \dfrac{\cancel{83}\,\cancel{mL}}{\underset{3}{\cancel{60}\,min}} \times \overset{1}{\cancel{20}}\,gtt/\cancel{mL} = \dfrac{83\,gtt}{3\,min} = 27.6\,gtt/min$

$= 28\,gtt/min$

35) $\dfrac{V}{T} \times C = \dfrac{\cancel{83}\,\cancel{mL}}{\underset{1}{\cancel{60}\,min}} \times \overset{1}{\cancel{60}}\,gtt/\cancel{mL} = 83\,gtt/min$

Remember, if drop factor is 60 gtt/mL, then

mL/h = gtt/min; so 83 mL/h = 83 gtt/min

48) $\dfrac{V}{T} \times C = R$; V is the unknown quantity

$\dfrac{V\,mL}{60\,min} \times 10\,gtt/mL = 25\,gtt/min$

$\dfrac{10V}{60} \;\;\diagdown\!\!\!\!=\!\!\!\!\diagup\;\; \dfrac{25}{1}$

$10V = 1500$

$\dfrac{10V}{10} = \dfrac{1500}{10}$

$V = 150\,mL$

49) $\dfrac{400\,\cancel{mL}}{75\,\cancel{mL}/h} = 5\dfrac{1}{3}$ h or 5 h and 20 min

$0730 + 0520 = 1250$ (or 12:50 PM)

Review Set 43 from pages 376–377

1) 0.68 **2)** 2.35 **3)** 0.69 **4)** 1.40 **5)** 2.03 **6)** 1 **7)** 1.66 **8)** 0.4 **9)** 1.69 **10)** 0.52 **11)** 1.11 **12)** 0.78 **13)** 0.15 **14)** 0.78 **15)** 0.39 **16)** 0.64 **17)** 0.25 **18)** 1.08 **19)** 0.5 **20)** 0.88

Solutions—Review Set 43

1) Household: BSA (m^2) $= \sqrt{\dfrac{ht\,(in) \times wt\,(lb)}{3131}} = \sqrt{\dfrac{36 \times 40}{3131}} = \sqrt{\dfrac{1440}{3131}} = \sqrt{0.46} = 0.678\,m^2 = 0.68\,m^2$

2) Metric: BSA (m^2) $= \sqrt{\dfrac{ht\,(cm) \times wt\,(kg)}{3600}} = \sqrt{\dfrac{190 \times 105}{3600}} = \sqrt{\dfrac{19{,}950}{3600}} = \sqrt{5.542} = 2.354\,m^2 = 2.35\,m^2$

Review Set 44 from pages 379–381

1) 1,640,000 **2)** 5.9; 11.8 **3)** 735 **4)** 15.84; 63.36 **5)** 250 **6)** 0.49; 122.5; Yes; 2.5 **7)** 0.89; 2.9; Yes; 1.2 **8)** 66; 22; Yes **9)** 198; Yes; 990 **10)** 612; 612; 1224; 2448 **11)** 8.1; 24.7 **12)** 67–167.5; 33.5–83.8; Yes **13)** 8–14.4; Yes **14)** 0.82; 2050; Yes; 2.7; 102.7; 51 **15)** 1.62; 4050; Yes; 5.4; 105.4; 53

Solutions—Review Set 44

1) $2{,}000{,}000\,U/\cancel{m^2} \times 0.82\,\cancel{m^2} = 1{,}640{,}000\,U$

2) $10\,mg/\cancel{m^2}/day \times 0.59\,\cancel{m^2} = 5.9\,mg/day$ (minimum safe dosage)

$20\,mg/\cancel{m^2}/day \times 0.59\,\cancel{m^2} = 11.8\,mg/day$ (maximum safe dosage)

3) $500\,mg/\cancel{m^2} \times 1.47\,\cancel{m^2} = 735\,mg$

4) $6\,mg/\cancel{m^2}/day \times 2.64\,\cancel{m^2} = 15.84\,mg/day$

$15.84\,mg/day \times 4\,days = 63.36\,mg$

6) Household: BSA (m^2) $= \sqrt{\dfrac{ht\,(in) \times wt\,(lb)}{3131}} =$

$\sqrt{\dfrac{30 \times 25}{3131}} = \sqrt{\dfrac{750}{3131}} = \sqrt{0.240} = 0.489\,m^2 = 0.49\,m^2$

$250\,mg/\cancel{m^2} \times 0.49\,\cancel{m^2} = 122.5\,mg$; dosage is safe

$\dfrac{D}{H} \times Q = \dfrac{122.5\,\cancel{mg}}{50\,\cancel{mg}} \times 1\,mL = 2.45\,mL = 2.5\,mL$

8) $150\,mg/\cancel{m^2}/day \times 0.44\,\cancel{m^2} = 66\,mg/day$

$\dfrac{66\,mg}{3\,doses} = 22\,mg/dose$; dosage is safe

9) $900\,mg/\cancel{m^2}/day \times 0.22\,\cancel{m^2} = 198\,mg/day$; dosage is safe

$198\,mg/day \times 5\,days = 990\,mg$

10) $600\,mg/\cancel{m^2} \times 1.02\,\cancel{m^2} = 612\,mg$, initially

$300\,mg/\cancel{m^2} \times 1.02\,\cancel{m^2} = 306\,mg$; for 2 doses:

$306\,mg \times 2 = 612\,mg$

q.12 h is 2 doses/day and 2 doses/day $\times$ 2 days = 4 doses

$306\,mg \times 4 = 1224\,mg$

$612\,mg + 612\,mg + 1224\,mg = 2448\,mg$ (total)

11) $10\,mg/\cancel{m^2} \times 0.81\,\cancel{m^2} = 8.1\,mg$ (bolus)

$30.5\,mg/\cancel{m^2}/day \times 0.81\,\cancel{m^2} = 24.7\,mg/day$

14) Metric: BSA (m^2) = $\sqrt{\dfrac{\text{ht (cm)} \times \text{wt (kg)}}{3600}}$ =

$\sqrt{\dfrac{100 \times 24}{3600}} = \sqrt{\dfrac{2400}{3600}} = \sqrt{0.667} = 0.816 \text{ m}^2 = 0.82 \text{ m}^2$

2500 U/m^2 × 0.82 m^2 = 2050 U; dosage is safe

$\dfrac{D}{H} \times Q = \dfrac{2{,}050 \text{ U}}{750 \text{ U}} \times 1 \text{ mL} = 2.7 \text{ mL}$

$\dfrac{102.7 \text{ mL}}{2 \text{ h}} = 51.3 \text{ mL/h} = 51 \text{ mL/h}$

15) Metric: BSA (m^2) = $\sqrt{\dfrac{\text{ht (cm)} \times \text{wt (kg)}}{3600}}$ =

$\sqrt{\dfrac{58.2 \times 162}{3600}} = \sqrt{\dfrac{9428.4}{3600}} = \sqrt{2.619} = 1.62 \text{ m}^2$

2500 U/m^2 × 1.62 m^2 = 4050 U; dosage is safe

$\dfrac{D}{H} \times Q = \dfrac{4050 \text{ U}}{750 \text{ U}} \times 1 \text{ mL} = 5.4 \text{ mL}$

Total volume: 100 mL IV fluid + 5.4 mL med. =

105.4 mL

$\dfrac{105.4 \text{ mL}}{2 \text{ h}} = 52.7 \text{ mL/h} = 53 \text{ mL/h}$

Review Set 45 from pages 384–385

1) 87; 2; 48 **2)** 75; 3; 57 **3)** 120; 3; 22 **4)** 80; 6; 44 **5)** 60; 1; 31; 180 **6)** 2; 23 **7)** 2; 8 **8)** 12; 45 **9)** 7.2; 36.8 **10)** 7.5; 88.5

Solutions—Review Set 45

1) Total volume: 50 mL + 15 mL = 65 mL

$\dfrac{V}{T} \times C = \dfrac{65 \text{ mL}}{45 \text{ min}} \times 60 \text{ gtt/mL} =$

$\dfrac{260 \text{ gtt}}{3 \text{ min}} = 86.6 \text{ gtt/min} = 87 \text{ gtt/min}$

$\dfrac{D}{H} \times Q = \dfrac{60 \text{ mg}}{60 \text{ mg}} \times 2 \text{ mL} = 2 \text{ mL (medication)}$

Volume IV fluid to add to chamber: 50 mL – 2 mL =

48 mL

4) Total volume: 50 mL + 30 mL = 80 mL

80 mL/60 min = 80 mL/h

$\dfrac{D}{H} \times Q = \dfrac{0.6 \text{ g}}{1 \text{ g}} \times 10 \text{ mL} = 6 \text{ mL (medication)}$

Volume IV fluid to add to chamber: 50 mL – 6 mL =

44 mL

6) $\dfrac{50 \text{ mL}}{60 \text{ min}} \bowtie \dfrac{X \text{ mL}}{30 \text{ min}}$

60X = 1500

$\dfrac{60X}{60} = \dfrac{1500}{60}$

X = 25 mL (total volume)

$\dfrac{D}{H} \times Q = \dfrac{250 \text{ mg}}{125 \text{ mg}} \times 1 \text{ mL} = 2 \text{ mL (medication)}$

Volume IV fluid to add to chamber: 25 mL – 2 mL =

23 mL

8) $\dfrac{85 \text{ mL}}{60 \text{ min}} \bowtie \dfrac{X \text{ mL}}{40 \text{ min}}$

60X = 3400

$\dfrac{60X}{60} = \dfrac{3400}{60}$

X = 56.6 mL = 57 mL (total volume)

$\dfrac{D}{H} \times Q = \dfrac{600 \text{ mg}}{50 \text{ mg}} \times 1 \text{ mL} = 12 \text{ mL (medication)}$

Volume IV fluid to add to chamber: 57 mL – 12 mL

= 45 mL

9) $\dfrac{66 \text{ mL}}{60 \text{ min}} \bowtie \dfrac{X \text{ mL}}{40 \text{ min}}$

60X = 2640

$\dfrac{60X}{60} = \dfrac{2640}{60}$

X = 44 mL (total volume)

$\dfrac{D}{H} \times Q = \dfrac{720 \text{ mg}}{1000 \text{ mg}} \times 10 \text{ mL} = \dfrac{720}{100} \text{ mL} = 7.2 \text{ mL (medication)}$

Volume IV fluid to add to chamber: 44 mL – 7.2 mL

= 36.8 mL

Hint: Add the medication to the volume control

chamber, and fill with IV fluid to the 44 mL mark.

The chamber measures whole (not fractional) mL.

10) 48 mL/h × 2 h = 96 mL (total volume)

$\dfrac{D}{H} \times Q = \dfrac{75 \text{ mg}}{100 \text{ mg}} \times 10 \text{ mL} = \dfrac{75}{10} \text{ mL} = 7.5 \text{ mL}$

Volume IV fluid to add to chamber: 96 mL – 7.5 mL

= 88.5 mL

Review Set 46 from page 387

1) 360 **2)** 250; Child will only receive 360 mL in a 24-hour period. The 500-mL bag would be hanging longer than 24 hours, which is not safe. **3)** 5 **4)** 2.5 **5)** 0.3 **6)** 7.2 **7)** 0.17; 6.8; No, not safe. Dosage as ordered would be too high. The physician should be called for clarification. **8)** 4.8; 2.4 **9)** 18; 9 **10)** 12.8; 6.4

Solutions—Review Set 46

1) $15 \text{ mL/h} \times 24 \text{ h/day} = 360 \text{ mL/day}$

3) $\dfrac{20 \text{ mEq}}{1000 \text{ mL}} \diagup\!\!\!\!\diagdown \dfrac{X \text{ mEq}}{250 \text{ mL}}$

$1000X = 5000$

$\dfrac{1000X}{1000} = \dfrac{5000}{1000}$

$X = 5 \text{ mEq}$

4) $\dfrac{5 \text{ mEq}}{2 \text{ mEq}} \times 1 \text{ mL} = 2.5 \text{ mL}$

5) Total volume: 250 mL ($D_5W \frac{1}{2} NS$) + 2.5 mL KCl = 252.5 mL

Per hour:

$\dfrac{5 \text{ mEq}}{252.5 \text{ mL}} \diagup\!\!\!\!\diagdown \dfrac{X \text{ mEq}}{15 \text{ mL}}$

$252.5X = 75$

$\dfrac{252.5X}{252.5} = \dfrac{75}{252.5}$

$X = 0.29 \text{ mEq} = 0.3 \text{ mEq (per hour)}$

6) $0.3 \text{ mEq/h} \times 24 \text{ h/day} = 7.2 \text{ mEq/day}$

7) $\text{BSA (m}^2) = \sqrt{\dfrac{\text{ht (in)} \times \text{wt (lb)}}{3131}} = \sqrt{\dfrac{18 \times 5}{3131}} = \sqrt{\dfrac{90}{3131}} = \sqrt{0.287} = 0.169 \text{ m}^2 = 0.17 \text{ m}^2$

Recommended maximum daily dosage:

$40 \text{ mEq/m}^2\text{/day} \times 0.17 \text{ m}^2 = 6.8 \text{ mEq/day}$

Ordered dosage is not safe. Dosage as ordered would be too high. The physician should be called for clarification.

8) $\dfrac{10 \text{ mEq}}{1000 \text{ mL}} \diagup\!\!\!\!\diagdown \dfrac{X \text{ mEq}}{480 \text{ mL}}$

$1000X = 4800$

$\dfrac{1000X}{1000} = \dfrac{4800}{1000}$

$X = 4.8 \text{ mEq}$

$\dfrac{D}{H} \times Q = \dfrac{\overset{2.4}{\cancel{4.8} \text{ mEq}}}{\underset{1}{\cancel{2} \text{ mEq}}} \times 1 \text{ mL} = 2.4 \text{ mL}$

Review Set 47 from pages 391–392

1) 4 **2)** 25 **3)** 1600; 67 **4)** 1150; 48 **5)** 1800; 75 **6)** 350; 15 **7)** 3.5 or 4; 11.6 or 12 **8)** 2.6 or 3; 65 **9)** 2.3 or 3; 35 **10)** This order should be questioned because Normal Saline is an isotonic solution and appears to be a continuous infusion for this child. This solution does not contribute enough electrolytes for the child and water intoxication may result. Hint: The equipment measures whole mL; therefore, round to the next whole mL.

Solutions—Review Set 47

1) $\dfrac{100 \text{ mg}}{1 \text{ mL}} \diagup\!\!\!\!\diagdown \dfrac{400 \text{ mg}}{X \text{ mL}}$

$100X = 400$

$\dfrac{100X}{100} = \dfrac{400}{100}$

$X = 4 \text{ mL}$

3) $\begin{aligned} 100 \text{ mL/kg/day} \times 10 \text{ kg} &= 1000 \text{ mL/day for first 10} \\ 50 \text{ mL/kg/day} \times 10 \text{ kg} &= 500 \text{ mL/day for next 10} \\ 20 \text{ mL/kg/day} \times 5 \text{ kg} &= \underline{100 \text{ mL/day for remaining}} \\ & \quad 1600 \text{ mL/day or per 24 h} \end{aligned}$

$\dfrac{1600 \text{ mL}}{24 \text{ h}} = 66.7 \text{ mL/h} = 67 \text{ mL/h}$

4) $\begin{aligned} 100 \text{ mL/kg/day} \times 10 \text{ kg} &= 1000 \text{ mL/day for first 10 kg} \\ 50 \text{ mL/kg/day} \times 3 \text{ kg} &= \underline{150 \text{ mL/day for next 10 kg}} \\ & \quad 1150 \text{ mL/day or per 24 h} \end{aligned}$

$\dfrac{1150 \text{ mL}}{24 \text{ h}} = 47.9 \text{ mL/h} = 48 \text{ mL/h}$

5) $77 \text{ lb} = \dfrac{77}{2.2} = 35 \text{ kg}$

$\begin{aligned} 100 \text{ mL/kg/day} \times 10 \text{ kg} &= 1000 \text{ mL/day for first 10} \\ 50 \text{ mL/kg/day} \times 10 \text{ kg} &= 500 \text{ mL/day for next 10} \\ 20 \text{ mL/kg/day} \times 15 \text{ kg} &= \underline{300 \text{ mL/day for remaining}} \\ & \quad 1800 \text{ mL/day or per 24 h} \end{aligned}$

$\dfrac{1800 \text{ mL}}{24 \text{ h}} = 75 \text{ mL/h}$

7)

$$\frac{100 \text{ mg}}{1 \text{ ml}} \times \frac{350 \text{ mg}}{X \text{ mL}}$$

$$100X = 350$$

$$\frac{100X}{100} = \frac{350}{100}$$

$$X = 3.5 \text{ or } 4 \text{ mL (min. dilution volume)}$$

$$\frac{30 \text{ mg}}{1 \text{ mL}} \times \frac{350 \text{ mg}}{X \text{ mL}}$$

$$30X = 350$$

$$\frac{30X}{30} = \frac{350}{30}$$

$$X = 11.6 \text{ or } 12 \text{ mL (max. dilution volume)}$$

Practice Problems—Chapter 15 from pages 393–399

1) 1.17; 1.8–2.3; Yes; 2; 0.5 **2)** 0.52; 42; 0.84 **3)** 0.43; 108 **4)** 2.2 **5)** 0.7 **6)** 350 **7)** 1 of each (one 100-mg capsule and one 250-mg capsule) **8)** 0.8; 2,000 **9)** 2.7 **10)** No **11)** 1.3; 26 **12)** 13 **13)** 1.69 **14)** 1.11 **15)** 0.32 **16)** 1.92 **17)** 1.63 **18)** 0.69 **19)** 1.67 **20)** 0.52 **21)** 560,000 **22)** 1085; 109 **23)** 1.9–3.8 **24)** 8 **25)** 40 **26)** 45; 90; 4.2; 25.8 **27)** 58.8 **28)** 60; 60; 1.9; 43.1 **29)** 22.8 **30)** 10; 33 **31)** 6.2; 37.8 **32)** 10.8; 5.4 **33)** 14; 7 **34)** 3.8; 1.9 **35)** 1520; 63 **36)** 1810; 75 **37)** 1250; 52 **38)** 240; 10 **39)** 1500–1875; 250–312.5; Yes; 2.8 **40)** 35; 2.8; 32.2 **41)** 12.3; 1230; 308; Yes; 6.2 **42)** 23; 6.2; 16.8 **43)** 330–495; 110–165; Yes; 3.3 **44)** 25; 3.3; 21.7 **45)** 1800–2700; 300–450; No; exceeds maximum dose; Do not give dosage ordered. **46)** Consult physician before further action. **47)** 25; 2,500,000-6,250,000; 416,667–1,041,667 **48)** Yes; 2.6 **49)** 20; 2.6; 17.4

50) Critical Thinking: Prevention.

The nurse made several assumptions in trying to calculate and prepare this chemotherapy quickly. The nurse assumed that the weight notation was the same on the two units without verifying that fact. The recording of the weights as 20/.45 was very confusing. Notice the period before the 45, which later the physician stated was the calculated BSA, 0.45 m². Because no unit of measure was identified, it was unclear what those numbers really meant. Never assume; always ask for clarification when notation is unclear. Also, a child who weighs 20 lb and a child who weighs 45 lb are quite different in size, yet the nurse failed to notice such a size difference. This nurse, though, is probably not used to discriminating small children's weight differences, but should have realized that weight in lb is approximately two times weight in kg. Additionally, the actual volume drawn up was probably very small in comparison to most adult dose volumes that this nurse prepares. The amount of 1.6 mL likely seemed reasonable to the nurse. Finally, this is an instance in which the person giving the medication, the physician, prevented a medication error by stopping and thinking what is a reasonable amount for this child and questioning the actual calculation of the dose. Remember, the person who administers the medication is the last point at which a potential error can be avoided.

Solutions—Practice Problems—Chapter 15

1) Household: BSA (m²) $= \sqrt{\dfrac{\text{ht (in)} \times \text{wt (lb)}}{3131}} = \sqrt{\dfrac{50 \times 85}{3131}} =$

$\sqrt{\dfrac{4250}{3131}} = \sqrt{1.357} = 1.165 \text{ m}^2 = 1.17 \text{ m}^2$

Recommended dosage range:

1.5 mg/m² × 1.17 m² = 1.75 mg = 1.8 mg

2 mg/m² × 1.17 m² = 2.34 mg = 2.3 mg

Ordered dosage is safe.

$\dfrac{D}{H} \times Q = \dfrac{2 \text{ mg}}{1 \text{ mg}} \times 1 \text{ mL} = 2 \text{ mL}$

Give 2 mL/min

$$\frac{2 \text{ mL}}{60 \text{ sec}} \times \frac{X \text{ mL}}{15 \text{ sec}}$$

$$60X = 30$$

$$\frac{60X}{60} = \frac{30}{60}$$

$$X = 0.5 \text{ mL (per 15 sec)}$$

2) BSA = 0.52 m²

80 mg/m²/day × 0.52 m² = 41.6 mg/day = 42 mg/day

$\dfrac{D}{H} \times Q = \dfrac{42 \text{ mg}}{50 \text{ mg}} \times 1 \text{ mL} = 0.84 \text{ mL}$

3) BSA = 0.43 m²

250 mcg/m²/day × 0.43 m² = 107.5 mcg/day

= 108 mcg/day

4) $\dfrac{D}{H} \times Q = \dfrac{108 \text{ mcg}}{500 \text{ mcg}} \times 10 \text{ mL} = 2.16 \text{ mL} = 2.2 \text{ mL}$

5) BSA = 0.7 m²

6) 0.5 g/m² × 0.7 m² = 0.35 g

0.35 g = 0.35 × 1000 = 350 mg

8) BSA = 0.8 m^2

2500 U/m^2 × 0.8 m^2 = 2000 U

9) $\dfrac{D}{H} \times Q = \dfrac{2000\ \cancel{U}}{750\ \cancel{U}} \times 1\ mL = 2.66\ mL = 2.7\ mL$

10) Dose amount exceeds child maximum IM volume per injection site; give in 2 injections.

11) Metric: BSA (m^2) = $\sqrt{\dfrac{ht\ (cm) \times wt\ (kg)}{3600}} = \sqrt{\dfrac{140 \times 43.5}{3600}} =$

$\sqrt{\dfrac{6090}{3600}} = \sqrt{1.69} = 1.3\ m^2$

20 mg/m^2 × 1.3 m^2 = 26 mg

12) $\dfrac{D}{H} \times Q = \dfrac{\overset{13}{\cancel{26\ mg}}}{\underset{1}{\cancel{2\ mg}}} \times 1\ mL = 13\ mL$

13) 5 ft 6 in = 66 inches (12 in/ft)

Household: BSA (m^2) = $\sqrt{\dfrac{ht\ (in) \times wt\ (lb)}{3131}} = \sqrt{\dfrac{66 \times 136}{3131}} =$

$\sqrt{\dfrac{8976}{3131}} = \sqrt{2.866} = 1.693\ m^2 = 1.69\ m^2$

15) Metric: BSA (m^2) = $\sqrt{\dfrac{ht\ (cm) \times wt\ (kg)}{3600}} = \sqrt{\dfrac{60 \times 6}{3600}} =$

$\sqrt{\dfrac{360}{3600}} = \sqrt{0.1} = 0.316\ m^2 = 0.32\ m^2$

19) 64 in = 64 × 2.5 = 160 cm (1 in = 2.5 cm)

Metric: BSA (m^2) = $\sqrt{\dfrac{ht\ (cm) \times wt\ (kg)}{3600}} = \sqrt{\dfrac{160 \times 63}{3600}} =$

$\sqrt{\dfrac{10,080}{3600}} = \sqrt{2.8} = 1.673\ m^2 = 1.67\ m^2$

22) 500 mg/m^2 × 2.17 m^2 = 1085 mg

1085 mg = 1085 ÷ 1000 = 1.085 g = 1.09 g

24) 6 mg/m^2 × 1.34 m^2 = 8.04 = 8 mg

25) 8.04 mg/day × 5 days = 40.2 mg = 40 mg

26) Total volume = 30 mL + 15 mL = 45 mL

Flow rate: $\dfrac{45\ mL}{\underset{1}{\cancel{30\ min}}} \times \dfrac{\overset{2}{\cancel{60\ min}}}{h} = 90\ mL/h$

$\dfrac{D}{H} \times Q = \dfrac{\cancel{420\ mg}}{\underset{100}{\cancel{500\ mg}}} \times \overset{1}{\cancel{5}}\ mL = \dfrac{420}{100}\ mL = 4.2\ mL\ (medication)$

30 mL total solution − 4.2 mL med = 25.8 mL D$_5$NS

Note: Add 4.2 mL med. to chamber and fill with D$_5$NS to 30 mL.

27) 4.2 mL/dose × 2 doses/day = 8.4 mL/day

8.4 mL/day × 7 days = 58.8 mL (total)

28) Total volume: 45 mL + 15 mL = 60 mL

Flow rate: $\dfrac{60\ mL}{60\ min} = 60\ mL/h$

$\dfrac{D}{H} \times Q = \dfrac{285\ \cancel{mg}}{75\ \cancel{mg}} \times 0.5\ mL = 1.9\ mL\ (med)$

Volume of IV fluid: 45 mL − 1.9 mL = 43.1 mL

29) 1.9 mL/dose × 3 doses/day = 5.7 mL/day

5.7 mL/day × 4 days = 22.8 mL (total)

30) $\dfrac{D}{H} \times Q = \dfrac{\overset{10}{\cancel{500\ mg}}}{\underset{1}{\cancel{50\ mg}}} \times 1\ mL = 10\ mL\ (med)$

$\dfrac{65\ mL}{60\ min} \quad \diagup\!\!\!\!\diagdown \quad \dfrac{X\ mL}{40\ min}$

60X = 2600

$\dfrac{60X}{60} = \dfrac{2600}{60}$

X = 43.3 mL = 43 mL

43 mL total solution − 10 mL med =

33 mL D$_5$ 0.33% NaCl

32) $\dfrac{30\ mEq}{1000\ mL} \quad \diagup\!\!\!\!\diagdown \quad \dfrac{X\ mEq}{360\ mL}$

1000X = 10,800

$\dfrac{1000X}{1000} = \dfrac{10,800}{1000}$

X = 10.8 mEq

$\dfrac{D}{H} \times Q = \dfrac{10.8\ \cancel{mEq}}{2\ \cancel{mEq}} \times 1\ mL = 5.4\ mL$

35) 100 mL/kg/day × 10 kg = 1000 mL/day for first 10 kg
50 mL/kg/day × 10 kg = 500 mL/day for next 10 kg
20 mL/kg/day × 1 kg = 20 mL/day for remaining 1 kg

1520 mL/day or per 24 h

$\dfrac{1520\ mL}{24\ h} = 63.3\ mL/h = 63\ mL/h$

36) 78 lb = 78 ÷ 2.2 = 35.45 = 35.5 kg
100 mL/kg/day × 10 kg = 1000 mL/day for first 10 kg
50 mL/kg/day × 10 kg = 500 mL/day for next 10 kg
20 mL/kg/day × 15.5 kg = 310 mL/day for remaining 15.5 kg

1810 mL/day or per 24 h

$\dfrac{1810\ mL}{24\ h} = 75.4\ mL/h = 75\ mL/h$

38) 2400 g = 2400 ÷ 1000 = 2.4 kg

100 mL/kg/day × 2.4 kg = 240 mL/day

$\dfrac{240\ mL}{24\ h} = 10\ mL/h$

39) Safe daily dosage range:
100 mg/kg × 15 kg = 1500 mg
125 mg/kg × 15 kg = 1875 mg

Safe single dosage range:

$\dfrac{1500\ mg}{6\ doses} = 250\ mg/dose$

$\dfrac{1875\ mg}{6\ doses} = 312.5\ mg/dose$

Yes, the dosage is safe.

1 g = 1000 mg

$\dfrac{D}{H} \times Q = \dfrac{275\ \cancel{mg}}{1000\ \cancel{mg}} \times 10\ mL = 2.75\ mL = 2.8\ mL$

40) IV fluid volume:

$$\frac{53 \text{ mL}}{60 \text{ min}} \underset{\times}{\overset{\times}{\rightleftarrows}} \frac{\text{X mL}}{40 \text{ min}}$$

$$60\text{X} = 2120$$

$$\frac{60\text{X}}{60} = \frac{2120}{60}$$

$$\text{X} = 35.3 \text{ mL} = 35 \text{ mL}$$

35 mL total – 2.8 mL med. = 32.2 mL D$_5$ 0.45% NaCl

45) Safe daily dosage range:

$$200 \text{ mg/kg} \times 9 \text{ kg} = 1800 \text{ mg}$$
$$300 \text{ mg/kg} \times 9 \text{ kg} = 2700 \text{ mg}$$

Safe single dosage range:

$$\frac{1800 \text{ mg}}{6 \text{ doses}} = 300 \text{ mg/dose}$$

$$\frac{2700 \text{ mg}}{6 \text{ doses}} = 450 \text{ mg/dose}$$

Dosage is *not* safe; exceeds maximum safe dosage.

Do not give dosage ordered; consult with physician.

47) $55 \text{ lb} = \frac{55}{2.2} = 25 \text{ kg}$

Safe daily dosage:

$$100,000 \text{ U/kg} \times 25 \text{ kg} = 2,500,000 \text{ U}$$
$$250,000 \text{ U/kg} \times 25 \text{ kg} = 6,250,000 \text{ U}$$

Safe single dosage:

$$\frac{2,500,000 \text{ U}}{6 \text{ doses}} = 416,666.6 = 416,667 \text{ U/dose}$$

$$\frac{6,250,000 \text{ U}}{6 \text{ doses}} = 1,041,666.6 = 1,041,667 \text{ U/dose}$$

48) Yes, dosage is safe.

$$\frac{\text{D}}{\text{H}} \times \text{Q} = \frac{525,000 \cancel{\text{U}}}{200,000 \cancel{\text{U}}} \times 1 \text{ mL} = 2.62 \text{ mL} = 2.6 \text{ mL}$$

49) $\frac{60 \text{ mL}}{60 \text{ min}} \underset{\times}{\overset{\times}{\rightleftarrows}} \frac{\text{X mL}}{20 \text{ min}}$

$$60\text{X} = 1200$$

$$\frac{60\text{X}}{60} = \frac{1200}{60}$$

$$\text{X} = 20 \text{ mL}$$

20 mL total – 2.6 mL med. = 17.4 mL D$_5$NS

Review Set 48 from pages 406–408

1) 40 **2)** 14 **3)** 10 **4)** 19 **5)** 48; consult physician **6)** 16 **7)** 75; 6000; 6; 1350; 14 **8)** 6000; 6; 1650; 17 **9)** 3000; 3; 1800; 18 **10)** Continue the rate at 1800 U/h or 18 mL/h **11)** 10 **12)** 50 **13)** 4 **14)** 20 **15)** 8

Solutions—Review Set 48

1) $\frac{\text{D}}{\text{H}} \times \text{Q} = \frac{1000 \cancel{\text{U}}/\text{h}}{\underset{25}{\cancel{25,000} \cancel{\text{U}}}} \times \overset{1}{\cancel{1000}} \text{ mL} = \frac{\overset{40}{\cancel{1000}}}{\underset{1}{\cancel{25}}} \text{ mL/h}$

$$= 40 \text{ mL/h}$$

4) $\frac{\text{D}}{\text{H}} \times \text{Q} = \frac{1500 \cancel{\text{U}}/\text{h}}{\underset{80}{\cancel{40000} \cancel{\text{U}}}} \times \overset{1}{\cancel{500}} \text{ mL} = 18.7 \text{ mL/h} = 19 \text{ mL/h}$

5) $\frac{\text{D}}{\text{H}} \times \text{Q} = \frac{1200 \cancel{\text{U}}/\text{h}}{\underset{25}{\cancel{25000} \cancel{\text{U}}}} \times \overset{1}{\cancel{1000}} \text{ mL} = 48 \text{ mL/h}$

The IV is infusing too rapidly. The physician should be called immediately for further action.

6) $\frac{\text{D}}{\text{H}} \times \text{Q} = \frac{800 \cancel{\text{U}}/\text{h}}{\underset{50}{\cancel{25000} \cancel{\text{U}}}} \times \overset{1}{\cancel{500}} \text{ mL} = \frac{\overset{16}{\cancel{800}}}{\underset{1}{\cancel{50}}} \text{ mL/h} = 16 \text{ mL/h}$

7) $165 \text{ lb} = \frac{165}{2.2} = 75 \text{ kg}$

Initial heparin bolus: $80 \text{ U/kg} \times 75 \text{ kg} = 6000 \text{ U}$

$$\frac{\text{D}}{\text{H}} \times \text{Q} = \frac{6000 \cancel{\text{U}}}{1000 \cancel{\text{U}}} \times 1 \text{ mL} = 6 \text{ mL}$$

Initial heparin infusion rate: $18 \text{ U/kg/h} \times 75 \text{ kg} = 1350 \text{ U/h}$

$$\frac{\text{D}}{\text{H}} \times \text{Q} = \frac{1350 \cancel{\text{U}}/\text{h}}{\underset{100}{\cancel{25,000} \cancel{\text{U}}}} \times \overset{1}{\cancel{250}} \text{ mL} = 13.5 \text{ mL/h} = 14 \text{ mL/h}$$

8) Rebolus: $80 \text{ U/kg} \times 75 \text{ kg} = 6000 \text{ U}$

$$\frac{\text{D}}{\text{H}} \times \text{Q} = \frac{6000 \cancel{\text{U}}}{1000 \cancel{\text{U}}} \times 1 \text{ mL} = 6 \text{ mL}$$

Reset infusion rate: $4 \text{ U/kg/h} \times 75 \text{ kg}$
$$= 300 \text{ U/h (increase)}$$

$$1350 \text{ U/h} + 300 \text{ U/h} = 1650 \text{ U/h}$$

$$\frac{\text{D}}{\text{H}} \times \text{Q} = \frac{1650 \cancel{\text{U}}/\text{h}}{\underset{100}{\cancel{25,000} \cancel{\text{U}}}} \times \overset{1}{\cancel{250}} \text{ mL} = 16.5 \text{ mL/h}$$

$$= 17 \text{ mL/h}$$

9) Rebolus: 40 U/kg × 75 kg = 3000 U

$$\frac{D}{H} \times Q = \frac{3000\ \cancel{U}}{1000\ \cancel{U}} \times 1\ mL = 3\ mL$$

Reset infusion rate: 2 U/kg/h × 75 kg

= 150 U/h (increase)

1650 U/h + 150 U/h = 1800 U/h

$$\frac{D}{H} \times Q = \frac{1800\ \cancel{U}/h}{\underset{100}{25,000\ \cancel{U}}} \times \overset{1}{\cancel{250}}\ mL = 18\ mL/h$$

11) $$\frac{D}{H} \times Q = \frac{10\ \cancel{U}/h}{\cancel{500}\ \cancel{U}} \times \cancel{500}\ mL = 10\ mL/h$$

13) $$\frac{D}{H} \times Q = \frac{5\ mg/h}{\underset{5}{125\ mg}} \times \overset{4}{\cancel{100}}\ mL = \frac{\overset{4}{\cancel{20}}}{\underset{1}{\cancel{5}}}\ mL/h = 4\ mL/h$$

14) $$\frac{D}{H} \times Q = \frac{10\ mg/h}{\underset{1}{125\ mg}} \times \overset{2}{\cancel{250}}\ mL = 20\ mL/h$$

Review Set 49 from pages 416–417

1) 2; 120 2) 1; 60 3) 1.5; 90 4) 90; 360; 0.4; 24 5) 1050; 0.66; 40 6) 142–568 7) 0.14–0.57 8) Yes 9) 4 10) Yes
11) 100; 25 12) 1 13) 0.025 14) 25 15) Yes

Solutions—Review Set 49

1) $$\frac{D}{H} \times Q = \frac{4\ mg/min}{\underset{2}{2000\ mg}} \times \overset{1}{\cancel{1000}}\ mL = \frac{\overset{2}{\cancel{4}}}{\underset{1}{\cancel{2}}}\ mL/min = 2\ mL/min$$

2 mL/min × 60 min/h = 120 mL/h

2) $$\frac{D}{H} \times Q = \frac{2\ mg/min}{\underset{2}{500\ mg}} \times \overset{1}{\cancel{250}}\ mL = \frac{\overset{1}{\cancel{2}}}{\underset{1}{\cancel{2}}}\ mL/min = 1\ mL/min$$

1 mL/min × 60 min/h = 60 mL/h

3) $$\frac{D}{H} \times Q = \frac{6\ mcg/min}{\underset{4}{2000\ mcg}} \times \overset{1}{\cancel{500}}\ mL = \frac{6}{4}\ mL/min$$

= 1.5 mL/min
1.5 mL/min × 60 min/h = 90 mL/h

4) 198 lb = $\frac{198}{2.2}$ = 90 kg; 4 mcg/kg/min × 90 kg = 360 mcg/min

360 mcg/min = 360 ÷ 1000 = 0.36 mg/min

$$\frac{D}{H} \times Q = \frac{0.36\ mg/min}{\underset{9}{450\ mg}} \times \overset{10}{\cancel{500}}\ mL = \frac{3.6}{9}\ mL/min$$

= 0.4 mL/min
0.4 mL/min × 60 min/h = 24 mL/h

5) 15 mcg/kg/min × 70 kg = 1050 mcg/min

1050 mcg/min = 1050 ÷ 1000 = 1.05 mg/min

$$\frac{D}{H} \times Q = \frac{1.05\ mg/min}{\underset{8}{800\ mg}} \times \overset{5}{\cancel{500}}\ mL = \frac{5.25}{8}\ mL/min$$

= 0.656 mL/min = 0.66 mL/min

0.66 mL/min × 60 min/h = 39.6 mL/h = 40 mL/h

6) 125 lb = $\frac{125}{2.2}$ = 56.81 = 56.8 kg

Minimum: 2.5 mcg/kg/min × 56.8 kg = 142 mcg/min
Maximum: 10 mcg/kg/min × 56.8 kg = 568 mcg/min

7) Minimum: 142 mcg/min = 142 ÷ 1000 =
0.14 mg/min
Maximum: 568 mcg/min = 568 ÷ 1000 =
0.57 mg/min

8)
$$\frac{500\ mg}{500\ mL} \underset{\diagup}{\overset{\diagdown}{=}} \frac{X\ mg/h}{15\ mL/h}$$

$$500X = 7500$$

$$\frac{500X}{500} = \frac{7500}{500}$$

$$X = 15\ mg/h$$

$$\frac{15\ mg/h}{60\ min/h} = 0.25\ mg/min$$

Yes, the order is within the safe range of

0.14– 0.57 mg/min.

9)
$$\frac{2000 \text{ mg}}{500 \text{ mL}} \times \frac{X \text{ mg/h}}{60 \text{ mL/h}}$$

$$500X = 120{,}000$$

$$\frac{500X}{500} = \frac{120{,}000}{500}$$

$$X = 240 \text{ mg/h}$$

$$\frac{240 \text{ mg/h}}{60 \text{ min/h}} = 4 \text{ mg/min}$$

10) Yes, 4 mg/min is within the normal range of 2–6 mg/min.

11) Bolus:
$$\frac{2 \text{ g}}{30 \text{ min}} \times \frac{X \text{ g}}{60 \text{ min}}$$

$$30X = 120$$

$$X = 4 \text{ g (per 60 min or 4 g/h)}$$

$$\frac{20 \text{ mg}}{500 \text{ mL}} \times \frac{4 \text{ g/h}}{X \text{ mL/h}}$$

$$20X = 2000$$

$$\frac{20X}{20} = \frac{2000}{20}$$

$$X = 100 \text{ mL/h}$$

Continuous:
$$\frac{20 \text{ mg}}{500 \text{ mL}} \times \frac{1 \text{ g/h}}{X \text{ mL/h}}$$

$$20X = 500$$

$$\frac{20X}{20} = \frac{500}{20}$$

$$X = 25 \text{ mL/h}$$

12) $1 \text{ mU} = 1 \div 1000 = 0.001 \text{ U}$

$$\frac{D}{H} \times Q = \frac{0.001 \text{ U/min}}{15 \text{ U}} \times 250 \text{ mL} = 0.017 \text{ mL/min}$$

$$0.017 \text{ mL/min} \times 60 \text{ min/h} = 1.02 \text{ mL/h} = 1 \text{ mL/h}$$

13)
$$\frac{10 \text{ mg}}{1000 \text{ mL}} \times \frac{X \text{ mg/h}}{150 \text{ mL/h}}$$

$$1000X = 1500$$

$$\frac{1000X}{1000} = \frac{1500}{1000}$$

$$X = 1.5 \text{ mg/h}$$

$$\frac{1.5 \text{ mg/h}}{60 \text{ min/h}} = 0.025 \text{ mg/min}$$

14) $0.025 \text{ mg/min} = 0.025 \times 1000 = 25 \text{ mcg/min}$

Review Set 50 from pages 420–422

1) 33; 19 **2)** 40; 42 **3)** 25; 32 **4)** 50; 90 **5)** 50; 40 **6)** 100; 100 **7)** 200; 76 **8)** 200; 122 **9)** 17; 21 **10)** 120; 112

Solutions—Review Set 50

1) Step 1. IV PB rate: $\frac{V}{T} \times C = \frac{100 \text{ mL}}{\overset{}{\underset{3}{30 \text{ min}}}} \times \overset{1}{10} \text{ gtt/mL} =$

$\frac{100}{3}$ gtt/min $= 33.3$ gtt/min $= 33$ gtt/min

Step 2. Total IV PB time: q.4h $\times$ 30 min $= 6 \times 30$ min $= 180$ min $= 180 \div 60 = 3$ h

Step 3. Total IV PB volume: 6×100 mL $= 600$ mL

Step 4. Total Regular IV volume: 3000 mL $-$ 600 mL $= 2400$ mL

Step 5. Total Regular IV time: 24 h $-$ 3 h $= 21$ h

Step 6. Regular IV rate:

$$\frac{2400 \text{ mL}}{21 \text{ h}} = 114 \text{ mL/h}$$

$$\frac{\text{mL/h}}{\text{drop factor constant}} = \text{gtt/min}; \frac{114 \text{ mL/h}}{6} = 19 \text{ gtt/min}$$

2) Step 1.   IV PB rate: When drop factor is 60 gtt/mL, then mL/h = gtt/min. Rate is 40 gtt/min.

     Step 2.   Total IV PB time: q.i.d. $\times$ 1 h = 4 $\times$ 1 h = 4 h

     Step 3.   Total IV PB volume: 4 $\times$ 40 mL = 160 mL

     Step 4.   Total Regular IV volume: 1000 mL – 160 mL = 840 mL

     Step 5.   Total Regular IV time: 24 h – 4 h = 20 h

     Step 6.   Total Regular IV rate: mL/h = $\frac{840 \text{ mL}}{20 \text{ h}}$ = 42 mL/h. When drop factor is 60 gtt/mL, then mL/h = gtt/min.

     Rate is 42 gtt/min.

3) Step 1.   IV PB rate: $\frac{V}{T} \times C = \frac{50 \text{ mL}}{\overset{30 \text{ min}}{2}} \times \overset{1}{15} \text{ gtt/mL} = \frac{50}{2} \text{ gtt/min} = 25 \text{ gtt/min}$

     Step 2.   Total IV PB time: q.6h $\times$ 30 min = 4 $\times$ 30 min = 120 min = 120 $\div$ 60 = 2 h

     Step 3.   Total IV PB volume: 4 $\times$ 50 mL = 200 mL

     Step 4.   Total Regular IV volume: 3000 mL – 200 mL = 2800 mL

     Step 5.   Total Regular IV time: 24 h – 2 h = 22 h

     Step 6.   Total Regular IV rate:

$\frac{2800 \text{ mL}}{22 \text{ h}} = 127 \text{ mL/h}$

$\frac{\text{mL/h}}{\text{drop factor constant}} = \text{gtt/min}; \frac{127 \text{ mL/h}}{4} = 31.7 \text{ gtt/min} = 32 \text{ gtt/min}$

4) Step 1.   IV PB rate: 50 mL/h or 50 gtt/min (because drop factor is 60 gtt/mL)

     Step 2.   Total IV PB time: q.6h $\times$ 1 h = 4 $\times$ 1 h = 4 h

     Step 3.   Total IV PB volume: 4 $\times$ 50 mL = 200 mL

     Step 4.   Total Regular IV volume: 2000 mL – 200 mL = 1800 mL

     Step 5.   Total Regular IV time: 24 h – 4 h = 20 h

     Step 6.   Regular IV rate: $\frac{1800 \text{ mL}}{20 \text{ h}}$ = 90 mL/h or 90 gtt/min (because drop factor is 60 gtt/mL)

5) Step 1.   IV PB rate: 50 mL/h or 50 gtt/min (because drop factor is 60 gtt/mL)

     Step 2.   IV PB time: q.8h $\times$ 1 h = 3 $\times$ 1 h = 3 h

     Step 3.   IV PB volume: 3 $\times$ 50 mL = 150 mL

     Step 4.   Total Regular IV volume: 1000 mL – 150 mL = 850 mL

     Step 5.   Total Regular IV time: 24 h – 3 h = 21 h

     Step 6.   Regular IV rate: $\frac{850 \text{ mL}}{21 \text{ h}}$ = 40.4 mL/h = 40 gtt/min (because drop factor is 60 gtt/mL)

6) Step 1.   IV PB rate

$\frac{50 \text{ mL}}{30 \text{ min}} \diagup\!\!\!\!\diagdown \frac{X \text{ mL}}{60 \text{ min}}$

$30X = 3000$

$\frac{30X}{30} = \frac{3000}{30}$

$X = 100 \text{ mL}; 100 \text{ mL/60 min} = 100 \text{ mL/h}$

     Step 2.   IV PB time: q.6h $\times$ 30 min = 4 $\times$ 30 min = 120 min = 120 $\div$ 60 = 2 h

     Step 3.   IV PB volume: 4 $\times$ 50 mL = 200 mL

     Step 4.   Total Regular IV volume: 2400 mL – 200 mL = 2200 mL

     Step 5.   Total Regular IV time: 24 h – 2 h = 22 h

     Step 6.   Regular IV rate: $\frac{2200 \text{ mL}}{22 \text{ h}}$ = 100 mL/h

7) Step 1.   IV PB rate:

$$\frac{100 \text{ mL}}{30 \text{ min}} \quad\times\quad \frac{X \text{ mL}}{60 \text{ min}}$$

$$30X \;=\; 6000$$

$$\frac{30X}{30} \;=\; \frac{6000}{30}$$

$$X \;=\; 200 \text{ mL}; \; 200 \text{ mL}/60 \text{ min} = 200 \text{ mL/h}$$

Step 2.   IV PB time: q.8h $\times$ 30 min = 3 $\times$ 30 min = 90 min = 90 $\div$ 60 = $1\frac{1}{2}$ h

Step 3.   IV PB volume: 3 $\times$ 100 mL = 300 mL

Step 4.   Total Regular IV volume: 2000 mL − 300 mL = 1700 mL

Step 5.   Total Regular IV time: 24 h − $1\frac{1}{2}$ h = $22\frac{1}{2}$ h

Step 6.   Regular IV rate: $\frac{1700 \text{ mL}}{22.5 \text{ h}}$ = 75.5 mL/h = 76 mL/h

8) Step 1.   IV PB rate

$$\frac{50 \text{ mL}}{15 \text{ min}} \quad\times\quad \frac{X \text{ mL}}{60 \text{ min}}$$

$$15X \;=\; 3000$$

$$\frac{15X}{15} \;=\; \frac{3000}{15}$$

$$X \;=\; 200 \text{ mL}; \; 200 \text{ mL}/60 \text{ min} = 200 \text{ mL/h}$$

Step 2.   IV PB time: q.6h $\times$ 15 min = 4 $\times$ 15 min = 60 min = 1 h

Step 3.   IV PB volume: 4 $\times$ 50 mL = 200 mL

Step 4.   Total Regular IV volume: 3000 mL − 200 mL = 2800 mL

Step 5.   Total Regular IV time: 24 h − 1 h = 23 h

Step 6.   Regular IV rate: $\frac{2800 \text{ mL}}{23 \text{ h}}$ = 121.7 mL/h = 122 mL/h

Practice Problems—Chapter 16 from pages 423–429

1) 60 **2)** 5 **3)** 20 **4)** 50 **5)** 1 **6)** 12 **7)** 50 **8)** 63 **9)** 35 **10)** 6; 15 **11)** 60 **12)** 45 **13)** 60 **14)** 24 **15)** Yes **16)** 17; 22 **17)** 100; 127 **18)** 102 **19)** 8 mEq **20)** 2 **21)** 15 **22)** 50; 50 **23)** 75; 75 **24)** 7.4 **25)** 12; 18 **26)** 150; 50 **27)** 2 **28)** 35 **29)** 8 **30)** 63 **31)** 80 **32)** 0.4 **33)** 4 **34)** 4 **35)** 100 **36)** 0.2; 200 **37)** 30 **38)** 200; 50 **39)** 5 **40)** 550 **41)** 2450 **42)** 19 **43)** 129 **44)** 13; 39 **45)** (Worksheet is on the next page.) 100; 80 **46)** 8000; 1000; 8 **47)** 18; 1800; 100; 18 **48)** 6; 4000; 4; increase; 200; 2; 20 **49)** Decrease rate by 2 U/kg/h; 18

50)   Critical Thinking Skill: Prevention.

The nurse who prepares any IV solution with an additive should *carefully* compare the order and medication three times: before beginning to prepare the dose, after the dosage is prepared, and just before it is administered to the patient. Further, the nurse should verify the safety of the dosage using the three-step method (convert, think, and calculate). It was clear that the nurse realized the error when a colleague questioned what was being prepared and the nurse verified the actual order. Also taking the time to do the calculation on paper helps the nurse to "see" the answer and avoid a potentially life-threatening error.

STANDARD WEIGHT-BASED HEPARIN PROTOCOL WORKSHEET

Round Patient's Total Body Weight to Nearest 10 kg: _100_ kg

DO NOT Change the Weight Based on Daily Measurements

FOUND ON THE ORDER FORM
Initial Bolus (80 U/kg) _8000_ U _8_ mL
Initial Infusion Rate (18 U/kg/h) _1800_ U/h _18_ mL/h

Make adjustments to the heparin drip rate as directed by the order form.

ALL DOSES ARE ROUNDED TO THE NEAREST 100 UNITS

Date	Time	APTT	Bolus	Rate Change U/h	Rate Change mL/h	New Rate	RN 1	RN 2
5/10/XX	1730	37 sec	4000 U (4 mL)	+200 U/h	+2 mL/h	20 mL/h	G.P.	M.S.
5/10/XX	2330	77 sec		−200 U/h	−2 mL/h	18 mL/h	G.P.	M.S.

Signatures	Initials
G. Pickar, R.N.	G.P.
M. Smith, R.N.	M.S.

Solutions—Practice Problems—Chapter 16

1) Volume control sets are microdrip infusion sets calibrated for 60 gtt/mL.

2) 1 g is ordered and it is prepared as a supply dosage of 1 g/5 mL. Add 5 mL.

3)
$$\frac{50 \text{ mL}}{60 \text{ min}} \diagdown\diagup \frac{X \text{ mL}}{30 \text{ min}}$$

$$60X = 1500$$

$$\frac{60X}{60} = \frac{1500}{60}$$

$$X = 25 \text{ mL total volume}$$

25 mL (total) − 5 mL (med) = 20 mL (D_5W)

4) $\dfrac{\text{mL/h}}{\text{drop factor constant}} = \dfrac{50 \text{ mL/h}}{1} = 50 \text{ gtt/min}$;

when drop factor is 60 gtt/mL, then mL/h = gtt/min

5) once (at 1200 hours)

6) $\dfrac{D}{H} \times Q = \dfrac{1200 \text{ U/h}}{\frac{25,000 \text{ U}}{100}} \times \overset{1}{\cancel{250}} \text{ mL} = \dfrac{\overset{12}{\cancel{1200}}}{\underset{1}{\cancel{100}}} \text{ mL/h} = 12 \text{ mL/h}$

7) $\dfrac{D}{H} \times Q = \dfrac{5 \text{ mg/h}}{\underset{1}{\cancel{100 \text{ mg}}}} \times \overset{10}{\cancel{1000}} \text{ mL} = 50 \text{ mL/h}$

ANSWERS

8) $\dfrac{D}{H} \times Q = \dfrac{500 \text{ mg/h}}{\underset{8}{4000 \text{ mg}}} \times \overset{1}{500} \text{ mL} = \dfrac{500}{8} \text{ mL/h} = 62.5 \text{ mL/h}$

$= 63 \text{ mL/h}$

9) $\dfrac{D}{H} \times Q = \dfrac{1400 \text{ U/h}}{\underset{40}{20000 \text{ U}}} \times \overset{1}{500} \text{ mL} = \dfrac{1400}{40} \text{ mL/h} = 35 \text{ mL/h}$

10) $1.5\text{L} = 1.5 \times 1000 = 1500 \text{ mL}$

$\dfrac{1500 \text{ mL}}{4 \text{ mL/min}} = 375 \text{ min}$

$375 \text{ min} \div 60 \text{ min/h} = 6.25 = 6\dfrac{1}{4} \text{ h} = 6 \text{ h } 15 \text{ min}$

11) $\dfrac{D}{H} \times Q = \dfrac{4 \text{ mg/min}}{\underset{4}{2000 \text{ mg}}} \times \overset{1}{500} \text{ mL} = \dfrac{4}{4} \text{ mL/min} = 1 \text{ mL/min},$

which is the same as 60 mL/60 min or 60 mL/h

12) $\dfrac{D}{H} \times Q = \dfrac{3 \text{ mg/min}}{\underset{4}{1000 \text{ mg}}} \times \overset{1}{250} \text{ mL} = \dfrac{3}{4} \text{ mL/min} = 0.75 \text{ mL/min}$

$0.75 \text{ mL/min} \times 60 \text{ min/h} = 45 \text{ mL/h}$

13) $\dfrac{D}{H} \times Q = \dfrac{2 \text{ mg/min}}{\underset{2}{1000 \text{ mg}}} \times \overset{1}{500} \text{ mL} = \dfrac{2}{2} \text{ mL/min} = 1 \text{ mL/min},$

which is the same as 60 mL/60 min or 60 mL/h

14) $5 \text{ mcg/kg/min} \times 80 \text{ kg} = 400 \text{ mcg/min}$

$400 \text{ mcg/min} = 400 \div 1000 = 0.4 \text{ mg/min}$

$\dfrac{D}{H} \times Q = \dfrac{0.4 \text{ mg/min}}{\underset{1}{250 \text{ mg}}} \times \overset{1}{250} \text{ mL} = 0.4 \text{ mL/min}$

$0.4 \text{ mL/min} \times 60 \text{ min/h} = 24 \text{ mL/h}$

15) $\dfrac{2000 \text{ mg}}{1000 \text{ mL}} \underset{\diagup\diagup}{\overset{X \text{ mg/h}}{\diagdown\diagdown}} \dfrac{X \text{ mg/h}}{75 \text{ mL/h}}$

$1000\text{X} = 150,000$

$\dfrac{1000\text{X}}{1000} = \dfrac{150,000}{1000}$

$\text{X} = 150 \text{ mg/h}$

$150 \text{ mg/h} \div 60 \text{ min/h} = 2.5 \text{ mg/min},$
within normal range of 1–4 mg/min

16) IV PB flow rate: $\dfrac{\text{mL/h}}{\text{drop factor constant}} = \dfrac{100 \text{ mL/h}}{6} =$

16.6 gtt/min = 17 gtt/min

Total IV PB time: q.6h $\times$ 1 h = 4 $\times$ 1 h = 4 h

Total IV PB volume: 4 $\times$ 100 mL = 400 mL

Total Regular IV volume: 3000 mL – 400 mL =
2600 mL

Total Regular IV time: 24 h – 4 h = 20 h

Regular IV rate: mL/h $= \dfrac{2600 \text{ mL}}{20\text{h}} = 130 \text{ mL/h};$

$\dfrac{\text{mL/h}}{\text{drop factor constant}} = \dfrac{130 \text{ mL/h}}{6} = 21.6 \text{ gtt/min} =$

22 gtt/min

17) IV PB rate:

$\dfrac{50 \text{ mL}}{30 \text{ min}} \underset{\diagup\diagup}{\overset{X \text{ mL}}{\diagdown\diagdown}} \dfrac{X \text{ mL}}{60 \text{ min}}$

$30\text{X} = 3000$

$\dfrac{30\text{X}}{30} = \dfrac{3000}{30}$

$\text{X} = 100 \text{ mL}; 100 \text{ mL}/60 \text{ min} = 100 \text{ mL/h}$

Total IV PB time: q.i.d. $\times$ 30 min = 4 $\times$ 30 min
= 120 min = 120 $\div$ 60 = 2 h

Total IV PB volume: 4 $\times$ 50 mL = 200 mL

Total Regular IV volume: 3000 mL – 200 mL =
2800 mL

Total Regular IV time: 24 h – 2 h = 22 h

Regular IV rate: $\dfrac{2800 \text{ mL}}{22 \text{ h}} = 127.2 \text{ mL/h} = 127 \text{ mL/h}$

18) $125 \text{ lb} = \dfrac{125}{2.2} = 56.81 \text{ kg} = 56.8 \text{ kg}$

$3 \text{ mcg/kg/min} \times 56.8 \text{ kg} = 170.4 \text{ mcg/min}$

$170.4 \text{ mcg/min} = 170.4 \div 1000 = 0.17 \text{ mg/min}$

$\dfrac{D}{H} \times Q = \dfrac{0.17 \text{ mg/min}}{\underset{1}{50 \text{ mg}}} \times \overset{10}{500} \text{ mL} = 1.7 \text{ mL/min}$

$1.7 \text{ mL/min} \times 60 \text{ min/h} = 102 \text{ mL/h}$

19) 1000 mL – 800 mL = 200 mL infused

$\dfrac{40 \text{ mEq}}{1000 \text{ mL}} \underset{\diagup\diagup}{\overset{X \text{ mEq}}{\diagdown\diagdown}} \dfrac{X \text{ mEq}}{200 \text{ mL}}$

$1000\text{X} = 8000$

$\dfrac{1000\text{X}}{1000} = \dfrac{8000}{1000}$

$\text{X} = 8 \text{ mEq}$

20) $\dfrac{125 \text{ mL}}{60 \text{ min}} = 2.1 \text{ mL/min} = 2 \text{ mL/min}$

21) $\dfrac{1500 \text{ mL}}{100 \text{ mL/h}} = 15 \text{ h}$

22)

$\frac{D}{H} \times Q = \frac{2 \text{ mEq/h}}{\underset{1}{40 \text{ mEq}}} \times \overset{25}{1000} \text{ mL} = 50 \text{ mL/h}$ or,

50 gtt/min, (because drop factor is 60 gtt/mL)

23)

$\frac{D}{H} \times Q = \frac{3750 \text{ U/h}}{\underset{50}{50,000 \text{ U}}} \times \overset{1}{1000} \text{ mL} = \frac{3750}{50} \text{ mL/h} = 75 \text{ mL/h};$

75 gtt/min, (because drop factor is 60 gtt/mL)

24)

$\frac{5 \text{ mg}}{1 \text{ mL}} \times \frac{37 \text{ mg}}{X \text{ mL}}$

$5X = 37$

$\frac{5X}{5} = \frac{37}{5}$

$X = 7.4 \text{ mL}$

25) 10 U = 10 × 1000 = 10,000 mU

$\frac{D}{H} \times Q = \frac{4 \text{ mU/min}}{\underset{20}{10,000 \text{ mU}}} \times \overset{1}{500} \text{ mL} = \frac{4}{20} \text{ mL/min} =$

0.2 mL/min (for first 20 min)

0.2 mL/min × 60 min/h = 12 mL/h

$\frac{D}{H} \times Q = \frac{6 \text{ mU/min}}{\underset{20}{10,000 \text{ mU}}} \times \overset{1}{500} \text{ mL} = \frac{6}{20} \text{ mL/min} =$

0.3 mL/min (for next 20 min)

0.3 mL/min × 60 min/h = 18 mL/h

26) Bolus:

$\frac{3 \text{ g}}{30 \text{ min}} \times \frac{X \text{ g}}{60 \text{ min}}$

$\frac{30X}{30} = \frac{180}{30}$

$X = 6 \text{ g}$

6 g/60 min = 6 g/h

$\frac{D}{H} \times Q = \frac{6 \text{ g/h}}{\underset{1}{20 \text{ g}}} \times \overset{25}{500} \text{ mL} = 150 \text{ mL/h}$

Continuous infusion:

$\frac{D}{H} \times Q = \frac{2 \text{ g/h}}{\underset{1}{20 \text{ g}}} \times \overset{25}{500} \text{ mL} = 50 \text{ mL/h}$

29)

$\frac{\overset{8}{4000 \text{ mg}}}{\underset{1}{500 \text{ mL}}} = 8 \text{ mg/mL}$

30)

$\frac{D}{H} \times Q = \frac{500 \text{ mg/h}}{\underset{8}{4000 \text{ mg}}} \times \overset{1}{500} \text{ mL} = \frac{500}{8} \text{ mL/h} = 62.5 \text{ mL/h}$

= 63 mL/h

31) 80 U = 8 × 1000 = 8000 mU

$\frac{\overset{80}{80,000 \text{ mU}}}{\underset{1}{1000 \text{ mL}}} = 80 \text{ mU/mL}$

33) 4 mg = 4 × 1000 = 4000 mcg

$\frac{\overset{4}{4000 \text{ mcg}}}{\underset{1}{1000 \text{ mL}}} = 4 \text{ mcg/mL}$

36)

$\frac{\overset{2}{20 \text{ mg}}}{\underset{10}{100 \text{ mL}}} = \frac{2}{10} \text{ mg/mL} = 0.2 \text{ mg/mL}$

0.2 mg/mL = 0.2 × 1000 = 200 mcg/mL

37) 1 mcg/kg/min × 100 kg = 100 mcg/min

$\frac{D}{H} \times Q = \frac{100 \text{ mcg/min}}{\underset{200}{20,000 \text{ mcg}}} \times \overset{1}{100} \text{ mL} = \frac{100}{200} \text{ mL/min}$

= 0.5 mL/min

0.5 mL/min × 60 min/h = 30 mL/h

38) IV PB rates:

$\frac{100 \text{ mL}}{30 \text{ min}} \times \frac{X \text{ mL}}{60 \text{ min}}$

$30X = 6000$

$\frac{30X}{30} = \frac{6000}{30}$

$X = 200 \text{ mL (per 60 min)}$

200 mL/60 min = 200 mL/h (ampicillin)

gentamycin: 50 mL/h

39) ampicillin: q.6h × 30 min = 4 × 30 min = 120 min

= 120 ÷ 60 = 2 h

gentamycin: q.8 h × 1 h = 3 × 1 h = 3 h

Total IV PB time: 2 h + 3 h = 5 h

40) ampicillin: 4 doses × 100 mL/dose = 400 mL
gentamycin: 3 doses × 50 mL/dose = 150 mL

Total IV PB volume: 400 mL + 150 mL = 550 mL

41) 3000 mL − 550 mL = 2450 mL

42) 24 h − 5 h = 19 h

43) $\frac{2450 \text{ mL}}{19 \text{ h}} = 128.9 \text{ mL/h} = 129 \text{ mL/h}$

44) $190 \text{ lb} = \dfrac{190}{2.2} = 86.36 \text{ kg} = 86.4 \text{ kg}$

$4 \text{ mcg/kg/min} \times 86.4 \text{ kg} = 345.6 \text{ mcg/min}$

$345.6 \text{ mcg/min} \times 60 \text{ min/h} = 20{,}736 \text{ mcg/h} =$

$20{,}736 \text{ mcg/h} = 20{,}736 \div 1000 = 20.736 \text{ mg/h} = 21 \text{ mg/h}$

$\dfrac{\text{D}}{\text{H}} \times \text{Q} = \dfrac{21 \text{ mg/h}}{\underset{8}{800 \text{ mg}}} \times \overset{5}{500} \text{ mL} = \dfrac{105}{8} \text{ mL/h} =$

$13.1 \text{ mL/h} = 13 \text{ mL/h (initial rate)}$

$12 \text{ mcg/kg/min} \times 86.4 \text{ kg} = 1036.8 \text{ mcg/min}$

$1036.8 \text{ mcg/min} \times 60 \text{ min/h} = 62{,}208 \text{ mcg/h}$

$62{,}208 \text{ mcg/h} = 62{,}208 \div 1000 = 62 \text{ mg/h}$

$\dfrac{\text{D}}{\text{H}} \times \text{Q} = \dfrac{62 \text{ mg/h}}{\underset{8}{800 \text{ mg}}} \times \overset{5}{500} \text{ mL} = \dfrac{310}{8} \text{ mL/h} =$

$38.7 \text{ mL/h} = 39 \text{ mL/h (after titration)}$

45) $225 \text{ lb} = \dfrac{225}{2.2} = 102.2 \text{ kg} = 100 \text{ kg (rounded)}$

$80 \text{ U/kg bolus dosage}$

46) $80 \text{ U/kg} \times 100 \text{ kg} = 8000 \text{ U}$

1000 U/mL

$\dfrac{\text{D}}{\text{H}} \times \text{Q} = \dfrac{8000 \text{ U}}{1000 \text{ U}} \times 1 \text{ mL} = 8 \text{ mL}$

47) 18 U/kg/h

$18 \text{ U/kg/h} \times 100 \text{ kg} = 1800 \text{ U/h}$

$25{,}000 \text{ U/250 mL or } 100 \text{ U/mL}$

$\dfrac{\text{D}}{\text{H}} \times \text{Q} = \dfrac{1800 \text{ U/h}}{100 \text{ U}} \times 1 \text{ mL} = 18 \text{ mL/h}$

48) q.6h

$40 \text{ U/kg} \times 100 \text{ kg} = 4000 \text{ U}$

$\dfrac{4000 \text{ U}}{1000 \text{ U}} \times 1 \text{ mL} = 4 \text{ mL}$

Increase rate: $2 \text{ U/kg/h} \times 100 \text{ kg} = 200 \text{ U/h}$

Increase rate: $\dfrac{\overset{2}{200 \text{ U/h}}}{\underset{1}{100 \text{ U}}} \times 1 \text{ mL} = 2 \text{ mL/h}$

$18 \text{ mL/h} + 2 \text{ mL/h} = 20 \text{ mL/h (new infusion rate)}$

49) Decrease rate by 2 U/kg/h.

$2 \text{ U/kg/h} \times 100 \text{ kg} = 200 \text{ U/h}$

$\dfrac{200 \text{ U/h}}{100 \text{ U}} \times 1 \text{ mL} = 2 \text{ mL/h}$

$20 \text{ mL/h} - 2 \text{ mL/h} = 18 \text{ mL/h (new infusion rate)}$

Section 4—Self-Evaluation from pages 430–433

1) 0.9% NaCl 2) 0.9 g NaCl/100mL 3) 0.45 g NaCl/100 mL 4) 50 5) 3.3 6) 2.25 7) 75 8) 6.75 9) mL/h 10) 21 11) 83 12) 1940 13) 1536 14) Give a total of 3000 mL IV solution per day to include 5% normal saline (0.9% NaCl) with 20 milliequivalents of potassium chloride added per liter (1000 mL) *and* a piggyback IV solution of 250 mg Kefzol added to 100 mL of normal saline (0.9% NaCl) every 8 hours. To administer the order each day, give 900 mL NS with KCl over $7\frac{1}{2}$ hours $\times$ 3 administrations and 100 mL NS with Kefzol over $\frac{1}{2}$ hour $\times$ 3 administrations, q.8h 15) 120 16) 200 17) Reset rate to 118 gtt/min, if policy and patient's condition permit. 18) 2.5 19) 1410 20) 59 21) 120 22) 5 23) 0.48 24) 1.30 25) 0.5 26) 18.5–37.5 27) Yes 28) 18.5 29) 37 mL 30) 120 31) 18.5 32) 0.8 33) 1.6 34) Yes 35) 1.6 36) 18; 2 37) 7.5 38) 43 39) 200 40) 43 41) 200 42) 50 43) 12 44) 15 45) 0.13 46) 8 47) 80 48) 20 49) 61 50) 38

Solutions—Section 4—Self-Evaluation

4) $\text{D}_5\ 0.33\%\ \text{NaCl} = 5\%\ \text{dextrose} =$

5 g dextrose/100 mL

$\dfrac{5 \text{ g}}{100 \text{ mL}} \overset{\nwarrow\nearrow}{\underset{\swarrow\searrow}{}} \dfrac{X \text{ g}}{1000 \text{ mL}}$

$100X = 5000$

$\dfrac{100X}{100} = \dfrac{5000}{100}$

$X = 50 \text{ g}$

5) $\text{D}_5\ 0.33\%\ \text{NaCl} = 0.33\%\ \text{NaCl} =$

0.33 g NaCl/100 mL

$\dfrac{0.33 \text{ g}}{100 \text{ mL}} \overset{\nwarrow\nearrow}{\underset{\swarrow\searrow}{}} \dfrac{X \text{ g}}{1000 \text{ mL}}$

$100X = 3300$

$\dfrac{100X}{100} = \dfrac{3300}{100}$

$X = 3.3 \text{ g}$

10) $\dfrac{2000 \text{ mL}}{24 \text{ h}} = 83.3 \text{ mL/h} = 83 \text{ mL/h}$

$\dfrac{\text{mL/h}}{\text{drop factor constant}} = \text{gtt/min}$

$\dfrac{83 \text{ mL/h}}{4} = 20.7 \text{ gtt/min} = 21 \text{ gtt/min}$

12) $\frac{V}{T} \times C = R: \frac{400 \text{ mL}}{T \text{ min}} \times 15 \text{ gtt/mL} = 24 \text{ gtt/min}$

$\frac{400}{T} \times 15 = 24$

$\frac{6000}{T} \underset{\diagdown}{\overset{\diagup}{\times}} \frac{24}{1}$

$24T = 6000$

$\frac{24T}{24} = \frac{6000}{24}$

$T = 250 \text{ min}$

$250 \text{ min} = 250 \div 60 = 4\frac{1}{6} \text{ h} = 4 \text{ h } 10 \text{ min}$

$\begin{array}{r} 1530 \text{ hours} \\ + 410 \text{ hours} \\ \hline 1940 \text{ hours} \end{array}$

13) $\frac{V}{T} \times C = R: \frac{V \text{ ml}}{60 \text{ min}} \times 10 \text{ gtt/mL} = 32 \text{ gtt/min}$

$\frac{10V}{60} \underset{\diagdown}{\overset{\diagup}{\times}} \frac{32}{1}$

$10V = 1920$

$\frac{10V}{10} = \frac{1920}{10}$

$V = 192 \text{ mL/h}; \ 192 \text{ mL/h} \times 8 \text{ h} = 1536 \text{ mL}$
(administered during your 8 h shift)

15) $\frac{2700 \text{ mL}}{22 \text{ h}} = 120 \text{ mL/h}$

16) $\frac{100 \text{ mL}}{30 \text{ min}} \underset{\diagdown}{\overset{\diagup}{\times}} \frac{X \text{ mL}}{60 \text{ min}}$

$30X = 6000$

$\frac{30X}{30} = \frac{6000}{30}$

$X = 200 \text{ mL}$

$200 \text{ mL/60 min} = 200 \text{ mL/h}$

17) $\frac{1200 \text{ mL}}{100 \text{ mL/h}} = 12 \text{ h}$ (total time ordered to infuse 1200 mL)

$\begin{array}{r} 2200 \text{ hours (current time)} \\ - 1530 \text{ hours (start time)} \\ \hline 0630 \ = 6 \text{ h } 30 \text{ min (elapsed time)} \end{array}$

$6\frac{1}{2} \text{ h} \times 100 \text{ mL/h} = 650 \text{ mL}$

After $6\frac{1}{2}$ h, 650 mL should have been infused, with 550 mL remaining. IV is behind schedule.

1200 mL − 650 mL = 550 mL (should be remaining)

$\frac{\text{remaining volume}}{\text{remaining time}} = \frac{650 \text{ mL}}{5.5 \text{ h}} = 118 \text{ mL/h}$ (adjusted rate)

$\frac{\text{Adjusted gtt/min − Ordered gtt/min}}{\text{Ordered gtt/min}} = \% \text{ of variation};$

$\frac{118 - 100}{100} = \frac{18}{100} = 0.18 = 18\%$ (variance is safe)

If policy and patient's condition permit, reset rate to 118 mL/h.

18) $\frac{20 \text{ mEq}}{1000 \text{ mL}} \underset{\diagdown}{\overset{\diagup}{\times}} \frac{X \text{ mEq}}{250 \text{ mL}}$

$1000X = 5000$

$\frac{1000X}{1000} = \frac{5000}{1000}$

$X = 5 \text{ mEq}$

$\frac{D}{H} \times Q = \frac{5 \text{ mEq}}{2 \text{ mEq}} \times 1 \text{ mL} = \frac{5}{2} \text{ mL} = 2.5 \text{ mL}$

19) $40 \text{ lb} = \frac{40}{2.2} = 18.18 \text{ kg} = 18.2 \text{ kg}$

1st 10 kg: $100 \text{ mL/kg/day} \times 10 \text{ kg} = \qquad 1000 \text{ mL/day}$

Remaining 8.2 kg: $50 \text{ mL/kg/day} \times 8.2 \text{ kg} = \underline{410 \text{ mL/day}}$
$\qquad\qquad\qquad\qquad\qquad\qquad\qquad\qquad 1410 \text{ mL/day}$

20) $\frac{1410 \text{ mL}}{24 \text{ h}} = 58.7 \text{ mL/h} = 59 \text{ mL/h}$

21) $1185 \text{ g} = 1185 \div 1000 = 1.185 \text{ kg} = 1.2 \text{ kg}$

1st 10 kg: $100 \text{ mL/kg/day} \times 1.2 \text{ kg} = 120 \text{ mL/day}$

22) $\frac{120 \text{ mL}}{24 \text{ h}} = 5 \text{ mL/h}$

23) Household:

$\text{BSA (m}^2) = \sqrt{\frac{\text{ht (in)} \times \text{wt (lb)}}{3131}} = \sqrt{\frac{30 \times 24}{3131}} = \sqrt{\frac{720}{3131}} = \sqrt{0.229} = 0.479 \text{ m}^2 = 0.48 \text{ m}^2$

24) Metric:

$\text{BSA (m}^2) = \sqrt{\frac{\text{ht (cm)} \times \text{wt (kg)}}{3600}} = \sqrt{\frac{155 \times 39}{3600}} = \sqrt{\frac{6045}{3600}} = \sqrt{1.679} = 1.295 \text{ m}^2 = 1.30 \text{ m}^2$

26) Minimum safe dosage: $37 \text{ mg/m}^2 \times 0.5 \text{ m}^2 = 18.5 \text{ mg}$

Maximum safe dosage: $75 \text{ mg/m}^2 \times 0.5 \text{ m}^2 = 37.5 \text{ mg}$

28) $\frac{D}{H} \times Q = \frac{18.5 \text{ mg}}{1 \text{ mg}} \times 1 \text{ mL} = 18.5 \text{ mL}$

29) $2 \text{ mL/mg} \times 18.5 \text{ mg} = 37 \text{ mL}$

30) $\frac{D}{H} \times Q = \frac{1 \text{ mg/min}}{18.5 \text{ mg}} \times 37 \text{ mL} = 2 \text{ mL/min}$

$2 \text{ mL/min} \times 60 \text{ min/h} = 120 \text{ mL/h}$

31) At 1 mg/min, 18.5 mg will infuse in 18.5 min.

$\frac{1 \text{ mg}}{1 \text{ min}} \underset{\diagdown}{\overset{\diagup}{\times}} \frac{18.5 \text{ mg}}{X \text{ min}}$

$X = 18.5 \text{ min}$

33) $2 \text{ mg/m}^2 \times 0.8 \text{ m}^2 = 1.6 \text{ mg}$

36) $\frac{D}{H} \times Q = \frac{\overset{2}{250 \text{ mg}}}{\underset{1}{125 \text{ mg}}} \times 1 \text{ mL} = 2 \text{ mL (Ancef)}$

$\frac{40 \text{ mL}}{60 \text{ min}} \underset{\diagdown}{\overset{\diagup}{=}} \frac{X \text{ mL}}{30 \text{ min}}$

$60X = 1200$

$\frac{60X}{60} = \frac{1200}{60}$

$X = 20 \text{ mL}$

20 mL (total IV solution) − 2 mL (Ancef) = 18 mL (NS)

37)

$$\frac{100 \text{ mg}}{1 \text{ mL}} \diagdown\diagup \frac{750 \text{ mg}}{X \text{ mL}}$$

$$100X = 750$$

$$\frac{100X}{100} = \frac{750}{100}$$

$$X = 7.5 \text{ mL}$$

7.5 mL IV solution to be used with the 750 mg of ticarcillin for minimal dilution.

38) Total IV PB volume: 100 mL × 6 = 600 mL

Regular IV volume: 1500 mL – 600 mL = 900 mL

Total IV PB time of q.4h × 30 min: 6 × 30 min = 180 min = 180 ÷ 60 = 3 h

Total Regular IV time: 24 h – 3 h = 21 h

Regular IV rate: mL/h = $\frac{900 \text{ mL}}{21 \text{ h}}$ = 42.8 mL/h = 43 mL/h

or 43 gtt/min because mL/h = gtt/min when drop factor is 60 gtt/mL.

$\frac{\text{mL/h}}{\text{drop factor constant}}$ = gtt/min; $\frac{43 \text{ mL/h}}{1}$ = 43 gtt/min

39)

$$\frac{100 \text{ mL}}{30 \text{ min}} \diagdown\diagup \frac{X \text{ mL}}{60 \text{ min}}$$

$$30X = 6000$$

$$\frac{30X}{30} = \frac{6000}{30}$$

X = 200 mL; 200 mL/60 min = 200 mL/h or 200 gtt/min (because drop factor is 60 gtt/mL)

40) See #38, Regular IV rate calculated at 42.8 mL/h or 43 mL/h.

41) See #39, IVPB rate calculated at 200 mL/h.

42) $\frac{\text{D}}{\text{H}} \times Q = \frac{\overset{1}{\cancel{2 \text{ mEq/h}}}}{\underset{20}{\cancel{40 \text{ mEq}}}} \times 1000 \text{ mL} = 50 \text{ mL/h}$

43) $\frac{25 \text{ mg}}{1 \text{ L}} = \frac{25.000.}{1.000.} = \frac{25,000 \text{ mcg}}{1000 \text{ mL}} = \frac{25,000 \text{ mcg}}{1000 \text{ mL}} = 25 \text{ mcg/mL}$

$\frac{\text{D}}{\text{H}} \times Q = \frac{\overset{}{\cancel{3 \text{ mcg/min}}}}{\underset{5}{\cancel{25 \text{ mcg}}}} \times 1 \text{ mL} = \frac{1}{5} \text{ mL/min} = 0.2 \text{ mL/min}$

0.2 mL/min × 60 min/h = 12 mL/h

44) $\frac{15 \text{ U}}{1 \text{ L}} = \frac{15.000.}{1.000.} = \frac{15,000 \text{ mU}}{1000 \text{ mL}} = 15 \text{ mU/mL}$

45) $\frac{\text{D}}{\text{H}} \times Q = \frac{2 \text{ mU/min}}{15 \text{ mU}} \times 1 \text{ mL} = \frac{2}{15} \text{ mL/min} = 0.13 \text{ mL/min}$

46) 0.13 mL/min × 60 min/h = 7.8 = 8 mL/h

47) $\frac{\overset{4}{\cancel{20 \text{ mU/min}}}}{\underset{3}{\cancel{15 \text{ mU}}}} \times 1 \text{ mL} = \frac{4}{3} \text{ mL/min} = 1.33 \text{ mL/min}$

1.33 mL/min × 60 min/h = 80 mL/h

48) 150 lb = $\frac{150}{2.2}$ = 68.18 kg = 68.2 kg;

4 mcg/kg/min × 68.2 kg = 272.8 = 273 mcg/min

273 mcg/min × 60 min/h = 16,380 mcg/h

0.5 L = 0.5 × 1000 = 500 mL

$\frac{400 \text{ mg}}{0.5 \text{ L}} = \frac{400 \text{ mg}}{500 \text{ mL}}$

= 0.8 mg/mL

0.8 mg/mL = 0.8 × 1000 = 800 mcg/mL

$\frac{\text{D}}{\text{H}} \times Q = \frac{16,380 \text{ mcg/h}}{800 \text{ mcg}} \times 1 \text{ mL} = 20.47 \text{ mL/h} = 20 \text{ mL/h}$

49) 12 mcg/kg/min × 68.2 kg = 818.4 mcg/min = 818 mcg/min

818 mcg/min × 60 min/h = 49,080 mcg/h

$\frac{\text{D}}{\text{H}} \times Q = \frac{49,080 \text{ mcg/h}}{800 \text{ mcg}} \times 1 \text{ mL} = 61.4 \text{ mL/h} = 61 \text{ mL/h}$

50) $\frac{\text{D}}{\text{H}} \times Q = \frac{750 \text{ U/h}}{\underset{20}{\cancel{10,000 \text{ U}}}} \times \overset{1}{\cancel{500}} \text{ mL} = \frac{750}{20} \text{ mL/h} =$

37.5 mL/h = 38 mL/h

Essential Skills Evaluation from pages 435–448

1)   0.5

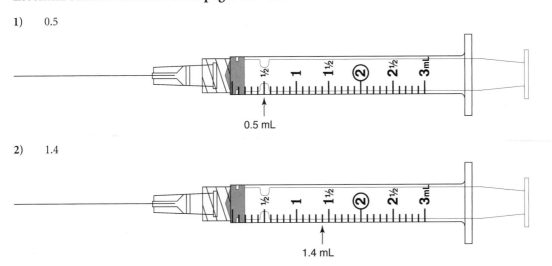

0.5 mL

2)   1.4

1.4 mL

3)   1, 1, 0.25

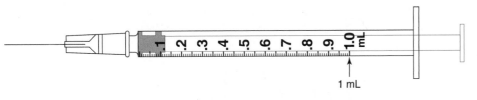

1 mL

4)   1

1 mL

5) $1\frac{1}{2}$
6)   0.5

0.5 mL

7) $\frac{1}{2}$
8)   1.4

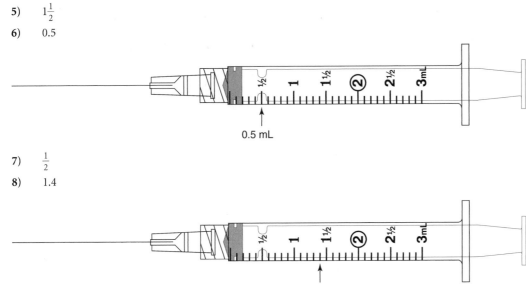

1.4 mL

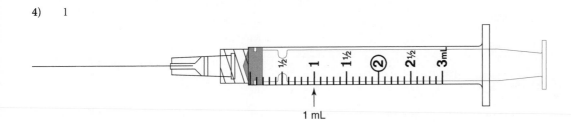

9)   68

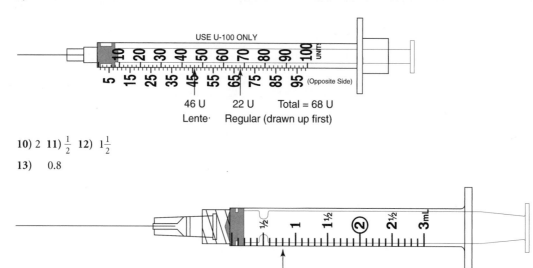

46 U   22 U   Total = 68 U
Lente·   Regular (drawn up first)

10) 2 **11)** $\frac{1}{2}$ **12)** $1\frac{1}{2}$

13)   0.8

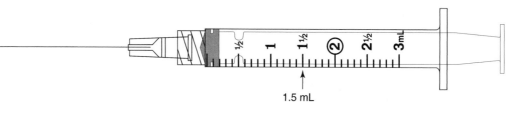

0.8 mL

14)   1.5

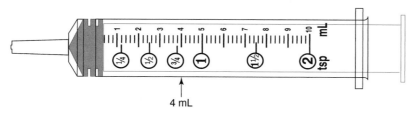

1.5 mL

15)   4

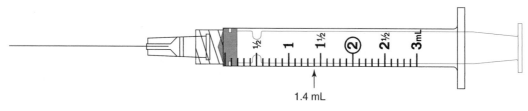

4 mL

16)   1.5

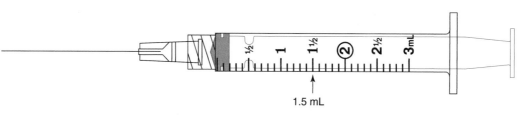

1.5 mL

17)   1.4; 75

1.4 mL

18) Yes. Her temperature is 102.2°F. Tylenol is indicated for fever > 101°F every 4 hours. It has been 5 hours and
5 minutes since her last dose.

19) 2 20) $\frac{1}{2}$ (one half)

21) Benadryl; 0.7

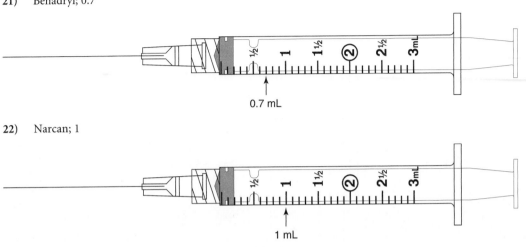

0.7 mL

22) Narcan; 1

1 mL

23) 18.8; 138 24) 138 25) 8; 2 26) 1; 0745, 1145, 1745, 2200

27) 18; subcutaneous

USE U-100 ONLY

18 U

28) 12 29) Yes. The usual dosage is 20–40 mg/kg/day divided into 3 doses q.8h, which is equivalent to 45–91 mg per dose
for a 15 lb (6.8 kg) child. 30) 1 31) $\frac{1}{2}$ dropperful to the 1 mL line; every 8 hours 32) 250–500; Yes; 1.7; 25 33) 1000

34) Yes 35) 4.8; dosage is safe 36) 38 37) 280–420 38) 13 39) 30; No 40) Do not administer; consult with physician
before giving drug. 41) 1 42) 50; 5 43) 30 44) 2030; 8:30 PM 45) 200 46) 10 47) 2000/10 48) 2.5

49)
> *1/30/XX, 1400, reconstituted as*
> *2 g/10mL. Expires 2/6/XX, 1400.*
> *Keep refrigerated. G.D.P.*

50) The importance of checking a medication label at least three times to verify supply dosage cannot be overemphasized.
It is also important NEVER to assume that the supply dosage is the same as a supply dosage used to calculate
previously. Always read the label carefully. Writing the calculation down will also help improve accuracy.

Solutions—Essential Skills Evaluation

1) $\dfrac{D}{H} \times Q = \dfrac{12.5 \text{ mg}}{25 \text{ mg}} \times 1 \text{ mL} = 0.5 \text{ mL}$

2) $\dfrac{D}{H} \times Q = \dfrac{\overset{7}{\cancel{35}} \text{ mg}}{\underset{5}{\cancel{25}} \text{ mg}} \times 1 \text{ mL} = \dfrac{7}{5} \text{ mL} = 1.4 \text{ mL}$

3) $\dfrac{D}{H} \times Q = \dfrac{50 \text{ mg}}{\dfrac{250 \text{ mg}}{50}} \times \overset{1}{\cancel{5}} \text{ mL} = \dfrac{\overset{1}{\cancel{50}}}{\underset{1}{\cancel{50}}} \times 1 \text{ mL} = 1 \text{ mL}$

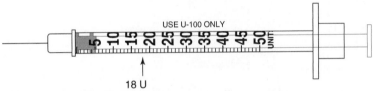

$$\dfrac{1 \text{ mL}}{60 \text{ sec}} \diagdown = \diagup \dfrac{X \text{ mL}}{15 \text{ sec}}$$

$$60X = 15$$

$$\dfrac{60X}{60} = \dfrac{15}{60}$$

$$X = 0.25 \text{ mL (per 15 sec)}$$

Note: 1 mL syringe is a better choice because
measurement of 0.25 mL increments is clearly visible.

4) $0.4 \text{ mg} = 0.4 \times 1000 = 400 \text{ mcg}$

$$\frac{D}{H} \times Q = \frac{\overset{200}{\cancel{200 \text{ mcg}}}}{\underset{200}{\cancel{400 \text{ mcg}}}} \times \overset{1}{\cancel{2}} \text{ mL} = \frac{\overset{1}{\cancel{200}}}{\underset{1}{\cancel{200}}} \times 1 \text{ mL} = 1 \text{ mL}$$

5) $\frac{D}{H} \times Q = \frac{7.5 \text{ mg}}{5 \text{ mg}} \times 1 \text{ tab} = 1.5 \text{ tab} = 1\frac{1}{2} \text{ tab}$

6) $0.125 \text{ mg} = 0.125 \times 1000 = 125 \text{ mcg}$

$$\frac{D}{H} \times Q = \frac{125 \text{ mcg}}{\underset{250}{\cancel{500 \text{ mcg}}}} \times \overset{1}{\cancel{2}} \text{ mL} = \frac{125}{\underset{2}{\cancel{250}}} \times 1 \text{ mL} = 0.5 \text{ mL}$$

7) $\text{gr } \frac{1}{8} = \frac{1}{8} \times \frac{60}{1} = \frac{60}{8} \text{ mg} = 7.5 \text{ mg}$

$$\frac{D}{H} \times Q = \frac{7.5 \text{ mg}}{15 \text{ mg}} \times 1 \text{ tab} = 0.5 \text{ tab} = \frac{1}{2} \text{ tab}$$

8) $\frac{D}{H} \times Q = \frac{\overset{7}{\cancel{350 \text{ mg}}}}{\underset{10}{\cancel{500 \text{ mg}}}} \times 2 \text{ mL} = \frac{14}{10} \text{ mL} = 1.4 \text{ mL}$

9) $46 \text{ U} + 22 \text{ U} = 68 \text{ U (total)}$

10) $0.3 \text{ mg} = 0.3 \times 1000 = 300 \text{ mcg}$

$$\frac{D}{H} \times Q = \frac{\overset{2}{\cancel{300 \text{ mcg}}}}{\underset{1}{\cancel{150 \text{ mcg}}}} \times 1 \text{ tab} = 2 \text{ tab}$$

11) $\frac{D}{H} \times Q = \frac{\overset{1}{\cancel{40 \text{ mg}}}}{\underset{2}{\cancel{80 \text{ mg}}}} \times 1 \text{ tab} = \frac{1}{2} \text{ tab}$

12) $\frac{D}{H} \times Q = \frac{\overset{3}{\cancel{375 \text{ mg}}}}{\underset{2}{\cancel{250 \text{ mg}}}} \times 1 \text{ tab} = \frac{3}{2} \text{ tab} = 1\frac{1}{2} \text{ tab}$

13) $\frac{D}{H} \times Q = \frac{\overset{4}{\cancel{40 \text{ mg}}}}{\underset{5}{\cancel{50 \text{ mg}}}} \times 1 \text{ mL} = \frac{4}{5} \text{ mL} = 0.8 \text{ mL}$

14) $\frac{D}{H} \times Q = \frac{3 \text{ mg}}{2 \text{ mg}} \times 1 \text{ mL} = \frac{3}{2} \text{ mL} = 1.5 \text{ mL}$

You will need 2 vials of the drug, because each vial contains 1 mL.

15) $\frac{D}{H} \times Q = \frac{\overset{4}{\cancel{100 \text{ mg}}}}{\underset{5}{\cancel{125 \text{ mg}}}} \times 5 \text{ mL} = \frac{4}{\cancel{5}} \times \overset{1}{\cancel{5}} \text{ mL} = 4 \text{ mL}$

16) $\text{gr } \frac{1}{100} = \frac{1}{100} \times \frac{60}{1} = \frac{60}{100} = \frac{6}{10} \text{ mg} = 0.6 \text{ mg}$

$$\frac{D}{H} \times Q = \frac{\overset{3}{\cancel{0.6 \text{ mg}}}}{\underset{2}{\cancel{0.4 \text{ mg}}}} \times 1 \text{ mL} = \frac{3}{2} \text{ mL} = 1.5 \text{ mL}$$

17) $\frac{D}{H} \times Q = \frac{\underset{25}{35 \text{ mg}}}{\underset{}{50 \text{ mg}}} \times \overset{1}{\cancel{2}} \text{ mL} = \frac{\overset{7}{\cancel{35}}}{\underset{5}{\cancel{25}}} \times 1 \text{ mL} = \frac{7}{5} \text{ mL} = 1.4 \text{ mL}$

$$\frac{V}{T} \times C = \frac{\overset{5}{\cancel{100 \text{ mL}}}}{\underset{1}{\cancel{20 \text{ min}}}} \times 15 \text{ gtt/mL} = 75 \text{ gtt/min}$$

18) $^\circ F = 1.8^\circ C + 32 = (1.8 \times 39) + 32 = 70.2 + 32 = 102.2^\circ F$

$102.2^\circ F > 101^\circ F; 2400 - 2110 = 0250 \text{ or } 2 \text{ h } 50 \text{ min};$
$0215 = 2 \text{ h } 15 \text{ min after } 2400; 2 \text{ h } 50 \text{ min } + 2 \text{ h } 15 \text{ min } = 5 \text{ h } 5 \text{ min}$

19) $\frac{D}{H} \times Q = \frac{\overset{2}{\cancel{650 \text{ mg}}}}{\underset{1}{\cancel{325 \text{ mg}}}} \times 1 \text{ tab} = 2 \text{ tab}$

20) $\frac{\overset{1}{\cancel{30 \text{ mg}}}}{\underset{2}{\cancel{60 \text{ mg}}}} = \frac{1}{2} \text{ (one half)}$

21) $\frac{D}{H} \times Q = \frac{\overset{7}{\cancel{35 \text{ mg}}}}{\underset{10}{\cancel{50 \text{ mg}}}} \times 1 \text{ mL} = \frac{7}{10} \text{ mL} = 0.7 \text{ mL}$

22) $\frac{D}{H} \times Q = \frac{\cancel{0.4 \text{ mg}}}{\cancel{0.4 \text{ mg}}} \times 1 \text{ mL} = 1 \text{ mL}$

23) $\frac{D}{H} \times Q = \frac{100 \text{ mg}}{\underset{16}{\cancel{80 \text{ mg}}}} \times \overset{3}{\cancel{15}} \text{ mL} = \frac{300}{16} \text{ mL} = 18.75 \text{ mL} = 18.8 \text{ mL}$

$50 \text{ mL} + 18.8 \text{ mL} = 68.8 \text{ mL}$

$$\frac{V}{T} \times C = \frac{68.8 \text{ mL}}{\underset{1}{\cancel{30 \text{ min}}}} \times \overset{2}{\cancel{60}} \text{ gtt/mL} = 137.6 \text{ gtt/min}$$

$= 138 \text{ gtt/min}$

24) $138 \text{ gtt/min} = 138 \text{ mL/h, because gtt/min} = \text{mL/h}$ when drop factor is 60 gtt/mL

25) $\frac{D}{H} \times Q = \frac{\overset{2}{\cancel{125 \text{ mg}}}}{\underset{1}{\cancel{62.5 \text{ mg}}}} \times 1 \text{ mL} = 2 \text{ mL}$

26) $\frac{D}{H} \times Q = \frac{\cancel{1 \text{ g}}}{\cancel{1 \text{ g}}} \times 1 \text{ tab} = 1 \text{ tab}$

29) $15 \text{ lb} = \frac{15}{2.2} = 6.81 \text{ kg} = 6.8 \text{ kg}$

Minimum dosage: $20 \text{ mg/kg/day} \times 6.8 \text{ kg} = 136 \text{ mg/day}$

$\frac{136 \text{ mg}}{3 \text{ doses}} = 45.3 \text{ mg/dose} = 45 \text{ mg/dose}$

Maximum dosage: $40 \text{ mg/kg/day} \times 6.8 \text{ kg} = 272 \text{ mg/day}$

$\frac{272 \text{ mg}}{3 \text{ doses}} = 90.6 \text{ mg/dose} = 91 \text{ mg/dose}$

30) $\frac{D}{H} \times Q = \frac{\cancel{50 \text{ mg}}}{\cancel{50 \text{ mg}}} \times 1 \text{ mL} = 1 \text{ mL}$

/22.2

32) $110 \text{ lb} = \frac{110}{2.2} = 50 \text{ kg}$

Minimum dosage: $20 \text{ mg/kg/day} \times 50 \text{ kg} = 1000 \text{ mg/day}$

$\frac{1000 \text{ mg}}{4 \text{ doses}} = 250 \text{ mg/dose}$

Maximum dosage: $40 \text{ mg/kg/day} \times 50 \text{ kg} = 2000 \text{ mg/day}$

$\frac{2000 \text{ mg}}{4 \text{ doses}} = 500 \text{ mg/dose}$

$\frac{D}{H} \times Q = \frac{\overset{5}{\cancel{250}} \text{ mg}}{\underset{6}{\cancel{300}} \text{ mg}} \times 2 \text{ mL} = \frac{\overset{5}{\cancel{10}}}{\cancel{6}} \text{ mL} = \frac{5}{3} \text{ mL} = 1.66 \text{ mL} = 1.7 \text{ mL}$

$\frac{V}{T} \times C = \frac{50 \text{ mL}}{\underset{2}{\cancel{20}} \text{ min}} \times \overset{1}{\cancel{10}} \text{ gtt/mL} = \frac{50 \text{ gtt}}{2 \text{ min}} = 25 \text{ gtt/min}$

33)
IV fluid =		200 mL
gelatin = ℥ iv = 4 × 30 =		120 mL
water = ℥ iii × 2 = (3 × 30) × 2 = 90 × 2 =		180 mL
apple juice = pt i =		500 mL
Total =		1000 mL

34) $40 \text{ lb} = \frac{40}{2.2} = 18.18 \text{ kg} = 18.2 \text{ kg}$

$40 \text{ mg/kg/day} \times 18.2 \text{ kg} = 728 \text{ mg/day}$

$\frac{728 \text{ mg}}{3 \text{ doses}} = 242.6 \text{ mg} = 243 \text{ mg}$; close approximation to ordered dosage of 240 mg; dosage is safe.

35) $\frac{D}{H} \times Q = \frac{240 \text{ mg}}{\underset{50}{\cancel{250}} \text{ mg}} \times \overset{1}{\cancel{5}} \text{ mL} = \frac{240}{50} \text{ mL} = 4.8 \text{ mL}$

36) $\text{mL/h} = \frac{\overset{150}{\cancel{600}} \text{ mL}}{\underset{1}{\cancel{4}} \text{ h}} = 150 \text{ mL/h}$

$\frac{V}{T} \times C = \frac{150 \text{ mL}}{\underset{4}{\cancel{60}} \text{ min}} \times \overset{1}{\cancel{15}} \text{ gtt/mL} = \frac{150 \text{ gtt}}{4 \text{ min}} = 37.5 \text{ gtt/min}$

$= 38 \text{ gtt/min}$

37) $61 \text{ lb } 8 \text{ oz} = 61.5 \text{ lb} = \frac{61.5}{2.2} = 27.95 \text{ kg} = 28 \text{ kg}$

Minimum dosage: $10 \text{ mg/kg} \times 28 \text{ kg} = 280 \text{ mg}$

Maximum dosage: $15 \text{ mg/kg} \times 28 \text{ kg} = 420 \text{ mg}$

38) $\frac{D}{H} \times Q = \frac{420 \text{ mg}}{80 \text{ mg}} \times 2.5 \text{ mL} = \frac{105}{8} \text{ mL}$

$= 13.1 \text{ mL} = 13 \text{ mL}$

39) $52 \text{ lb} = \frac{52}{2.2} = 23.63 \text{ kg} = 23.6 \text{ kg}$

$5 \text{ mg/kg/day} \times 23.6 \text{ kg} = 118 \text{ mg/day}$

$\frac{118 \text{ mg}}{4 \text{ doses}} = 29.5 \text{ mg/dose} = 30 \text{ mg/dose}$; dosage is too low to be therapeutic and is not safe.

41) $\frac{D}{H} \times Q = \frac{10 \text{ mg}}{\underset{10}{\cancel{300}} \text{ mg}} \times \overset{1}{\cancel{30}} \text{ mL} = \frac{\overset{1}{\cancel{10}}}{\underset{1}{\cancel{10}}} \text{ mL} = 1 \text{ mL}$

42) $10 \text{ mg/dose} \times 5 \text{ doses} = 50 \text{ mg}$

$1 \text{ mL/dose} \times 5 \text{ doses} = 5 \text{ mL}$

43) $\frac{\frac{\overset{30}{\cancel{300}} \text{ mg}}{\underset{1}{\cancel{10}} \text{ mg/dose}}}{} = 30 \text{ doses}$

44) $\frac{30 \text{ doses}}{5 \text{ doses/h}} = 6 \text{ h}$

$\begin{array}{r} 1430 \text{ h} \\ + 600 \text{ h} \\ \hline 2030 \text{ h} \end{array} \qquad \begin{array}{r} 2030 \\ - 1200 \\ \hline 8:30 \text{ PM} \end{array}$

45) $\frac{100 \text{ mL}}{30 \text{ min}} \,\diagdown\!\!\!\!\diagup\, \frac{X \text{ mL}}{60 \text{ min}}$

$30X = 6000$

$\frac{30X}{30} = \frac{6000}{30}$

$X = 200 \text{ mL}$

$200 \text{ mL/60 min} = 200 \text{ mL/h}$

Comprehensive Skills Evaluation from pages 449–462

1) 2 2) Sublingual. The medication is to be administered under the tongue. 3) 2; 2; 0.5 4) 1

5)   1; 1; 0.25

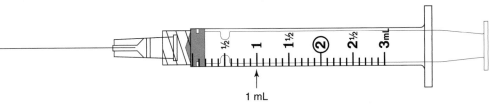

1 mL

6) $\frac{1}{2}$ 7) 80

8)   5

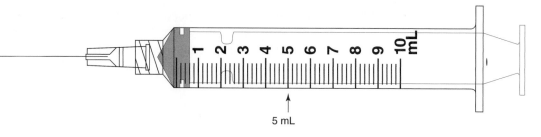

5 mL

9) 0.8 **10)** 1920 **11)** 0500; 9/4/XX **12)** 2 **13)** 80 **14)** all: nitroglycerin, furosemide, digoxin, KCl, and acetaminophen

15)   5

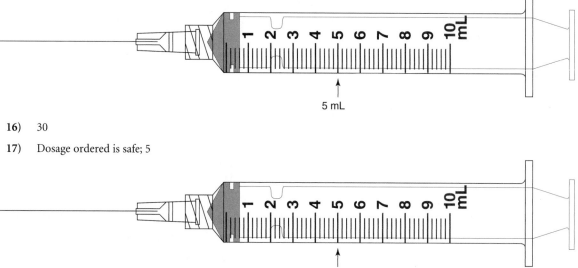

5 mL

16)   30

17)   Dosage ordered is safe; 5

5 mL

18) 19 **19)** 30,000; 30 **20)** 60 **21)** Yes, the recommended dosage for this child is 225 mg/day in 3 divided doses or 75 mg/dose. This is the same as the order; 2; 23; 40 **22)** 12 **23)** Yes, safe dosage for this child is 300 mg/dose, which is the same as the order; 6; 44; 1200 **24)** 5; 2.5 **25)** 19

26)

> 2/6/xx, 0800, reconstituted as 1 g in
> 10 mL (100 mg/mL). Expires 2/7/xx, 0800.
> Keep at room temperature. G.D.P.

27)   5; 45

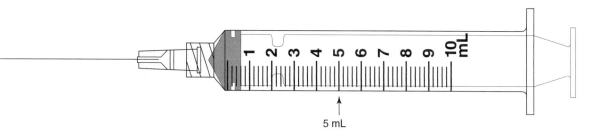

5 mL

28)   65

29) 2; 60

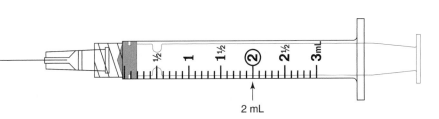

2 mL

30) 56.8; 4544; 4.6; 1022; 10 **31)** Decrease rate by 2 U/kg/h; 908; 9

32) 8; 0.08

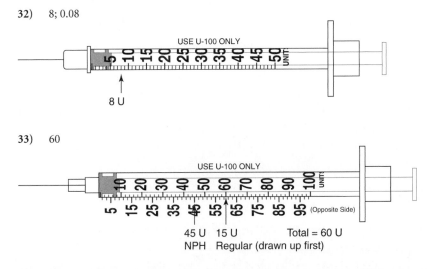

8 U

33) 60

USE U-100 ONLY

(Opposite Side)

45 U   15 U   Total = 60 U
NPH   Regular (drawn up first)

34) 20 **35)** 720; 960 **36)** 730; 30 **37)** 1.43 **38)** 14.3–28.6; Yes; 0.5; 56; 5.6; 1.4 **39)** 50; 3.3 **40)** 8; 4 **41)** 2.2; 47.8 **42)** Yes; the minimal amount of IV fluid to safely dilute this med is 13.5 mL. The order calls for 50 mL total, or 47.8, almost 48 mL of IV fluid. **43)** 1,600,000; Yes, the minimum daily dosage is 1,500,000 U/day and the maximum is 2,500,000 U/day. The ordered dosage falls within this range; 1.8; 500,000; 0.8

Reconstitution Label

> 1/14/xx; 0800, reconstituted as
> 500,000 U/mL. Expires 1/21/xx; 0800.
> Keep refrigerated. G.D.P.

44) 101 **45)** 2145 **46)** 0.5; 0.5; 0.13 **47)** 7.5 **48)** 200

49)   Either the route or the frequency of this order is missing or is unclear. If the student actually gave this medication in the eye, it would cause a severe reaction. The medication particles could scratch the eyes, or cause a worse reaction, such as blindness.

To prevent this from occurring, the student/nurse should always ensure that each medication order is complete. Every order should include the name of the drug, the dose, the route, and the time. When any of these are missing, the order should be clarified. The student/nurse should also look medications up and know the safe use for each medication ordered. Had this student looked Lanoxin up in a drug guide, it would have been discovered that the medication is never given in the eye.

50)   The student nurse took the correct action with this order. The nurses who had given the medication previously should have looked up the medication if they were unfamiliar with it to safely identify whether it was ordered by an appropriate route, correct dose, and correct time. There was also an error made by the pharmacist who supplied the medication to the nursing unit. It is extremely important to be familiar with the medications being given. If there's a question or any doubt, the medication should be looked up in a drug guide and/or the prescriber questioned. Also, close reading of the label and matching it to the order is also extremely important. Remember the six rights of medication administration.

Solutions—Comprehensive Skills Evaluation

1) $\dfrac{D}{H} \times Q = \dfrac{\overset{2}{\cancel{13} \text{ mg}}}{\underset{1}{\cancel{6.5} \text{ mg}}} \times 1 \text{ cap} = 2 \text{ cap}$

3) $\dfrac{D}{H} \times Q = \dfrac{\overset{2}{\cancel{20} \text{ mg}}}{\underset{1}{\cancel{10} \text{ mg}}} \times 1 \text{ mL} = 2 \text{ mL}$

$\dfrac{40 \text{ mg}}{2 \text{ min}} \diagdown \diagup \dfrac{20 \text{ mg}}{X \text{ min}}$

$40X = 40$

$\dfrac{40X}{40} = \dfrac{40}{40}$

$X = 1 \text{ min}$ Give 2 mL over 1 min

$\dfrac{2 \text{ mL}}{60 \text{ sec}} \diagdown \diagup \dfrac{X \text{ mL}}{15 \text{ sec}}$

$60X = 30$

$\dfrac{60X}{60} = \dfrac{30}{60}$

$X = 0.5$ Give 0.5 mL over 15 sec

4) $\dfrac{D}{H} \times Q = \dfrac{\overset{1}{\cancel{20} \text{ mcg}}}{\underset{1}{\cancel{20} \text{ mcg}}} \times 1 \text{ tab} = 1 \text{ tab}$

5) $0.25 \text{ mg} = 0.25 \times 1000 = 250 \text{ mcg}$

$\dfrac{D}{H} \times Q = \dfrac{\overset{1}{\cancel{250} \text{ mcg}}}{\underset{2}{\cancel{500} \text{ mcg}}} \times 2 \text{ mL} = \dfrac{\overset{1}{\cancel{2}}}{\underset{1}{\cancel{2}}} \text{ mL} = 1 \text{ mL}$

$0.25 \text{ mg} = 1 \text{ mL}$ added to 4 mL NS = 5 mL total

$\dfrac{\overset{1}{\cancel{5} \text{ mL}}}{\underset{1}{\cancel{5} \text{ min}}} = 1 \text{ mL/min}$

$\dfrac{1 \text{ mL}}{60 \text{ sec}} \diagdown \diagup \dfrac{X \text{ mL}}{15 \text{ sec}}$

$60X = 15$

$\dfrac{60X}{60} = \dfrac{15}{60}$

$X = 0.25 \text{ mL (per 15 sec)}$

6) $0.125 \text{ mg} = 0.125 \times 1000 = 125 \text{ mcg}$

$\dfrac{D}{H} \times Q = \dfrac{\overset{1}{\cancel{125} \text{ mcg}}}{\underset{2}{\cancel{250} \text{ mcg}}} \times 1 \text{ tab} = \dfrac{1}{2} \text{ tab}$

"q.d." means once per day; will need $\dfrac{1}{2}$ tab per 24 h

7) $\dfrac{\text{mL/h}}{\text{drop factor constant}} = \text{gtt/min}$

$\dfrac{80 \text{ mL/h}}{1} = 80 \text{ gtt/min}$ or

80 mL/h = 80 gtt/min (because drop factor is

60 gtt/mL)

8) $\dfrac{D}{H} \times Q = \dfrac{\overset{5}{\cancel{10} \text{ mEq}}}{\underset{1}{\cancel{2} \text{ mEq}}} \times 1 \text{ mL} = 5 \text{ mL}$

9) The total fluid volume is:

1000 mL $D_5 \frac{1}{2}$ NS + 5 mL KCl = 1005 mL

$\dfrac{10 \text{ mEq}}{1005 \text{ mL}} \diagdown \diagup \dfrac{X \text{ mEq/h}}{80 \text{ mL/h}}$

$1005X = 800$

$\dfrac{1005X}{1005} = \dfrac{800}{1005}$

$X = 0.8 \text{ mEq/h}$

10) $80 \text{ mL/}\cancel{h} \times 24 \cancel{h} = 1920 \text{ mL}$

11) $\dfrac{1000 \cancel{\text{ mL}}}{80 \cancel{\text{ mL}}/h} = 12.5 \text{ h} = 12 \text{ h } 30 \text{ min}$

1630 hours + 12 h 30 min later = 0500 hours the next

day

12) 1 g = 1000 mg

$\dfrac{D}{H} \times Q = \dfrac{\overset{2}{\cancel{1000} \text{ mg}}}{\underset{1}{\cancel{500} \text{ mg}}} \times 1 \text{ tab} = 2 \text{ tab}$

13) Order is for 80 cc/h or 80 mL/h.

15) $\dfrac{D}{H} \times Q = \dfrac{\overset{5}{\cancel{50} \text{ mg}}}{\underset{1}{\cancel{10} \text{ mg}}} \times 1 \text{ mL} = 5 \text{ mL}$

16) $\dfrac{D}{H} \times Q = \dfrac{\overset{1}{\cancel{2} \text{ mg/min}}}{\underset{4}{\cancel{2000} \text{ mg}}} \times \overset{1}{\cancel{500}} \text{ mL} = \dfrac{\overset{1}{\cancel{2}}}{\underset{2}{\cancel{4}}} = 0.5 \text{ mL/min}$

$0.5 \text{ mL/}\cancel{\text{min}} \times 60 \cancel{\text{min}}/h = 30 \text{ mL/h}$

17) $110 \text{ lb} = \dfrac{110}{2.2} = 50 \text{ kg}$

Minimum: $5 \text{ mcg/kg/min} \times 50 \cancel{\text{kg}} = 250 \text{ mcg/min}$

Maximum: $10 \text{ mcg/kg/min} \times 50 \cancel{\text{kg}} = 500 \text{ mcg/min}$

Ordered dosage is safe.

$\dfrac{D}{H} \times Q = \dfrac{\overset{5}{\cancel{400} \text{ mg}}}{\underset{1}{\cancel{80} \text{ mg}}} \times 1 \text{ mL} = 5 \text{ mL}$

18) $500 \text{ mcg/min} = 500 \div 1000 = 0.5 \text{ mg/min}$

$\dfrac{D}{H} \times Q = \dfrac{0.5 \text{ mg/min}}{\underset{8}{\cancel{400} \text{ mg}}} \times \overset{5}{\cancel{250}} \text{ mL} = \dfrac{2.5 \text{ mL}}{8 \text{ min}}$

$= 0.312 \text{ mL/min} = 0.31 \text{ mL/min}$

$0.31 \text{ mL/}\cancel{\text{min}} \times 60 \cancel{\text{min}}/h = 18.6 \text{ mL/h} = 19 \text{ mL/h}$

19) $500 \text{ mcg/}\cancel{\text{min}} \times 60 \cancel{\text{min}}/h = 30{,}000 \text{ mcg/h}$

$30{,}000 \text{ mcg/h} = 30{,}000 \div 1000 = 30 \text{ mg/h}$

20) $\dfrac{D}{H} \times Q = \dfrac{\overset{1}{\cancel{4 \text{ mg/min}}}}{\underset{4}{\cancel{2000 \text{ mg}}}} \times \overset{1}{\cancel{500}} \text{ mL} = \dfrac{\overset{1}{\cancel{4}}}{\underset{1}{\cancel{4}}} = 1 \text{ mL/min}$

$1 \text{ mL/}\cancel{\text{min}} \times 60 \text{ }\cancel{\text{min}}\text{/h} = 60 \text{ mL/h}$

21) $33 \text{ lb} = \dfrac{33}{2.2} = 15 \text{ kg}$

$15 \text{ mg/}\cancel{\text{kg}}\text{/day} \times 15 \text{ }\cancel{\text{kg}} = 225 \text{ mg/day}$

Maximum: $\dfrac{225 \text{ mg}}{3 \text{ doses}} = 75 \text{ mg/dose}$

The order is safe.

$\dfrac{D}{H} \times Q = \dfrac{\overset{1}{\cancel{75 \text{ mg}}}}{\underset{1}{\cancel{75 \text{ mg}}}} \times 2 \text{ mL} = 2 \text{ mL}$

25 mL total IV solution − 2 mL Kantrex = 23 mL

$D_5 \frac{1}{2} \text{ NS}$

25 mL total solution + 15 mL flush = 40 mL total in 1 h

40 mL over 1 h is 40 mL/h.

22) $\dfrac{D}{H} \times Q = \dfrac{\overset{3}{\cancel{15 \text{ mg/h}}}}{\underset{25}{\cancel{125 \text{ mg}}}} \times 100 \text{ mL} = \dfrac{3 \text{ h}}{\cancel{25}} \times \overset{4}{\cancel{100}} \text{ mL} = 12 \text{ mL/h}$

23) $66 \text{ lb} = \dfrac{66}{2.2} = 30 \text{ kg}$

$40 \text{ mg/}\cancel{\text{kg}}\text{/day} \times 30 \text{ }\cancel{\text{kg}} = 1200 \text{ mg/day}$

$\dfrac{1200 \text{ mg}}{4 \text{ doses}} = 300 \text{ mg/dose}$

$\dfrac{D}{H} \times Q = \dfrac{300 \text{ mg}}{\underset{50}{\cancel{500 \text{ mg}}}} \times \overset{1}{\cancel{10}} \text{ mL} = \dfrac{300}{50} \text{ mL} = 6 \text{ mL}$

50 mL (total IV volume) − 6 mL (Vancocin) =

44 mL ($D_5 \frac{1}{2}$ NS); 50 mL/$\cancel{h} \times 24 \cancel{h} = 1200$ mL

24) $\dfrac{20 \text{ mEq}}{1000 \text{ mL}} \diagdown\diagup \dfrac{X \text{ mEq}}{250 \text{ mL}}$

$1000X = 5000$

$\dfrac{1000X}{1000} = \dfrac{5000}{1000}$

$X = 5 \text{ mEq}$

$\dfrac{D}{H} \times Q = \dfrac{5 \text{ mEq}}{2 \text{ mEq}} \times 1 \text{ mL} = \dfrac{5}{2} \text{ mL} = 2.5 \text{ mL}$

25) Select smallest quantity diluent (19 mL) to obtain most concentrated solution because 50 mL IV fluid is ordered for each Prostaphlin dose.

27) $\dfrac{D}{H} \times Q = \dfrac{500 \text{ mg}}{\underset{100}{\cancel{1000 \text{ mg}}}} \times \overset{1}{\cancel{10}} \text{ mL} = \dfrac{500}{100} \text{ mL} = 5 \text{ mL}$

50 mL (total IV volume) − 5 mL (Prostaphlin) =

45 mL (D_5W)

28) 50 mL (total IV solution) + 15 mL (flush) =

65 mL (total)

65 mL over 60 min = 65 mL/h

29) $\dfrac{D}{H} \times Q = \dfrac{\overset{2}{\cancel{10,000 \text{ U}}}}{\underset{1}{\cancel{5000 \text{ U}}}} \times 1 \text{ mL} = 2 \text{ mL}$

$\dfrac{D}{H} \times Q = \dfrac{1200 \text{ U/h}}{\underset{20}{\cancel{10,000 \text{ U}}}} \times \overset{60}{\cancel{500}} \text{ mL} = \dfrac{\overset{60}{\cancel{1200}}}{\underset{1}{\cancel{20}}} \text{ mL/h} = 60 \text{ mL/h}$

30) $125 \text{ lb} = \dfrac{125}{2.2} = 56.81 \text{ kg} = 56.8 \text{ kg}$

$80 \text{ U/}\cancel{\text{kg}} \times 56.8 \text{ }\cancel{\text{kg}} = 4544 \text{ U}$

$\dfrac{D}{H} \times Q = \dfrac{4544 \text{ U}}{1000 \text{ U}} \times 1 \text{ mL} = 4.554 \text{ mL} = 4.6 \text{ mL}$

$18 \text{ U/}\cancel{\text{kg}}\text{/h} \times 56.8 \text{ }\cancel{\text{kg}} = 1022.4 \text{ U/h} = 1022 \text{ U/h}$

$\dfrac{D}{H} \times Q = \dfrac{1022 \text{ U/h}}{\underset{100}{\cancel{25000 \text{ U}}}} \times \overset{1}{\cancel{250}} \text{ mL} = 10.22 \text{ mL/h}$

$= 10 \text{ mL/h}$

31) Decrease rate by 2 U/kg/h

$2 \text{ U/}\cancel{\text{kg}}\text{/h} \times 56.8 \text{ }\cancel{\text{kg}} = 113.6 \text{ U/h} = 114 \text{ U/h}$

1022 U/h − 114 U/h = 908 U/h

$\dfrac{D}{H} \times Q = \dfrac{908 \text{ U/h}}{\underset{100}{\cancel{25000 \text{ U}}}} \times \overset{1}{\cancel{250}} \text{ mL} = 9.08 \text{ mL/h} = 9 \text{ mL/h}$

32) $\dfrac{100 \text{ U}}{1 \text{ mL}} \diagdown\diagup \dfrac{8 \text{ U}}{X \text{ mL}}$

$100X = 8$

$\dfrac{100X}{100} = \dfrac{8}{100}$

$X = 0.08 \text{ mL}$

33) 15 U + 45 U = 60 U

34) U 100 insulin: 100 U/mL

$$\frac{100\ U}{1\ mL} \diagup\!\!\!\!\!\!= \diagdown \frac{300\ U}{X\ mL}$$

$$100X = 300$$

$$\frac{100X}{100} = \frac{300}{100}$$

$$X = 3\ mL$$

Total IV volume: 150 mL NS + 3 mL insulin = 153 mL

$$\frac{300\ U}{153\ mL} \diagup\!\!\!\!\!\!= \diagdown \frac{X\ U/h}{10\ mL/h}$$

$$153X = 3000$$

$$\frac{153X}{153} = \frac{3000}{153}$$

$$X = 19.6\ U/h = 20\ U/h$$

35) $8\ oz = 8 \times 30 = 240\ mL$

$$D \times Q = X$$

$$\frac{1}{4} \times Q = 240\ mL$$

$$\frac{1}{4}Q = 240\ mL$$

$$\frac{\frac{1}{4}Q}{\frac{1}{4}} = \frac{240}{\frac{1}{4}}$$

$$Q = 240 \times \frac{4}{1}$$

$$Q = 960\ mL\ (\text{total volume of reconstituted } \tfrac{1}{4} \text{ strength Isomil})$$

960 mL (total solution) – 240 mL (solute or Isomil) = 720 mL (solvent or water)

36) $16\ lb = \dfrac{16}{2.2} = 7.27\ kg = 7.3\ kg$

$100\ mL/kg/day \times 7.3\ kg = 730\ mL/day$

$730\ mL/day \div 24\ h/day = 30.4 = 30\ mL/h$

37) $5\ ft = 5 \times 12 = 60\ in;\ 60\ in + 2\ in = 62\ in$

Household:

$$BSA\ (m^2) = \sqrt{\frac{ht\ (in) \times wt\ (lb)}{3131}} = \sqrt{\frac{62 \times 103}{3131}} = \sqrt{2.03} = 1.428\ m^2 = 1.43\ m^2$$

38) $10\ mg/m^2 \times 1.43\ m^2 = 14.3\ mg$

$20\ mg/m^2 \times 1.43\ m^2 = 28.6\ mg$

Yes, the order is safe.

Concentration: 40 mg/80 mL = 0.5 mg/mL

$$\frac{D}{H} \times Q = \frac{28\ mg}{0.5\ mg} \times 1\ mL = 56\ mL$$

$$\frac{56\ mL}{10\ min} \diagup\!\!\!\!\!\!= \diagdown \frac{X\ mL}{1\ min}$$

$$10X = 56$$

$$\frac{10X}{10} = \frac{56}{10}$$

$$X = 5.6\ mL/min$$

$$\frac{5.6\ mL}{60\ sec} \diagup\!\!\!\!\!\!= \diagdown \frac{X\ mL}{15\ sec}$$

$$60X = 84$$

$$\frac{60X}{60} = \frac{84}{60}$$

$$X = 1.4\ mL\ (\text{per 15 sec})$$

39) Dextrose:

$$\frac{5\ g}{100\ mL} \diagup\!\!\!\!\!\!= \diagdown \frac{X\ g}{1000\ mL}$$

$$100X = 5000$$

$$\frac{100X}{100} = \frac{5000}{100}$$

$$X = 50\ g$$

NaCl:

$$\frac{0.33\ g}{100\ mL} \diagup\!\!\!\!\!\!= \diagdown \frac{X\ g}{1000\ mL}$$

$$100X = 330$$

$$\frac{100X}{100} = \frac{330}{100}$$

$$X = 3.3\ g$$

40)

$$\frac{20\ mEq}{1000\ mL} \diagup\!\!\!\!\!\!= \diagdown \frac{X\ mEq}{400\ mL}$$

$$1000X = 8000$$

$$\frac{1000X}{1000} = \frac{8000}{1000}$$

$$X = 8\ mEq$$

$$\frac{D}{H} \times Q = \frac{8\ mEq}{40\ mEq} \times 20\ mL = \frac{4}{2}\ mL = 4\ mL$$

41) $\dfrac{D}{H} \times Q = \dfrac{540\ mg}{250\ mg} \times 1\ mL = 2.16\ mL = 2.2\ mL$

50 mL – 2.2 mL = 47.8 mL IV fluid. Note: Add the med to the chamber, and then add IV fluid up to 50 mL.

42)

$$\frac{40\ mg}{1\ mL} \diagup\!\!\!\!\!\!= \diagdown \frac{540\ mg}{X\ mL}$$

$$40X = 540$$

$$\frac{40X}{40} = \frac{540}{40}$$

$$X = 13.5\ mL$$

43) 400,000 U/dose $\times$ 4 doses/day = 1,600,000 U/day

Minimum: 150,000 U/kg/day $\times$ 10 kg = 1,500,000 U/day

Maximum: 250,000 U/kg/day $\times$ 10 kg = 2,500,000 U/day

Reconstitute with 1.8 mL for a concentration of 500,000 U/mL. This concentration is selected because it will be further diluted.

$$\frac{D}{H} \times Q = \frac{400{,}000\ \cancel{U}}{500{,}000\ \cancel{U}} \times 1\ \text{mL} = 0.8\ \text{mL penicillin}$$

44) 100 mL (NS) + 0.8 mL (penicillin) = 100.8 or 101 mL to be infused in 60 min or 1 h. Set IV pump at 101 mL/h.

45) The primary IV will infuse for 8 hours. The IVPB will infuse for 30 minutes. Therefore, the primary IV will be interrupted by the IVPB and then will resume. The IV will be completely infused in 8 hours and 30 min.

(1315 + 8 h 30 min = 1315 + 0830 = 2145)

46) $$\frac{D}{H} \times Q = \frac{\overset{1}{\cancel{25}\ \cancel{mg}}}{\underset{2}{\cancel{50}\ \cancel{mg}}} \times 1\ \text{mL} = 0.5\ \text{mL}$$

Give 0.5 mL/min or

$$\frac{0.5\ \text{mL}}{60\ \text{sec}} \,\diagdown\!\!\!\!\!\diagup = \frac{X\ \text{mL}}{15\ \text{sec}}$$

$$60X = 7.5$$

$$\frac{60X}{60} = \frac{7.5}{60}$$

$$X = 0.125\ \text{or}\ 0.13\ \text{mL (per 15 sec)}$$

47) $$\frac{D}{H} \times Q = \frac{\overset{3}{\cancel{1500}\ \cancel{mg}}}{\underset{4}{\cancel{2000}\ \cancel{mg}}} \times 10\ \text{mL} = \frac{3}{\underset{2}{\cancel{4}}} \times \overset{5}{\cancel{10}}\ \text{mL} = \frac{15}{2}\ \text{mL} = 7.5\ \text{mL}$$

48) $$\frac{100\ \text{mL}}{\underset{1}{\cancel{30}\ \text{min}}} \times \frac{\overset{2}{\cancel{60}\ \cancel{min}}}{1\ \text{h}} = 200\ \text{mL/h}$$

Index

Getting Started with the *Dosage Calculations User Tutorial, 7th edition* CD-ROM

System Requirements

Operating system: Microsoft, Windows™ 98, Me, NT 4.0, 2000, XP, or newer
Processor: Pentium II processor or faster
Memory: 32–64 MB
Hard disk space: 16 MB
Monitor: SVGA-compatible color
Graphics adapter: SVGA or higher; 800 x 600, True Color (24-bit or 32-bit) or High Color (16-bit) modes
CD-ROM drive: 8x or faster

An Internet connection and Netscape Navigator 6.2 or Microsoft Internet Explorer 5.5, or newer, are required.

Microsoft, is a registered trademark and Windows, and Windows NT, are trademarks of Microsoft Corporation.

Set Up Instructions

1. Insert disc into CD-ROM player. The program should start. If it does not, go to step 2.
2. From My Computer, double click the icon for the CD drive.
3. Double click the *index.htm* file to start the program.

License Agreement for Delmar Learning, a division of Thomson Learning, Inc.

Educational Software/Data

You the customer, and Delmar Learning, a division of Thomson Learning, Inc. incur certain benefits, rights, and obligations to each other when you open this package and use the software/data it contains. BE SURE YOU READ THE LICENSE AGREEMENT CAREFULLY, SINCE BY USING THE SOFTWARE/DATA YOU INDICATE YOU HAVE READ, UNDERSTOOD, AND ACCEPTED THE TERMS OF THIS AGREEMENT.

Your rights:

1. You enjoy a non-exclusive license to use the software/data on a single microcomputer in consideration for payment of the required license fee, (which may be included in the purchase price of an accompanying print component), or receipt of this software/data, and your acceptance of the terms and conditions of this agreement.
2. You acknowledge that you do not own the aforesaid software/data. You also acknowledge that the software/data is furnished "as is," and contains copyrighted and/or proprietary and confidential information of Delmar Learning, a division of Thomson Learning, Inc. or its licensors.

There are limitations on your rights:

1. You may not copy or print the software/data for any reason whatsoever, except to install it on a hard drive on a single microcomputer and to make one archival copy, unless copying or printing is expressly permitted in writing or statements recorded on the diskette(s).
2. You may not revise, translate, convert, disassemble or otherwise reverse engineer the software/data except that you may add to or rearrange any data recorded on the media as part of the normal use of the software/data.
3. You may not sell, license, lease, rent, loan or otherwise distribute or network the software/data except that you may give the software/data to a student or and instructor for use at school or, temporarily at home.

Should you fail to abide by the Copyright Law of the United States as it applies to this software/data your license to use it will become invalid. You agree to erase or otherwise destroy the software/data immediately after receiving note of termination of this agreement for violation of its provisions from Delmar Learning.

Delmar Learning, a division of Thomson Learning, Inc gives you a LIMITED WARRANTY covering the enclosed software/data. The LIMITED WARRANTY follows this License.

This license is the entire agreement between you and Delmar Learning, a division of Thomson Learning, Inc. interpreted and enforced under New York law.

LIMITED WARRANTY

Delmar Learning, a division of Thomson Learning, Inc. warrants to the original licensee/purchaser of this copy of microcomputer software/data and the media on which it is recorded that the media will be free from defects in material and workmanship for ninety (90) days from the date of original purchase. All implied warranties are limited in duration to this ninety (90) day period. THEREAFTER, ANY IMPLIED WARRANTIES, INCLUDING IMPLIED WARRANTIES OF MERCHANTABILITY AND FITNESS FOR A PARTICULAR PURPOSE, ARE EXCLUDED. THIS WARRANTY IS IN LIEU OF ALL OTHER WARRANTIES, WHETHER ORAL OR WRITTEN, EXPRESS OR IMPLIED.

If you believe the media is defective please return it during the ninety day period to the address shown below. Defective media will be replaced without charge provided that it has not been subjected to misuse or damage.

This warranty does not extend to the software or information recorded on the media. The software and information are provided "AS IS." Any statements made about the utility of the software or information are not to be considered as express or implied warranties.

Limitation of liability: Our liability to you for any losses shall be limited to direct damages, and shall not exceed the amount you paid for the software. In no event will we be liable to you for any indirect, special, incidental, or consequential damages (including loss of profits) even if we have been advised of the possibility of such damages.

Some states do not allow the exclusion or limitation of incidental or consequential damages, or limitations on the duration of implied warranties, so the above limitation or exclusion may not apply to you. This warranty gives you specific legal rights, and you may also have other rights which vary from state to state. Address all correspondence to: Delmar Learning, a division of Thomson Learning, Inc., 5 Maxwell Drive, P.O. Box 8007, Clifton Park, NY 12065-8007. Attention: Technology Department